PROGRESS IN BIOMEDICAL OPTICS AND IMAGING

Vol. 3, No. 22

Medical Imaging 2002

Image Processing

Milan Sonka
J. Michael Fitzpatrick
Chairs/Editors

24–28 February 2002
San Diego, USA

Sponsored and Published by
SPIE—The International Society for Optical Engineering

Cooperating Organizations
AAPM—American Association of Physicists in Medicine
APS—American Physiological Society
FDA Center for Devices and Radiological Health (USA)
IS&T—The Society for Imaging Science and Technology
NEMA—National Electrical Manufacturers Association/Diagnostic Imaging
   and Therapy Systems Division (USA)
RSNA—Radiological Society of North America
SCAR—Society for Computer Applications in Radiology (USA)

Proceedings of SPIE
Volume 4684
Part Two of Three Parts

SPIE is an international technical society dedicated to advancing engineering and scientific applications of optical, photonic, imaging, electronic, and optoelectronic technologies.

Please use the following format to cite material from this book:

   Author(s), "Title of paper," in *Medical Imaging 2002: Image Processing*, Milan Sonka, J. Michael Fitzpatrick, Editors, Proceedings of SPIE Vol. 4684, page numbers (2002).

ISSN 1605-7422
ISBN 0-8194-4429-4

Published by
SPIE—The International Society for Optical Engineering
P.O. Box 10, Bellingham, Washington 98227-0010 USA
Telephone 1 360/676-3290 (Pacific Time) • Fax 1 360/647-1445
http://www.spie.org/

Printed in the United States of America.

Contents

SESSION 11   REGISTRATION II/MODELS

SESSION 12   COMPUTER-AIDED DIAGNOSIS I

Part Two

SESSION 14   COMPUTER-AIDED DIAGNOSIS III

POSTER SESSION I

Part Three

POSTER SESSION II

Automated Lung Nodule Segmentation Using Dynamic Programming and EM Based Classification

Ning Xu[a], Narendra Ahuja[a] and Ravi Bansal[b]

[a]ECE Department and Beckman Institute, University of Illinois at Urbana-Champaign, IL 61801
[b]Siemens Corporate Research, Inc. Princeton, NJ 08540

ABSTRACT

In this paper we present a robust and automated algorithm to segment lung nodules in three dimensional (3D) Computed Tomography (CT) volume dataset. The nodule is segmented out in slice–per–slice basis, that is, we first process each CT slice separately to extract two dimensional (2D) contours of the nodule which can then be stacked together to get the whole 3D surface. The extracted 2D contours are optimal as we utilize dynamic programming based optimization algorithm. To extract each 2D contour, we utilize a shape based constraint. Given a physician specified point on the nodule, we blow a circle which gives us rough initialization of the nodule from where our dynamic programming based algorithm estimates the optimal contour. As a nodule can be calcified, we pre–process a small region–of–interest (ROI), around the physician selected point on the nodule boundary, using the Expectation Maximization (EM) based algorithm to classify and remove calcification. Our proposed approach can be consistently and robustly used to segment not only the solitary nodules but also the nodules attached to lung walls and vessels.

Keywords: Lung nodule, Segmentation, Dynamic Programming, Expectation Maximization, Calcification Pattern

1. INTRODUCTION

Mortality due to lung cancer is a leading cause for the cancer related deaths in the country. One of the main cause for such a high rate of mortality is the fact that it is very difficult to detect malignant lung nodules. Usually by the time nodules are detected, it is too late. The nodules are either too large or too advanced to be effectively cured. Thus, there is a need for lung screening with the motivation for early detection of the malignant lung nodule at a stage where it can be effectively treated. Conventional chest X–rays (CXR)[1,2] have been utilized for long time. However, CXR are of limited use as using CXR only large lung nodules can be detected. With the advances in the X–ray Computed Tomography (CT) technology, there is a potential for screening of nodules which can be malignant. Using thin section multi–slice helical CT (hCT) scans, it is now possible to detect nodules which are as small as 3 mm in diameter.[3,4] Usage of high resolution CT (HRCT) image dataset allows for quantitative measurements, such as, size, shape and density, for each nodule to be made.

However, each helical CT scan of a patient leads to a volume consisting of 500 to 600 slices with 512×512 voxels in each slice. Thus, the advantages of having high resolution CT over CXR can be fast lost without the help of efficient image analysis and interpretation methods. Computer–assisted nodule detection[4–7] has already transformed the way lung cancer screening is done by providing better ways for visualization, detection and characterization of lung nodules.

Physical characteristics of the nodules,[8,9] such as rate of growth, pattern of calcification, type of margins are very important in the investigation of the lung nodules. Every lung nodules grows in volume over time. However, the malignant nodules grow at an exponential rate, which is usually expressed as tumor's doubling time. Malignant nodules have a doubling time of between 25 to 450 days where as the benign nodules are stable and have a doubling time of more than 500 days.[8] In addition to the rate of growth of the nodules, the pattern

---

E-mail: {ningxu,ahuja}@vision.ai.uiuc.edu, ravi.bansal@scr.siemens.com

Medical Imaging 2002: Image Processing, Milan Sonka, J. Michael Fitzpatrick,
Editors, Proceedings of SPIE Vol. 4684 (2002) © 2002 SPIE · 1605-7422/02/$15.00

of the calcification is an important indicator whether the nodule is benign or malignant. Nodules which are centrally or diffuse calcified are usually benign.

Before the nodules can be characterized, it is necessary to detect them in the volume of 3D CT image dataset that is being acquired. Manual lung nodule detection, which was possible while using CXR, is no longer possible. It is necessary to have automated tools that can assist a physician in quickly detecting the nodules. A number of automated lung nodule systems have already been proposed in the literature.[4, 6, 10–15] While the automated detection of the lung nodules is very important task, segmenting the nodules once they have been detected remains to be equally challenging task. The difficulty of the task comes from the fact that some of the nodules maybe sitting on the chest wall or on the lung vessels. Accurate and consistent segmentation of the lung nodule over time acquired CT volume datasets is necessary to study the rate of growth of the nodules and hence to predict whether the nodule is malignant or benign.

In this paper we present an automated method of segmenting the lung nodules from CT images on a per slice method. Once the nodules have been segmented in each slice, a 3D surface of the nodule can then be reconstructed using surface reconstruction methods.[16] Our approach allows for human interaction to correct for any errors in the automated technique. In addition, our method allows, naturally, to extract a pattern on the calcification of each nodule which can further be used to classify the nodules.

2. BACKGROUND

Since accurate and robust segmentation of lung nodule is very important in accurately measuring the volume, various of methods to segment nodules have been proposed in the literature.

Fuzzy clustering algorithm[14] is used to extract both the lung and pulmonary blood vessel region and then use feature based diagnostic rules to determine the candidate nodule locations. Zhao et al.[17] propose a method to process the CT volume data in a slice–by–slice manner. They also propose a set of multiple criteria, such as density, gradient strength and a shape constraint, to separate the nodule from the surroundings. In their approach, a whole region of interest need to be selected prior to the segmentation. They extend their approach to segment nodules directly in 3D volume.[18] Fan et al.[6] propose an adaptive histogram threshold followed by connected component analysis based approach to detect and segment isolatory nodules. A series of 3D morphological operators[5, 19, 20] are proposed to segment the nodules from the lung vessels. Armato et al.[15] utilize a *rolling ball* algorithm to define the segmented lung region after the lungs have been segmented from the thorax region using gray–level thresholding. After that Armato et al. utilize a 10–point connectivity scheme to identify contiguous 3D structures.

While all the approaches in the literature have their merits, there is no one single approach which can robustly and consistently segment all types of nodules, that is, nodules on the lung walls, nodules attached to the vessels or the isolated nodules. In this paper we present a shape based approach which can segment lung nodules consistently and robustly. Our approach uses dynamic programming[21, 22] to find the optimal lung nodule boundary. However, due to the calcification of the lung nodules, many times the initialization of the shape based approach fails. Thus, to overcome this problem we first pre–process the CT volume dataset, locally around the nodule selected by the physician, using *Expectation Maximization* (EM)[23–25] algorithm to detect and remove the calcification from the nodules. This approach can also feasibly give information about the pattern of calcification of the nodules. Our approach is completely automated and requires only an initial point from the physician on the surface of the nodule. However, since any completely automated algorithm may fail in a complicated case, in our approach we have provided efficient user interaction for corrections of the segmentation results, if desired.

3. OUR APPROACH

3.1. A shape model based framework for segmenting object boundary

In our framework, the object to be segmented has a defined shape, such as a circle or an ellipse. The task of segmentation is to estimate the parameters $\beta = [O, s]^T$ of the shape in an image and estimate the optimal boundary based on these parameters. Here O is the position of the shape and s is the scale of the shape. Since the real world objects are far more complicated than those simple shapes, we need to allow certain degree of shape morphology. Also, in real world images, object may be occluded, or some part of the object boundary may be indistinguishable from the background. All these make the object boundary to be discontinuous. In our framework, we are trying to solve the segmentation problem of objects with discontinuous boundaries. An object boundary, B, is represented as $B = (\bigcup_i B_{ci}) \bigcup (\bigcup_j B_{dj})$, where B_{ci}, for $i = 1, \ldots, M$, represents parts of the visible object boundary and B_{dj}, for $j = 1, \ldots, N$, represents the parts of the object boundary which are occluded. Note that we model the object boundary to be a union of $N + M$ contours where some, N, of the contours are visible and the other M are occluded, forming discontinuities in the object boundary. We initialize β and then determine the discontinuous parts of the object contour, find out the optimal segments of the continuous parts and estimate β based on our results. This procedure is carried out iteratively until β converges. Then the estimated segments of the continuous parts of the object boundary, i.e. B_{ci}'s, are linked by straight lines to give an optimal estimate of the object boundary. The whole procedure is described as follows:

1. Initialize β;

2. Determine discontinuities in the object boundary;

3. Find out the optimal realization for continuous parts:

$$\hat{B_{ci}} = \arg\max_{B_{ci}} p(B_{ci}|I, \beta)$$

4. Link all those continuous parts, $B_{ci} \forall i$, using straight lines to get the object boundary along the discontinuous parts, $B_{dj} \forall j$, of the object boundary;

$$\hat{B_{di}} = f(B_{ci})$$

5. Estimate new parameters of the shape

$$\hat{\beta} = \arg\min_{\beta} g(\beta, B),$$

where $g(\beta, B)$ is a distance measurement between the resulting object boundary B and the shape β;

6. If β converges then stop; otherwise go to step 2;

In our nodule segmentation problem, we model a nodule as a circle shaped object with some deformation and iteratively apply dynamic programming algorithm to find out the optimal contour of the nodule. After each iteration, we fit a circle onto the result and estimate the center and radius of the circle. The parameters β of the circular shape are center O and radius r. The probability $p(B_{ci}|\beta, I)$ is set as

$$p(B_{ci}|\beta, I) = \frac{1}{C_f} \exp(-f_\beta(B_{ci})),$$

where

$$f_\beta(B_{ci}) = w_{shape} \cdot f_{shape}(B_{ci}) + w_{smooth} \cdot f_{smooth}(B_{ci}),$$

and

$$f_{smooth}(B_{ci}) = \sum_{B_{ci}} (w_1 |B_{ci}^k - B_{ci}^{k-1}|^2 + w_2 |B_{ci}^{k+1} - 2B_{ci}^k - B_{ci}^{k-1}|^2)$$

and $f_{shape}(B_{ci}) = \frac{1}{N_c}\sum_k f_{shape}(B_{ci}^k)$, where N_c is the number of pixels on B_{ci}. f_{shape} consists of four parts as

$$f_{shape}(B_{ci}^k) = w_z f_z(B_{ci}^k) + w_g f_g(B_{ci}^k) + w_d f_d(B_{ci}^k) + w_v f_v(B_{ci}^k),$$

where f_z is a Laplacian zero-crossing measurement at B_{ci}^k,

$$f_z(B_{ci}^k) = \begin{cases} 0, & \text{if} \quad \nabla^2 G \otimes I(B_{ci}^k) = 0 \\ 1, & \text{if} \qquad else \end{cases},$$

f_g is the gradient magnitude of pixel B_{ci}^k

$$f_g(B_{ci}^k) = 1 - \frac{\|\nabla G \otimes I(B_{ci}^k)\|}{\max_i \|\nabla G \otimes I(B_{ci}^k)\|},$$

f_d is the gradient direction of pixel B_{ci}^k

$$f_d(B_{ci}^k) = \arccos(\frac{< \nabla I(B_{ci}^k), B_{ci}^k - O >}{\|\nabla I(B_{ci}^k)\| \cdot \|B_{ci}^k - O\|}),$$

f_v is a heuristic gray value criterion based on the shape and the intensity of pixel B_{ci}

$$f_v(B_{ci}^k) = \|I(B_{ci}^k - k(O - B_{ci}^k)) - I_{in}\| + \|I(B_{ci}^k + k(O - B_{ci}^k)) - I_{out}\|,$$

where I_{in} is the intensity value inside the object and I_{out} is the intensity value outside of the object.

3.2. Computing optimal object boundary using dynamic programming

Given initial parameters or estimated parameters from previous iteration, i.e. β, the following steps estimate the optimal nodule boundary:

1. Detect discontinuous parts of the object boundary,

2. estimate B_{ci} $\forall i$ using dynamic programming,

3. link all segments of continuous parts by straight lines to obtain the optimal object boundary, B. Then, B_{dj} $\forall j$ are the straight lines required to link B_{ci} $\forall i$ to form a closed nodule boundary.

3.2.1. Detecting discontinuity directions

From the center of the given circle, defined by β, we draw N rays which divide the circle into N equally spaced directions. The number N is set according to the length of the radius R of the circle. An area of interest is set to be a ring shaped area whose inner circle radius is $R - r$ and outer circle radius is $R + r$. Both inner circle and outer circle have the same center as the original circle. For each direction i, we check each pixel p from $R - r$ to $R + r$ and evaluate

$$f_i(p) = w_z \times f_z(p) + w_g \times f_g(p) + w_d \times f_d(p).$$

We set a threshold $\mathcal{T}$ and if $\min_p f_i(p) > \mathcal{T}$, there is a discontinuity on the object boundary in this direction.

This first step will detect object boundary discontinuities directions around the circle defined by β. If the object boundary is detected to be discontinuous, the dynamic programming procedures in the next step are then well defined. If no discontinuities in the object boundary are detected, we can either detect the weakest radial direction or detect a direction with a very high gradient pixel that can be a starting pixel and break the circle at this direction. Again, the dynamic programming procedure in the next step is well defined.

3.2.2. Using dynamic programming to compute continuous parts segments of object boundary

For each segment of those continuous parts of the object boundary, we use time-delayed discrete dynamic programming to compute an optimal boundary segment B_{ci} $\forall i$. Suppose there are n directions within this segment, $v_1, v_2, ..., v_n$, and in each direction, there are m candidate pixels. For each direction $k > 2$, keep an $m \times m$ matrix for each entry within this direction.

$$f_\beta(v_1, v_2, ..., v_n) = f_{\beta 1}(v_1, v_2, v_3) + f_{\beta 2}(v_2, v_3, v_4) + ... + f_{\beta(n-2)}(v_{n-2}, v_{n-1}, v_n),$$

where $f_{\beta(k-1)}(v_{k-1}, v_k, v_{k+1}) = f_{shape}(v_k) + f_{smooth}(v_{k-1}, v_k, v_{k+1})$ for each direction $k > 2$, an m^2 matrix $m_k(v_k, v_{k-1})$ is calculated and the best value of v_{k-2} is kept together with the calculated value

$$m_k(v_k, v_{k-1}) = \min_{v_{k-2}}(m_{k-1}(v_{k-1}, v_{k-2}) + f_{\beta(k-2)}(v_{k-2}, v_{k-1}, v_k)).$$

Finally, the optimal path can be derived by back tracking from the last direction to the first direction. Once we have estimated each segment, B_{ci} $\forall i$, we link them using straight lines to get the final optimal object boundary. Again, note that since B_{ci} $\forall i$ are linked by straight lines to get the optimal closed boundary of the nodule, B_{dj} $\forall j$ are these straight lines.

3.2.3. User interaction

If the result is not satisfactory, user can interactively select a pixel p to be on the following resulting contours. No matter whether this pixel p is inside a continuous part or a discontinuous part, we just set $f_{shape}(p) = 0$, and set the shape function of all the other pixels at the same direction to be a very large value. Then the resultant optimal boundary will pass through this pixel p selected by the user.

3.3. Initialization and circle fitting

3.3.1. Initialization by blowing a circle

In our approach, initial center and radius, i.e. an initial estimate of β, is required before we can start. At the very beginning, we only need the user to select a point near the nodule boundary. This initializing point can be detected manually by an expert or by an automated algorithm. Then we get an estimate of the initial contour by blowing a circle from a nearby points with a highest intensity, which means the point should be a soft tissue point. We first use Canny's edge detection method to generate an edge map of the original image data and proceed with our circle blowing algorithm as follows:

1. Select a pixel P in a region with highest intensity, set $O^0 = P$;

2. Set $radius = 0$;

3. Set $radius = radius + 1$, check whether there is any point on the circle is an edge point in the edge map. If none, repeat this step;

4. Suppose a set of points $P_i, i = 1, 2, \ldots, m$, on the circle are edge points, and the shortest curve which consists of all these points is shorter than half a circle, then set

$$O^{n+1} = O^n + \frac{(O^n - (P_1 + P_m)/2)}{(\|O^n - (p_1 + p_m)/2\|)};$$

5. Go to step 3 until the shortest curve mentioned in step 4 is longer than half a circle;

3.3.2. Circle fitting

After we link all the continuous segments, i.e. $B_{ci} \, \forall i$, computed using dynamic programming to obtain a closed contour, we fit a circle to this contour by trying to find a center and radius which will minimize some kind of distance measurement. First, express all the pixels $p_i, i = 1, 2, ..., N$ on the contour to be $[x_i, y_i]^T$. To improve numerical stability, we need to subtract the mean of the pixels and then scale them by the range of the resulting values. The equation of a circle can be expressed as

$$a_1 x^2 + a_1 y^2 + a_2 x + a_3 y + a_4 = 0.$$

If given $[a_1, a_2, a_3, a_4]^T$, then

$$O = [-a_2/(2a_1), -a_3/(2a_1)]^T,$$

and

$$r = \sqrt{a_4/a_1 - \|O\|^2},$$

where O is the center of the circle and r is the radius.

In our approach, we use approximated Euclidean distance to measure the distance. If we try to minimize the Euclidean distance

$$\min \frac{1}{N} \sum_{i=1}^{N} \frac{f(R)^2}{\|\nabla f(R_i)\|^2},$$

the desired solution is the minimum eigenvalue of the system $L\vec{a} = \lambda S\vec{a}$, where

$$L = \frac{1}{N} \sum_{i=1}^{N} B(R_i) \cdot B(R_i)^T,$$

$$S = \frac{1}{N} \sum_{i=1}^{N} D(R_i) \cdot D(R_i)^T,$$

and

$$B(R_i) = [x_i^2 + y_i^2, x_i, y_i, 1]^T,$$

$$D(R_i) = \begin{pmatrix} 2x_i & 2y_i \\ 1 & 0 \\ 0 & 1 \\ 0 & 0 \end{pmatrix}.$$

3.4. Pre-processing using EM based classification

In our approach described above, a circle is blown from the initial physician selected point on the nodule boundary. The radius of the initial circle is slowly increased as proposed above. Such an approach leads to a nodule segmentation approach which is quite independent of the initial selected point on the boundary. However, a nodule can be calcified in a variety of locations, which will cause problems when blowing a circle or looking for optimal contours. To overcome this problem, we propose to first pre-process the CT volume, in the region of interest around the physician selected point using *Expectation Maximization* (EM)[24, 25] based algorithm. In the volume of interest, the voxel values can be due to three tissue types, air, soft tissue or calcified. Using EM algorithm, we classify each voxel to be one of these three classes. The voxels which are labeled as calcified are then removed from the volume and the removed voxels are interpolated from its neighborhood.

The EM algorithm has been successfully used to estimate parameters which maximizes the likelihood of the observed data, in the presence of missing data. The EM based maximum likelihood classification algorithm consists of two steps, the *E–Step* and the *M–Step*, as the name suggests. In the *E–Step*, the algorithm estimates the expected value of the missing information. In the *M–step*, the algorithm utilizes the expected values of the missing information from the *E–step* to estimate the optimal parameters. The two steps are computed iteratively till convergence.

3.4.1. Mathematical formulation

Consider random variables $\mathbf{x}$ and $\mathbf{y}$ to be defined over the sample spaces, $\mathcal{X}$ and $\mathcal{Y}$ respectively, and there is a many–to–one mapping from $\mathcal{Y}$ to $\mathcal{X}$. $\mathcal{Y}(\mathbf{y})$ denotes the subset in $\mathcal{Y}$ from which the observed data $\mathbf{x}$ can be obtained. The observed data $\mathbf{x}$, called *incomplete data*, is a realization of $\mathcal{X}$. The corresponding $\mathbf{y}$, called *complete data* in $\mathcal{Y}$ is not observed. Let $\mathcal{Y}(\mathbf{x})$ denote the subset in $\mathcal{Y}$ from which the observed data $\mathbf{x}$ can be obtained. If $p_{\mathbf{x}}(x|\theta)$ is the probability density function of the observed data over the sample space $\mathcal{X}$, and $p_{\mathbf{y}}(y|\theta)$ is the corresponding probability density function of the complete data over the sample space $\mathcal{Y}$, the two density functions are related as follows:

$$p_{\mathbf{x}}(x|\theta) = \int_{\mathcal{Y}(\mathbf{x})} p_{\mathbf{y}}(y|\theta) \, dy$$

Notice that for a given incomplete data specification $p_{\mathbf{x}}(x|\theta)$, there are many possible complete data statistics $p_{\mathbf{y}}(y|\theta)$ that will generate $p_{\mathbf{x}}(x|\theta)$. The EM algorithm aims at estimating the value of θ which maximizes $p_{\mathbf{x}}(x|\theta)$ given the observed data, but in doing so it uses the associated family $p_{\mathbf{y}}(y|\theta)$. Then, the two steps in the EM algorithm to compute the parameters θ are derived to be:

E Step: Compute

$$Q(\theta|\theta^k) = E[\ln p(y|\theta)|x, \theta^k]$$

where the expected value is evaluated with respect to the density function $p(y|x, \theta^k)$.

M step: Estimate

$$\theta^{k+1} = \arg\max_\theta Q(\theta|\theta^k)$$

The E–step requires evaluation of the expected value of $\ln p(y|\theta)$, the reason being to *integrate out* the missing data, and thus, to write the objective function only in terms of observed data and the parameters to be estimated. Taking the expectation with respect to the density function $p(y|x, \theta^k)$ is of core importance to the iterative nature of the algorithm. Note that as the expectation is taken with respect to the density function with parameters estimated from the previous iteration, θ^k, this helps give an iterative nature to the algorithm.

3.4.2. Classification using EM

In our model, we assume that the pixel intensities from the three tissue classes are Gaussian distributed. Thus, the problem of classification is then a maximum likelihood problem of estimating the parameters of these three Gaussian distribution. However, a nodule may or may not be calcified. Thus, in addition to classifying the voxels to a class, we also need to find out how many classes there are. In our case there can be either two or three classes only. To estimate both the number of classes and the parameters of the component mixture densities, we utilize fully Bayesian mixture modeling.[26] The basic formulation for observations x_i, using a mixture model can be written as

$$x_i \equiv \sum_{j=1}^{k} w_j \; f(.|\theta_j)$$

where the weight, w_j, are called the *component weights* such that $\sum_{j=1}^{k} w_j = 1$, θ_j are the component mixture density parameters and k is the number of components which are also unknown.

In our implementation of the EM algorithm to find the number of component densities k and the mixture density parameters, we always assumed that the number of components are three and then estimate the parameters for three mixtures from the given image data. If the mean of the distribution for the class *calcified* is in between the means for the other two classes, then we assume that there are only two classes in the mixture model. Otherwise there are three classes.

Once the pixels have been labeled to belong to one of the three classes, *soft tissue*, *air* or *calcified*, the pixels belonging to the *calcified* class are removed from the volume of interest and the corresponding pixels are replaced with bilinear interpolation of the neighboring pixels.

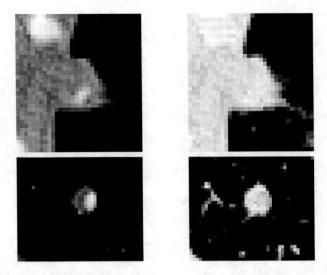

Figure 1. Images in the left column show the ROI before pre–processing using the EM based algorithm. Images in the right column show the results obtained after running the EM algorithm to classify and removed the detected calcified nodules.

4. RESULTS

In this section we present the results of our proposed lung nodule segmentation framework. Our algorithm starts with user selected point near the boundary of the nodule, in each slice in CT. Thus, our algorithm assumes that the nodule detection has already been done, either manually by an expert or by an automated algorithm. Once a user selects a point near the nodule boundary, we grow a circle to give us a rough initialization of the nodule boundary. This initial rough estimate of the nodule boundary forms the initialization of our algorithm. Note that this initialization makes our algorithm robust to the variability in user selection of the point. We tested our algorithm with various initial selected point near a nodule and our algorithm estimated the same initial circle. However, calcification of a nodule can effect the circle growing step. Thus, to overcome this problem, we first pre–process a region–of–interest (ROI) around the selected point to remove the calcification. Fig.1 shows the effects of removing the calcification in a nodule. The images in the left column of Fig.1 shows the ROI around the user selected point near two example nodules. The images in the right column of Fig.1 shows the results obtained after removing the calcification. Note that once the calcification has been removed, the pixel intensity within the nodule is more uniform. This estimated calcification of the nodules can then, in addition to the estimated volume and surface characteristics, be used to classify the nodule as benign or malignant.

Fig.2 shows the results obtained using our algorithm for a variety of nodules. These are the results obtained after running our algorithm completely automatically, with no corrections. In Fig.2, the initial expert selected point near the nodule boundary is shown as a single point. The initial grown circle is shown in black cross marks and the final nodule estimated boundary is shown as a white curve. In the images in the top and the third row show the segmentation results obtained for segmenting the nodules which are attached to lung wall. The images in third row show that even if a nodule appears as a small bump in the lung wall, our algorithm does a very reasonable job in segmenting it from the wall. Images in the second row of Fig.2 show the results obtained for segmenting the nodule that is attached to a vessel. Note that in this case the vessel is actually passing through the nodule. Still our algorithm is able to automatically segment the nodule from the vessel. The fourth row of the Fig.2 shows that we can segment the isolated nodule also with our proposed segmentation framework. These results show that visually our algorithm is able to segment the lung nodules accurately. However, in some of the obtained results, it feels that corrections might be needed.

We feel that a completely segmentation algorithm, including our proposed algorithm, might fail in some of the cases. This motivated us to provide a mechanism to an expert to correct an estimated nodule boundary. In

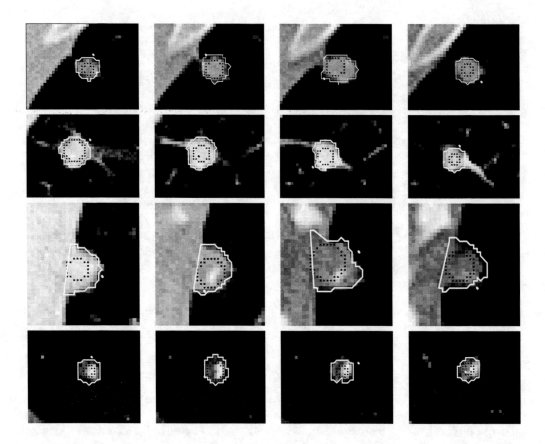

Figure 2. These results are obtained after an expert selects a point, shown as a single point near the nodule boundary. The initial blown circle is shown in black cross marks and the final estimated boundary of the nodule is shown as a white curve. The results shown are the estimated nodule boundary obtained after running our algorithm completely automatically, with no corrections. Note that while our algorithm did a very good job in segmenting the nodules, corrections might be needed in some of the results.

our nodule segmentation framework, corrections to the estimated boundary has been incorporated as a single-click mechanism. An expert selects a point through which the estimated nodule boundary must pass and our algorithm takes that as a hard constraint and automatically updates the estimated nodule boundary. Results obtained after expert corrections are shown in Fig.3. Images in Fig.3 show the results obtained after corrections to the results in Fig.2. Note that only one or two corrections, for only two images, were required. The final estimated boundaries are shown as white curve. Note that after these corrections, the lung nodule has been perfectly segmented in all the cases.

5. DISCUSSION

In this paper we presented an automated lung nodule segmentation algorithm where the segmentation of the nodule is carried out on a per slice basis from the initial physician selected point. We implemented our algorithm in Matlab, and for each slice, the automated algorithm took less than 5 seconds to compute the optimal contour. Once the 2D contours of a nodule have been segmented out of the CT volume dataset, the surface fitting algorithm[16] can be used to fit a surface. All the surface features have been preserved which can then be used to visually characterize a nodule. The preprocessing step using EM algorithm classifies those pixels within the region of interest as one of the three classes: soft tissue, air or calcified. This information can then, in addition to the volume and surface features of the segmented nodule, be utilized for further calcification of the nodule. Our proposed algorithm can be used to segment not only isolated nodules but also the nodules on the lung walls and the vessels without any modifications. As we utilize dynamic programming to estimate nodule boundary, based

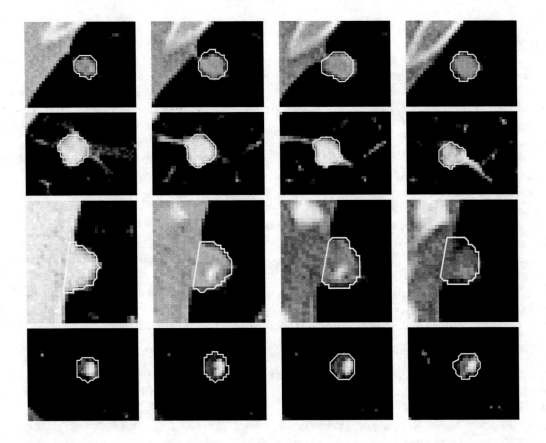

Figure 3. Final estimated lung nodule boundaries after corrections to the results obtained automatically, shown in Fig.2.

on external image information, such as gradient and the internal energy of the estimated contour, the estimated nodule boundary is optimal. For our future work, we will like to do further validations of our approach and to extend this method to directly segment nodules in 3D, i.e. without having to first segment 2D contours in each slice.

REFERENCES

1. M. Carreira, D. Cabello, *et al.*, "Computer-aided lung nodule detection in chest radiography," *Lecture Notes in Computer Science, Image Analysis Applications and Computer Graphics* **1024**, pp. 331–338, 1995.

2. B. van Ginneken, *Computer–Aided Diagnosis in Chest Radiography.* PhD thesis, University of Utrecht, 1970.

3. M. Brown, D. Aberle, *et al.*, "Model-based segmentation architecture for lung nodule detection in CT," *Radiology* **217**(P), 2000.

4. M. Brown, D. Aberle, *et al.*, "Computer-aided method for lung micronodule detection in CT," *Radiology* **217**(P), 2000.

5. A. P. Reeves and W. J. Kostis, "Computer–aided diagnosis of small pulmonary nodules," *Seminars in Ultrasound, CT, and MRI* **21**(2), pp. 116–128, 2000.

6. L. Fan *et al.*, "Automatic detection of cellular necrosis in epithelial cell cultures," *SPIE Medical Imaging* , Feb 2001.

7. P. F. Judy and F. L. Jacobson, "Evaluation of segmentation using lung nodule phantom CT images," *SPIE Medical Imaging* , Feb 2001.

8. G. A. Lillington, "Management of solitary pulmonary nodules," *Postgraduate Medicine* **101**(3), 1997.

9. S. G. Armato, M. L. Giger, and H. MacMahon, "Analysis of a three-dimensional lung nodule detection method for thoracic CT scans," *SPIE Medical Imaging* **3979**, pp. 103–109, 2000.

10. M. Penedo, A. Cabello, *et al.*, "Computed-aided diagnosis: A neural network based approach to lung nodule detection," *IEEE Transactions on Medical Image* **17**(6), pp. 872–880, 1998.

11. Y. Lee, T. Hara, *et al.*, "Nodule detection on chest helical CT scans by using a genetic algorithm," *Proceedings of the 1997 IASTED International Conference on Intelligent Information*, 1997.

12. G. Cox, F. Hoare, and G. Jager, "Experiments in lung cancer nodule detection using texture analysis and neural network classifiers," *citeseer.nj.nec.com/cox92experiments.html*, 1992.

13. G. Gonzalez *et al.*, "Application of computer-performed holographic recognition to lung nodule detection and evaluation in thoracic CT scans," *European Congress of Radiology (ECR)*, 2000.

14. K. Kanazawa *et al.*, "Computer–aided diagnosis for pulmonary nodules based on helical CT images," *Comput. Med. Imaging Graph.* **22**, pp. 157–167, 1998.

15. S. G. Armato, M. L. Giger, *et al.*, "Three-dimensional approach to lung nodule detection in helical CT," *SPIE Medical Imaging* **3661**, pp. 553–559, 1999.

16. B. Geiger, *Three–Dimensional Modelling of Human Organs and its Application to Diagnosis and Surgical Planning*. PhD thesis, INRIA, France, 1993. Number 2105.

17. Z. B, Y. DF, *et al.*, "2-D multi-criteria automatic segmentation of pulmonary nodules of helical CT images," *Medical Physics* **26**(6), pp. 889–895, 1999.

18. Z. B, R. A, *et al.*, "3-D multi-criteria automatic segmentation of pulmonary nodules of helical CT images," *Optical Engineering*, 1999.

19. W. Kostis *et al.*, "Three–dimensional segmentation of solitary pulmonary nodules from helical CT scans," *Proc. of Comp. Asst. Rad. and Surg. (CARS)*, pp. 203–207, 1999.

20. D. Yankelevitz *et al.*, "Small pulmonary nodules: Volumetrically determined growth rates based on CT evaluation," *Radiology* **217**, pp. 251–256, 2000.

21. A. Amini *et al.*, "Using dynamic programming for solving variational problems in vision," *IEEE Trans. on PAMI* **12**, September 1990.

22. D. Geiger, A. Gupta, L. A. Costa, and J. Vlontzos, "Dynamic programming for detecting, tracking, and matching deformable contours," *IEEE Trans. on PAMI* **17**, March 1995.

23. T. K. Moon, "The expectation–maximization algorithm," in *IEEE Signal Processing Magazine*, pp. 47–60, IEEE, November 1996.

24. A. P. Dempster, N. M. Laird, and D. B. Rubin, "Maximum likelihood from incomplete data via EM algorithm," *J. Royal Statistical Soc., Ser. B* **39**, pp. 1–38, 1977.

25. R. A. Redner and H. F. Walker, "Mixture densities, maximum likelihood and the EM algorithm," *SIAM Review* **26**(2), pp. 195–239, 1984.

26. S. Richardson and P. Green, "On Bayesian analysis of mixtures with an unknown number of components," *J. R. Statist. Soc. B* **59**(4), pp. 731–792, 1997.

Computer aided lung nodule detection
on high resolution CT data

Rafael Wiemker[a], Patrik Rogalla[b], André Zwartkruis[c], Thomas Blaffert[a]

[a] Philips Research Laboratories Hamburg, Germany
[b] Dept. of Radiology, Charité Hospital, Humboldt University Berlin, Germany
[c] Philips Medical Systems Best, The Netherlands

ABSTRACT

Most of the previous approaches to computer aided lung nodule detection have been designed for and tested on conventional CT with slice thickness of 5–10 mm. In this paper, we report results of a specifically designed detection algorithm which is applied to 1 mm slice data from multi-array CT. We see two prinicipal advantages of high resolution CT data with respect to computer aided lung nodule detection: First of all, the algorithm can evaluate the fully isotropic three dimensional shape information of potential nodules and thus resolve ambiguities between pulmonary nodules and vessels. Secondly, the use of 1 mm slices allows the direct utilization of the Hounsfield values due to the absence of the partial volume effect (for objects larger than 1 mm).

Computer aided detection of small lung nodules (≥ 2 mm) may thus experience a break-through in clinical relevance with the use of high resolution CT. The detection algorithm has been applied to image data sets from patients in clinical routine with a slice thickness of 1 mm and reconstruction intervals between 0.5 and 1 mm, with hard- and soft-tissue reconstruction filters. Each thorax data set comprises 300–500 images. More than 20 000 CT slices from 50 CT studies were analyzed by the computer program, and 12 studies have so far been reviewed by an experienced radiologist. Of 203 nodules with diameter ≥ 2 mm (including pleura-attached nodules), the detection algorithm found 193 (sensitivity of 95%), with 4.4 false positives per patient. Nodules attached to the lung wall are algorithmically harder to detect, but we observe the same high detection rate. The false positive rate drops below 1 per study for nodules ≥ 4 mm.

Keywords: Computer aided detection, CAD, lung nodules, segmentation, shape analysis, high resolution CT, HRCT, lung cancer screening

1. INTRODUCTION

The detection and diagnosis of pulmonary nodules in CT data sets of the thorax is a standard procedure in radiological practise. Pulmonary nodules are often benign, but they may also be an indication for lung cancer, or may be metastases from other cancer types. In any case, early detection of lung nodules is crucial, either for close observation or biopsy to differentiate between benign or malignant nodules, or for timely therapy. There are clear indications that early detection of lung cancer can improve the survival rate. Moreover, it is hoped that lung cancer screening of high risk patient groups may significantly increase the rate of lung cancer cases which are diagnosed before the cancer has metastasized.

Lung nodules can be detected particularly well by CT, since they show good contrast in the lung parenchyma and — in contrast to projection X-ray — cannot be hidden by ribs etc. However, although in principle detectable in CT, a non negligible fraction of small nodules may be overlooked by the radiologist, particularly if they are located centrally and hidden in a maze of vessels of similar size. Therefore, computer assistance for detecting lung nodules in CT data sets has been suggested and investigated as early as 1989.[1-3] The underlying idea is not that the diagnosis is delegated to a machine, but rather that a machine algorithm acts as a support to the radiologist and points out locations of suspicious objects, so that the overall sensitivity (detection rate) is raised. This could be important particularly in screening situations, with a massive reviewing load of CT studies.

The overwhelming majority of computer aided lung nodule detection approaches has been designed for and tested on conventional 5–10 mm CT slice thickness.[3-12] However, the reported sensitivity and specificity rates were often

Rafael.Wiemker@philips.com, Röntgenstr. 24, 22335 Hamburg
Patrik.Rogalla@charite.de, Schumannstr. 20, 10117 Berlin

low and have so far failed to reach the level of clinical acceptance and usefulness. On the one hand, the detection rate was often disappointing, and on the other hand the false positive rate sometimes so high that the annoyance and tiring-out of the radiologist might possibly cancel out any potential gain in sensitivity. E.g. the 10 mm slice study of Fiebich et al. (2001)[7] reports 38% sensitivity (on 68 nodules) with 6 false positives per patient. Lee et al. (2001)[5] report 72% sensitivity (on 98 nodules) with 31 false positives per patient. Moreover, both studies have restricted themselves to nodules with size $\geq$ 5 mm.

The principal problem of computerized nodule detection in thick slices of 5–10 mm is that the opacity of nodules which are smaller than the slice thickness is thinned out by the partial volume effect. Therefore it is impossible to set a certain Hounsfield value as a threshold for potential nodules. Rather, many different thresholds have to be tried,[8] and false positives cannot be rejected simply due to a low Hounsfield value. Another approach to cope with the unkown Hounsfield level caused by the partial volume effect is to apply a morphological tophat- or Quoit-filter[13,14] which measured the difference in attenuation between the center and surrounding of a possible nodule. This is quite costly as the filters have to applied in each possible size (diameter). Another problem of thick CT slices is that a reasoning mechanism is required to recognize constellations where a small nodule is overshadowed by a vessel of similar size within the 10 mm projection.[12] Also thin vessels may appear disconnected when running obliquely through the slice images and thus be mistaken for nodules.

High resolution CT data with slice thickness $\leq$1 mm allows the detection of very small nodules. High resolution CT (HRCT) has so far been used mainly for characterization and classification of already singled-out individual nodules.[15–19] Only recently HRCT data has been used for the nodule *detection* within a complete thorax data set.[20,21] Fan et al. (2001)[20] evaluated 112 nodule candidates $\geq$ 2 mm, but no sensitivity (detection rate) was specified, and pleural nodules were not considered. The obvious advantage of HRCT data is that with voxel dimensions of e.g. $0.7 \times 0.7 \times 0.7$ mm^3 the partial volume effect can be neglected for nodules of size $>$ 1 mm. The Hounsfield values can be evaluated as absolute attenuation values, and the fully isotropic three dimensional shape information of potential nodules can be utilized to resolve ambiguities between pulmonary nodules and vessels.

The utilization of high resolution CT (HRCT) for computer aided nodule detection holds the promise of increasing sensitivity and specificity in such a way as to achieve a break-through for CAD in clinical practise.

2. HIGH RESOLUTION CT IMAGE DATA

The image data evaluated in this paper was recorded in the years 2000–2001 during clinical routine in the radiology department of the Charité university hospital, Berlin, by multi slice CT (Toshiba Aquillion, 4 slices per half-second rotation). Each thorax data set comprises 300–500 slice images with 512 $\times$512 pixels. The x-y-resolution (in-slice) varies between 0.5–1.0 mm, and also the z-resolution (reconstruction interval) varies between 0.5–1.0 mm, with a slice thickness of 1 mm (overlapping slices). The scans were recorded over the entire thorax at 120 kV and 100 mAs. More than 20 000 CT slices from 50 thoracic scans were analyzed by our nodule detection program, and 12 scans have so far been reviewed by a radiologist.

3. NODULE DETECTION ALGORITHM

3.1. Lung segmentation

Prior to the nodule detection, some approaches at first segment the lung out of the overall thorax data set in order to reduce the amount of image data to be analyzed[20] (Fig. 1, left-hand). However, this removes as well nodules which are attached to the lung wall (pleural nodules, see Fig. 4, right-hand). Other approaches include these lung wall attached nodules by a morphological opening of the lung volume,[8] or by correcting the lung circumference by enforcing convexity at locations of rapidly changing curvature.[22] In our experience this may induce many false positive candidates which have to rejected in a later stage. Moreover, the morphologically included objects have a completely artificial surface at the cut-off boundary (the convex envelope of the lung volume) which may complicate the subsequent spatial shape analysis of the potential nodule candidates. Therefore we have chosen an approach where in a binary mask image the airspace around the patient body is filled (thereby also eliminating the tray and objects on the outside of the body) but the voxels outside of the lung are not removed (Fig. 1, right-hand). Rather, the full extent of each slice image is analyzed in the search of seed points for possible nodule candidates. In each binary mask image slice, a 2D filter is applied which identifies all structures similar to circles or half-circles.

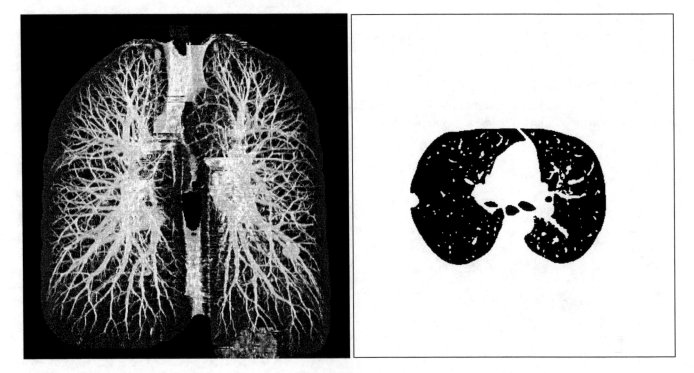

Figure 1. Left: Lung structures segmented out of the overall thorax data (coronal MIP).
Right: In our approach, the whole slice image is scanned for circular or semi-circular structures (after thresholding and filling of the surrounding airspace) in order to include also nodules attached to the lung wall (see pleural nodule in the right lung).

3.2. Isotropic resolution and the missing partial volume effect

In earlier approaches to lung nodule detection on thick slices (5–10 mm) the nodule candidates are often identified on thresholded binary images by virtue of the criterion that at a certain HU-threshold the nodule is a connected component (blob) which is confined to a small volume. In other words, a region growing (or connected component labeling) would eventually come to a stop after the nodule is filled, in contrast to a vessel (tubular structure) in which the growth would continue throughout the vessel tree. The nodules may be connected to vessels as well, of course (see Fig. 4). The underlying idea of multiple thresholding,[8,23] or the Quoit-filter[13,14] is that the thin vessels connecting to the nodule show lower Hounsfield values than the nodule itself, due to the partial volume effect. So there would always be a difference in Hounsfield value which could be measured (Quoit-filter) or exploited by an appropriate HU-threshold to separate the nodule from the connecting vessels.

For one thing, the use of multiple thresholding with high resolution CT (HRCT) would be very time-consuming since we have to deal with the 10-fold amount of image data. More important, however, is that the whole detection paradigm does not work on thin CT slices. For the case of nodule and connecting vessels thicker than 1 mm in diameter, the missing partial volume effect means that we often encounter the situation that there is no possible HU-threshold which would actually cut off the connecting vessels from the nodule. Hence, nodule detection algorithms on HRCT data need to concentrate on shape analysis rather than on finding appropriate thresholds. The principal criterion for nodules in HRCT is whether all vessels connecting to a nodule candidate are significantly smaller in diameter than the nodule itself. This can be determined e.g. by a region growing scheme.[20] The shape analysis of our algorithm evaluates compactness, thickness of connecting vessels, and average Hounsfield value and HU distribution within the nodule candidate. The average Hounsfield value is particularly useful for rejction of false positive candidates.

The 3-dimensional shape analysis can be carried out on binary threshold images. Due to the absence of the partial volume effect the HU-threshold can be a global one for the whole CT data set. In our analysis of nodule candidates from 36 of the CT studies we have found that the average Hounsfield value is almost independent of the nodule size (Fig. 2). The average Hounsfield values of all nodule candidates are clearly above −400 HU. The bulk of all nodule candidates has an average Hounsfield values between –200 and –100 HU (Fig. 3, left-hand.). We have also measured the optimal HU-threshold in local volumes of interest around 129 nodule candidates. The optimality is defined in such a way as to maximize the mean gradient at the HU-isosurface between nodule and the surrounding parenchyma.[24] The results (Fig. 3, right-hand) suggest that the strongest contrast between nodule and background is reached around –300 HU.

The efficiency of the lung nodule detection algorithm is based on the fact that in HRCT a single Hounsfield threshold suffices to identify all seed points for near circular or semi-circular nodule candidates.

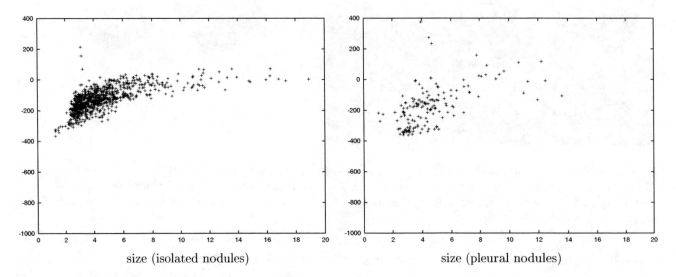

size (isolated nodules)   size (pleural nodules)

Figure 2. Mean Hounsfield value [HU] of nodule candidates vs. nodule diameter [mm] of 941 nodule candidates from 36 CT studies. The mean Hounsfield value is only weakly correlated with the nodule size, and all nodules are clearly above –400 HU.
Right: Nodule candidates in CT data reconstructed with a soft tissue reconstruction filter (157 nodule candidates from 15 CT studies).

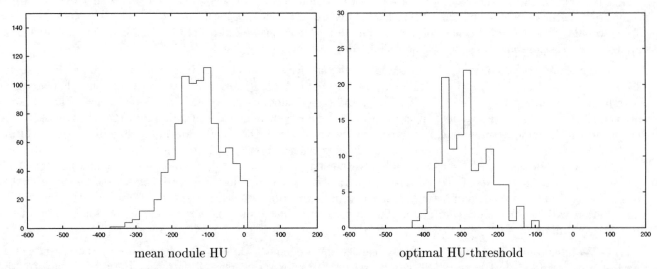

mean nodule HU   optimal HU-threshold

Figure 3. Left: Histogram of the mean Hounsfield value of 941 nodule candidates (see data of Fig. 2, left-hand). Right: Histogram of the optimal HU-threshold value of 129 local volumes of interest around nodule candidates.

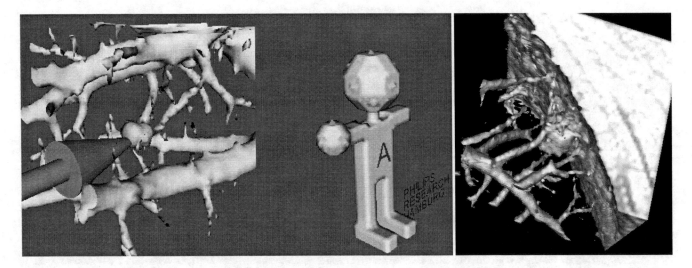

Figure 4. Left: Example of a small nodule (surface rendering at threshold −500 HU; with arrow pointing at nodule, and dummy figure to indicate viewing direction).
Right: Example of a nodule attached to the lung wall with connecting vessels (volume rendering of a local volume of interest of 50×50×50 voxels).

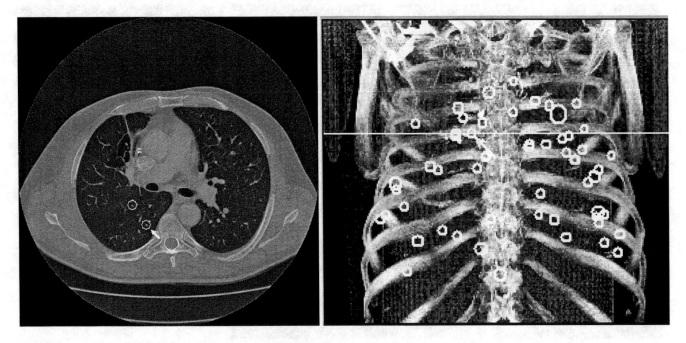

Figure 5. Evaluation of the nodules by the radiologist:
Left: Axial slice with two nodules (arrow-marked nodule is of 2 mm size).
Right: Overview image (coronal MIP), with currently displayed slice (left) indicated as white line. The overview image can be chosen between various projections: MIP, DRR, blended MIP / DRR, or segmented lung volume. Mouse click on marked nodule candidates sets the currently displayed axial view to the appropriate slice image, and vice versa. The nodule candidates are also accessible through a list which can be ordered according to slice location, diameter, likelihood, and average Hounsfield value.

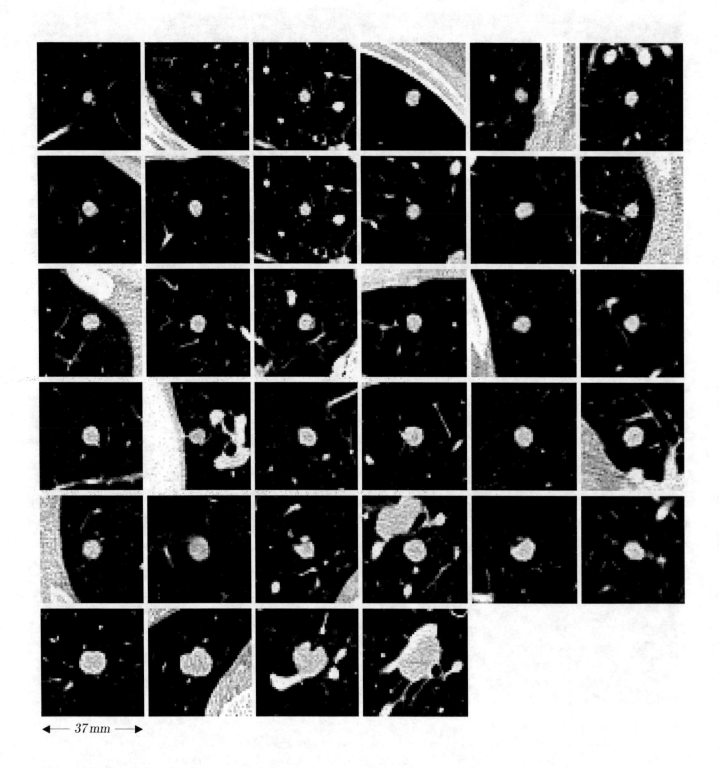

← 37 mm →

Figure 6. Examples of pulmonary nodules
(out of a single thorax study; ordered in ascending size, the smallest 3 mm, top left).

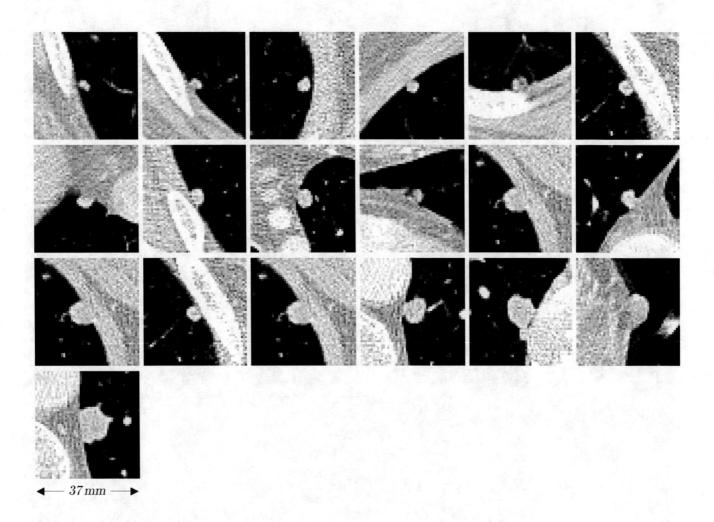

← 37 mm →

Figure 7. Examples of nodules attached to the pleural surface (out of a single thorax study, ordered in ascending size).

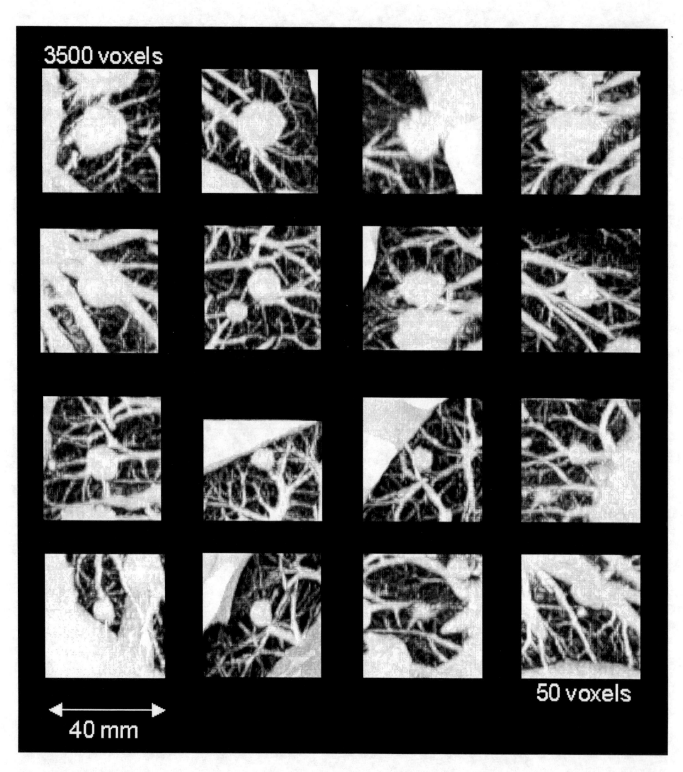

Figure 8. Maximum intensity projections (MIPs) of a local volume of interest of $50 \times 50 \times 50$ voxels centered around the nodules. The nodules are ordered in descending size, with the largest (top left) consisting of 3 500 voxels down to the smallest consisting of only 50 voxels (ca. 3 mm).

4. RESULTS

4.1. Evaluation of detection rate and false positive rate

The nodule detection algorithm is a fully automatic offline-program which starts out from the input of the high resolution CT data set (as described in section 2) and does not require any interaction. The program runs typically 3–5 minutes for 300–500 slices per thorax scan on a SUN Sparc Ultra processor (300 MHz) and produces a list of nodule candidates. A variety of detected nodules are depicted in Fig. 6–8. The nodule candidates are presented to the radiologist in a graphical user interface (see Fig. 5). Each nodule candidate is annotated with a likelihood, size, HU average, and geometrical descriptors. The nodule candidates are marked in the axial slice images. They are also accessible by mouse click into an coronal overview image or by a candidate list which can be ordered according to slice location, diameter, likelihood, and average Hounsfield value.

An experienced radiologist then reviewed each thorax data set and classified the computer marked nodule candidates as true or false positives. Moreover, the radiologist marked nodules which have been missed entirely by the detection algorithm (false negatives). From 12 CT studies (patients) which have been reviewed as of yet, we observe the following results for sensitivity and false positive rate (a specificity cannot be computed as there is no meaningful definition of true negative candidates) :

size	nodules	detected	missed	false positives
≥ 1 mm	271	234	37	59
		86% sensitivity		**4.9 FP per study**

size	nodules	detected	missed	false positives
≥ 2 mm	203	193	10	53
		95% sensitivity		**4.4 FP per study**

without pleural nodules

size	nodules	detected	missed	false positives
≥ 2 mm	157	149	8	40
		95% sensitivity		**3.3 FP per study**

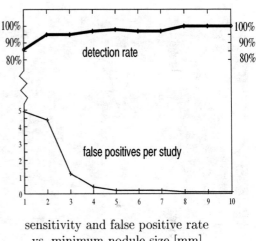

sensitivity and false positive rate
vs. minimum nodule size [mm]

The graph shows the dependence of the detection rate from the minimum nodule size (i.e. the sensitivity for the set of all nodules with size $\geq d$ mm is plotted as a function of d). We observe that the sensitivity is ca. 95% and quite independent of the nodule size once they are larger or equal to 2 mm, and that there are no missed nodules at all larger than 8 mm. The false positive candidates are essentially all smaller than 5 mm, and thus the false positive rate drops below 1 per study for nodules ≥ 4 mm.

4.2. Limiting detection size

We observe that a reliable detection and shape analysis becomes possible if a minimum number of ca. 30 voxels is available for analysis. On high resolution CT data with a voxel resolution of $0.7 \times 0.7 \times 0.7$ mm^3, say, a nodule of 2 mm diameter corresponds approximately to a $3 \times 3 \times 3$ block of voxels (for comparison see a nodule with 50 voxels in Fig. 8, bottom right).

4.3. Lung wall attached nodules

More than half of the computation time of the lung nodule detection program is spent on the search for nodules attached to the lung wall. The detection of hemi-spherical objects is conceptually as well as numerically more demanding since there a more degrees of freedom than for isolated nodules which are completely surrounded by the lung parenchyma. Different possible orientations of the lung wall have to tested (see examples in Fig. 7). Our results indicate that the detection rate for pleural nodules is equally high as for the parenchyma surrounded nodules.

4.4. Principal cases of false positive candidates

We have observed two principal cases of false positive candidates:

▶ Vessels which are running close to the heart and seemingly disrupted by caridac motion, and thus appear as a series of small isolated nodules (Fig. 9).

▶ Hilus vessels which branch out of the mediastinum and decrease rapidly in diameter so that they are mistaken as lung wall attached nodules with connecting vessels (Fig. 10).

Other false positive candidates are caused by thick vessel bifurcations and bronchial wall thickenings.

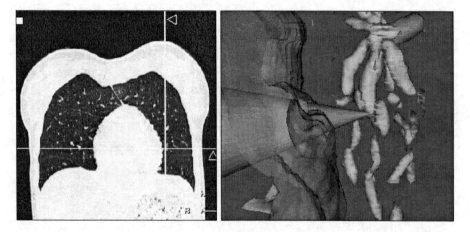

Figure 9. Left: False positive candidates from cardiac motion artifacts in the left lung.
Right: Enlarged surface rendering (with arrow indicating the false positive candidates).

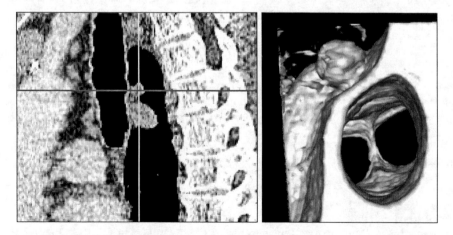

Figure 10. One true positive nodule (cross hair), and one false positive candidate (below), both close to the trachea.
Left: Sagittal cut-plane; the upper nodule is true, whereas the lower candidate is a strongly curved vessel.
Right: Volume rendering of the true positive nodule seen along the trachea close to the carina.

5. CONCLUSIONS

We are presenting results from computer aided lung nodule detection on high resolution CT (HRCT) image data. Most previous approaches to computer aided detection of pulmonary nodules have been designed for and applied to conventional CT image data with slice thickness of 5–10 mm. Then the sensitivity and specificity of automatic nodule detection is compromised by the partial volume effect for small nodules.

Nodule detection algorithms for HRCT data must be designed in a different way: They must be efficient since they have to cope with the ca. 10-fold amount of image data, and they cannot cut off small vessels from nodules by means of their difference in Hounsfield values, due to the missing partial volume effect. On the other hand, they have the crucial advantage that the absolute Hounsfield values can be directly used for recognition of nodules and rejection of false positive candidates. Moreover, the fine isotropic resolution allows a fully three dimensional shape analysis for nodules larger than 2 mm.

We have processed more than 20 000 slices from 50 thoracic high resolution CT scans with 1 mm slice thickness and on average 0.7 mm reconstruction interval, recorded during clinical routine at the radiology department of the Charité university hospital, Berlin. Each data set consists of 300–500 slices. 12 data sets have so far been reviewed by an experienced radiologist. Isolated nodules surrounded by the lung parenchyma as well as nodules attached to the lung wall (pleural nodules) have been taken into account. Out of 203 nodules with diameter ≥ 2 mm (including pleural nodules), the detection algorithm found 193 (sensitivity of 95%), with 4.4 false positives per patient.

We observe that with HRCT reliable automatic detection seems feasible for nodules larger or equal to 2 mm in diameter. The false positive rate drops below 1 per study for nodules ≥ 4 mm. The use of high resolution CT may raise the levels of sensitivity and specificity significantly, and thus bring the break-through for acceptance of CAD in clinical routine, particularly with respect to cancer screening.

REFERENCES

1. F. Preteux, N. Merlet, P. Grenier, and M. Mouellhi, "Algorithms for automated evaluation of pulmonary lesions by high resolution CT via image analysis," in *Proc. Radiol. Soc. of North America RSNA'89*, p. 416, 1989.

2. F. Preteux, "A non-stationary Markovian modeling for the lung nodule detection in CT," in *Proceedings of the International Conference on Computer Assisted Radiography CAR'91*, pp. 199–204, Springer, ISBN 3-540-54143-8, 1991.

3. M. Giger, K. Bae, and H. MacMahon, "Computerized detection of pulmonary nodules in computed tomography images," *Investigative Radiology* **29**(4), pp. 459–465, 1994.

4. Y. Lee, T. Hara, H. Fujita, S. Itoh, and T. Ishigaki, "Nodule detection on chest helical CT scans by using a genetic algorithm," in *Proc. Intel. Inf. Systems*, pp. 67–70, 1997.

5. Y. Lee, T. Hara, H. Fujita, S. Itoh, and T. Ishigaki, "Automated detection of pulmonary nodules in helical CT images based on an improved template-matching technique," *IEEE Trans. Medical Imaging* **20**, pp. 595–604, July 2001.

6. M. Fiebich, C. Wietholt, B. Renger, S. Armato, K. Hoffmann, D. Wormanns, and S. Diederich, "Automatic detection of pulmonary nodules in low-dose screening thoracic CT examinations," in *Proceedings of the SPIE Medical Imaging Conference 1999, San Diego*, vol. SPIE-3661, pp. 1434–1439, 1999.

7. M. Fiebich, D. Wormanns, and W. Heindel, "Improvement of method for computer-assisted detection of pulmonary nodules in CT of the chest," in *Proceedings of the SPIE Medical Imaging Conference 2001, San Diego*, vol. SPIE-4322, pp. 702–709, 2001.

8. S. Armato, M. Giger, C. Moran, J. Blackburn, K. Doi, and H.MacMahon, "Computerized detection of pulmonary nodules on CT scans," *RadioGraphics* **19**, pp. 1303–1311, 1999.

9. S. Armato, M. Giger, J. Blackburn, K. Doi, and H.MacMahon, "Three-dimensional approach to lung nodule detection in helical CT," in *Proceedings of the SPIE Medical Imaging Conference 1999, San Diego*, vol. SPIE-3661, pp. 553–559, 1999.

10. S. Armato, M. Giger, and H. MacMahon, "Analysis of a three-dimensional lung nodule detection method for thoracic CT scans," in *Proceedings of the SPIE Medical Imaging Conference 2000, San Diego*, vol. SPIE-3979, pp. 103–109, 2000.

11. H. Satoh, Y. Ukai, N. Niki, K. Eguchi, K. Mori, H. Ohmatsu, R. Kakinuma, M. Kaneko, and N. Moriyama, "Computer aided diagnosis system for lung cancer based on retrospective helical CT image," in *Proceedings of the SPIE Medical Imaging Conference 1999, San Diego*, vol. SPIE-3661, pp. 1324–1335, 1999.

12. H.Takizawa, G. Fukano, S. Yamamoto, T. Matsumoto, Y. Tateno, T. Iinuma, and M. Matumoto, "Recognition of lung cancers from X-ray CT images considering 3-D structure of objects and uncertainty of recognition," in *Proceedings of the SPIE Medical Imaging Conference 2000, San Diego*, vol. SPIE-3979, pp. 998–1007, 2000.

13. S. Yamamoto, M. Matsumoto, and Y. Tateno, "Quoit filter: a new filter based on mathematical morphology to extract the isolated shadow, and its application to automatic detection of lung cancer in X-ray CT," in *International Conference on Pattern Recognition ICPR'96*, vol. 2, pp. 3–7, 1996.

14. S. Yamamoto, H. Takizawa, H. Jiang, T. Nakagawa, T. Matsumoto, Y. Tateno, T. Iinuma, and M. Matsumoto, "A CAD system for lung cancer screening test by X-ray CT," in *Proceedings of the International Conference on Computer Assisted Radiography and Surgery CARS'01, Berlin*, pp. 605–610, Elsevier, 2001.

15. A. Reeves, W. Kostis, D. Yankelewitz, and C. Henschke, "Three-dimensional shape characterization of solitary pulmonary nodules from helical CT scans," in *Proceedings of the International Conference on Computer Assisted Radiography and Surgery CARS'99, Paris*, pp. 83–87, Elsevier, ISBN 0-444-50290-4, 1999.

16. W. Kostis, A. Reeves, D. Yankelewitz, and C. Henschke, "Three-dimensional segmentation of solitary pulmonary nodules from helical CT scans," in *Proceedings of the International Conference on Computer Assisted Radiography and Surgery CARS'99, Paris*, pp. 203–207, Elsevier, ISBN 0-444-50290-4, 1999.

17. Y. Kawata, N. Niki, H. Ohmatsu, M. Kusumoto, R. Kakinuma, K. Mori, H. Nishiyama, K. Eguchi, M. Kaneko, and N. Moriyama, "Curvature based characterization of shape and internal intensity structure for classification of pulmonary nodules using thin-section CT images," in *Proceedings of the SPIE Medical Imaging Conference 1999, San Diego*, vol. SPIE-3661, pp. 541–552, 1999.

18. Y. Kawata, N. Niki, H. Ohmatsu, M. Kusumoto, R. Kakinuma, K. Mori, H. Nishiyama, K. Eguchi, M. Kaneko, and N. Moriyama, "Computer aided differential diagnosis of pulmonary nodules based on a hybrid classification approach," in *Proceedings of the SPIE Medical Imaging Conference 2001, San Diego*, vol. SPIE-4322, pp. 1796–1806, 2001.

19. M. McNitt-Gray, E. Hart, N. Wyckoff, J. Sayre, J. Goldin, and D. Aberle, "A pattern classification approach to characterizing solitary pulmonary nodules imaged on high resolution CT: Preliminary results," *Medical Physics* **26**(6), pp. 880–888, 1999.

20. L. Fan, C. Nowak, J. Qian, G. Kohl, and D. Naidich, "Automatic detection of lung nodules from multi-slice low-dose CT images," in *Proceedings of the SPIE Medical Imaging Conference 2001, San Diego*, vol. SPIE-4322, pp. 1828–1835, 2001.

21. C. Novak, L. Fan, J. Qian, G. Kohl, and D. Naidich, "An interactive system for CT lung nodule identification and examination," in *Proceedings of the International Conference on Computer Assisted Radiography and Surgery CARS'01, Berlin*, pp. 599–604, Elsevier, 2001.

22. K. K. amd Y. Kawata, N. Niki, H. Satoh, H. Ohmatsu, R. Kakinuma, M. Kaneko, N. Moriyama, and K. Eguchi, "Computer aided diagnosis for pulmonary nodules based on helical CT images," *Computerized Medical Imaging and Graphics* **22**, pp. 157–167, 1998.

23. B. Zhao, D. Yankelevitz, A. Reeves, and C. Henschke, "Two-dimensional multi-criterion segmentation of pulmonary nodules on helical CT-images," *Medical Physics* **26**(6), pp. 889–895, 1999.

24. R. Wiemker and A. Zwartkruis, "Optimal thresholding for 3D segmentation of pulmonary nodules in high resolution CT," in *Proceedings of the International Conference on Computer Assisted Radiography and Surgery CARS'01, Berlin*, pp. 653–658, Elsevier, 2001.

Knowledge-based Automatic Detection of Multi-type Lung Nodules from Multi-detector CT Studies

Jianzhong Qian[a], Li Fan[a], Guo-Qing Wei[a], Carol L. Novak[a], Benjamin Odry[a], Hong Shen[a],

Li Zhang[a], David P. Naidich[b], Jane P. Ko[b], Ami N. Rubinowitz[b], Georgeann McGuinness[b],

Gerhard Kohl[c], Ernst Klotz[c]

[a] Siemens Corporate Research, Inc. Princeton, NJ 08540, USA

[b] New York University Medical Center, New York City, NY 10016, USA

[c] Siemens Medical Solutions, 91301 Forchheim, Germany

Email: {qian, li.fan, guo-qing.wei, corol.novak, bodry, hong.shen, li.zhang} @scr.siemens.com

ABSTRACT

Multi-slice computed tomography (CT) provides a promising technology for lung cancer detection and treatment. To optimize automatic detections of a more complete spectrum of lung nodules on CT requires multiple specialized algorithms in a coherently integrated detection system. We have developed a knowledge-based system for automatic lung nodule detection and analysis, which coherently integrates several robust novel detection algorithms to detect different types of nodules, including those attached to the chest wall, nodules adjacent to or fed by vessels, and solitary nodules, simultaneously. The system architecture can be easily extended in the future to include a still greater range of nodule types, most importantly so-called ground-glass opacities (GGOs). In addition, automatic local adaptive histogram analysis, dynamic cross-correlation analysis, and the automatic volume projection analysis by using by data dimension reduction method, are used in nodule detection. The proposed system has been applied to 10 patients screened with low-dose multi-slice CT. Preliminary clinical tests show that (1) the false positive rate averages about 3.2 per study; and (2) by using the system radiologists are able to detect nearly twice the number of nodules as compared with working alone.

Keywords: CT lung nodule, automatic detection, knowledge-based image analysis, computer-aided diagnosis.

1. INTRODUCTION

Computed tomography (CT) provides a promising technology for lung cancer detection. State of the art multi-slice CT imaging has been reported as extremely useful for non-invasive detection of peripheral lung cancers at an early stage[6].

Several automatic lung nodule detection algorithms have been published in recent years [2-5, 7-8]. Nodules in these studies have been noted to vary considerably in size, shape, location, density, and in relation to adjacent structures, in particular, vessels and the chest wall[6]. To date, this variability has not been sufficiently emphasized. One single algorithm usually can only detect one type of nodules optimally. Even though the algorithm could be robust for a certain type of nodules, it still suffers from considerable failures on other types of nodules. The need to correctly develop and apply specific algorithms for specific types of nodules, and to systematically integrate them to achieve optimal nodule detection represents a challenging problem yet to be solved.

In this paper, we propose a knowledge-based system that is able to automatically detect and analyze lung nodules from multi-slice CT images obtained during a single breath-hold. In principle, without *a priori* knowledge human vision system could not see anything meaningful. In this sense, the knowledge-based image analysis, which aims at making the computer "see" something meaningful by the help of domain-specific knowledge, is a long-term research subject and has many potential new applications. Visual information to be processed in the real world of medical image analysis is often (a) partial or incomplete, (b) locally ambiguous, and (c) conflict from different viewers. Since none of the currently existing low-level image processing operators is perfect, some important features are not extracted and erroneous features are detected. This even may introduce more uncertainty in medical image analysis. How to cope with uncertainties and variations is the key issue in solving real world medical image analysis and processing problems, such as lung nodule detection. We believe that knowledge-based image analysis [9-10, 13-15, 18-19], incorporated with reasoning about multiple-visual evidence [11-12, 16-17], is a promising approach to solving such problems.

Based upon knowledge, humans may infer many properties of a visual scene that may not be strongly or directly supported by the visual data. That relates research in medical image analysis to some research areas in which large amount of problem-specific knowledge is used to obtain constrained solutions. By systematically utilizing domain specific knowledge, including physical knowledge about the imaging process, semantic knowledge about the target object being analyzed, and perceptual knowledge about viewing the object, knowledge-based image analysis would be able to provide better solutions for complex medical image analysis problems, which were considered not possible before. This is the guideline for us to develop the automatic detection system to cope with the challenges of lung CT nodule detection. The detailed description of the system is given in the next section and preliminary experimental results and analysis are given in Section 3.

2. METHODS AND SYSTEM DESCRIPTION

A "divide and conquer" approach is used in the development of this knowledge-based automatic detection system. The system block diagram is shown in Figure 1. First we divide the task of nodule detection into several subtasks. Then we develop dedicated solutions for each of these subtasks. Using anatomical knowledge, three new robust algorithms are developed for three major sub-types of nodules: nodules attached to the chest wall; nodules connected to vessels, and solitary nodules. These three detection algorithms can be viewed as three Expert Processing Modules (EPMs), each with optimal detection capability for one specific type of nodule.

For each defined Volume Of Interest (VOI), the EPMs are applied sequentially. Each EPM outputs the detection result, as well as an information map that contains analysis information that is passed to the next EPM as additional evidence for further processing or exclusion. Each EPM is activated by both the input VOI and its valid information map. Diagnostic information about nodules, such as size, shape, and density, is fused when the detection process proceeds from one EPM to another. In this way, the system is extendable to allow even more expert processing modules. The system is designed to be transparent to users, with the reasons for each decision explained by providing multiple diagnostically meaningful measurements and 3-D visualization. The automatic detection system is interfaced to an Interactive CAD (ICAD) system (see Figure 2) for optimal clinical workflow integration [1].

The system reported in this paper has three main EPMs, and one dedicated false positive reduction module to reduce the false positives due to thickenings of the bronchial wall. These three main EPMs are Data Dimension Reduction (DDR) for detection of vessel-feeding nodules, Automatic Local Histogram Analysis (ALOHA) for detection of solitary nodules, and dynamic cross-correlation analysis (DCA) for detection of nodules on chest wall.

2.1 Vessel-Feeding Nodule Detection by Data Dimension Reduction (DDR)
Existing methods of nodule detection are based on radiometric and/or morphological features of the volume of interest. However, when there are other anatomic structures attached to a nodule, such as vessels, these features will inevitably involve contributions from non-nodule structures, depending on the degree of attachment. A direct consequence of this is that there will be either too many false negatives or too many false positives. When contributions of the non-nodule structures cannot be separated from those of the nodules, one has to either lower the acceptance criteria for those nodules to be detected and increase the number of false positives, or risk missing them altogether.

In our system, we use a principal component analysis method to reduce the data dimension, so that the features of the nodules can be well extracted even with the presence of vessel attachment. The features we use include both the patterns of nodule shape and the intensity distribution of nodules in the reduced data space. A set of sequential classifiers is built to filter different non-nodule structures. Nodule candidates that meet all the classification criteria are determined as nodules.

2.2 Automatic Local Histogram Analysis (ALOHA) for Detection of Solitary Nodules

ALOHA is used as a core technology for the segmentation of target structures. As we previous reported [2], segmentation is very sensitive to threshold and there is a tradeoff in setting this value. If the threshold is set too high, vessels will lose some weak parts and appear to be nodule-like. However, if the threshold is set too low, noise will be enhanced and may make a nodule appear to be a vessel. Both problems may be exacerbated in low-dose images used for screening. ALOHA is our solution for this problem.

The local histogram of intensity of the defined VOI ideally has two distinct peaks, which correspond to the relatively bright anatomical structure and its dark surroundings. The valley between the peaks then can be chosen as the threshold to segment the target structure. However, the situation is more complicated in many cases due to the partial volume effect. This occurs frequently with small vessels. In either case, there will be no distinct valley in the histogram.

Instead, we adaptively set the threshold for target structure segmentation by finding the curvature extrema of the local histogram. Noticing that peaks in the curvature plot correspond to sharp drops in the histogram, and reflect abrupt changes in intensity distribution, the threshold can be set as the intensity value where the sharpest change occurs. ALOHA is able to cope with almost all these complicated situations.

A classifier is applied to the output of ALOHA using a few geometric properties that characterize the structure after it has been segmented. These properties include five geometric features: diameter, volume, sphericity, mean intensity value and standard deviation of intensity.

2.3 Dynamic Cross-Correlation Analysis (DCA) for Detection of Nodules on Chest Wall

The DCA EPM can automatically segment and detect lung nodules from high resolution multi-slice CT images by dynamically initializing and adjusting a 3D template and analyzing its cross correlation with the structure of interest. First, thresholding is used to extract the structure of interest, which comprises a candidate nodule and its possibly connected anatomies such as vessels or the chest wall. Then, the proposed segmentation method finds the core of the structure of interest, which corresponds to the nodule, analyzes its orientation and size, and initializes a 3D template accordingly. Next, the template gradually expands, with the cross correlation to the original structure of interest computed at each step. The template is then optimized based on the analysis of the cross correlation curve.

A segmentation of the nodule is first roughly obtained by doing an 'AND' operation between the optimal template and the extracted structure, and then refined by a spatial reasoning method. Template parameters can be recorded and recalled in later diagnosis so that reproducibility and consistency can be achieved. A chest wall removal algorithm is embedded in the EPM for any given VOI with part of the chest wall. Note that this EPM can be expanded for accurate segmentation of nodules on vessels as well [5].

2.4 Reduction of False Positive Caused by Thickening of the Bronchial Wall

In automated lung nodule detection, false-positives may be caused by bronchial wall thickening. The partial volume effect makes them appear as solitary nodules since the walls of the airway are in many cases too thin to be completely imaged [2]. Accordingly, a processing module with a dedicated bronchial wall thickening detection technique is used in our system so that the false-positive ratio can be substantially reduced.

The basic idea is to test if the nodule candidate is anatomically connected to any airway cavities. Because of the different geometric features of two types of airway branches, two complementary approaches are used to detect them. The first approach, called perpendicular test, detects airway branches that are perpendicular or nearly perpendicular to the scan plane using features derived from perpendicular airways. Similarly, the other approach is called parallel test that recognizes parallel or nearly parallel airways. For a nodule candidate, the module performs both perpendicular test and parallel test on examination planes that comprise different spin planes, sagittal planes, and coronal planes. If either the perpendicular test or parallel test on any of the examination planes leads to a decision that this nodule candidate is located on an airway, the candidate is considered as a false positive.

The final outputs of this module can either be directly provided on the display devices so that physicians can mark them by visual checking or these candidates can be automatically removed by the automatic knowledge-based detection system to decrease the false positive rate.

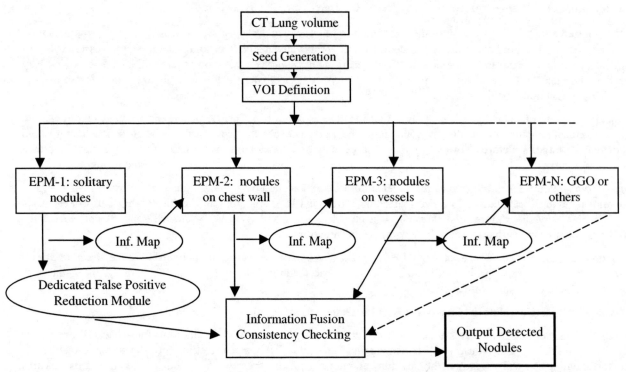

Figure 1.The block diagram of the Knowledge-based Automatic Detection System with multiple EPMs.

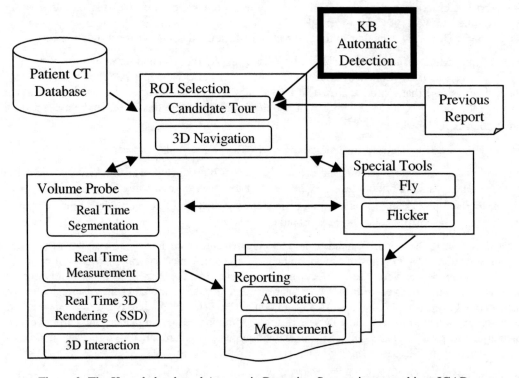

Figure 2: The Knowledge-based Automatic Detection System integrated into ICAD
for nodule identification and examination.

3. PRELIMINARY RESULTS

In this section, we first briefly discuss the materials and methods used for testing the proposed lung nodule detection method. Then the preliminary results are presented and discussed.

3.1. Materials

We applied the proposed lung nodule detection method to 10 patient studies acquired using Siemens Volume Zoom multi-slice CT scanner. The data was collected at New York University Medical Center for a screening project of current and former smokers who were asymptomatic. The data sets were all obtained using low dose, only 20 to 40 mAs, at high resolution over the entire lung volume, with a slice collimation of 1mm. The data was reconstructed with a slice thickness of 1.25 mm and an overlap of 0.25 mm. The number of thin sections ranged from 245 to 319 slices, and each slice contained 512 by 512 pixels, with the pixel size ranging from 0.57 to 0.67 mm. Some typical slices are shown in Figure 3, with a nodule indicated on each.

3.2. Methods

There were three phases in the preliminary clinical evaluation. First, three chest radiologists read the 10 patient studies separately using 7 mm thick reconstructions on hard copies. Their marks were documented and later transferred into coordinates in pixel unit. Meanwhile, the proposed lung nodule detection method was applied to 1.25mm reconstructions. The automatic detection results were also recorded. Finally, two experienced chest radiologists examined all the marks made by both radiologists and computer. At this stage, an interactive computer-aided diagnosis system (ICAD) which can provide real time segmentation, quantification, and detection, and other assistant tools for pulmonary nodule analysis, was employed to improve radiologists' confidence in interpretation. Consensus was made on all marked suspicious structures and was used as the gold standard to evaluate performance.

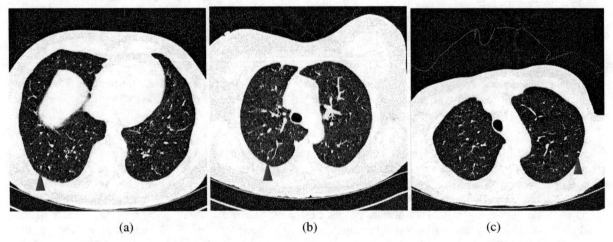

(a)   (b)   (c)

Figure 3. Three typical slices of the screening CT data used, with a nodule on each indicated by an arrow.

(a) A solitary nodule; (b) A nodule attached to vessel; (c) A nodule attached to the chest wall.

3.3. Preliminary Results

Three types of nodules, solitary nodules, nodules attached to vessels, and nodules attached to the chest wall, were detected by applying the proposed automatic detection method. Some typical examples are shown in Figure 4.

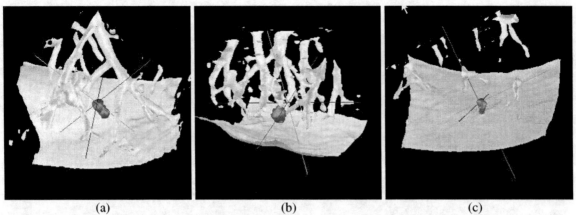

(a)   (b)   (c)

Figure 4. Some typical examples of the detected nodules. (a) A solitary nodule;
(b) A nodule attached to vessels; (c) A nodule attached to the chest wall.

The overall experimental results are listed in Table 1. Analysis has shown that there were in total 50 nodules detected and confirmed by radiologists and the proposed lung nodule detection method together, of which 2 were ground glass opacities (GGOs). The three radiologists detected 21, 17, and 14 nodules, representing sensitivities of 42.0%, 34.0% and 28.0%, respectively. The automatic detection algorithm detected 37 nodules, achieving a sensitivity of 74.0%, with a mean false positive rate of 3.2 per patient study. The computer detection result had significant overlap with that of the individual radiologist, ranging from 64.3% to 71.4%. With the help of the proposed automatic detection system, radiologists would detect an average of 147% more nodules than alone, and reach sensitivities of 86.0%, 80.0% and 84.0%, respectively.

Since it is very hard for radiologists to detect nodules smaller than 3 mm on 7mm thickness sections, we then excluded all confirmed nodules that were smaller than 3 mm in diameter, resulting in 33 confirmed nodules, and computed the statistics again. Radiologists detected 19, 15, and 13 nodules, achieving sensitivities of 57.6%, 45.5% and 39.4%, respectively. Obviously, radiologists' performance increased. The computer detected 27 nodules greater than or equal to 3mm in diameter, achieving a sensitivity of 81.8%, with a mean false positive rate of 2.5 per patient study. The computer detection result overlap with that of the individual radiologist ranged from 69.2% to 80.0%. It would help radiologists detect an average of 101% more nodules than alone, and reach sensitivities of 93.9%, 90.9% and 93.9%, respectively.

As we have described in the previous section, the proposed automatic detection algorithm has three different Expert Processing Modules (EPMs) to detect three different types of nodules: solitary nodules, nodules on chest wall, and nodules attached to vessels. However, it does not yet possess the ability to detect ground glass opacities (GGOs). Therefore, we excluded the GGOs and analyzed the experimental results again. There were in total 48 confirmed non-GGO nodules. Radiologists detected 19, 16, and 12 nodules, achieving sensitivities of 39.6%, 33.3% and 25.0%, respectively. The computer detected 37 non-GGO nodules, achieving a sensitivity of 77.1%, with a mean false positive of 3.2 per patient study. The computer detection result overlap with that of the individual radiologist ranged from 75.0% to 87.5%, and can help radiologists detect an average of 164% more nodules and reach sensitivities of 85.4%, 81.3% and 83.3%, respectively.

If excluding GGOs and nodules smaller than 3mm, there were in total 31 confirmed nodules. Radiologists detected 17, 14, and 11 nodules, achieving sensitivities of 54.8%, 45.2% and 35.5%, respectively. The computer detected 27 non-GGO nodules that are greater than or equal to 3mm in diameter, achieving a sensitivity of 87.1%, with a mean false positive of 2.5 per patient study. The computer detection result overlap with that of individual radiologist ranged from 81.8% to 88.2%, and can help radiologists detect an average of 114% more nodules and reach sensitivities of 93.5%, 93.5% and 93.5%, respectively. The experimental results are also illustrated in Figure 5.

We also compared the size distribution of the nodules detected by the automatic detection algorithm and by radiologists. Figure 6 shows them separately. It can be observed that for nodules smaller than 3mm in diameter, the automatic detection algorithm performs significantly better than the radiologists. The reasons lie in two aspects. First, it is harder for radiologists to pick them up on thick sections. Secondly, analysis has shown that most of the small nodules missed by radiologists are located in central area of the lungs, which has many more anatomical structures than the peripheral area. In such situation, it is very difficult for radiologists to identify the small opacities using only 2D information.

It can also be observed that even for middle-sized nodules up to 6 mm, the proposed automatic detection approach can detect more than radiologists. This is mainly because radiologists are sensitive to peripherally located nodules yet less sensitive to centrally located ones. In addition, some middle-sized nodules are also attached to vessels on 2D slices, which makes them less eye-catching to radiologists. However, as the nodule sizes go up and the nodules become more eye-catching, radiologists' performances increase.

All nodules confirmed: 50					
	Nodules detected	*Sensitivity %*	*New sensitivity* %*	*Overlap with computer*	*Overlap rate %*
Radiologist 1	21	42.0	86.0	15	71.4
Radiologist 2	17	34.0	80.0	14	82.4
Radiologist 3	14	28.0	84.0	9	64.3
Automatic detection	37	74.0	-	*FPs/patient study:* 3.2	

All nodules ≥ 3mm: 33					
	Nodules detected	*Sensitivity %*	*New sensitivity* %*	*Overlap with computer*	*Overlap rate %*
Radiologist 1	19	57.6	93.9	15	78.9
Radiologist 2	15	45.5	90.9	12	80.0
Radiologist 3	13	39.4	93.9	9	69.2
Automatic detection	27	81.8	-	*FPs/patient study:* 2.5	

All non-GGO nodules: 48					
	Nodules detected	*Sensitivity %*	*New sensitivity* %*	*Overlap with computer*	*Overlap rate %*
Radiologist 1	19	39.6	85.4	15	78.9
Radiologist 2	16	33.3	81.3	14	87.5
Radiologist 3	12	25.0	83.3	9	75.0
Automatic detection	37	77.1	-	*FPs/patient study:* 3.2	

All non-GGO nodules ≥ 3mm: 31					
	Nodules detected	*Sensitivity %*	*New sensitivity* %*	*Overlap with computer*	*Overlap rate %*
Radiologist 1	17	54.8	93.5	15	88.2
Radiologist 2	14	45.2	93.5	12	85.7
Radiologist 3	11	35.5	93.5	9	81.8
Automatic detection	27	87.1	-	*FPs/patient study:* 2.5	

Table 1. Experimental results of the proposed lung nodule detection method.

*: New sensitivity refers to the sensitivities that radiologists can achieve with the help of the automatic nodule detection algorithm.

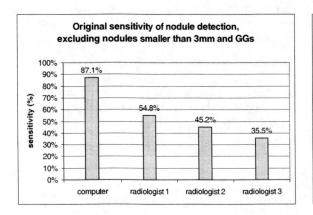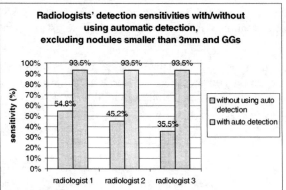

Figure 5. Some experimental results of the proposed automatic lung nodule detection method,
when nodules smaller than 3mm in diameter and GGOs are excluded.
(Left): the original sensitivities of the automatic detection algorithm and radiologists;
(Right): the sensitivities radiologists can reach with the help of the automatic detection algorithm.

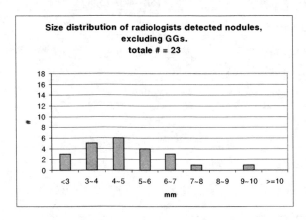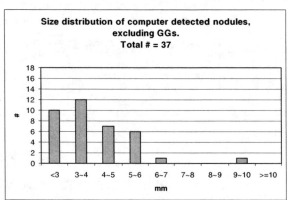

Figure 6. Size distribution of nodules detected by radiologists (left) and computer (right).

CONCLUSION

To optimize the automatic detection of a more complete spectrum of lung nodules identified from CT requires multiple specialized algorithms in a coherently integrated detection system. We describe a novel approach for development of such a system with several new robust automatic detection algorithms. First, the system can simultaneously detect different types of nodules, including those attached to the chest wall, nodules adjacent to or fed by vessels, and solitary nodules. Secondly, the system architecture can be easily extended in the future to include a still greater range of nodules, most importantly so-called ground-glass opacities (GGOs). In addition, automatic local adaptive histogram analysis, dynamic cross-correlation analysis, and the automatic volume projection analysis by using data dimension reduction method, are all new system features used in nodule detection. Preliminary clinical tests using multi-slice CT data sets have shown encouraging results for practical application to lung nodule screening.

ACKNOWLEDGEMENTS

The authors wish to thank Prof. Aaron Bobick of Georgia Institute of Technology for his various helpful discussions and suggestions , and to acknowledge Emilio Vega and Fiona Feeley of NYU for their invaluable technical assistance.

REFERENCES

1. C.L. Novak, L. Fan, J. Qian, G. Kohl, D.P. Naidich, "An interactive System for CT lung nodule identification and examination", *Computer Assisted Radiology and Surgery 2001 (CARS 2001)*, pp. 599-604, 2001.
2. L. Fan, C.L. Novak, J. Qian, G. Kohl, and D.P. Naidich, "Automatic detection of lung nodules from multi-slice low-dose CT images," *Proceedings of SPIE Medical Imaging 2001, Image Processing*, vol 4322, pp. 1828-1835, 2001.
3. L. Fan, C.L. Novak, J.Qian, B. Odry, D.P. Naidich, J.P. Ko, A.N. Rubinowitz, G. McGuinness, "An automatic nodule detection system for complementing radiologists' interpretation of low-dose multi-detector lung CT studies", *Radiological Society of North America (RSNA) Annual Meeting*, 2001.
4. M.L. Giger, K.T. Bae, and H. MacMahon, "Computerized detection of pulmonary nodules in computed nodule detection in helical CT", *Proceedings of SPIE Medical Imaging 1999*, vol. 3661, pp. 553-559, 1999.
5. L. Fan, J. Qian, B. Odry, H. Shen, D. P. Naidich, Gerhard Kohl, Ernst Klotz, "Automatic Segmentation of Pulmonary Nodules by Using Dynamic 3D Cross-correlation for Interactive CAD Systems" to appear in *Proceedings of SPIE Medical Imaging 2002, Image Processing, 2002*
6. P. Croisille, M. Souto, M. Cova, S. Wood, Y. Afework, J.E. Kuhlman, and E.A. Zerhouni, "Pulmonary nodules: tomography images", *Investigative Radiology*, vol. 29, pp. 459-465, 1994.
7. S.G. Armato III, M.L. Giger, C.J. Moran, J.T. Blackburn, K. Doi, and H. MacMahon, "Computerized detection of pulmonary nodules on CT scans", Imaging & Therapeutic Technology, vol. 19, pp. 1303-1311, 1999.
8. S.G. Armato III, M.L. Giger, J.T. Blackburn, K. Doi, and H. MacMahon, "Three-dimensional approach to lung improved detection with vascular segmentation and extraction with spiral CT", *Radiology*, vol. 197, pp. 397-401, 1995.
9. J. Qian, "Uncertain Reasoning Based-upon Directional Topographic Features for Medical Image Analysis," Proc. IEEE International Conference on Systems, Man, and Cybernetics, Chicago, Oct. 1992. Pp.129-135.
10. Andress, K. and A. Kak, ``A Production System Environment for Integrating Knowledge with Vision Data,'' Proceedings of Workshop on Spatial Reasoning, pp. 1--12, 1987.
11. Bhatnagov, R. and L. N. Kanal, "Handling Uncertain Information: A Review of Numeric and Non-Numeric Methods," In Uncertainty in AI, L. N. Kanal and J. F. Lemmer (Eds.). New York: Elsevier Science Publishers B. V., pp. 3--26, 1986.
12. Brooks, R., ``Symbolic Reasoning Among 3-D Models and 2-D Images," Artificial Intelligence (17), pp. 285--348, August 1981.
13. Lehrer, N., G. Reynolds, and J. Griffith, `` A Method for Initial Hypothesis Formation in Image Understanding," Proceedings of IEEE First Int. Conf. on Computer Vision, pp. 578--585, 1987.
14. Li Z. and L. Uhr, ``Pyramid Vision Using Key Features to Integrate Image-Driven Bottom-Up and Model-Driven Top-Down Processes," IEEE Trans. on Sys., Man, and Cyb. (17), No. 2, pp. 250--263, March/April 1987.
15. Lowe, D., ``Perceptual Organization and Visual Recognition." New York: Kluwer Academic Publishers, 1985.
16. Pearl, J., "On Evidential Reasoning in a Hierarchy of Hypotheses," Artificial Intelligence (28), pp. 9--15, February 1986.
17. Qian, J. and R. Ehrich, "A Framework for Uncertainty Reasoning in Hierarchical Visual Evidence Space," Proceedings of The 10th International Conference on Pattern Recognition, June 1990.
18. Shapiro, L. G. and R. M. Haralick, "Structural Descriptions and Inexact Matching," IEEE Trans. on PAMI (3), No. 5, pp. 504--519, September 1981.
19. Wesley, L. P., ``Evidential Knowledge-based Computer Vision," Optical Engineering, (25), No. 3, pp. 363--379, March 1986.

Enhanced Lung Cancer Detection in Temporal Subtraction Chest Radiography Using Directional Edge Filtering Techniques

Hui Zhao[a,b], Shih-Chung Ben Lo[a], Matthew T. Freedman[a], and Yue Wang[b]

[a]ISIS Center, Radiology Department,Georgetown University Medical Center, Washington DC, 20007
[b]Electrical Engineering and Computer Science Department, The Catholic University of America, Washington DC, 20064

ABSTRACT

We have developed a series of directional edge enhancement and edge extraction methods that can accurately segment posterior and anterior ribs in chest radiography. These methods can also separate the lower and upper edges of ribs. The edges were first enhanced by two sets of proximate parabola curve models for left and right sides of the image. We used a directional edge filtering technique to remove low signals and noises on the edge enhanced image in the multiresolution domain. Finally, we employed a rib curve projection and reasoning method to reconstruct the rib edges and remove false edges for the upper and lower bound of the rib edges independently. A two-step registration, corresponding to global and local matching, is applied for current and prior images assisted by their corresponding edge images. The subtraction images were then processed by a rule-based CAD system. The FROC results were compared to that obtained by the original image using a CAD system consisting of rule-based and convolution neural network processing. The majority of lung cancer in temporal subtraction images were lit-up. The FROC results were significantly improved using the subtraction image with the rule-based CAD.

Keywords: Directional edge filtering, temporal subtraction, radiography.

1. INTRODUCTION

Lung cancer is the leading cause of cancer deaths in the United States in both men and women and is a leading cause of cancer deaths throughout the world. While preventive methods (smoking cessation and diminution) are having some success, the long (10-15 year) latency of deleterious effect that continue after smoking cessation and the failure of successful treatment of nicotine addiction in most smokers indicates that there will be a long term need for improved techniques for early detection. The most common detection techniques currently known include chest radiography, cytologic analysis of sputum samples, fiberoptic examination of bronchial airways, and computerized tomography (CT) scans. Among these, chest radiography remains the most cost-effective and widely used detection. We estimate that more than 90% of lung cancer detection now takes place on chest radiographs. The chest radiograph is non-invasive, relatively inexpensive, and routinely available. In the 1980s, Stitik and his colleagues found that a single radiologist did miss 32% of all lung nodules viewed retrospectively and that two radiologists working with an arbiter missed only 15%. Motivated by these clinical reports, we began to develop computer techniques to enhance the cancer visibility in the chest radiography. Specifically, we attempt to remove the lung structures such as ribs, and vessels. At the same time, the growing abnormalities including the lung cancer can be enhanced.

Further author information: (Send correspondence to Hui Zhao or Shih-Chung B. Lo.)
Hui Zhao: E-mail: zhao@isis.imac.georgetown.edu, Telephone: 202 687 5135
Shih-Chung B. Lo: E-mail: lo@isis.imac.georgetown.edu, Telephone: 202 687 1659, Address: ISIS Center, Radiology Department, Georgetown University Medical Center, 2115 Wisconsin Ave. Suite 603, N.W. Washington, DC, 20007

Medical Imaging 2002: Image Processing, Milan Sonka, J. Michael Fitzpatrick, Editors, Proceedings of SPIE Vol. 4684 (2002) © 2002 SPIE · 1605-7422/02/$15.00

2. METHOD

We first filtered the ribs and structures in the lung. The filter image would facilitate delineation of the lung field. In this study, our effort has been concentrated on the detection of rib and registration of ribs for temporal chest radiography. Approximately one hundred chest radiographs were randomly selected by the third author who is a senior radiologist. All the selected radiographs were 14" × 17" postero-anterior (PA) view films. These films were digitized by a Vidar film digitizer (Model: VXR-12 Plus) at 12 bits depth with a resolution at 150 pixels per inch. In this study, the images were averaged and resized to 525 × 637 pixels.

The rib frame is the one of most prominent structures on chest radiographs. They sometimes are obstacles in clinical chest radiology. On the other hand, the ribs can facilitate position identification in the lung. Technically, upper and middle ribs are reliable landmarks for comparing temporal and contralateral lung images. Accurate rib delineation and registration would be a technical backbone for the development of automatic computer-aided tools to assist the radiologists in the detection of lung cancer, tuberculosis, interstitial lung diseases, etc. It would also make quantitative analysis of chest image possible.

Vogelsang et al[1] and Sanada et al[2] have used model based segmentation methods to delineate the ribs on chest radiographs. In this study, we created an initial rib curve model and performed the directional filtering along the curves. The filtered image was processed by a directional rib extraction technique in multi-resolution domains. Based on these curves, broken segmented ribs could be reconstructed using a rib curve projection technique. Finally, an active line model was used to confirm and label the ribs. This whole process could be repeated twice, with the initial generic ribs model in the first run, and refined the ribs model for the second run. We could split our algorithm into three major parts, rib enhancement, rib extraction, and rib confirmation and labelling.

2.1. Directional filtering

By visually inspecting the rib curves on many chest radiographs, we found that posterior ribs showed as the convex curves on the film. Since a generic edge detector would produce all edges, we selectively extracted ribs by applying directional filters along the rib curves. We started with a posterior rib modelling (i.e., Eq.(1). Two sets of proximate parabola functions were used to represent the left and right lung rib curvatures respectively. Rib orientations were modelled in such as way that the flat segment is on the central side of the lung and tilt region is on the lateral side of the lung. This quantitative description can be proximately expressed by:

$$y - y_{o,k} = a_{k,[y]}(x - x_{o,k})^p \tag{1}$$

where $a_{k,[y]}$ is a function of y and $p = 2 \sim 3$. The norm orientations can be computed by taking first derivative of the curves,

$$\frac{dy}{dx} = pa_{k,[y]}(x - x_{o,k})^{p-1} \tag{2}$$

and the angle with respect to x axis is

$$\theta(x,y) = \arctan(\frac{dy}{dx}) \tag{3}$$

We interpolated the norm orientation value of the ribs for the whole lung area and saved them to a map file. Then we picked up our edge detector as the first derivative of Gaussian(DoG). The DoG filter is a very effective edge detector.[3] It is natural weighted kernel, and easy to implement. Also it shows the symmetric in two-dimensional, we could modified the DoG as the function of the orientation, as

$$\begin{aligned} DoG(\theta, x, y) &= \Re(DoG(x,y)) \\ &= DoG(x\sin\theta - y\cos\theta, x\cos\theta + y\sin\theta) \end{aligned} \tag{4}$$

If we force the edge enhancement to be performed in directions of our modelled rib norm map , only the posterior rib edges will get fully enhanced. Our directional filtering finally could be expressed as

$$\begin{aligned} g(x,y) &= f(x,y)\bar{\otimes}DoG(u,v,\theta(x,y)) \\ &= \sum_{u,v} f(x+u, y+v) \bullet DoG(u,v,\theta(x,y)) \end{aligned} \tag{5}$$

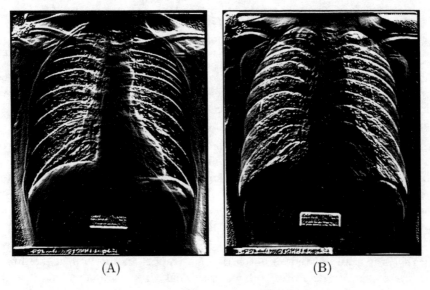

(A)   (B)

Figure 1. (A) The enhanced upper edge of ribs by directional filtering;and (B) The enhanced lower edge of ribs by directional filtering.

where $f(x, y)$ denotes the intensity of original image, and $g(x, y)$ denotes the filtered image, $\bar{\otimes}$ represents this kind of non-conventional convolution.. At each pixel, the operation between the two vectors is a typical inner product. DoG operator rotates based on the position of the center pixel and guided by the rib norm orientation map of the posterior ribs. Kernel changes from one pixel to another, the operation is not a typical convolution. Fig.(1) shows the results after we performed the directional filtering. Since the first derivative kernel could detect the rising and following edge, we got the upper edge of the ribs and lower edge of the ribs at the same time.

2.2. Directional extraction

Although the directional filtering can enhance the posterior rib edges, the edges running relatively the same directions were also shown high signals in the enhanced image. Since we use the generic rib norm orientation map for all the chest radiographs, some orientations on the map do not closely align with the rib curves on a specific case. Therefore, a part of rib edges may not be enhanced. In order to handle various conditions of the enhanced edges, we developed a set of edge detection algorithms called directional extraction (DirE) to incorporate with the DirF for extract the ribs. The DirE consists of three components. Firstly, we extracted high intensity DirF values in multi-resolution domains. All the small images are filtered independently and then aggregated to formed the results. Secondly we perform directional non-maxima suppression obtaining only the points where the DirF value is at maximum along the direction of the norm of the predefined curvatures. Finally, we perform the rib projection along the rib orientation to connect the broken edges and remove the branches.

Most of the false ribs could be removed using the DirE. In some situations, one side of the rib has double edges. This is due to the structure of the ribs. The ribs could be modelled as a cylinder with spongy bone in the core and the compact bone as the ring. Since these two kinds of bone have different attenuation coefficients for the X-rays, they will generate a pair of edges with distance within a few millimeters: stronger and weaker edges at the outer and inner sides of the rib, respectively. Because they are close and parallel to each other, we could take advantage of this phenomenon to consolidate the ribs. In some situations, they could be used to recover a part of the rib edges.

2.3. Confirmation and labelling

Having applied the DirF and DirE, we could extract most of the posterior ribs. However, two problems remain unsolved: (1) some of the rib edges were still disconnected, and (2) identification of ribs. Since we planned to

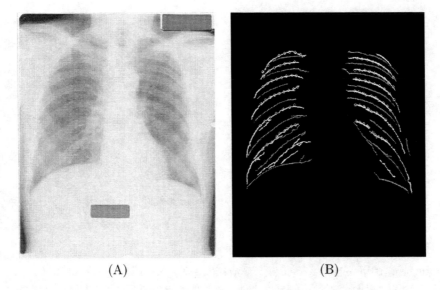

(A)   (B)

Figure 2. (A) The original image; (B) The ribs extracted image. The lower edge of the ribs are shown in bright white, and upper edge of the ribs are shown in darker lines. The active line confirmation and labelling procedure was done on the lower edge of the ribs. The tags of confirmation appear as small circles on the image.

use the rib as the registration landmarks, it is essential to identify the anatomic indices of the ribs. In order to address these issues, we developed an active curve method to link the small segments if they belong to the same rib edge and label the ribs according to their relative positions. The active line model is derived from the snake model.[4] By adding a push force, the active curve could move along its norm direction up and down to search for potential rib edge on the DirE processed image. Whenever it hits a pixel associated with a rib edge, it stops there and the active curve will extend to find the other points following the curvature of the rib map. By automatically adjusting the elastic and bending parameters, the active curve will maintain the smoothness while moving. The distance and shape between adjacent ribs are also estimated to form the rules that would help the active curves follow the rib edge segments instead of being stuck on a wrong place.

2.4. Anterior ribs detection

Since the posterior rib signals are much stronger than anterior rib signals, it is a challenge to extract the anterior ribs without including the posterior ribs. In this study, we also applied the DirF and DirE methods to extract the anterior ribs in corresponding directions. The parameters used in the orientation map for extracting the anterior ribs are conjugate to the parameters used in detecting the posterior ribs. Although the posterior and anterior ribs are not perpendicular, edge signals along the anterior can be modelled and effectively extracted by the same techniques with the predefined orientation map associated with the anterior rib curves. As far as implementation is concerned, we need to change the curvatures of the rib model and a part of rule bases to open different angle range for the edge extraction. Otherwise, the software implementation is pretty much the same. We consider that this is a great feature of the proposed DirF and DirE methods.

2.5. Image registration

We defined that a pair of temporal images consisting of prior and current chest radiographs obtained from the same patient with the same x-ray procedure at two different occasions (typically one or two years apart). Before subtracting the prior image from the current image, the prior image was transformed to align with the current image. The transformation processes consists of two steps: (1) global matching and (2) local registration. Since the upper part of the chest and lung field borders are quite steady when taking chest x-ray, the global similar between the prior and current images could be matched by applying translation and rotation transformations. In practice, only a pair of critical points was used to perform translation and rotation. The critical points are obtained by using two crossing points (one for each side) of the lung field borders and the most prominent ribs

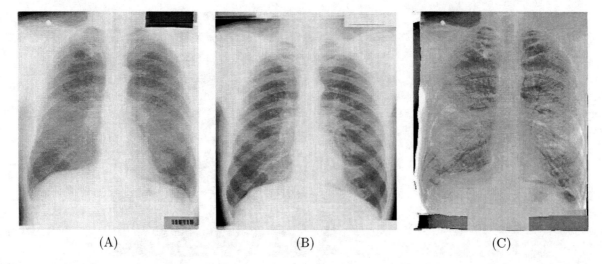

(A)   (B)   (C)

Figure 3. (A) current image; (B) prior image; and (C) subtraction image. There is a cancer located in the upper right lobe of the lung. Since it is beneath the clavicle bone, it is not very apparent in the original images. It becomes more noticeable in the subtraction image.

in the upper lobe of the lung region. The control points were assigned by using equal distance sampling on the rib edges and along the lung and heart borders. Finally, the thin plate splines technique[5] was employed to perform the warping based on the local control points.

3. TEMPORAL SUBTRACTION AND CAD EVALUATION

We subtracted the warped prior image from the current image to get the subtraction image. In the subtraction image, as one shown in Fig.(3), we found that the normal structures such as ribs and aligned large vessels were cancelled out on the images. The bright spots in the subtraction image are either growing patterns or artifacts. By reviewing many subtraction images, we found that artifacts are close to the diaphragm, heart, clavicle bones, etc. Typically, their shapes are associated with the anatomic borders and are not round.

We modified our existing CAD system[6] to detect only circular spot on the subtraction. The convolution neural network was not involved in the detection process. The aim of the modified CAD system was only to detect the bright and round patches. As a preliminary study, we collected approximately 32 pairs of chest radiographs to perform the evaluation study using a simplified CAD method on the subtraction images. Each case has only one single cancer spot. The sizes of cancer vary from 7mm to 20mm. The suspicious regions were evaluated by the CAD system specifically in the analysis of circularity and contrast. By varying the circularity and contrast criterion, we obtained three points of the FROC performance. Table (1) shows the results of the experiment.

Sensitivity	56.67%	78.28%	81.61%
FPs (number of false positives/image)	0.85	1.82	2.58

Table 1: FROC results for CAD on subtraction image

4. CONCLUSIONS

The DirF incorporated with DirE is an effective method for rib extraction for both posterior and anterior ribs. We found that the proposed method is quite robust in extracting rib edges on chest radiographs with and without prominent ribs. We also demonstrated that accurate registration method based on rib edges and chest wall can be done automatically. In addition, the lung cancer detection results using contrast and circularity assessment on temporal subtraction images showed a significant improvement over the current CAD method on the original chest images.

ACKNOWLEDGMENTS

Zhao was supported in part by Deus Technology LLC. The authors are grateful for Ms. Lisa Kinnard's editorial assistance.

REFERENCES

1. F. Vogelsang, M. Kohnen, J. Mahlke, F. Weiler, M. W. Kilbinger, B. B. Wein, and R. W. Günther, "Model based analysis of chest radiographs," in *SPIE Medical Imaging 2000, Image Processing*, K. M. Hanson, ed., **3979**, pp. 1040–1052, 2000.
2. S. Sanada, K. Doi, and H. MacHahon, "Image feature analysis and computer-aided diagnosis in digital radiography: Automated delineation of posterior ribs in chest images," *Med. Phys.* **18**, pp. 964–971, Sep/Oct 1991.
3. J. Canny, "A computational approach to edge detection," *IEEE Trans. Pattern Anal. Mach. Intell.* **8**, pp. 679–698, 1986.
4. M. Kass, A. Witkin, and D. Terzopoulos, "Active contour models," *International Journal of Computer Vision* **1**(4), pp. 321–331, 1987.
5. F. L. Bookstein, "Principal warps: Thin-plate splines and the decomposition of deformations," *IEEE Trans. Pattern Anal. Mach. Intell.* **11**, pp. 567–585, 1989.
6. S.-C. B. Lo, H. Chan, J. Lin, M. Freedman, and S. Mun, "Artificial conveolution neural network for medical image pattern recognition," *Neural Networks* **8**(7/8), pp. 1201–1214, 1995.

Computer-aided classification of pulmonary nodules in surrounding and internal feature spaces using three-dimensional thoracic CT images

Y. Kawata, N. Niki, H. Ohmatsu[a], M. Kusumoto[b], R. Kakinuma[a], K. Mori[c],
H. Nishiyama[d], K. Eguchi[e], M. Kaneko[b], N. Moriyama[b]

Dept. of Optical Science, Univ. of Tokushima, Tokushima ,
[a]National Cancer Center Hospital East, [b]National Cancer Center Hospital,
[c]Tochigi Cancer Center, Tochigi , [d]The Social Health Insurance Medical Center,
[e]National Shikoku Cancer Center Hospital

ABSTRACT

The detection rate of small pulmonary lesions has recently increased due to the advances in imaging technology such as Multi-slice CT scanner. In assessing the malignant potential of small pulmonary nodules in thin-section CT images, it is important to examine the nodule internal structure. In our previous work, we found that internal structure features derived from CT density and curvature indexes such as shape index and curvedness were useful for differentiating malignant and benign nodules in 3-D thoracic CT images. This may be attributed to the texture changes in the nodule region due to a developing malignancy. The relationship between nodules and their surrounding structures such as vessel, bronchi, and pleura are another important cue to classification between malignant and benign nodules. We therefore develop a scheme to analyze surrounding structures of the nodule using differential geometry based vector fields in 3-D thoracic images. In addition we present a joint histogram-based representation approach of the internal and surrounding structures of the nodule to visualize the characteristics between nodules. In the present study, we explore the feasibility of combining internal and surrounding structure features for classification of pulmonary nodules.

Keywords: computer-aided diagnosis, pulmonary nodule, internal structure, surrounding structure, joint histogram-based representation, visualization

1. INTRODUCTION

Lung cancer is the leading cause of cancer deaths for men in Japan. Early detection and treatment of lung cancers are crucially important to achieve high survival rate for lung cancer. There is hope in the possibility of early detection of lung cancer with the promising scientific advanced of low-dose CT[1]. Computer-aided diagnosis (CAD) is a promising approach to detect suspicious lesions on the thoracic CT images and alert physicians to these regions[5]. The detailed examinations of the small nodule lesions depend on the malignant potential. The differential diagnosis is ordinarily concluded by histological diagnosis from biopsy. It is often the case that the differential diagnosis by means of biopsy becomes difficult due to nodule size. It becomes important to increase specificity for differentiation between malignant and benign nodules preventing unnecessary biopsies. In order to provide physicians with objective information for making diagnostic decisions, it is desirable to develop CAD techniques for extracting image features from region of interests (ROIs) and estimating the likelihood of malignancy for a given lesion.

There has been a considerable amount of interest in the use of thin-section CT images to observe small pulmonary nodules for differential diagnosis [1-4]. In assessing the malignant potential of small pulmonary nodules in thin-section CT images, it is important to examine the nodule margin, the nodule internal intensity, and the relationships between nodules and surrounding structures such as vessels, bronchi, and spiculation[1-4]. A number of investigators have developed a feature extraction and a classification methods for characterizing pulmonary nodules. Siegelman investigated CT density in the center of a nodule on two-dimensional (2-D) CT images[6]. Other groups also presented nodule density analysis with a special reference phantom to improve measurement accuracy[7]. Cavouras demonstrated that multiple features including nodule density and texture were useful to classify malignancies from other lesions[8]. Following his work, McNitt-Gray proposed pattern classification approach incorporating multiple features, including

Medical Imaging 2002: Image Processing, Milan Sonka, J. Michael Fitzpatrick,
Editors, Proceedings of SPIE Vol. 4684 (2002) © 2002 SPIE · 1605-7422/02/$15.00

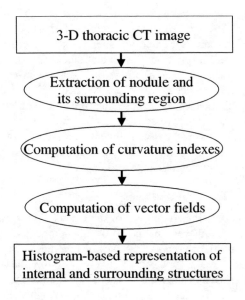

Figure 1 Block diagram of the nodule representation scheme of the internal and surround structures.

measures of density, size measures, and texture of nodules on CT slice images[9]. One promising area of recent researches has been the analysis of three-dimensional (3-D) pulmonary nodule images.

We quantified the concave and convex surfaces by using surface curvatures to characterize surface condition of malignant and benign nodules[10]. Hirano presented an index to quantify how a nodule evolved the surrounding vessels[11]. Tozaki proposed a classification approach between pulmonary artery and vein to characterize the relationships between nodules and surrounding structures[12]. Kitaoka developed mathematical models of bronchial displacements caused by nodules to discriminate cancers from inflammatory pulmonary nodules[13]. Although the performances of these algorithms are expected to depend on data set, they indicate their potential of using 3-D CAD techniques to improve the diagnostic accuracy of differentiating malignant and benign pulmonary nodules.

In our previous work, we found that internal structure features derived from CT density and curvature indexes such as shape index and curvedness were useful for differentiating malignant and benign nodules in 3-D thoracic CT images[14]. This may be attributed to the texture changes in the nodule region due to a developing malignancy. The usefulness of curvature based measures in differentiating malignant and benign nodules was further demonstrated by introducing topological features with respect to morphology of the nodule internal structure[15] In assessing the malignant potential of pulmonary nodules, the relationship between nodules and their surrounding structures such as vessel, bronchi, and pleura are another important cue. We therefore develop a scheme to analyze surrounding structures of the nodule using differential geometry based vector fields in 3-D thoracic images. In order to design a nodule classifier, it is important to observe the difference patterns between benign and malignant cases with respect to the internal and surrounding structures. In this paper we present a method to represent the nodule using the extracted features of the internal and surrounding structures. We are then showing the representation results of benign and malignant nodules and potential usefulness of the representation for the nodule classification.

2. METHODS

The block diagram of the representation scheme of the internal and surrounding structures of the nodule is shown in Figure 1. Each steps is described next.

2.1 3-D thoracic CT images

The 3-D thoracic images used in this paper were reconstructed from thin-section CT images obtained by the helical CT scanner (Toshiba TCT900S Superhelix and Xvigor). The thin-section CT images were measured under the following conditions; beam width: 2mm, table speed: 2mm/sec, tube voltage: 120kV, tube current: 250mA or 200mA. For the scan duration, patients held their breath at full inspiration. Per patient, about CT slices at 1mm intervals were obtained to observe whole nodule region and its surroundings. The range of pixel size in each square slice of 512 pixels was between 0.3x0.3 mm² and 0.4x0.4 mm², and the slice contains an extended region of the lung area. The 3D chest image was reconstructed from the thin-section CT images by a linear interpolation technique to make each voxel isotropic. The data set in this study included 248 3-D chest images from 248 patients provided by National Cancer Center Hospital East and Tochigi Cancer Center. Of the 248 cases, 179 contained malignant nodules, and 69 contained benign nodules. Whole malignant nodules were histologically diagnosed. In benign cases lesions showed no change or decreased in size over a 2-year period were considered benign nodules.

2.2 Extraction of nodule and its surrounding region

The segmentation of the 3D pulmonary nodule image consists of three steps[10];1)extraction of lung area, 2) selection of the region of interest (ROI) including the nodule region, and 3) nodule segmentation based on a geometric approach. The lung area extraction step plays an essential role when the part of a nodule in the peripheral lung area touches the chest wall. The ROI including the nodule was selected interactively. A pulmonary nodule was segmented from the selected ROI image by the geometric approach proposed by Caselles[16]. The nodule surrounding region was computed by the distance from the nodule surface. The distance was obtained by applying the Euclidean distance trance formation approach proposed by Saito et al. [17] to the nodule surrounding region.

2.3 Computation of curvature indexes

Each voxel in the region of interest (ROI) including the pulmonary nodule was locally represented by two curvature indexes that represented the shape index and the curvedness. By assuming that each voxel in the ROI lies on the surface which has the normal corresponding to the 3-D gradient at the voxel, we computed directly the curvatures on each voxel from the first and the second derivatives of the gray level image of the ROI by using an approach proposed by Thirion[18]. Let $I(\mathbf{x})$ be a ROI image. To compute the partial derivatives of the ROI images $I(x)$, the ROI images were blurred by convolving with a 3-D Gaussian function with width σ. The computation of the blurred derivatives were efficiently performed by using the recursive implementation of the Gaussian function[19]. The Gaussian curvature $K(x; \sigma)$ and mean curvature $H(x; \sigma)$ were computed and then the principal curvatures and directions were obtained. The principal curvatures $\kappa_1(x; \sigma)$ and $\kappa_2(x; \sigma)$ ($\kappa_1(x; \sigma) \geq \kappa_2(x; \sigma)$) are obtained by

$$\kappa_i = H(\mathbf{x};\sigma) \pm \sqrt{H^2(\mathbf{x};\sigma) - K(\mathbf{x};\sigma)} \quad (i = 1, 2). \tag{1}$$

The voxel $\mathbf{x}$ in the ROI image is locally described by curvature indexes and CT value. The curvature indexes consist of the shape index and the curvedness[20, 21]. The shape index $S(\mathbf{x}; \sigma)$ with scale σ at the voxel $\mathbf{x}$ is given by

$$S(\mathbf{x};\sigma) = \frac{1}{2} + \frac{1}{\pi} \arctan \frac{\kappa_1(\mathbf{x};\sigma) + \kappa_2(\mathbf{x};\sigma)}{\kappa_1(\mathbf{x};\sigma) - \kappa_2(\mathbf{x};\sigma)}. \tag{2}$$

This index maps the surface shape on the continuous number between zero and one. Voxels that belong to the peak surface type have values around 0; ridge surface type, around 0.25; saddle surface type, around 0.5; and pit surface type, around 1.0. The shape index contributes to describe subtle shape variation. The curvedness $R(\mathbf{x}; \sigma)$ with scale σ at the voxel $\mathbf{x}$ is given by

$$R(\mathbf{x};\sigma) = \sqrt{\frac{\kappa_1(\mathbf{x};\sigma)^2 + \kappa_2(\mathbf{x};\sigma)^2}{2}}. \tag{3}$$

The curvedness is a measure of how highly curved a surface and its dimension is that of the reciprocal of length. The selection of the width σ of the Gaussian function is a critical issue. When the curvature indexes with width σ was utilized to characterize the internal structure of pulmonary nodules, we assigned the value 2.0 to the width, which provided high accuracy of classification between malignant and benign nodules for discrete width values using a data set. In this present study, we also assigned the value 2.0 to the width.

2.4 Computation of vector fields

In order to quantify the relationship between the nodule and its surrounding structure such as vessel and pleura, we focus on two indicators of malignancy, which are denoted as vascular convergence and pleural retraction[1-4]. In the 3-D thoracic CT images, these findings are observed so that the vessel and pleura images are drawn in the nodule. We assumed that the shape of the vessel and the pleura images are similar to cylindrical or conic structures. Therefore, we measure an amount of the vascular convergence and pleural retraction by computing the absolute value of the inner product of the directions of cylindrical or conic structures and the normal directions of the nodule surface. For the representation of the directions, we compute two vector fields that consist of the directions of the maximum principal curvature and normal vector of nodule surface. In this section we present the computation of the vector fields.

The principal curvatures are computed by Eq. (1) and then the directions of them are derived from the first and second partial derivatives of the gray scale 3-D image using the formulae proposed by Thirion[18]. The principal directions $\mathbf{v}_1$ and $\mathbf{v}_2$ for the principal curvatures $\kappa_1(\boldsymbol{x}; \sigma)$ and $\kappa_2(\boldsymbol{x}; \sigma)$ are defined by

$$\mathbf{v}_i(\mathbf{x};\sigma) = \mathbf{a} \pm \sqrt{H^2(\mathbf{x};\sigma) - K(\mathbf{x};\sigma)} \ \mathbf{b} \quad (i = 1, 2). \tag{4}$$

where $\mathbf{b} = (I_z - I_y, I_x - I_z, I_y - I_x)$ and the x component of the vector $\mathbf{a}$ is obtained by

$$\begin{aligned}
\mathbf{a} \cdot \mathbf{x} = -\frac{1}{2h^{3/2}}[& -2I_z^3 I_{xy} + I_y^3 I_{zz} + 2I_y^3 I_{xz} - 2I_y^2 I_z I_{xy} \\
& + 2I_z^2 I_x I_{yz} + 2I_z^2 I_y I_{xz} - 2I_y^2 I_x I_{yz} - 2I_z I_x I_y I_{zz} \\
& + 2I_x I_y I_z I_{yy} + I_y^2 I_z I_{xx} - 2I_z^2 I_x I_{xz} + I_z I_x^2 I_{zz} \\
& - I_x^2 I_z I_{yy} + 2I_z^2 I_y I_{yz} - I_z I_y^2 I_{zz} + I_z^3 I_{xx} - I_z^3 I_{yy} \\
& - I_y^2 I_x I_{xz} + 2I_x^2 I_y I_{yz} - I_y^3 I_{xx} + 2I_x I_z^2 I_{xy} - I_y I_z^2 I_{xx} \\
& - 2I_z I_y^2 I_{yz} + I_y I_z^2 I_{yy} - 2I_z I_x^2 I_{yz} + 2I_x I_y^2 I_{xy} + I_x^2 I_y I_{zz} - I_x^2 I_y I_{yy}]
\end{aligned} \tag{5}$$

The y and z components are obtained by circular permutation of x, y, and z. In tube-like structures such as vessel and pleura, axial directions of them are approximately parallel to the direction of maximum principal curvature of the central part of isointensity surface of the structure. Therefore, a vector field of the nodule surrounding was represented by the direction of the maximum principal curvature. We denote this vector field as the maximum principal curvature vector (MPV) field.

The normal directions of the nodule surface at the vicinity of the nodule was estimated by the following procedure. This procedure was based on the idea which was proposed by Xu[22] to improve the segmentation accuracy of the snake model. Let g(x) be an edge map defined and $f(\mathbf{x}) : \mathbf{R}^3 \rightarrow \mathbf{R}$ be a segmented 3-D binary image of the nodule. The edge map was derived from the segmented 3-D binary image of the nodule having property that it is larger near the nodule edges. The edge map was represented as

$$g(\mathbf{x}) = G_\sigma * |\nabla f(\mathbf{x})| \tag{6}$$

where G_σ is 3-D Gaussian function with the width σ. The edge map has the following three properties; (1) the gradient of an edge map $\nabla g(\mathbf{x})$ has vector toward the edges, which are normal to the edge, (2) these vectors have large magnitudes in the vicinity of the edge, and (3) in the homogeneous region $f(\mathbf{x})$ is nearly constant and $\nabla g(\mathbf{x})$ is nearly zero. Because of the first property, the normal directions of the nodule surface are approximated by the gradient of the edge map in the vicinity of the edges. Since this property is utilized to measure the relationship between nodule surface and surrounding structures, the first property is a desirable property. The capture range will be small due to the second property. The homogenous regions at the surrounding nodule will have zero. The last two properties are undesirable. The approach is to keep the desirable property of the gradients near the nodule edges, but to expand the gradient away from the edges into homogeneous regions of the nodule surrounding using a computational diffusion process. A vector field obtained by the computational diffusion process is denoted as gradient vector (GV) field. The GV field was defined as the vector field $\mathbf{h}(\mathbf{x})$ that minimized the energy functional

$$E = \int_{\mathbf{R}^3} \mu |\nabla \mathbf{h}|^2 + |\nabla g|^2 |\mathbf{h} - \nabla g|^2 d\mathbf{x} \tag{7}$$

where the gradient operator ∇ is applied to each component of $\mathbf{h}$ separately. Minimizing Eq. (7) makes the vector field smooth when there is no data. When $|\nabla g|$ is small, the first term dominates the energy. On the other hand the second term dominates the energy as $|\nabla g|$ is large. In this study, we assigned the term of $|\nabla g|$ to the constant value of one to expand the gradient away from the edges. The parameter μ is a regularization parameter controlling the tradeoff between the first term and the second term. Using the calculus of variations, it is found that the GV field must satisfy the Euler equation. We implemented the iteration technique presented by Xu[22] to solve the Eq. (7).

2.5 Joint histogram-based representation

In order to characterize the distribution pattern of the CT density and the shape index inside nodule, we compute two joint histograms using the distance value from the nodule center. To compute the distance value at each voxel, we apply the Euclidean distance transformation technique [8] to the segmented nodule image and obtain the maximum distance value (D_M) inside the nodule. Since the distance value (v_d) at each voxel is the distance from the nodule surface, the maximum distance value seems to be assigned to the voxel at the nodule center area. To obtain the distance from the nodule center, we compute the value ($D_M - v_d$) at each voxel inside the nodule. Let $I(\mathbf{x})$ and $D(\mathbf{x})$ be respectively the CT density value and the distance value at the voxel $\mathbf{x}$ in the nodule image. The joint histogram of $I(\mathbf{x})$ and $D(\mathbf{x})$ is expressed as

$$H(d_1 = \frac{k_1}{B_1}, d_2 = \frac{k_2}{B_2}) = \frac{1}{N} \sum_{j=1}^{N} \sum_{i=1}^{N} K_{k_1, k_2}(I(\mathbf{x}_i), D(\mathbf{x}_i)) \tag{8}$$

with

$$K_{k_1, k_2}(t_1, t_2) \begin{cases} 1 & \frac{k_1 - 1}{B_1} \le t_1 < \frac{k_1}{B_1}, \frac{k_2 - 1}{B_2} \le t_2 < \frac{k_2}{B_2} \\ 0 & otherwise \end{cases} \tag{9}$$

where B_1 and B_2 are the numbers of bins for the CT density value and the distance value, respectively, and N is the number of voxels inside the nodule. Statistically, the normalized joint histogram denotes the joint probability of the CT density value and the distance value. It measures how the CT density value distributes inside the nodule with respect to the distance from the nodule center. The similar equation for the joint histogram of the shape index value and the density value is obtained. In the preliminary study, the domain of CT density, distance value, and shape index values were specified to [-1000, 500] (HU), [0, 50] (mm), [0, 1], respectively. The number of bins was set to 50 for each value.

Additionally, we compute the absolute value (F) of the inner product between MPV and GV fields at each voxel in surrounding region of the nodule and then, compute a joint histogram of the distance value from he nodule surface and the absolute value of the inner product. The joint histogram is used as the representation of the nodule surrounding structure. To select the part of cylindrical or conic structures in the surrounding region, we specified two threshold values T_{SH} for the shape index value (SH) and then obtained the region consisting of voxels which satisfied with a condition of $SH < T_{SH}$. The value of T_{SH} was set to 0.5. The joint histogram was computed for the selected region in the similar equation of the computation the joint histogram of the CT density value and the distance value. This process means that the surface types of cylindrical or conic structures are extracted by the shape index value.

3. EXPERIMENTAL RESULTS

In this section we present an example of application result of the representation scheme to a malignant case and then show the representation results of benign and malignant nodules in our data set.

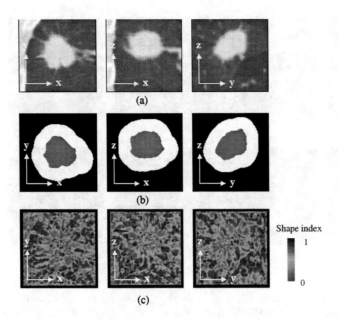

Figure 2 Extraction results of a nodule and its surrounding region and shape index distribution. (a) Slice images of the ROI Including the malignant nodule. Form left to right : x-y plan, x-z plan, y-z plan. (b) Extraction results of the nodule and its surrounding. Gray region: nodule region. White region: surrounding region. (c) Shape index distribution.

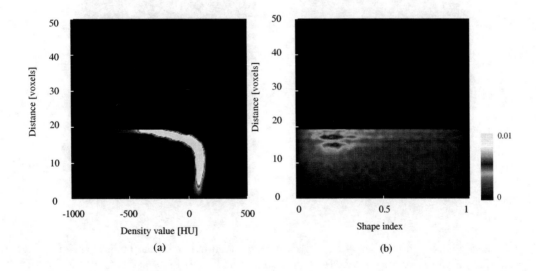

Figure 3 Joint histogram-based representation of the inner structure of the nodule shown in Figure 2. (a) Joint histogram of the density value and the distance value. (b) Joint histogram of the shape index value and the distance value.

Figure 2 presents the ROI image, the extraction result of nodule and surrounding region, and the shape index image of the malignant case, respectively. Figure 3 presents the joint histogram-based representation inside the nodule with respect to CT density value and shape index value.

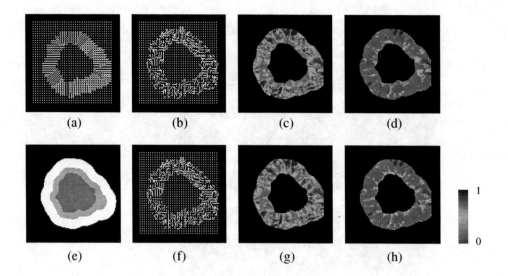

Figure 4 Computation results of F value in the surrounding region of the nodule shown in Figure 2. (a) Slice image of the GV field. (b) Slice image of the MPV field. (c) Computation result of the absolute value of inner product between the GV and MPV field. (d) Slice image of F value. (e) The nodule boundary region for modification of the maximum principal curvature direction. (f) Modification result of the MPV field. (g) Modification result of the absolute value of inner product between the GV and the modified MPV field. (h) Slice image of the F value computed by using the modified MPV field.

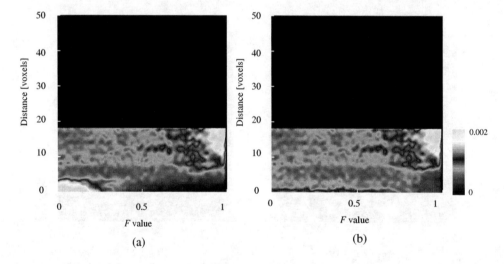

Figure 5 Joint histogram-based representation of the surrounding structure of the nodule shown in Figure 2. (a) Joint histogram of the F value and the distance from the nodule surface. (b) Joint histogram of the modified F value and the distance from the nodule surface.

Figure 4 presents the slice images of the computation results of F value in the surrounding region of the nodule shown in Figure 2. Figure 4 (c) is the computation result between the GV and MPV fields as shown in (a) and (b), respectively. Using shape index value, Figure 4 (d) is extracted from the F value image. Compared Figure 4 (d) with Figure 2 (a), it is observed that the part of cylindrical or conic structures such as vessels and speculations are corresponding to the extracted regions in Figure 4 (d). However, when observing the part with the vessels and speculations at the vicinity of the nodule boundary, there are some parts in which the directions of the maximum

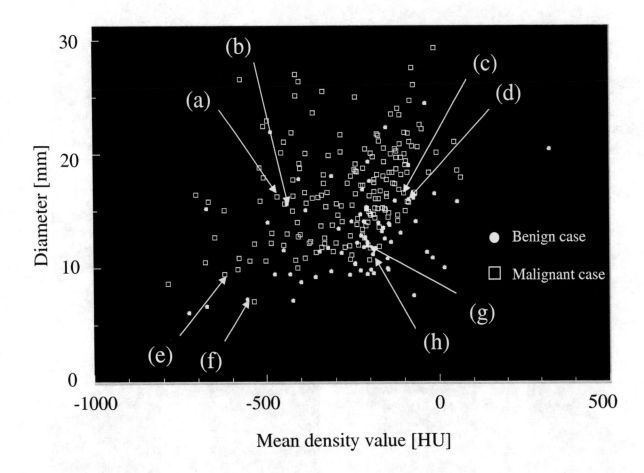

Figure 6 Plot of the data set in the feature space of mean density value against the nodule diameter. Rectangle mark : malignant case. Filled circle mark: benign case. The eight cases denoted by arrows from (a) to (h). Each nodule is denoted as follows: (a): A_m, (b): A_b, (c): B_m, (d): B_b, (e) C_m, (f): C_b, (g): D_m, (h): D_b.

principal curvature are away from the direction along the vessels and speculations. It seems that the nodule boundary density affects the computation of the directions. To avoid the problem, we specified the nodule boundary region as shown in Figure 4 (e) and then recomputed the MPV field from ones of the region of the nodule surrounding except for the specified boundary region. The specification of the nodule boundary region is computed using the Euclidean distance value in the nodule surrounding as shown in Figure 4 (e), and the computation of the MPV field at the nodule boundary region is performed by the diffusion process in the similar manner mentioned in Section 2.4. Compared Figure 4 (d) with (h), it is observed that the F values along the vessels and speculations become closer to one value at the vicinity of the nodule boundary. Figure 5 presents the joint histogram-based representation of the nodule surrounding region. Figure 5 (a) and (b) are obtained by using the F value distributions shown in Figure 4 (d) and (h), respectively. Compared Figure 5 (a) with (b), the modification of the direction of the MPV field at the vicinity of the nodule boundary decrease the frequency of the F value around zero and increase the frequency of the F value round one.

Figure 6 presents the plot of our data set in the feature space of mean density value inside the nodule against the nodule diameter. To observe the differentiation of such nodule representation, we selected four samples with different diameter and mean density value. The nodules A_m and A_b present the malignant and benign cases with low mean density value and large diameter, respectively. The nodules B_m and B_b present the malignant and benign with high mean density value and large diameter, respectively. The nodules C_m and C_b present the malignant and benign cases with low mean

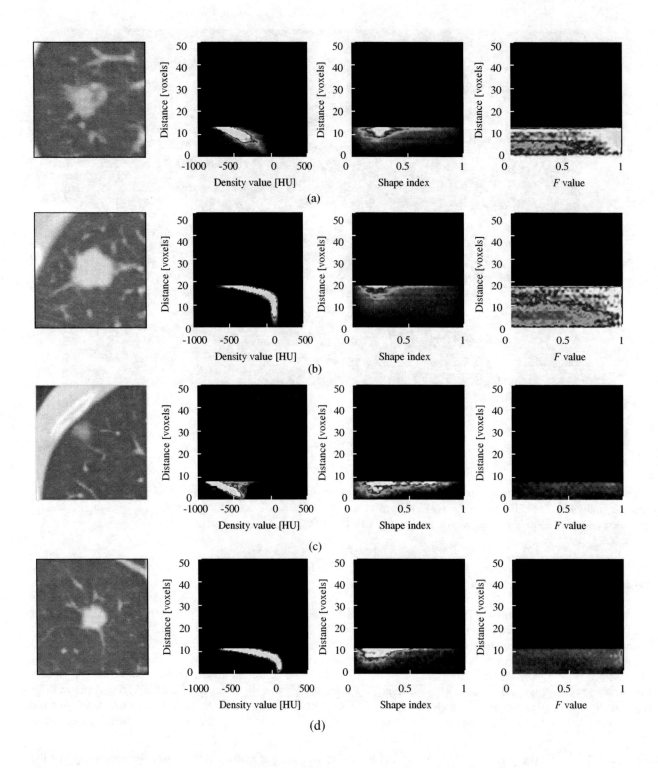

Figure 7   Joint histogram-based representation of malignant cases denoted in Figure 6. (a) :A_m, (b): B_m, (c): C_m, (d) D_m. From left to right, slice image of ROI image including the nodule, joint histograms with respect to CT density value, shape index value, and F value, respectively.

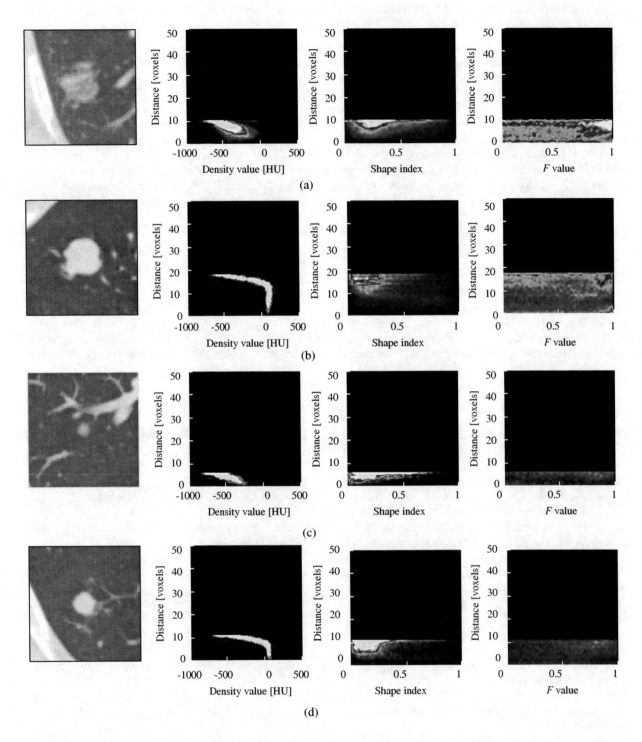

Figure 8 Joint histogram-based representation of benign cases denoted in Figure 6. (a) :A_b, (b): B_b, (c): C_b, (d) D_b. From left to right, slice image of ROI image including the nodule, joint histograms with respect to CT density value, shape index value, and F value, respectively.

density value and small diameter, respectively. The nodules D_m and D_b present a case with high mean density value and small diameter, respectively.

Figures 7 and 8 respectively presents the joint histogram-based representations of the malignant and benign nodules denoted in Figure 6. Compared malignant with benign cases, it can be observed that there are difference patterns of the joint histogram-based representations concerning the shape index and the F value. Compared A_m with A_b, A_m has larger amount of the component radiating from the nodule than A_b. Compared B_m with B_b, B_b has extremely high frequency of the shape index value around zero. This means that peak surface type occupies the inner structure of the B_b. Owning to the component of vessels and speculations, it seems that B_m has larger amount of the component radiating from the nodule than B_b. Compared C_m with C_b, C_b has higher frequency of the shape index value around zero than C_m. Compared D_m with D_b, D_b has also higher frequency of the shape index value around zero than D_m. Though the amount of the difference of the distribution pattern in the representation concerning the F value between malignant and benign case is smaller as the nodule size becomes smaller, the malignant cases (C_m and D_m) have higher frequency of the F value around one than the benign cases (C_b and D_b). From the observation of the nodule representation, it is desired to design multiple classifiers for nodule patterns with respect to the nodule size and density.

4. COMCLUSION

We have presented a scheme to analyze surrounding structures of the nodule using differential geometry based vector fields in 3-D thoracic images. In addition we presented a joint histogram-based representation approach of inner and surrounding structures of the nodule to visualize the characteristics between nodules. We demonstrated the difference pattern of the representation between benign and malignant cases using our data set. We believe that this representation approach will visualize the difference patterns of nodule characterizations and help to design the nodule classifier for the CAD scheme.

REFERENCES

1. M.Kaneko, K.Eguchi, H.Ohmatsu, R.Kakinuma,T.Naruke, K.Suemasu, N. Moriyama, "Peripheral lung cancer: Screening and detection with low-dose spiral CT versus radiography," *Radiology*, **201**, pp.798-802, 1996.
2. K.Mori, Y.Saitou, K.Tominaga, K.Yokoi, N.Miyazawa, A.Okuyama, M.Sasagawa, "Small nodular legions in the lung periphery: New approach to diagnosis with CT," *Radiology*, **177**, pp.843-849, 1990.
3. C.V. Zwirewich, S.Veda, R.R.Miller, N.L.Muller, "Solitary pulmonary nodule: High-resolution CT and radiological pathologic correlation," *Radiology*, **179**, pp.469-476, 1991.
4. K.Kuriyama, R. Tateishi, O. Doi, K. Kodama, M. Tatsuta, M. Matsuda, T. Mitani, Y. Narumi, M. Fujita, "CT-pathologic correlation in small peripheral lung cancers," *AJR*, **149**, pp.1139-1143, 1987.
5. K. Kanazawa, Y. Kawata, N. Niki, H. Satoh, H. Ohmatsu, R. Kakinuma, M. Kaneko, N. Moriyama, K. Eguchi, "Computer-aided diagnosis for pulmonary nodules based on helical CT images," *Computerized Medical Imaging and Graphics*, **22**, pp.157-167, 1998.
6. S.S.Siegelman, E.A.Zerhouni, F.P.Leo, N.F. Khouri, F.P. Stitik, "CT of the solitary pulmonary nodule," AJR, vol.135, pp.1-13, 1980.
7. A.V.Proto and S.R.Thomas, "Pulmonary nodules studied by computed tomography," *Radiology*, **156**, pp.149-153, 1985.
8. D. Cavouras, P. Prassopoulos and N. Pantelidis, "Image analysis methods for solitary pulmonary nodule characterization by computed tomography," *European Journal of Radiology*, **14**, pp.169-172, 1992.
9. M.F. McNitt-Gray, E.M.Hart, J. Goldin, C.-W, Yao, and D.R. Aberle, " A pattern classification approach to characterizing solitary pulmonary nodules imaged on high resolution computed tomography," *Proc. SPIE*, **2710**, pp.1024-1034, 1996.
10. Y.Kawata, N.Niki, H.Ohmatsu, R.Kakinuma, K.Eguchi, M.Kaneko, N.Moriyama, "Quantitative surface characterization of pulmonary nodules based on thin-section CT images," *IEEE Trans. Nuclear Science*, **45**, pp.2132-2138, 1998.
11. Y.Hirano, Y.Mekada, J.Hasegawa, J. Toriwaki, H.Ohmatsu, and K.Eguchi, "Quantification of vessels convergence in three-dimensional chest X-ray CT images with three-dimensional concentration index," *Medical Imaging Technology*, **15**, pp.228-236, 1997.

12. T.Tozaki, Y.Kawata, N.Niki, H.Ohmatsu, R. Kakinuma, K.Eguchi, N. Moriyama, "Pulmonary organs analysis for differential diagnosis based on thoracic thin-section CT images," *IEEE Trans. Nuclear Science*, **45**, pp.3075-3082, 1998.

13. H. Kitaoka and R. Takaki, "Simulations of bronchial displacement owing to solitary pulmonary nodules," *Nippon Acta Radiologica*, **59**, pp. 318-324, 1999.

14. Y.Kawata, N.Niki, H.Ohmatsu, R.Kakinuma, K.Mori, K.Eguchi, M.Kaneko, N. Moriyama, "Curvature based analysis of internal structure of pulmonary nodules using thin-section CT images," *Proc. IEEE Int. Conf. on Image Processing*, Chicago, **3**, pp.851-855, 1998.

15. Y. Kawata, N.Niki, H.Ohmatsu, M. Kusumoto, R. Kakinuma, K. Mori, K. Eguchi, M. Kaneko, N. Moriyama, "Potential usefulness of curvature based description for differential diagnosis of pulmonary nodules" *Proc. Medical Image Computing and Computer-Assisted Intervention*, pp.386-393, 1999.

16. V.Caselles, R.Kimmel, G.Sapiro, and C.Sbert, "Minimal surfaces based object segmentation," *IEEE Trans. Pattern Analysis Machine Intelligence*, **19**, pp.394-398, 1997.

17. T. Saito and J. Toriwaki, "Euclidean distance transformation for three-dimensional digital images," IEICE Trans, **J76-D-II**, pp.445-453, 1993.

18. J.-P, Thirion and A. Gourdon, "Computing the differential characteristics of isointensity surfaces," *Computer Vision and Image Understanding*, **61**, pp.190-202, 1995.

19. R. Deriche, "Recursively implementing the gaussian and its derivatives," *INRIA Research Report*, **1893**, 1993

20. J. J. Koenderink and A.J.V. Doorn, "Surface shape and curvature scales," *Image and Vision Computing*, **10**, pp.557-565,1992.

21. C.Dorai and A.K. Jain, " COSMOS-A representation scheme for 3D free-form objects," *IEEE Trans. Pattern Analysis Machine Intelligence*, **19**, pp.1115-1130,1997.

22. C. Xu, J. L. Prince, "Snakes, shapes, and gradient vector flow," *IEEE Trans. Image Processing*, **7**, pp.359-369, 1998.

Recognition of Lung Nodules from X-ray CT Images Using 3D Markov Random Field Models

Hotaka Takizawa[a], Shinji Yamamoto[a],
Tohru Matsumoto[b], Yukio Tateno[b], Takeshi Iinuma[b], Mitsuomi Matsumoto[c]

[a] Toyohashi Univ. of Tech., Toyohashi, Aichi, Japan
[b] National Institute of Radiological Science, Chiba, Japan
[c] Tokyo Metropolitan Univ. of Health Sciences, Tokyo, Japan

ABSTRACT

In this paper, we propose a new recognition method of lung nodules from X-ray CT images using 3D Markov random field (MRF) models. Pathological shadow candidates are detected by our Quoit filter which is a kind of mathematical morphology filter, and volume of interest (VOI) areas which include the shadow candidates are extracted. The probabilities of the hypotheses that the VOI areas come from nodules (which are candidates of cancers) and blood vessels are calculated using nodule and blood vessel models evaluating the relations between these object models using 3D MRF models. If the probabilities for the nodule models are higher, the shadow candidates are determined to be abnormal. Otherwise, they are determined to be normal. Experimental results for 38 samples (patients) are shown.

Keywords: X-ray CT images, recognition of lung nodules, 3D nodule and blood vessel models, 3D Markov random field models

1. INTRODUCTION

We proposed a lung cancer screening system by CT (LSCT) for the mass screening[1]. In this system, one problem is the increase of the number of the images to be diagnosed by a doctor to about 30 slices per patient from 1 X-ray film. To overcome such a problem, we have to develop a recognition algorithm of the pathological shadow candidates which can reduce the images to be diagnosed by a doctor.

There are several works on recognition of pathological shadow candidates[234]. They utilize image filters which respond selectively only to isolated shadows to detect the pathological shadow candidates. In these methods, however, normal shadows whose characteristics are similar to those of the abnormal ones are also detected as false positives.

We have also developed an image filter called *Quoit* filter[56] which is a kind of mathematical morphology filter. This filter can detect pathological shadows with the sensitivity over 95[%], but it also detects a lot of false positives yet.

For example, if a shadow candidate is too small as shown in Fig.1(a), it cannot be determined to be a nodule or not. In this case, we pay attentions not only to the shadow candidate but also the shadows around it. If ridge shadows related to the shadow candidate are newly found as shown in Fig.1(b), it can be determined to be a blood vessel(normal).

In this paper, we propose a new recognition method of abnormalities of shadow candidates evaluating the relations between the shadow candidates and the shadows around them by using 3D Markov random field (MRF) models with geometrical object models such as nodules (which are candidates of cancers) and blood vessels.

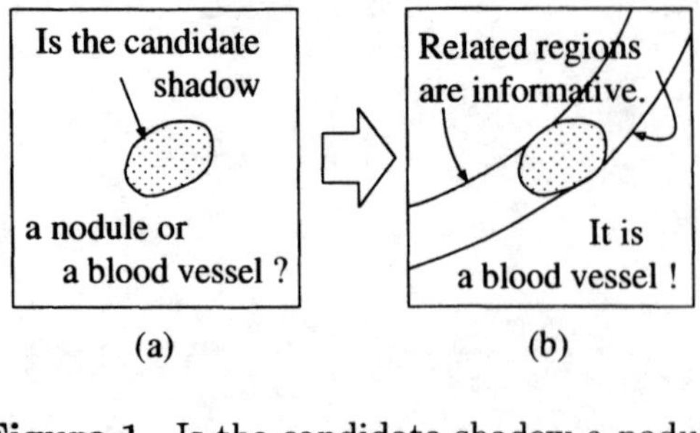

Figure 1. Is the candidate shadow a nodule or not ?

E-mail: {takizawa,yamamoto}@parl.tutkie.tut.ac.jp; URL: http://www.parl.tutkie.tut.ac.jp/~takizawa/

2. RECOGNITION PROCESS

Fig.2 shows the recognition process described in this paper. First, a pathological shadow candidate is detected by our Quoit filter. Next, a VOI area including the shadow candidate is extracted, and is divided into some rectangle regions. A 3D partial space corresponding to each rectangle region is called a *cell*. For each cell, some possible geometrical object models (such as nodules and blood vessels) are generated considering the correspondence with the VOI area. By combining these object models, a set of object model combinations is generated. From these object model combinations, artificial CT images are generated using computer graphics techniques. By comparing the VOI area of the observed CT image and the generated artificial CT images, the most possible object model combination is searched for evaluating the relationship between the cells in each object model combination by MRF models. If the most possible combination includes any nodule models, the shadow candidate is determined to be abnormal. Otherwise, it is determined to be normal.

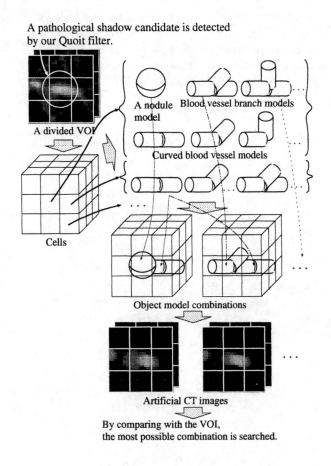

Figure 2. Recognition process.

3. DIVISIONS OF VOI AREAS

We extract VOI areas whose centers are located at candidate shadows detected by our quoit filter and whose sizes are N[pixel] $\times$ N[pixel] $\times$ M[slice]. The VOI areas are divided into $n \times n \times m$ rectangle regions(in this experiment, $N = 30$, $M = 3$, $n = 3$ and $m = 3$). A 3D partial space corresponding to each rectangle region is called a cell, and each neighboring cell which connects to a cell is called a *neighbor* of the cell.

In this paper, we suppose that each cell has only one of object models described in the next section, and that the state of each cell depends only on the neighbors(26 neighbors).

4. DEFINITIONS OF OBJECT MODELS

4.1. Nodules

We represent a nodule as a sphere model whose radius is r. The radius varies within a certain range. We represent the variation by describing the radius as a normal distribution $g_{ND}^r(r)$. The priori probability of the hypothesis that a cell has a nodule is represented as $p_{ND} \cdot g_{ND}^r(r)$, where p_{ND} is the probability of appearance of a nodule.

4.2. Curved blood vessels

We represent curved parts of blood vessels using two connected cylinder models as shown in Fig.3. The vessel which is nearer to the heart is called a *parent vessel*, the other a *child vessel*. r, θ and ds represent a radius of the cylinder model, a curving angle and a difference between the areas of the cross sections, respectively. We suppose that they are independent each other, and that the variations of them are represented by normal distributions.

We define two kinds of the priori probabilities of the hypotheses that cells have curved blood vessel models considering the positions of the models in tree structure of blood vessels. (1) If a curved blood vessel model is the root of a tree structure in a VOI area, the priori probability of it is defined to be $p_{CB1} \cdot g_{CB}^r(r) \cdot g_{CB}^\theta(\theta) \cdot g_{CB}^{ds}(ds)$, (2) if a model is not the root, the priori probability is defined to be $p_{CB2} \cdot g_{CB}^\theta(\theta) \cdot g_{CB}^{ds}(ds)$, where p_{CB1} and p_{CB2} represent the probabilities of the appearance of curved blood vessel models, respectively.

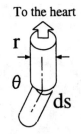

Figure 3. A curved blood vessel model.

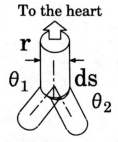

Figure 4. A blood vessel branch model.

4.3. Blood vessel branches

We also represent branch parts of blood vessels using three connected cylinder models as shown in Fig.4. The priori probabilities for the blood vessel branch models are also defined in the same way as curved blood vessel models.

4.4. Air

A cell is filled with air. The priori probability is represented as p_{AR}.

4.5. Relation between object models

We define two kinds of relationship between object models in neighboring cells considering knowledge about anatomy of human bodies(lungs). One is *consistent* relationship, the other is *inconsistent* relationship.

1. Relationship between two neighboring air models is consistent.

2. Next, relationship between an air model and a blood vessel model(a curved blood vessel model or a blood vessel branch model) is defined as follows:

    (a) If an end point of the blood vessel is in the cell of the air model as shown in Fig.5, it is inconsistent, because it indicates that the end point is isolated.

    (b) Otherwise, it is consistent.

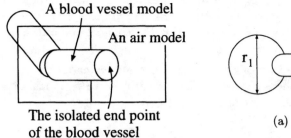

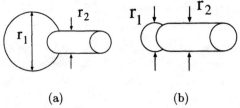

(a)   (b)

Figure 5. An isolated end point of a blood vessel model.

Figure 6. Relation between a radius of a nodule and that of a blood vessel.

3. Relationship between an air model and a nodule model is consistent.

4. Relationship between two neighboring blood vessel models is defined as follows:

   (a) If these blood vessel models are connected each other, it is consistent.
   (b) If the end point of one of these blood vessel models is isolated, it is inconsistent.
   (c) If they are parallel, it is consistent.

5. Finally, relationship between a blood vessel model and a nodule model is defined. Let r_1 be a radius of the nodule, r_2 be a radius of the blood vessel model and $R_r = r_1/r_2$ be the ratio of them, respectively.

   (a) If they are connected each other, and
      i. if the ratio R_r is greater than a threshold R_r^B as shown in Fig.6 (a), then it is consistent because the blood vessel can be regarded as a spicule of the nodule;
      ii. else if the ratio is less than another threshold R_r^S as shown in Fig.6(b), then it is inconsistent because it is unusual;
      iii. else if $R_r^S < R_r < R_r^B$, then we define the middle evaluation between consistent and inconsistent depending on the ratio value R_r.

   (b) If they are not connected, it is consistent.

5. GENERATION OF OBJECT MODEL COMBINATIONS

We list a set of the possible object models for each cell. And by combining them, a set of object model combinations is generated.

Generally, the number of the combinations is large, and it needs a lot of calculation time. In order to reduce the number, we determine the promising object models whose possibilities are high in each cell before combination. The possibilities of the object models are obtained from degrees of the correspondence of the object models with the rectangle regions of the VOI areas. In this section we explain how to determine the promising object models in each cell.

5.1. Determination of promising object models

5.1.1. Nodules

A sphere model whose center is at that of a cell and radius is the average of that of the cancer is generated. An artificial CT image is generated using the sphere model in the same way as the previously proposed method[7] , and a SSD (Sum of Squared Difference) value between the artificial CT image and the rectangle region of the VOI area is calculated. The optimal parameters (of the sphere model such as the position of the center and the radius) minimizing the SSD value are searched for. The sphere model which has such optimal parameters is promising and is used to generate object model combinations.

5.1.2. Curved blood vessels

In order to generate a curved blood vessel model, we prepare two cylinder models whose radii are the averages of those of blood vessels. Ones of the end points of these cylinder parts are connected at the center of a cell. The others are located at the centers of the different neighboring cells. By changing the combination of the neighboring cells, 26×25 possible curved blood vessel models are generated.

From these models, we generate artificial CT images, calculate SSD values and search for the optimal parameters of the curved blood vessel models which minimize the SSD values. The curved blood vessel models whose SSD values are less than a threshold are listed as the promising object models.

5.1.3. Blood vessel branches

$26 \times {}_{25}C_2$ possible blood vessel branch models are generated and the promising object models are listed in the same way as curved blood vessel models.

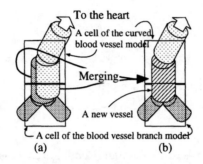

Figure 7. The vessels are merged.

5.2. Generation of object model combinations

A set of object model combinations is generated by combining the object models selected from each cell. If the neighboring blood vessel models satisfy the following two conditions, they are merged as shown in Fig.7.

Condition 1 : The cylinder parts of the blood vessel models faces each other.

Condition 2 : One of these cylinder parts is a parent vessel, and the other is a child vessel.

For each object model combination, a sum of the SSD values over the cells is calculated. And the combinations are sorted by the sum of the SSD values. We use N_{mc}(int this experiment, $N_{mc} = 20$) smallest combinations which have the nodule models and N_{mc} smallest combinations which have no nodule models for recognition process which is described in the next section.

6. RECOGNITION OF OBJECT MODEL COMBINATIONS USING 3D MRF MODELS

In this section, we describe a recognition method of the generated object model combinations by evaluating the possibilities of them using 3D MRF models. In MRF, the optimal states over the whole random variables can be obtained by calculating the optimal states of local areas. In the research fields of computer vision, MRF models are used for image segmentation[89] , object recognition[10] and so on. In this paper, we compute the optimal states over the cells from the relationship of the neighboring cells by using MRF techniques.

6.1. Formulation of possibilities of combinations using 3D MRF models

Let O^s be a random variable indicating an object model in a cell L^s located at a 3D position s, and the value of the random variable O^s be $o^s = \{ND, CB, BB, AR\}$, where ND represents a nodule model, CB a curved blood vessel, BB a blood vessel branch, AR an air model, respectively. Let $L^{n(s)}$ be a neighbor of a cell L^s. The state of O^s depends only on $O^{n(s)}$. An object model combination is represented as $o = \{o^1, o^2, ...\} \in O$. Specially, let a combination including nodule models be $o_A \in O_A$, a combination without any nodule models be $o_N \in O_N$, respectively.

Given a VOI area whose pixel values are $v = v_1, v_2, ...$, the most possible object model combination o^* can be obtained by minimizing the following potential energy function:

$$U(o \in O | v) = \sum_{c \in C} V_c(o) - T \cdot \log p(v|o), \qquad (1)$$

where C is a set of cliques of neighboring variables in the MRF(or Gibbs distribution), $V_c(o)$ is a potential energy of a clique c of the object model combination o, $p(v|o)$ is the likelihood and T is a constant value.

The likelihood $p(v|o)$ represents the conditional probability of the hypothesis that a VOI area v comes from an object model combination o. This probability is calculated in the same way as[7].

Next, the potential energies of the cliques are needed to be specified. For efficiency concerns, we only consider 1- and 2-cliques when computing the energy function(in other words, $V_c(o) = 0, c > 2$).

For 1-clique, clique c consists of a single MRF variable. The 1-clique energies of $c = \{o^s\}$ correspond to the prior probabilities, $V_1(o^s \in O^s) = -\log p(o^s)$.

For 2-clique, clique c consists of two neighboring MRF variables: $c = \{o^s, o^{n(s)}\}$, and the potential energy $V_2(o^s \in O^s, o^{n(s)} \in O^{n(s)})$ is defined considering the relationship between the two neighboring object models described in Sec. 4.5.

- $V_2(AR \in O^s, AR \in O^{n(s)}) = OK.$ $\qquad (2)$

- $V_2(AR \in O^s, CB \in O^{n(s)}) = \begin{cases} NG & \text{(if the end point of the blood vessel} \\ & \text{models is in the cell of the air model),} \\ OK & \text{(otherwise).} \end{cases}$ $\qquad (3)$

- $V_2(AR \in O^s, BB \in O^{n(s)})$ is defined in the same way as $V_2(AR \in O^s, CB \in O^{n(s)})$. $\qquad (4)$

- $V_2(AR \in O^s, ND \in O^{n(s)}) = OK.$ $\qquad (5)$

- $V_2(CB \in O^s, CB \in O^{n(s)}) = \begin{cases} NG & \text{(if the end point of the blood vessel is isolated),} \\ OK & \text{(otherwise).} \end{cases}$ $\qquad (6)$

- $V_2(CB \in O^s, BB \in O^{n(s)})$ is defined in the same way as $V_2(CB \in O^s, CB \in O^{n(s)})$. $\qquad (7)$

- $V_2(CB \in O^s, ND \in O^{n(s)}) = \begin{cases} OK & \text{(if the blood vessel and the cancer are} \\ & \text{connected each other, and } R_r > R_r^B), \\ NG & \text{(if they are connected and } R_r < R_r^S), \\ NG + (OK - NG) * \dfrac{R_r - R_r^S}{R_r^B - R_r^S} \\ & \text{(if they are connected and } R_r^S < R_r < R_r^B), \\ OK & \text{(if they are not connected).} \end{cases}$ $\qquad (8)$

- $V_2(BB \in O^s, ND \in O^{n(s)})$ is defined in the same way as $V_2(CB \in O^s, ND \in O^{n(s)})$. $\qquad (9)$

In these equations, OK and NG indicate the consistent relationship and inconsistent relationship, respectively. They are defined $OK = -1, NG = 10$ in this experiment.

6.2. Searching for the most possible object model combination

We search for two kinds of the most possible object model combinations which minimize the potential energy described in Eq.(1) by changing the parameters of the object models such as the radii of the blood vessel models. One is the combination o_A^* including nodule models, and the other is o_N^* not including any nodule models. They are formulated as follows:$o_A^* = \arg \min_{o_A \in O_A} U(o_A|v)$ and $o_N^* = \arg \min_{o_N \in O_N} U(o_N|v)$.

If the ratio between these potential energies of o_N^* and o_A^*

$$\gamma = \frac{U(o_A^*|v)}{U(o_N^*|v)} \tag{10}$$

is less than a certain value T_γ(in this experiment, $T_\gamma = 1$), then the VOI areas are determined to be abnormal. Otherwise they are determined to be normal.

7. RESULTS

We use 38 samples (patients) for the experiment. A sample is composed of about 30 slices per patient. One slice cross section has 512x512 pixels (resolution of 0.625[mm]) and thickness of 10[mm]. The sample CT images include 41 typical lung cancer regions which include 20 ground glass opacities (GGO).

First, we apply our quoit filter[56] to these sample images, and 540 pathological shadow candidates are extracted with the sensitivity over 95[%].

Next, by applying our new method described in this paper to these extracted shadows, the total number of pathological shadow candidates is decreased to 181 without any new false negatives. The ratio of false positives is 3.74[shadow/patient].

Table.1 shows the sensitivity and the average number of the false positives finally obtained by the quoit filter[56] and the new recognition method described in this paper.

Table 1. The final result of our recognition methods.

Sensitivity	over 95[%]
False positives	3.74[shadow/patient]

7.1. Examples

7.1.1. Example 1

Fig.8 shows an example of a VOI area of a candidate shadow detected by our quoit filter. Fig.9(a) and (b) show the most possible object model combinations including a nodule and not including any nodules, respectively. Fig.10 shows the artificial CT images generated from these object model combinations. The ratio of the potential energies $\gamma = 1.24$, and the candidate shadow is successfully determined to be normal.

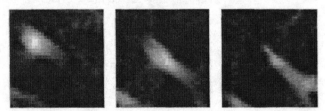

Figure 8. A shadow candidate(at the center in the middle image) and its VOI.

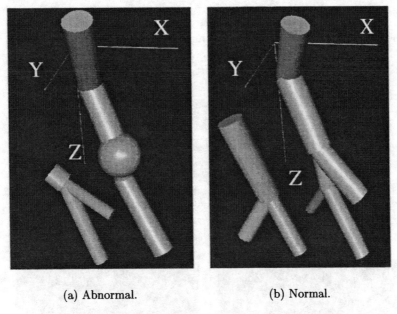

(a) Abnormal.   (b) Normal.

Figure 9. The most possible object model combinations.

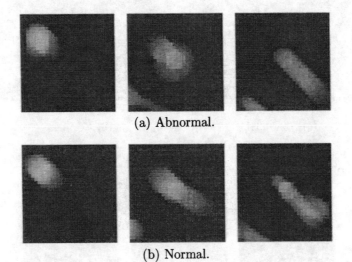

(a) Abnormal.

(b) Normal.

Figure 10. Artificial CT images generated from the object model combinations(Fig.9).

7.1.2. Example 2

Fig.11 shows another example of a VOI area of a candidate shadow detected by our quoit filter. Fig.12(a) and (b) show the most possible object model combinations including a nodule and not including any nodules, respectively. Fig.13 shows the artificial CT images generated from these object model combinations. The ratio of the potential energies $\gamma = 0.655$, and the candidate shadow is successfully determined to be normal.

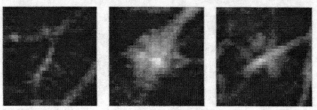

Figure 11. Another shadow candidate and its VOI.

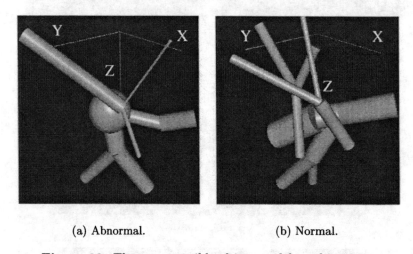

(a) Abnormal. (b) Normal.

Figure 12. The most possible object model combinations.

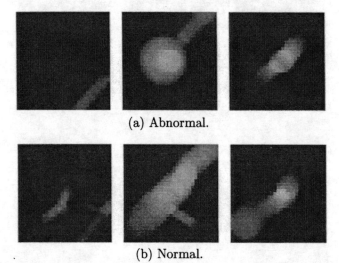

(a) Abnormal.

(b) Normal.

Figure 13. Artificial CT images generated from the object model combinations(Fig.12).

8. CONCLUSION

In this paper, we proposed a new recognition method of lung nodules from X-ray CT images using 3D Markov random field (MRF) models. First, pathological shadow candidates were detected by our Quoit filter which is a kind of mathematical morphology filter. Next, VOI areas which include the shadow candidates were extracted. The probabilities of the hypotheses that the VOI areas come from nodules and blood vessels were calculated using nodule and blood vessel models evaluating the relations between these object models using 3D MRF models. If the probabilities for the nodule models were higher, the shadow candidates were determined to be abnormal. Otherwise, they were determined to be normal.

By applying our new method to actual CT images (38 patient images), good results has been acquired.

REFERENCES

1. S. Yamamoto, I. Tanaka, M. Senda, Y. Tateno, T. Iinuma, T. Matsumoto, and M. Matsumoto, "Image Processing for Computer-Aided Diagnosis of Lung Cancer by CT(LSCT)" *Systems and Computers in Japan* **25**(2), pp. 67–80, 1994.

2. H.Kobatake, Y.Yoshinaga, and M.Murakami, "Automatic Detection of Malignant Tumor on Mammogram" in *Proc. Int. Conf. on Image Processing I*, pp. 407–410, 1994.

3. S. Hideo and I. Noriko, "Development of a computer-aided detection system for lung cancer diagnosis" in *SPIE 1652*, pp. 567–571, 1992.

4. A. Shimizu, M. Hagai, J. Hasegawa, and J. Toriwaki, "Performance Evaluation of 3D Enhancement Filters for Detection of Lung Cancer from 3D Chest X-ray CT Images (in japanese)" *Medical Imaging Technology* **13**(6), pp. 853–863, 1995.

5. S. Yamamoto, M. Matsumoto, Y. Tateno, T. Iinuma, and T. Matshmoto, "Quoit Filter: A New Filter Based on Mathematical Morphology to Extract the Isolated Shadow, and Its Application to Automatic Detection of Lung Cancer in X-Ray CT" in *Proc. 13th Int. Conf. Pattern Recognition II*, pp. 3–7, 1996.

6. T. Okumura, T. Miwa, J. Kako, S. Yamamoto, M. Matsumoto, Y. Tateno, T. Iinuma, and T. Matshmoto, "Variable N-Quoit filter applied for automatic detection of lung cancer by X-ray CT" in *Computer Assisted Radiology and Surgery(CAR'98)*, pp. 242–247, 1998.

7. H. Takizawa, S. Yamamoto, G. Fukano, T. Matsumoto, Y. Tateno, T. Iinuma, and M. Matsumoto, "Recognition of Lung Cancers from X-ray CT Images Considering 3-D Structure of Objects and Uncertainty of Recognition" in *Proc. of Image Processing, part of SPIE*, vol. 1, pp. 998–1007, 2000.

8. S. Geman and D. Geman, "Stochastic Relaxation, Gibbs Distribution, and the Bayesian Restoration of Images" *IEEE Trans. on pattern analysis and Machine Intelligence(PAMI)* **PAMI-6**(6), pp. 721–742, 1984.

9. P. B. Chou and C. M. Brown, "The Theory and Practice of Baysian Image Labeling" *International Journal of Computer Vision* **4**, pp. 185–210, 1990.

10. M. D. Wheeler and K. Ikeuchi, "Sensor Modeling, Probabilistic Hypothesis Generation, and Robust Localization for Object Recognition" *IEEE Trans. on pattern analysis and Machine Intelligence(PAMI)* **17**(3), pp. 252–265, 1995.

Incorporation of negative regions in a knowledge-based computer-aided detection scheme

Yuan-Hsiang Chang[*], Xiao-Hui Wang, Lara A. Hardesty, Christiane M. Hakim,
Bin Zheng, Walter F. Good, David Gur
Department of Radiology, University of Pittsburgh, and Magee-Womens Hospital of the
University of Pittsburgh Medical Center Health System, Pittsburgh, PA 15213

ABSTRACT

The purpose was to evaluate the effect of incorporating negative but suspicious regions into a knowledge-based computer-aided detection (CAD) scheme of masses depicted in mammograms. To determine if a suspicious region is "positive" for a mass, the region was compared not only with actually positive regions (masses), but also with known negative regions. A set of quantitative measures (i.e., a positive, a negative, and a combined likelihood measure) was computed. In addition, a process was developed to integrate two likelihood measures that were derived using two selected features. An initial evaluation with 300 positive and 300 negative regions was performed to determine the parameters associated with the likelihood measures. Then, an independent set of 500 positive and 500 negative regions was used to test the performance of the CAD scheme. During the training phase, the performance was improved from Az = 0.83 to 0.87 with the incorporation of negative regions and the integration process. During the independent test, the performance was improved from Az = 0.80 to 0.83. The incorporation of negative regions and the integration process was found to add information to the scheme. Hence, it may offer a relatively robust solution to differentiate masses from normal tissue in mammograms.

Keywords. Breast cancer, computer-aided detection (CAD), knowledge-based approach, mammography, receiver-operating characteristic (ROC)

1. INTRODUCTION

Mammography is the most common image modality for breast cancer detection and diagnosis.[1-3] Because of increasing volumes of mammograms being performed each year and the expected low yield in a screening environment (only 3 to 8 cases in every 1,000 women screened[4]), detecting early breast cancers from complex breast tissue background with high efficiency and accuracy remains a challenging task. The problem is also compounded by human interpretation errors due to sub-optimal viewing conditions, outside distractions, lack of a systematic approach, oversight of subtle lesions, lack of knowledge of other clinical findings, imprecise correlation with results of other studies, and nonbelief.[5] As a result, the rate of false-negative mammograms has been reported to be in the range of 4%-34%.[6-9]

Computer-aided diagnosis (CAD) schemes have been investigated with the hope that they may serve as an aid to radiologists in order to increase detection sensitivity and/or specificity.[10-12] Recent studies have demonstrated that CAD schemes can serve as an excellent tool in aiding radiologists to improve their performance.[13-15] In a prospective study of 12,860 patients, the use of CAD results in the interpretation process of screening mammograms has been shown to increase the detection of malignancies without undue effect on the recall rate or positive predictive value for biopsy.[16] Although these results are quite encouraging, continuous efforts to improve CAD performances and to assess various issues that may be limiting factors in this area such as limited sensitivity or specificity,[17,18] false-positive reduction,[19] robustness of CAD due to case mix or film digitization,[20,21] mammographic feature selection,[22-24] and assessment of observer performance with and without CAD schemes,[25,26] remain desirable if CAD schemes are to be widely used in a clinical environment.

---

[*] ychang@mail.magee.edu; phone 1 412 641-2573; fax 1 412 641-2582; http://www.upmc.edu; Imaging Research, Suite 4200 MWH, Department of Radiology, University of Pittsburgh, 300 Halket Street, Pittsburgh, PA, USA 15213-3180

During the development and evaluation of a CAD scheme, the process to differentiate between "positive" (abnormal) regions and "negative" regions is an important step during the final decision by the scheme. A classifier is generally trained or derived to differentiate between positive and negative regions on mammograms.[27-30] Therefore, the design of an effective classifier becomes one of the most important issues for these schemes. To define these classifiers, a limited number of positive and negative regions are typically used for training purposes.[30] Significant efforts have been expanded in most instances to include mainly positive regions, and these regions are routinely the major contributor to the detection performances. Most classifiers are generally optimized in a manner where both positive and negative regions are presented and analyzed simultaneously (e.g., interconnecting weights of an artificial neural network to minimize an error function derived from misclassifications of both the positive and negative regions). As a result, despite various strategies for the selection of positive and negative regions, the possible role of each type and its independent contributions to the overall detection performance of a scheme is generally ambiguous. A separate analysis of negative regions may be of great interest in this case because of the potential to provide valuable independent information that may improve detection.

Previously, we have investigated a knowledge-based CAD scheme[31] that served as a region-pruning approach with an effort to reduce a number of false positive regions while maintaining reasonable sensitivity. During this study, the region was first compared (correlated) with a number of verified mass regions (i.e., a "positive" knowledge base) using a set of "similarity" measures. Then, one "likelihood" measure was derived from the set of "similarity" measures to determine the region's likelihood to be positive for a mass. In this study, we attempted to include a set of regions that were considered suspicious, but actually negative regions, to establish a "negative" knowledge base. Alternatively, to determine if a suspicious region was positive for a mass, the suspicious region was compared not only with actually positive regions, but also with known negative regions. Then, one positive, one negative, and one combined "likelihood" measure for both were derived. As a result, the contributions of either positive or negative regions to the detection process can be developed, optimized, and evaluated independently in two independent settings.

2. MATERIAL

Since 1994, a large clinical database (>2000 images) of pathology-verified mammograms has been collected at the University of Pittsburgh Medical Center under an IRB-approved protocol. All mammograms were digitized at our laboratory using a laser film digitizer (Lumisys, Sunnyvale, CA) with a pixel pitch of 0.1mm and 12-bit digital value resolution. The digitizer was routinely calibrated to assure that film optical density (OD) was linearly translated into pixel digital values (DV) in the range of 0.2 to 3.8 OD (1 DV $\equiv$ 0.001 OD). For the purpose of this study, all images were sub-sampled after digitization by a factor of 4 in both dimensions. Hence, the digitized mammograms were approximately 600 × 450 pixels in size with an effective pixel size of 0.4 mm × 0.4 mm.

To establish the two knowledge bases, a total of 300 positive regions (verified masses) were included in a "positive" knowledge base, and a total of 300 suspicious but actually negative regions were included in a "negative" knowledge base. Both the positive and negative regions in this study had been previously detected in digitized mammograms using a different rule-based CAD scheme.[31] All 300 positive regions had been verified (134 malignant and 166 benign masses). Similarly, 500 different verified mass regions and 500 suspicious, but actually negative regions, were randomly selected from our clinical database for the purpose of independent testing. These 1000 regions were not used for any scheme development tasks.

3. METHODOLOGY

Figure 1 shows a flow diagram of the knowledge-based approaches, where (I) only a "positive" knowledge base was used (Approach I); and (II) both "positive" and "negative" knowledge bases were used (Approach II) to determine if a suspicious region is likely to be positive for a mass. Technical approaches are described as follows.

3.1 Positive and negative "Similarity" measures

Each region was first quantitatively characterized using region growing routines and feature extractions that have been described previously[31]. Then, a number of "known" and verified masses (termed N_P) were characterized to establish a "positive" knowledge base. In addition, a number of suspicious, but actually negative, regions (termed N_N) were characterized to establish a "negative" knowledge base. To determine if a suspicious region is similar to a "known" region in quantitative terms, "similarity" measures were computed using distance measures as defined as:

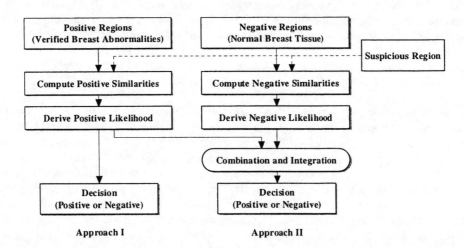

Figure 1. A flow diagram of the knowledge-based approaches, where (I) only a "positive" knowledge base was used (Approach I); and (II) both "positive" and "negative" knowledge bases were used (Approach II), to determine if a suspicious region is likely to be positive for a mass.

$$d = \min \sum_i \frac{|f(w(i)) - \hat{f}(i)|}{\hat{f}(i)} Modulation(i), \tag{1}$$

where $f(\bullet)$ and $\hat{f}(\bullet)$ are the feature profiles for the suspicious region and the "known" region, respectively, and $w(i)$ is a constrained warping function that was intended to achieve better correspondence between feature profiles. The *Modulation(i)* function was selected in a manner that only feature profiles from the interior area of a known region were compared.

Using the positive knowledge base, a set of N_P positive "similarities" (termed $\{d_j^P, j = 1, \cdots N_P\}$) is computed for all pairs consisting each of the "known" masses and the suspicious (unknown) region. Similarly, using the negative knowledge base, a set of N_N negative "similarities" (termed $\{d_j^N, j = 1, \cdots N_N\}$) is computed for all possible pairs consisting each of the negative regions and the suspicious (unknown) region.

3.2 Positive and negative "Likelihood" measures

After all "positive" and "negative" similarity measures are computed, we computed one positive "likelihood" estimate and one negative "likelihood" estimate for each suspicious region as follows:

Positive likelihood: The positive likelihood measure is defined as the sum of "similarity" measures with respect to k_P-th nearest known masses (or positive regions) as:

$$Likelihood^P(k_P) = \sum_j d_j^P, \quad if \ Rank(d_j^P) = 1, \cdots, k_P, \tag{2}$$

where $Rank(d_j^P)$ is the rank in an ascending order of all the positive "similarity" measures. Here, the positive likelihood is derived from positive similarity measures where the suspicious region is compared with all known masses in the positive knowledge base only. The numerical value of positive likelihood measure implies that the suspicious region is likely (or not) to be positive for a mass.

Negative Likelihood: Alternatively, the negative likelihood is defined as the sum of "similarity" measures with respect to k_N-th nearest "known" negative regions as:

$$Likelihood^N(k_N) = \sum_j d_j^N, \quad if \ Rank(d_j^N) = 1, \cdots, k_N,$$ (3)

where $Rank(d_j^N)$ is the rank in an ascending order of all the negative "similarity" measures. The numerical value of the negative likelihood measure is expected to imply that the suspicious region is likely (or not) to be negative for a mass.

3.3 Combination and Integration

To combine information from both positive and negative knowledge bases, a combined likelihood is defined as:

$$Likelihood^C(k_P, k_N) = \frac{Likelihood^P(k_P)}{Likelihood^N(k_N)},$$ (4)

where both the aforementioned positive and negative likelihood measures are used. Here, the two parameters k_P, k_N can be different. The number of likelihood measures that can be computed for each suspicious (unknown) region is $k_P \times k_N$. The numerical value of the combined likelihood measure relates to the likelihood that a region is (or is not) positive for a mass.

To further explore if the use of additional features can improve overall performances, an integration process was designed to incorporate results as acquired from two separate selected features. Here, the two features we selected were circularity[20] and compactness,[32] respectively. For each region, two feature profiles were computed using each of the features. Similarity and likelihood measures were then computed using the two different feature profiles. As a result, two independent combined likelihood measures, termed $Likelihood^C_{Circularity}$ and $Likelihood^C_{Compactness}$, were derived. Finally, an overall likelihood was determined as:

$$Likelihood^I = \sqrt{[\Phi(Likelihood^C_{Circularity})]^2 + [\Phi(Likelihood^C_{Compactness})]^2},$$ (5)

where $\Phi(\bullet)$ is a normalization function to assure that the resulting combined likelihood measures lie in the range of [0, 1] prior to integration. Therefore, the resulting likelihood was defined as the Euclidean distance to the origin in the two-dimensional feature space.

3.4 Performance evaluation and comparison

During the initial evaluation, 300 verified masses and 300 suspicious, but actually negative regions, were assessed using a leave-one-out method. That is, one region was excluded from the knowledge base, and the operation was repeated until all 600 regions (both "positive" and "negative") were evaluated. Then, receiver-operating characteristic (ROC) analyses[33,34] were performed, and the areas (Az) under the ROC curves were computed. Using the three likelihood (one positive, one negative, and one combined) measures, we plotted the areas (Az) under the ROC curves as functions of both parameters k_P and k_N.

To evaluate the effects of incorporating negative regions into the knowledge-based CAD scheme, we performed the ROC analyses using the "positive" and "negative" likelihood measures in two independent settings. In the first setting, the positive likelihood measure was used to determine if the suspicious region was likely to be "positive" for a mass. Alternatively, in the second setting, the negative likelihood measure was used to determine if the suspicious region was likely to be "not negative" for a mass. The parameters associated with the two likelihood measures were selected for the optimal performance (highest Az) within each independent setting, using the initial "training" set.

Once the two knowledge bases were established, we performed a second independent validation test using a different data set that included 500 regions depicting verified masses and 500 regions suspected for masses but proven to be actually negative.

4. RESULTS

Figure 2(a) shows the performance levels in the "training" set as measured by the areas under the ROC curves (A_z), before and after the incorporation of negative regions. As seen in Figure 2, using the positive knowledge base alone (Approach I), we achieved a performance plateau at the ranges of Az = 0.83 ($k_p = 10$ was selected for comparison). After incorporating the negative regions, the performance was improved to above Az = 0.84 ($k_p = 80, k_N = 290$ were selected for comparison). Figure 2(b) shows the performance levels as measured by the area under the ROC curves (Az) for the negative regions alone. As seen, the performance monotonically increased with the increase in the value of the parameter k_N.

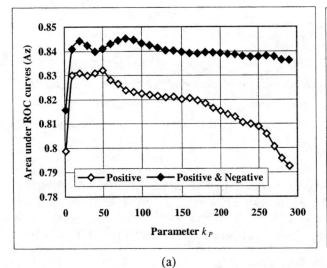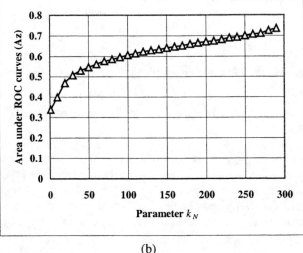

(a)   (b)

Figure 2: Preliminary results of the knowledge-based CAD performance as measured by the areas under the ROC curves (Az), where (a) results before and after the incorporation of negative regions; and (b) results using solely negative regions, are shown. The parameters k_p and k_N were associated with the positive and negative likelihood measures, respectively. A set of 300 positive and 300 negative regions, each characterized with one feature profile (circularity), was evaluated using a leave-one-out method.

Table 1 summarizes the highest performances achieved with both approaches during the initial ("training") phase, as well as during the independent test. During the initial evaluation, the highest performances were improved from Az = 0.828 to Az = 0.844 after incorporating negative regions, and further to 0.867 (P < 0.1) after integrating the two features. During the independent test, the comparable performances improved from Az = 0.798 to Az = 0.83 (P = 0.18).

Table 1

Summary of the highest CAD performances (Az) using the knowledge-based approach after the incorporation of negative regions and the integration of two features is shown. Here, 300 positive and 300 negative regions were evaluated during the initial development phase, while 500 positive and 500 negative regions were evaluated during the independent test.

	Positive Regions Only	Incorporation of Negative Regions	Integration of Two Features
Initial Evaluation (Az)	0.828	0.844 (P = 0.46)	0.867 (P < 0.1)
Independent Test (Az)	0.798	N/A	0.83 (P = 0.18)

5. DISCUSSION AND CONCLUSION

In this study, the incorporation of negative regions in the CAD decision processes has been shown to improve CAD performance as compared with the performance when only positive regions are used. Therefore, the approach to use a classifier that includes not only "positive" mass regions, but also "negative" regions, was proven beneficial. Our preliminary results also demonstrated that the performance characteristic using solely negative regions is quite different from the performance characteristic using solely positive regions. These findings clearly indicated that positive and negative regions could potentially provide independent information and their contributions to detection performance should be evaluated and optimized in two different settings. In addition, despite that only shape-based information was used, integration of the two selected features has been shown to improve the overall performance. Therefore, an effective combination could be of interest if one uses a knowledge-based CAD decision processes.

Our results, while encouraging, are quite preliminary in nature and only limited information from negative regions was incorporated, because only a small set of 300 negative regions was used. In addition, only two features were evaluated, and the method to combine information from positive and negative regions, as well as from multiple features, remains sub-optimal.

ACKNOWLEDGMENTS

This study was supported in part by Grants CA77850, CA82912, and CA85241 from the National Cancer Institute, National Institutes of Health, and IMG 2000-362 from the Susan G. Komen Breast Cancer Foundation.

REFERENCES

1. C. R. Smart, R. E. Hendrick, J. H. Rutledge, R. A. Smith, "Benefit of mammography screening in women aged 40-49: current evidence from randomized controlled trials," *Cancer* **75,** pp. 1619-1626, 1995.
2. D. S. May, N. C. Lee, M. R. Nadel, R. M. Henson, D. S. Miller, "The national breast and cervical cancer early detection program: Report on the first 4 years of mammography provided to medically underserved women," *AJR Am. J. Roentgenol* **178**, pp. 178:97-104, 1998.
3. E. A. Sickles, "Breast Imaging: From 1965 to the present," *Radiology* **215**, pp. 1-16, 2000.
4. E. A. Sickles, "Quality assurance: how to audit your own mammography practice," *Radiol. Clin. North. Am.* **30**, pp. 265-275, 1992.
5. P. T. Huynh, A. M. Jarolimek, S. Daye, "The false-negative mammogram," *RadioGraphics* **18**, pp. 1137-1154, 1998.
6. M. G. Wallis, M. T. Walsh, J. R. Lee, "Review of false negative mammography in a symptomatic population," *Clin. Radiol.* **44**, pp. 13-15, 1991.
7. R. E. Burd, T. W. Wallace, B. C. Yankaskas, "Analysis of cancers missed at screening mammography," Radiology **184**, pp. 613-617, 1992.
8. S. K. Goergen, J. Evans J, G. P. B. Cohen, J. H. MacMillan, "Characteristics of breast carcinomas missed by screening radiologists," *Radiology* **204**, pp. 131-135, 1997.
9. D. Laming, R. Warren, "Improving the detection of cancer in the screening of mammograms," *J. Med. Screen.* **7**, pp. 24-30, 2000.
10. S. Nawano, K. Murakami, N. Moriyama, H. Kobatake, H. Takeo, K. Shimura, "Computer-aided diagnosis in full digital mammography," *Invest. Radiol.* **34**, pp. 310-316, 1999.
11. H. P. Chan, B. Sahiner, M. A. Helvie, et al, "Improvement of radiologists' characterization of mammographic masses by using computer-aided diagnosis: an ROC study," *Radiology* **212**, pp. 817-827, 1999.
12. C. J. Vyborny, M. L. Giger, R. M. Nishikawa, "Computer-aided detection and diagnosis of breast cancer," *Radiol. Clin. North. Am.* **38**, pp. 725-740, 2000.
13. Y. Jiang, R. M. Nishikawa, R. A. Schmidt, C. E. Metz, M. L. Giger, K. Doi, "Improving breast cancer diagnosis with computer-aided diagnosis," *Acad. Radiol.* **6**, pp. 22-33, 1999.

14. L. J. Warren Burhenne, S. A. Wood, C. J. D'Orsi, S. A. Feig, D. B. Kopans, K. F. O'Shaughnessy, E. A. Sickles, L. Tabar, C. J. Vyborny CJ, R. A. Castellino, "Potential contribution of computer-aided detection to the sensitivity of screening mammography," *Radiology* **215**, pp. 554-562, 2000.

15. I. Leichter, S. Buchbinder, P. Bamberger, B. Novak, S. Fields, R. Lederman, "Quantitative characterization of mass lesions on digitized mammograms for computer-assisted diagnosis," *Invest. Radiol.* **35**, pp. 366-372, 2000.

16. T. W. Freer, M. J. Ulissey, "Screening mammography with computer-aided detection: prospective study of 12,860 patients in a community breast center," *Radiology* **220**, pp. 781-786, 2001.

17. N. Karssemeijer, J. H. Hendriks, "Computer-assisted reading of mammograms," *Eur. Radiol.* **7**, pp. 743-748, 1997.

18. E. Thurfjell, M. G. Thurfjell, E. Egge, N. Bjurstam, "Sensitivity and specificity of computer-assisted breast cancer detection in mammography screening," *Acta. Radiol.* **39**, pp. 384-388, 1998.

19. L. Li, Y. Zheng, L. Zhang, R. A. Clark, "False-positive reduction in CAD mass detection using a competitive classification strategy," *Med. Phys.* **28**, pp. 250-258, 2001.

20. Z. Huo, M. L. Giger, C. J. Vyborny, D. E. Wolverton, C. E. Metz, "Computerized classification of benign and malignant masses on digitized mammograms: A study of robustness," *Acad. Radiol.* **7**, pp. 1077-1084, 2000.

21. A. Malich, T. Azhari, T. Bohm, M. Fleck, W. A. Kaiser. Reproducibility--an important factor determining the quality of computer-aided detection (CAD) systems. *Eur. J. Radiol.* **36**, pp. 170-174, 2000.

22. B. Sahiner, H. P. Chan, D. Wei, N. Petrick, M. A. Helvie, D. D. Adler, M. M. Goodsitt, "Image feature selection by a genetic algorithm: application to classification of mass and normal breast tissue," *Med. Phys.* **23**, pp. 1671-1684, 1996.

23. B. Zheng, Y. H. Chang, X. H. Wang, W. F. Good, D. Gur, "Feature selection for computerized mass detection in digitized mammograms by using a genetic algorithm," *Acad. Radiol.* **6**, pp. 327-332, 1999.

24. I. Leichter, R. Lederman, S. Buchbinder, P. Bamberger, B. Novak, S. Fields, "Optimizing parameters for computer-aided diagnosis of microcalcifications at mammography," *Acad. Radiol.* **7**, pp. 406-412, 2000.

25. R. F. Brem, J. M. Schoonjans, "Radiologist detection of microcalcifications with and without computer-aided detection: a comparative study," *Clin. Radiol.* **56**, pp. 150-154, 2001.

26. B. Zheng, M. A. Ganott, C. A. Britton, C. M. Hakim, L. A. Hardesty, T. S. Chang, D. Gur, "Soft-display mammographic readings under different computer-assisted diagnosis cueing environments: preliminary findings," *Radiology* **221**, pp. 633-640, 2001.

27. B. Sahiner, H. P. Chan, N. Petrick, M. A. Helvie, M. M. Goodsitt, "Design of a high-sensitivity classifier based on a genetic algorithm: application to computer-aided diagnosis," *Phys. Med. Biol.* **43**, pp. 2853-2871, 1998.

28. Z. Huo, M. L. Giger, C. E. Metz, "Effect of dominant features on neural network performance in the classification of mammographic lesions," *Phys. Med. Biol.* **44**, pp. 2579-2595, 1999.

29. F. Schmidt, E. Sorantin, C. Szepesvari, E. Graif, M. Becker, H. Mayer, K. Hartwagner, "An automatic method for the identification and interpretation of clustered microcalcifications in mammograms," *Phys. Med. Biol.* **44**, pp. 1231-1243, 1999.

30. H. P. Chan, B. Sahiner, R. F. Wagner, N. Petrick, "Classifier design for computer-aided diagnosis: effects of finite sample size on the mean performance of classical and neural network classifiers," *Med. Phys.* **26**, pp. 2654-2668, 1999.

31. Y. H. Chang, L. A. Hardesty, C. M. Hakim, T. S. Chang, W. F. Good, D. Gur, "Knowledge-based computer-aided detection of masses on digitized mammograms: A preliminary assessment," *Med. Phys.* **28**, pp. 455-461, 2001.

32. A. Rosenfeld, "Compact figures in digital pictures," *IEEE Trans. Syst. Man. Cybern.* **SMC-4**, pp. 394-396, 1974.

33. Y. Jiang, C. E. Metz, R. M. Nishikawa, "A receiver operating characteristics partial area index for highly sensitive diagnostic tests," *Radiology* **201**, pp. 745-750, 1996.

34. C. E. Metz, B. A. Herman, J. Shen, "Maximum-likelihood estimation of receiver operating characteristic (ROC) curves from continuously-distributed data," *Stat. Med.* **17**, pp. 1033-1053, 1998.

Separation of Malignant and Benign Masses using Maximum-Likelihood Modeling and Neural Networks

Lisa Kinnard[a,b], Shih-Chung B. Lo[a], Paul Wang[c], Matthew Freedman[a], Mohamed Chouikha[b]

[a]ISIS Center, Department of Radiology, Georgetown University Medical Center, Washington, D.C.
[b]Department of Electrical Engineering, Howard University, Washington, D.C., USA
[c]Biomedical NMR Laboratory, Department of Radiology, Howard University, Washington, D.C.

ABSTRACT

This study attempted to accurately segment the masses and distinguish malignant from benign tumors. The masses were segmented using a technique that combines pixel aggregation with likelihood analysis. We found that the segmentation method can delineate the tumor body as well as tumor peripheral regions covering typical mass boundaries and some spiculation patterns. We have developed a multiple circular path convolution neural network (MCPCNN) to analyze a set of mass intensity, shape, andtexture features for determination of the tumors as malignant or benign. The features were also fed into a conventional neural network for comparison. We also used values obtained from the maximum likelihood values as inputs into a conventional backpropagation neural network. We have tested these methods on 51 mammograms using a grouped Jackknife experiment incorporated with the ROC method. Tumor sizes ranged from 6mm to 3cm. The conventional neural network whose inputs were image features achieved an A_z value of 0.66. However the MCPCNN achieved an A_z value of 0.71. The conventional neural network whose inputs were maximum likelihood values achieved an A_z value of 0.84. In addition, the maximum likelihood segmentation method can identify the mass body and boundary regions, which is essential to the analysis of mammographic masses.

Keywords: Computer-assisted diagnosis, breast cancer, convolution neural networks, feature extraction

1. INTRODUCTION

While many breast cancer diagnostic systems have been developed, fully-automated mass segmentation continues to be a major challenge in this area. Several investigators exploited methods using intensity values to decide if a pixel should be placed in the region of interest (ROI) or background [14,9,5,7]. Petrick[12] et al. developed the density weighted contrast enhancement (DWCE) method which applies a series of filters to the image in an attempt to extract masses. Li[6] et al. developed a competetitive classification strategy, which uses a combined soft and hard classification method for deciding if segmented regions are true or false positives. Li[7] et al. developed a segmentation method that uses probability to determine segmentation contours. Most of these methods are successful at segmenting the tumor body, however, they sometimes do not properly obtain the extended boundaries of the tumor. While conventional region-growing is an excellent pixel-based segmentation method, it may not suitable to use this method alone. It produces many segmentation contours for one tumor image, but does not decide which segmentation contour is the best. Based on the above reasons, we have developed a tumor segmentation method that combines region-growing with probability assessment to determine final segmentation contours for various breast tumor images.

The most recognized obstacles in breast cancer diagnosis are (1) difficulties of diagnostic decision making in calling back patient for further breast examination, (2) the large number of suspected lesions of which only part

Further author information: (Send correspondence to Lisa M. Kinnard)

Lisa M. Kinnard: E-mail: kinnard@isis.imac.georgetown.edu, Telephone: 1 202 687 5135

S.C. Ben Lo: E-mail: lo@isis.imac.georgetown.edu, Telephone: 1 202 687 1659,

Address: ISIS, Georgetown University, 2115 Wisconsin Avenue, NW, Washington DC, USA

of them are malignant lesions; and (3) missed diagnosis of breast cancer. The callback rates vary from 5% to 20% in today's breast cancer screening programs[1,16]. At some medical centers, the positive predictive rate can be 30% to 35%[4,1]while at others this rate can be as low as 10% to 15%. It is well known that effective treatment of breast cancer calls for early detection of cancerous lesions (e.g., clustered microcalcifications and masses associated with malignant cellular processes)[16,11,15] Tumors can be missed because they are obscured by glandular tissue and it is therefore difficult to observe their boundaries. We were motivated by this clinical obstacle and have developed a computer-assisted diagnostic system attempted to tackle this issue as demonstrated in the following sections.

2. METHODS

Computer-assisted breast cancer diagnosis is divided into three parts, namely, image segmentation, feature calculation, and classification. The next several section will theoretically describe the methods used in the study.

2.1. Segmentation

It is well known that lesion segmentation is one of the most important aspects of computer-assisted diagnosis (CAD_x) because one of the main characteristics of malignant tumors is ill-defined, and/or spiculated borders. Conversely, benign tumors typically have well-defined, rounded borders. Segmentation is therefore extremely important because the diagnosis of a tumor can strongly depend upon image features.

Pixel aggregation is an automated segmentation method in which the region of interest begins as a single pixel and grows based on surrounding pixels with similar properties, e.g., grayscale level or texture.[2] It is a commonly used method[13,14,9]due to its simplicity and accuracy. The computer will use the maximum intensity as the "seed point" -a pixel that is similar to the suspected lesion and is located somewhere inside the suspected lesion. The next 4- or 8-neighboring pixel is checked for similarity so that the region can grow. If pixels in the 4- or 8-neighboring region are similar, they are added to the region. The region continues to grow until there are no remaining similar pixels that are 4- or 8-neighbors of those in the grown region.

Our implementation of this method checks the 4-neighbors of the seed pixel and uses a graylevel threshold as the similarity criterion. If a 4-neighbor of a pixel has an intensity value greater than or equal to a set threshold, it is included in the region of interest. The 4-neighbors were checked instead of the 8-neighbors so that surrounding tissue will not be included. The intensity threshold was used as a similarity criterion due to its simplicity and effectiveness.

By using the same seed point with multiple intensity threshold values we obtained between 150 and 300 of gray level change per lesion; however, the computer did not have the ability to choose the best partition. We added a maximum-likelihood component to the region-growing algorithm. The algorithm can be summarized in five steps. The image was first multiplied by a 2D shadow, whose size was approximately the same size as the ROI. We will henceforth refer to the image to which the 2D shadow has been applied as the "fuzzified" image. We started the threshold value at the maximum intensity in the image and decreased the intensities in successive steps. Consequently, we obtained a sequence of growing contours (S_i), where intensity value was the similarity criterion. There was an inverse relationship between intensity value and contour size, i.e., the lower the intensity value, the larger the contour. Next, we calculated the composite probability (P_i) for each contour (S_i):

$$P_i = p(S_i|pdf_i) \times p(outside S_i|ROI). \tag{1}$$

where $p(S_i|pdf_i)$ is the probability density function (pdf) of the ROI subject to the fuzzified image (see Fig. 1). This pdf is calculated *inside* the contour, S_i, where i is the thresholding step. The quantity $p(outside S_i|ROI)$ is the pdf of the ROI subject to the original image. This pdf is calculated *outside* the contour, S_i. Next we find the logarithm of the composite probability, P_i in the following way:

$$log(P_i) = log(p(S_i|pdf_i)) + log(p(outside S_i|ROI)), \tag{2}$$

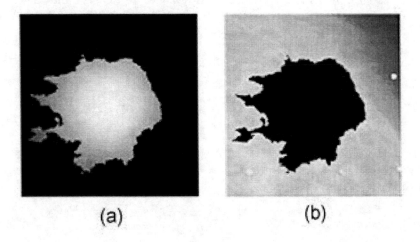

(a)　　　(b)

Figure 1: Figure (a) is used to calculate $p(S_i|pdf_i)$. Figure (b) is used to calculate $p(outsideS_i|ROI)$

Finally, we determine the likelihood that the contour represents the tumor body by assessing the maximum likelihood function:

$$argmax(Log(P_i)), \tag{3}$$

Equation 3 intends to find the maximum value of the aforementioned likelihood values as a function of intensity threshold. We assess (so as other investigators[5]) that the intensity value corresponding to this maximum likelihood value is the optimal intensity for the tumor body contour. We also determine the likelihood that the contour represents the tumor extended borders by assessing the maximum change of the likelihood function:

$$argmax(\frac{dLog(P_i)}{di}), \tag{4}$$

i.e., find the steepest jump on the aforementioned function. An intensity value between this jump and the maximum value on the function produces the best contour of the tumor body and its extended borders.

2.2. Feature Calculation

One extremely important task in the separation of malignant and benign tumors is feature selection and calculation. Benign tumors can be lucent at the center and can have well-defined borders; while malignant tumors can have spiculated and/or fuzzy borders. We used the following features:

Global Features

$$Skewness = \frac{1}{N}\frac{\sum_{i,j=0}^{N-1}[g(i,j) - \overline{g(i,j)}]^3}{\sqrt{\sum_{i,j=0}^{N-1}[g(i,j) - \overline{g(i,j)}]^3}} \tag{5}$$

where $g(i,j)$ is intensity value and $\overline{g(i,j)}$ is average intensity value.

$$Kurtosis = \frac{1}{N}\frac{\sum_{i,j=0}^{N-1}[g(i,j) - \overline{g(i,j)}]^4}{\sqrt{\sum_{i,j=0}^{N-1}[g(i,j) - \overline{g(i,j)}]^4}} \tag{6}$$

$$Circularity = \frac{A_1}{A}, \tag{7}$$

where A is the area of the actual ROI; A_1 is the area of the overlapped region of A and the effective circle A_c, which is defined as the circle whose area is equal to A and is centered at the corresponding centroid of A.

$$Compactness = \frac{p^2}{a},\tag{8}$$

where, p=tumor perimeter and a=tumor area

$$perimeter = tumor\ perimeter.\tag{9}$$

Local Features

These intensity features were calculated on the 10° ROI as it was divided into 10° sectors in the polar coordinate system, therefore each tumor contained 36 sectors.

$$\overline{g(i,j)} = \frac{1}{N}\sum_{i,j=0}^{N-1}g(i,j),\tag{10}$$

where Mean $= \overline{g(i,j)}$, N is the total pixel number inside the ROI

$$Contrast = \frac{P_f - P_b}{P_f},\tag{11}$$

where P_f is the average gray-level inside the ROI's and P_b is the average gray-level surrounding the ROI.

$$\sigma_f^2 = \frac{1}{N}\sum_{i=1}^{N}(g(i,j) - \overline{g(i,j)})^2,\tag{12}$$

where $\sigma_f^2 =$ standard deviation.

$$Area = tumor\ area\tag{13}$$

$$\sigma_n = \frac{1}{N_b}\sum_{i=1}^{N_b}(r_i - \bar{r})^2,\tag{14}$$

where $\sigma_n =$ Deviation of the Normalized Radial Length, N_b is the total number of pixels located on the boundary of the ROI, r_i is the value of the normalized radial length from the boundary coordinate (x_i, y_i) to the centroid of the ROI; $\bar{r}$ is the mean of r_i.

$$Roughness = ([\frac{1}{N_b}\sum_{i=1}^{N_b}(r_i - \bar{r})^4]^{\frac{1}{4}} - [\frac{1}{N_b}\sum_{i=1}^{N_b}(r_i - \bar{r})^2]^{\frac{1}{2}})/\bar{r}.\tag{15}$$

$$radial\ length = length\ of\ radius,\tag{16}$$

where *length of radius* is the distance from the center of the tumor to its edge.

Given a second-order joint probability matrix $P_{d,\theta}(i,j)$, where $P_{d,\theta}(i,j)$ is the joint gray level distribution of a pixel pair (i,j) with the distance d and in the direction θ, six texture features are defined as follows:

$$E_{d,\theta}(i,j) = \sum_{i=1}^{L}\sum_{j=1}^{L}P_{d,\theta}(i,j)^2,\tag{17}$$

where $E_{d,\theta}(i,j)$ = energy.

$$I_{d,\theta}(i,j) = \sum_{i=1}^{L} \sum_{j=1}^{L} (i-j)^2 P_{d,\theta}(i,j), \qquad (18)$$

where $I_{d,\theta}(i,j)$ = inertia.

$$E = \sum_{i=1}^{L} \sum_{j=1}^{L} P_{d,\theta}(i,j) log_2 P_{d,\theta}(i,j), \qquad (19)$$

where E = entropy.

$$IDM_{d,\theta} = \sum_{i=1}^{L} \sum_{j=1}^{L} \frac{1}{1+(i-j)^2} P_{d,\theta}(i,j), \qquad (20)$$

where, $IDM_{d,\theta}$ = Inverse Difference Moment.

$$DE_{d,\theta} = -\sum_{k=0}^{n-1} P_{x-y}(k) log_2 P_{x-y}(k), \; P_{x-y}(k) = \sum_{i=0}^{n-1} \sum_{j=0}^{n-1} P_{d,\theta}(i,j), \qquad (21)$$

for $|i-j| = k, k = 0, 1, ..., n-1$ where, $DE_{d,\theta}$ = Difference Entropy.

2.3. Classifiers

We used a conventional backpropagation neural network for two of the three studies described in this paper. It is comprised of an input layer, one hidden layer, and one output. We used the multiple circular path neural network[8] for the third study described in this paper. It is comprised of 3 input layers, one hidden layer and one output. The first input layer is fully connected, i.e., all inputs connect to all hidden nodes. The second input layer is called a self correlation path, i.e., each node on the layer connects to a single set of the 18 image features for the fan-in and fully connects to the hidden nodes for fan-out. The third input layer is called a neighborhood correlation path, i.e., each node on the layer connects to the input nodes of adjacent sectors for the fan-in and fully connects to the hidden nodes for fan-out. Our study used 18 hidden layer nodes. A more detailed explanation of the MCPCNN can be found the work done by Lo et. al.[8].

3. EXPERIMENT

The image samples were chosen from several databases compiled by the ISIS Center of the Georgetown University (GU) Radiology Department and the University of Florida's Digital Database for Screening Mammography (DDSM).[3] They are a mixture of "obvious" cases and "not obvious" cases. The "obvious" cases contain tumors that are easily identifiable as malignant or benign while the "not obvious" cases are those that radiologists find difficult to observe and/or classify. Forty malignant and forty benign tumors were tested during this experiment. The GU films were digitized at a resolution of 100μm using a Lumiscan digitizer. The DDSM films were digitized at 43 and 50 μm's using both the Lumiscan and Howtek digitizers. We compensated for this difference in resolution by reducing the DDSM images to half their normal sizes. The images were of varying contrasts and the tumors were of varying sizes. There were 28 malignant cases and 23 benign cases.

The experiment was subdivided into three studies as shown in table 1 below.

Experiments 1 and 2 used 6 global and 12x36 sector features to yield a total of 438 image features per tumor. There were 18 hidden nodes and 1 output for both the BP and MCPCNN classifiers. The training and testing method used was the jackknife method. Experiment 3 used 19 likelihood feature values per tumor. There were 15 hidden nodes and 1 output for the BP classifier. The training and testing method used was the jackknife method. The results were analyzed using the LABROC4 program.[10]

Experiment	Features	Neural Network
1	Image Features	Conventional NN
2	Image Features	MCPCNN
3	ML-curve as features	Conventional NN

Table 1: This table summarizes the studies presented in this paper.

4. RESULTS

Here are two examples of segmentation results for both malignant (see Fig. 2) and benign (see Fig. 4) cases. Each example gives the segmentation result produced by the maximum likelihood value on the curves described in section 2.1.

The following is a table, which gives the A_z values produced by the neural network.

Experiment	Features	Neural Network	Az
1	Image Features	Conventional NN	0.66
2	Image Features	MCPCNN	0.71
3	ML-curve as features	Conventional NN	0.84

Table 2: Results from Experiments 1-3.

5. CONCLUSION AND DISCUSSION

In analyzing the segmentation results we drew several conclusions. We discovered that there was a marked difference between the likelihood functions in malignant cases and the likelihood functions in benign cases. The likelihood function in the benign case often experiences a sharp drop, while the likelihood function in the malignant case is often smoother. In the image, a sharp drop value in the likelihood function represents an abrupt change in the area as well as likelihood value. We observed thatin benign cases, the likelihood function sharp changes are much more evident because benign tumors usually have well-defined borders. Conversely, in many malignant cases, the likelihood functions are smoother because many of their the borders are ill-defined. In analyzing the likelihood functions for malignant cases we recognized that those curves with very sharp changes were produced from tumors with well-defined borders and vice versa; i.e., there were malignant tumors that could be mistaken as benign and vice versa.

The maximum likelihood curves used as inputs to the BP neural network produced the best performance overall. The image features used as inputs to the MCPCNN produced the second best performance. The image features used as inputs to the BP produced the worst performance. Since we received the best results by using the likelihood functions as features, we expect that the MCPCNN may improve the overall results by giving the likelihood functions in every sector.

ACKNOWLEDGMENTS

This work has been supported by the following grants: DAMD17-00-1-0291, DAAG55-98-1-0187, and DAMD17-00-1-0267.

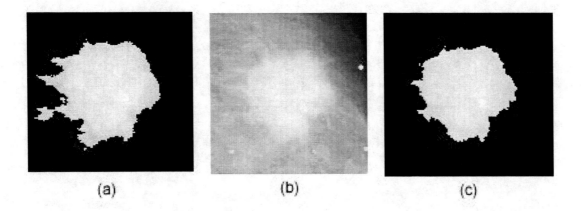

(a)   (b)   (c)

Figure 2. The segmentation results for a malignant tumor. Part (a) shows the segmentation result produced by the maximum likelihood change intensity choice, part (b) shows the original image, and part (c) shows the segmentation result produced by the maximum likelihood intensity choice.

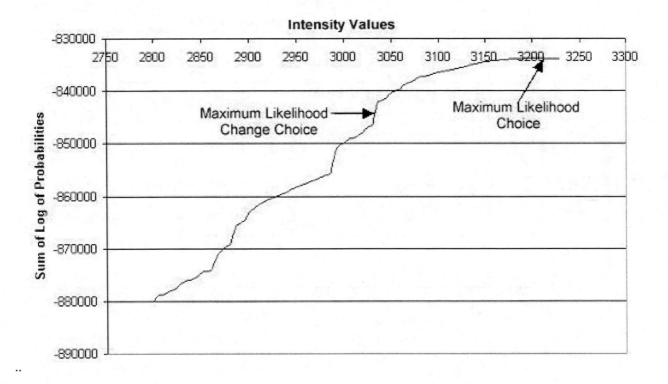

Figure 3. A likelihood function with respect to threshold values for all segmentation steps (malignant case) shown in Fig. 2.

REFERENCES

1. Frankel SD, Sickel EA, Curpen BN, Sollito RA, Ominsky SH, Galvin HB, *Initial versus subsequent screening mammography: Comparison of findings and their prognostics significance*. AJR, 1995, vol. 164, pp. 1107-1109.
2. Gonzalez RC, Woods RE. Digital Image Processing Reading, MA: Addison Wesley, 1992.

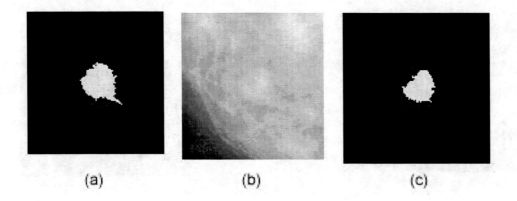

(a)   (b)   (c)

Figure 4. The segmentation results for a benign tumor. Part (a) shows the segmentation result produced by the maximum likelihood change intensity choice, part (b) shows the original image, and part (c) shows the segmentation result produced by the maximum likelihood intensity choice.

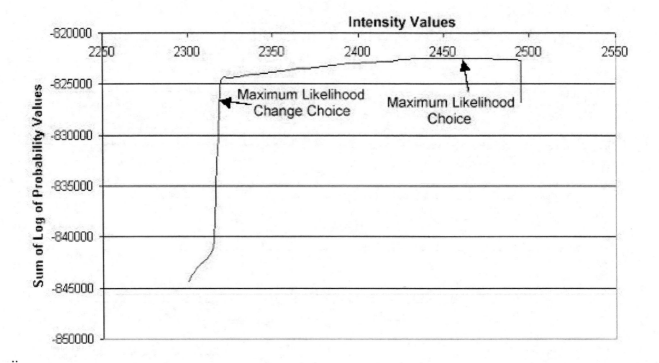

Figure 5. A likelihood function with respect to threshold values for all segmentation steps (benign case) shown in Fig. 4.

3. Heath M, Bowyer KW, Kopans D et al, *Current status of the Digital Database for Screening Mammography*, Digital Mammography, Kluwer Academic Publishers, 1998, pp. 457-460.

4. Kopans DB. *The positive predictive value of mammography*, AJR, 1991, vol. 158, pp. 521-526.

5. Kupinski MA, Giger ML, *Automated Seeded Lesion Segmentation on Digital Mammograms*, IEEE Transactions on Medical Imaging, 1998, vol. 17, no. 4, pp. 510-517.

6. Li L, Zheng Y, Zhang L, Clark R, *False-positive reduction in CAD mass detection using a competitive classification strategy*, Medical Physics, 2001, Vol. 28, no. 2, pp. 250-258.

7. Li H, Wang Y, Liu KJR, Lo S-C, Freedman MT, *Computerized Radiographic Mass Detection - Part I: Lesion Site Selection by Morphological Enhancement and Contextual Segmentation*, IEEE Transactions on Medical Imaging, 2001, vol. 20, no. 4, pp. 289-301.

8. Lo SC, Li H, Wang J, Kinnard L, Freedman MT, *A Multiple Circular Path Convolution Neural Network System for Detection of Mammographic Masses*, IEEE Transactions on Medical Imaging, 2002, vol. 21, No. 2, (Accepted for publication).

9. Mendez AJ, Tahoces PG, Lado MJ, Souto M., Vidal JJ, *Computer-aided diagnosis: Automatic detection of malignant masses in digitzed mammograms*, Medical Physics, 1998, vol. 25, no. 6, pp. 957-964.

10. Metz C, LABROC Program, ftp://radiology.uchicago.edu/roc.

11. Nystrom L, Rutqvist LE, Wall S, Lindgren A, Lindqvist M, Ryden S, et. al., *Breast cancer screening with mammography: Overview of Swedish randomized trials*, Lancet, 1993, vol. 341, pp. 973-978.

12. Petrick N, Chan H-P, Sahiner B, Wei D, *An Adaptive Density-Weighted Contrast Enhancement Filter for Mammographic Breast Mass Detection*, IEEE Transactions on Medical Imaging, 1996, vol. 15, no. 1, pp. 59-67.

13. Pohlman S, Powell KA, Obuchowski NA, Chilcote WA, Grundfest-Broniatowski S, *Quantitative classification of breast tumors in digitized mammograms*, Medical Physics, 1996, vol. 23, no. 8, pp. 1336-1345.

14. Sahiner B, Chan HP, Wei D, Petrick N, Helvie MA, Adler DD, Goodsit MM, *Image feature selection by a genetic algorithm: Application to classification of mass and normal breast tissue*, Medical Physics, 1996, vol. 23, no. 10, pp. 1671-1684.

15. Shapiro S, *Screening: Assessment of current studies*, Cancer, 1994, vol. 74, pp.231-238.

16. Tabar L, Fagerberg G, Duffy S, Day NE, Gad A, Grontoft O. *Update of the Swedish two-country program of mammographic screening for breast cancer*, Radiology Clinics of North America: Breast Imaging - Current Status and Future Directions, 1992, vol. 30, pp. 187-210.

Change of Region Conspicuity in Bilateral Mammograms: Potential Impact on CAD Performance

Bin Zheng, Xiao-Hui Wang, Yuan-Hsiang Chang, Lara A. Hardesty, Marie A. Ganott,
Walter F. Good, David Gur, Department of Radiology, University of Pittsburgh and
Magee-Womens Hospital of the University of Pittsburgh Medical Center Health System,
Pittsburgh, PA 15213

ABSTRACT

In this study, we test a new method to automatically search for matched regions in bilateral digitized mammograms and to compute differences in region conspicuities in pairs of matched regions. One hundred pairs of bilateral images of the same view were selected for the experiment. Each pair of images depicted one verified mass. These 100 mass regions, along with 356 suspicious but actually negative mass regions, were first detected by a single-image-based CAD scheme. To find the matched regions in the corresponding bilateral images, a Procrustean-type technique was used to register the two images, which corrects the deformation of tissue structure between images by guaranteeing the registration of nipples, skin lines, and chest walls. Then, a region growth algorithm was applied to generate a growth region in the matched area, which has the same effective size as the suspicious region in the abnormal image. The conspicuities in the two matched regions, as well as their differences, were computed. Using the conspicuity in the original mass regions and the difference of conspicuities in the two matched regions as two identification indices to classify this set of 456 suspicious regions, the computed areas under the ROC curves (A_Z) were 0.77 and 0.75, respectively. This preliminary study indicates that by comparing the difference of conspicuities in two matched regions that a very useful feature for the CAD schemes can be extracted.

Key Words: Computer-assisted detection, mass detection, image registration, region conspicuity.

1. INTRODUCTION

Mammography is a common and the most effective method used for the early detection of breast cancers [1,2]. With the current recommendations for annual screening of women over 40 years of age and with gradually increased compliance, the total number of mammograms obtained each year is increasing [3]. Because of the large volume of mammograms performed and the low yield of abnormalities in screening environments, detecting a subtle abnormality (e.g., masses) surrounded by complex normal anatomy is a difficult and time-consuming task [4,5]. Hence, there is a growing interest in the development of computer-assisted detection (CAD) schemes for digitized mammograms. Many studies have demonstrated that CAD systems could have great potential to provide radiologists a valuable "second opinion" and improve the diagnostic accuracy in detecting breast cancers at an early stage [6-10]. Although significant improvements in CAD schemes have been made in the last two decades, many issues remain unsolved (such as the relatively high false-positive rate and the low reproducibility [11]). The performance level of current CAD schemes may not be optimal for some clinical applications. One study found that high false-positive cues generated from the CAD system influenced radiologists not to have sufficient confidence in the CAD cues and changed their original interpretation of the mammograms [12].

To improve CAD performance, significant effort has been expanded in recent years by a large number of research groups, which includes, but is not limited to: 1) searching for more effective classifiers [13-15]; 2) optimizing feature selection and network architecture [16-18]; 3) using adaptive optimization methods [19,20]; and 4) combining detection results from independent classifiers [20,21]. Despite these efforts, many current CAD schemes still produce a large number of false-positive detections (e.g., more than one per image) in order to maintain a reasonable case-based sensitivity (e.g., above 80%) in a laboratory environment with a limited image database [18-21]. Most current CAD schemes are single image-based and only use the pixel-values and feature-based information from a single image to classify true-positive and false-positive regions. Studies have shown that in the clinical environment the lack of related

Medical Imaging 2002: Image Processing, Milan Sonka, J. Michael Fitzpatrick,
Editors, Proceedings of SPIE Vol. 4684 (2002) © 2002 SPIE · 1605-7422/02/$15.00

images (e.g., bilateral images from left and right breasts, or the images from previous examinations) for comparison lead radiologists to produce significantly greater false-positive detections (or "call-back" rate) [22]. Without comparison of related feature changes in other images, the single-image based CAD schemes have an obvious disadvantage in this regard. Recently, several new methods to automatically locate corresponding regions in different images (e.g., CC and MLO views [23,24]) and temporal images (current and previous examinations [25]) have been reported. These studies demonstrated that the performance of CAD schemes could be improved by incorporating information related to feature changes of the same abnormality depicted in different images into the schemes [24,25].

In this study, we tested a new method to automatically search for the "matched" regions in bilateral images (the same view of the left and right breasts) and computed the feature difference between the pairs of matched regions. The potential performance improvements of the CAD scheme by incorporating feature changes into the scheme were also analyzed. The feature examined in this preliminary experiment is "region conspicuity," which was originally defined as the "region contrast" divided by the "surrounding complexity" [26] and has also been shown to be an effective feature in our CAD scheme for mass detection [17].

2. METHODS

Image Database

From the image database established in our laboratory and assembled under an approved IRB protocol, one hundred pairs of bilateral digitized mammograms were selected for this experiment. Among these 100 pairs of images, half were cranio-caudal (CC) image pairs and half were mediolateral oblique (MLO) image pairs. The original mammograms were digitized in our laboratory using a Lumisys laser-film digitizer with a pixel size of 100 μm × 100 μm and 12 bit gray-level resolution. For mass detection, the images were then sub-sampled (pixel digital value average) by a factor of 4 in both directions to generate images of approximately 600 × 450 pixels. Each image pair includes one positive image and one negative image. The positive image depicts one pathology verified mass region. Hence, a total of 100 mass regions were tested in this study.

Each positive image was first processed by a single-image-based CAD scheme previously developed in our laboratory [27]. In brief, this scheme uses three distinct stages to identify mass regions. The first stage uses dual kernel filtering, subtraction, and labeling to locate suspicious regions, and the second stage used an adaptive region growth algorithm to define a growth region for each suspicious "mass." For each suspicious region, a set of image features is automatically computed by the scheme. In the third stage of the scheme, a multi-feature based classifier (i.e., an artificial neural network [28]) is used to further classify the suspicious regions into positive and negative regions. In this experiment, 100 positive mass regions as well as 356 suspicious but actually negative regions (false-positive) were initially detected by the CAD scheme at the second stage. All of these regions were used in this study.

Global Image Registration

Searching for "matched" regions in each of these 456 suspicious "mass" regions in the corresponding bilateral images included two steps, global image registration and local region adjustment. Global image registration depends on the automated detection of several image fiducials, such as the skin line, nipple, and chest wall. The computing algorithms are described below.

Skin line detection

Due to a variety of clinical reasons and in some cases the saturation (clipping) of the film digitizer at high optical densities, the skin line (skin-air interface) could be very fuzzy or indistinguishable in a number of images. To develop an efficient computing algorithm, we assumed that a transition curve with the smoothest curvature between the breast tissue and air background represented the skin line. An iterative method was applied to search for an optimal threshold that could generate the smoothest transition boundary of the tissue-air interface. Since a digitized mammogram typically includes a multi-modal gray level histogram [29], the algorithm first detected the deepest valley in the low end of the histogram. We defined the gray level in the valley and air background peak in the histogram as d_v and d_{air}, respectively. A series of thresholds is selected as $T_i = T_{i-1} + 16, i = 2,3,\ldots,n$, where the first one is $T_1 = d_v$, and the last one is $T_n < d_{air} - 16$. At each threshold level, the program tracks the "tissue-air interface." Then, the smoothness of all tracked boundaries was determined and defined as the "skin line."

Chest wall detection

Because the chest wall is usually invisible in CC view images, we assume that the chest wall is parallel to the edge of the film and 5mm beyond it. For MLO view images, a computer algorithm was developed to identify the chest wall. From the top of the image, the computer program scans horizontally from the edge of the film to the skin line and searches for the maximum gradient before reaching the skin line. The program computes the gray level change (or gradient) for each pixel. The point with the maximum gradient is the candidate for the intercept between the horizontal scanning line and the chest wall. Scanning is terminated when the point with the maximum gradient is very close to the edge of the film (e.g., 10 pixels away). A regression method is then applied to fit all the identified maximum gradient points into a line, which is defined as the "chest wall."

Nipple detection

Similar to the skin line, the visibility of the nipples varies across images. To develop an automatic algorithm for detecting or estimating the nipple position in a variety of clinical images, the following hypotheses are used.

1. A small and obvious protruding area in a smooth skin boundary (interface between breast and background) can indicate the location of a not in profile nipple [30].
2. If a nipple is in profile, it is likely to be located in an area where the pixel values are not only relatively unchanged, but also significantly smaller than that of any other tissue regions near the skin boundary [30].
3. For a nipple that is invisible on an image, a point in the skin line that has the maximum distance to the chest wall is assumed as the location of the nipple [31].

Based on these three assumptions, a three-step automatic algorithm was designed to detect nipple locations. The first step is a search for a possible protruding area along the skin line, with the computer program scanning along the skin line. In each scanned point (x_i, y_i), the program selects another point that is 40 tracking points away (x_{i+40}, y_{i+40}). A line is then drawn between these two points and the area (e.g., the number of pixels) between this line and the computed skin line is computed. After scanning the entire skin line, if the maximum size of the areas is larger than a pre-trained value, this protruding area is identified as the nipple area. If the nipple location is not detected in the first step, the algorithm scans the skin line and computes the gray levels in the tissue side using a square window of 20×20 pixels. Then, the program selects one area with the smallest medium gray level inside the scanning window and computes (1) the difference between this mean gray level and the gray level at the skin line as well as (2) the standard deviation of gray levels inside the window. If both the gray level difference and the standard deviation can pass through the predetermined thresholds (or rules), this area is an identified "nipple" area. If both steps fail to identify a nipple location, it often means that the nipple is not visible and the algorithm computes the distance of every point on the skin line to the computed chest wall. The point with the maximum distance is used to represent the location of the nipple.

The detailed procedure for training and testing of these algorithms for the detection of the skin line, chest wall, and nipple has been reported elsewhere [32]. The performance of these algorithms was evaluated based on the distance of the target locations (e.g., nipple and chest wall) between the computer assignment and the visual identification. For some cases where the nipples were not visible, the locations were estimated based on the maximum distance from the chest wall [31]. In but a few cases, the procedure failed requiring that a visual inspection be used to assign the "nipple location."

Image coordinate for the registration

For the global image registration and in order to identify matched regions in the corresponding images, a polar coordinate was established in each image as shown in Figure 1. The baseline axis ($\alpha = 0$) starts from the nipple and is perpendicular to the chest wall. Suppose that a suspicious "mass" region with polar coordinate (α, ρ) is detected in one image (see Figure 1). To find the corresponding "matched" region (α', ρ') in another image, the following equations were used. $\alpha' = \alpha$, and, $\rho' = d' \times \rho / d$, where d and d' are the distance from the nipple to the chest wall along the line passing through the center of the regions. Using this Procrustean technique [33], we corrected the deformation of tissue structure between two images by guaranteeing the registration of the nipples and chest walls in the two images. The polar coordinate (α', ρ') is transposed to the regular Cartesian coordinate (x', y'), which originates from the top-left edge of the image.

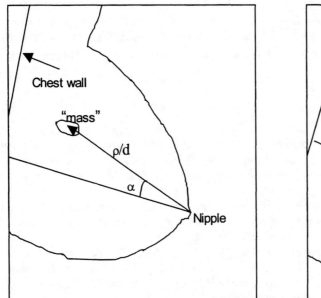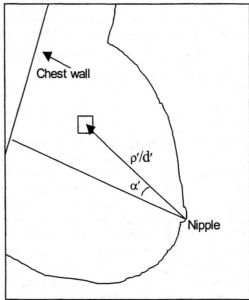

Figure 1: Illustration of finding matched regions in bilateral images.

Local Match and Feature Extraction

Unlike matching two mass regions (representing the same mass) in two views (CC and MLO) [24] or temporal sequential images [25], we tried to match one abnormal region in one image to a negative region in the corresponding contralateral image. To define the "matched" region, the following local adjustments were performed. From the initial center (x', y') located during the global image registration procedure, a square window of 30×30 pixels (or equivalent to 1.2 cm $\times$ 1.2 cm) centered at (x', y') is opened (see Figure 1). The computer algorithm searches for a pixel that had the minimum digital value inside the window. Using this pixel as a growth seed, a region growth algorithm was applied to force the seed to grow into a region that had the same size as the suspicious "mass" identified in the original contralateral image. Region conspicuity was computed for this "matched" region. The conspicuity difference between an original "mass" region (C_o) and its corresponding "matched" region (C_m) was also computed as $CC = (C_o - C_m)/C_o$. The two features (C_o and CC) were applied as two classification indices to identify the 100 true-positive mass regions and 356 false-positive regions in this dataset. The classification performance was analyzed and compared using the ROCFIT program [34]. The comparison included the areas under two ROC curves (A_z) as well as their correlation coefficient ($\rho_{C_0,CC} = \dfrac{COV(C_0, CC)}{\sigma_{C_0} \sigma_{CC}}$).

3. RESULTS

Of the 200 images, 118 had relatively visible skin lines and nipples by changing the image display parameters (window size and level). After applying our previously trained algorithm to these 200 new images (which were not a part of the development phase), nipples in 162 images (81%) were correctly detected by the computer algorithm. The largest deviations between the nipple locations and the "assigned locations" happened in the images where the nipples and skin lines were not visible (31 of 38 images). For the 100 MLO images, the chest walls were correctly detected in 92 images.

Using conspicuity of the original suspicious regions and the relative conspicuity differences between the original suspicious "mass" regions and their "matched" regions as classification indices, the areas under these ROC curves (A_z) were 0.77 ±0.01 and 0.75 ±0.01, respectively. Either one was significantly (*p < 0.01*) better than random assignment ($A_z = 0.5$). The correlation coefficient between the two sets of feature values (C_o and CC) was 0.18.

4. DISCUSSION

Information regarding asymmetry between corresponding areas in bilateral images plays an important role during radiologists' interpretation of mammograms. In order to improve CAD performance, researchers have attempted to incorporate such information into the schemes. To facilitate this approach, significant effort has been made in an attempt to improve the accuracy of image registration [35]. However, due to differences in positioning breast compression and variation of image quality, accurate registration of mammograms remains a challenge. In this preliminary study, we tested a simple multi-stage algorithm to automatically detect the skin line, nipple, and chest wall. The result of this test is encouraging, albeit far from being perfect. For the cases where the nipple positions can be visually located, the algorithm achieved very high accuracy (94% or 111 / 118 images). For the cases where the nipple positions were not easily visible, using the maximum distance between skin boundary and the chest wall to estimate the nipple location yielded a reasonable, but significantly lower accuracy (62.2% or 51 / 82 images). Clearly, the algorithm needs to be further improved and tested using a much larger image database.

Even with a reasonable success in image registration, it may still be difficult to accurately map one suspicious region (e.g., a mass region in an MLO mammogram of the left breast) into the corresponding image (MLO image of the right breast). Hence, to compensate for such difficulty, in our algorithm, we compared regional differences by enabling the center to be shifted within a certain region (e.g., 30 × 30 pixels in the subsampled image or 1.2 cm × 1.2 cm) to assign an appropriate growth seed. The two "matched" regions in this study could have large differences in their geometric shape and pixel value distribution. This provides us an opportunity to compare the change of a number of features in these two matched regions. In this preliminary study, we only compared the feature differences of conspicuity in "matched" regions. Using the conspicuity in the original suspicious "mass" regions and the conspicuity differences as two classification indices, we obtained similar performances. Both yield results that are significantly better than random assignment ($A_z = 0.5$). The relatively low correlation between the classification results generated by these two indices is also encouraging, indicating that incorporation of the conspicuity difference into the schemes as a feature is likely to add significantly independent information, hence, an overall performance improvement of the scheme.

ACKNOWLEDGEMENTS

This work was partially supported from grants CA77850, CA85241 and CA80836 from the National Cancer Institute of the National Institutes of Health and from grant IMG 2000 362 from the Susan G. Komen Breast Cancer Foundation.

REFERENCES

1. AB Miller, "Mammography: reviewing the evidence-epidemiology aspects," Can Fam Physician **39**, 85-90 (1993)
2. RA Smith, "Breast cancer screening among women younger than age 50: A current assessment of the issues," CA Cancer J Clin **50**, 312-336 (2000).
3. SA Feig, CJ D'Orsi, RE Hendrick, "American College of Radiology guidelines for breast cancer screening," AJR **171**, 29-33 (1998).
4. RE Bird, TW Wallace, BC Yankaskas, "Analysis of cancers missed at screening mammography," Radiology **184**, 613-617 (1992).
5. EL Thurfjell, KA Lernevall, AS Taube, "Benefit of independent double reading in a population-based mammography screening program," Radiology **191**, 241-244 (1994).
6. I Leichter, S Fields, R Nirel, "Improved mammographic interpretation of masses using computer-aided diagnosis," Eur Radiol **10**, 377-383 (2000).
7. LJ Burhenne, SA Wood, CJ D'Orsi, SA Feig, DB Kopans, KF O'Shaughnessy, EA Sickles, L Tabar, CJ Vyborny, RA Castellino, "Potential contribution of computer-aided detection to the sensitivity of screening mammography," Radiology **215**, 554-562 (2000).
8. TW Freer, MJ Ulissey, "Screening mammography with computer-aided detection: Prospective study of 12,860 patients in a community breast center," Radiology **220**, 781-786 (2001).
9. RL Birdwell, DM Ikeda, KF O'Shaughnessy, EA Sickles, "Mammographic characteristics of 115 missed cancers later detected with screening mammography and the potential utility of computer-aided detection," Radiology **219**, 192-202 (2001).
10. B Zheng, MA Ganott, CA Britton, CM Hakim, LA Hardesty, TS Chang, D Gur, "Soft-copy mammographic readings under different computer-assisted detection cueing environments: Preliminary findings," Radiology **221**, 633-640 (2001).
11. A Malich, T Azhari, T Bohm, M Fleck, WA Kaiser, "Reproducibility – an important factor determining the quality of computer aided detection (CAD) systems," Euro Radiology **36**, 170-174 (2000).
12. K Moberg, N Bjurstam, B. Wilczek, L Rostgard, E Egge, C Muren, "Computed assisted detection of interval breast cancers," Euro Radiology **39**, 104-110 (2001).
13. L Li, W Qian, LP Clarke, "Computer-assisted diagnosis method for mass detection with multiorientation and multiresolution wavelet transforms," Acad Radiol **4**; 724-731 (1997).
14. R Rymon, B Zheng, YH Chang, D Gur, "Incorporation of a set enumeration tree-based classifier into a hybrid computer-assisted diagnosis scheme for mass detection," Acad Radiol **5**, 181-187 (1998).
15. XH Wang, B Zheng, WF Good, JL King, YH Chang, "Computer-assisted diagnosis of breast cancer using a data-driven Bayesian belief network," International J Med Informatics **54**, 115-126 (1999).
16. MA Anastasio, H Yoshida, RM Nishikawa, "A genetic algorithm-based method for optimizing the performance of a computer-aided diagnosis scheme for detection of clustered microcalcifications in mammograms," Med Phys **25**, 1613-1620 (1998).
17. B Zheng, YH Chang, XH Wang, WF Good, D Gur, "Feature selection for computerized mass detection in digitized mammograms by using a genetic algorithm," Acad Radiol **6**, 327-332 (1999).
18. MN Gurcan, B Sahiner B, Chan HP, L Hadjiiski, N Petrick, "Selection of an optimal network architecture for computer-aided detection of microcalcifications – comparison of automated optimization techniques," Med Phys **28**, 1937-1948 (2001).
19. W Qian, L Li, L Clarke, RA Clark, J Thomas, "Digital mammography: comparison of adaptive and nonadaptive CAD schemes for mass detection," Acad Radiol **6**, 471-480 (1999).
20. B Zheng, YH Chang, WF Good, D Gur, "Performance gain in computer-assisted detection schemes by averaging scores generated from artificial neural networks with adaptive filtering," Med Phys **28**, 2302-2308 (2001).
21. L Li, Y Zheng, L Zhang, RA Clark, "False-positive reduction in CAD mass detection using a competitive classification strategy," Med Phys **28**, 250-258 (2001).
22. MP Callaway, CR Boggis, SA Astley, "Influence of previous films on screening mammographic interpretation and detection of breast carcinoma," Clin Radiol **52**, 527-529 (1997).
23. YH Chang, WF Good, JH Sumkin, B Zheng, D Gur, "Computerized localization of breast lesions from two views: An experimental comparison of two method," Invest Radiol **34**, 585-588 (1999).

24. WF Good, B Zheng, YH Chang, XH Wang, GS Maitz, D Gur, "Multi-image CAD employing features derived from ipsilateral mammographic views," Proc SPIE on Image Processing **3361**, 474-485 (1999).

25. L Hadjiiski, HP Chan, B Sahiner, N Petrick, MA Helvie, "Automated registration of breast lesions in temporal pairs of mammograms for interval change analysis – local affine transformation for improved localization," Med Phys **28**, 1070-1079 (2001).

26. HL Kundel, and G. Revesz, "Lesion conspicuity, structure noise, and film reader error," Am. J. Roentgen. **126**, 1233-1238 (1977).

27. B Zheng, YH Chang, D Gur, "Computerized detection of masses in digitized mammograms using single-image segmentation and a multilayer topographic feature analysis," Acad Radiol **2**, 959-966 (1995).

28. B Zheng, YH Chang, WF Good, D Gur, "Adequacy testing of training set sample sizes in the development of a computer-assisted diagnosis scheme," Acad Radiol **4**, 497-502 (1997).

29. JJ Heine, SR Deans, RP Velthuizen, LP Clarke, "On the statistical natural of mammograms," Med Phys **26**, 2254-2265 (1999).

30. R Chandrasekhar, Y Attikiouzel, "A simple method for automatically locating the nipple on mammograms," IEEE Trans on Med Imaging **16**, 483-494 (1997).

31. AJ Mendez, PG Tahoces, MJ Lado, M Souto, JL Correa, JJ Vidal, "Automatic detection of breast border and nipple in digital mammograms," Comput Methods Programs Biomed **49**, 253-262 (1996).

32. B Zheng, XH Wang, YH Chang, WF Good, "Automatic detection of nipple and chest wall in digitized mammograms," Proc Computer Assisted Radiology and Surgery, 13th International Symposium and Exhibition, Paris, France, June 23-26 (1999).

33. WF Good, B Zheng, YH Chang, XH Wang, GS Maitz, "Procrustean image deformation for bilateral subtraction of mammograms," Proc SPIE on Image Processing **3661**, 1526-1573 (1999).

34. CE Metz, BA Herman, JH Shen, "Maximum likelihood estimation of receiver operating characteristic (ROC) curves from continuously-distributed data," Stat. Med. **17**, 1033-1053 (1998).

35. MY Sallam, KW Bowyer, "Registration and difference analysis of corresponding mammogram images," Med Image Anal **3**, 103-118 (1999).

Computer-aided characterization of malignant and benign microcalcification clusters based on the analysis of temporal change of mammographic features

Lubomir Hadjiiski, Heang-Ping Chan, Berkman Sahiner, Nicholas Petrick,
Mark A. Helvie, Marilyn Roubidoux, Metin Gurcan

Department of Radiology, The University of Michigan, Ann Arbor, MI 48109-0904

ABSTRACT

We have previously demonstrated that interval change analysis can improve differentiation of malignant and benign masses. In this study, a new classification scheme using interval change information was developed to classify mammographic microcalcification clusters as malignant and benign. From each cluster, 20 run length statistic texture features (RLSF) and 21 morphological features were extracted. Twenty difference RLSF were obtained by subtracting a prior RLSF from the corresponding current RLSF. The feature space consisted of the current and the difference RLSF, as well as the current and the difference morphological features. A leave-one-case-out resampling was used to train and test the classifier using 65 temporal image pairs (19 malignant, 46 benign) containing biopsy-proven microcalcification clusters. Stepwise feature selection and a linear discriminant classifier, designed with the training subsets alone, were used to select and merge the most useful features. An average of 12 features were selected from the training subsets, of which 3 difference RLSF and 7 morphological features were consistently selected from most of the training subsets. The classifier achieved an average training A_z of 0.98 and a test A_z of 0.87. For comparison, a classifier based on the current single image features achieved an average training A_z of 0.88 and test A_z of 0.81. These results indicate that the use of temporal information improved the accuracy of microcalcification characterization.

Keywords: Computer-Aided Diagnosis, Interval Changes, Classification, Feature analysis, Mammography, Malignancy.

1. INTRODUCTION

Mammography is currently the most effective method for early breast cancer detection[1,2]. Radiologists routinely compare mammograms from a current examination with those obtained in previous years, if available, for identifying interval changes, detecting potential abnormalities, and evaluating breast lesions. It is widely accepted that analysis of interval changes in mammographic features is very useful for both detection and classification of abnormalities[3,4]. A variety of computer-aided diagnosis (CAD) techniques have been developed to detect mammographic abnormalities and to distinguish between malignant and benign lesions. We are studying the use of CAD techniques to assist radiologists in interval change analysis.

Commonly used classification methods for CAD use information from a single image. These methods have been shown to perform well in lesion classification problems[5-11]. However, when multiple-year mammograms of a lesion are available, it is not trivial to design computer vision methods to use the temporal information for computer-aided classification and to improve the differentiation between benign and malignant masses.

The goal of our research is to develop a technique for computerized analysis of temporal differences between a microcalcification cluster on the most recent mammogram and a prior mammogram of the same view. The computer algorithm can be used to assist radiologists in evaluating interval changes and thus distinguishing between malignant and benign microcalcification clusters for CAD. In our previous studies we have demonstrated that interval change analysis can improve differentiation of malignant and benign masses[12,13]. In this study we will introduce a new classification scheme using interval change information to classify mammographic microcalcification clusters as malignant and benign. Additionally, we will compare this method with a classification method based on information extracted from the current mammogram alone.

2. CLASSIFICATION TECHNIQUE

A new classification scheme was developed to classify mammographic microcalcification clusters as malignant and benign by using interval change information. The technique is based on the design of features that will represent the temporal information and will discriminate between malignant and benign microcalcification clusters.

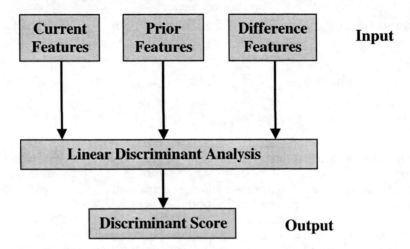

Figure 1. Block-diagram of the classification method.

The clusters to be analyzed can either be identified manually by a radiologist or automatically by a computerized detection program. In this study, the microcalcification clusters were identified by an MQSA radiologist on each mammogram. The locations of the individual microcalcifications from the clusters on both the current and the prior mammograms have been determined manually. Features such as texture features, morphological features and the number of microclacifications in a cluster were extracted from each microcalcification cluster. Additionally, the interval change of a given feature of the cluster is determined as the difference between its current feature value and the corresponding prior feature value. The feature space consisted of current, prior, and difference features. Stepwise feature selection applied to linear discriminant analysis (LDA) was used to select the most useful features. The selected features were then used as the input predictor variables of the LDA classifier (Figure 1). A leave-one-case-out resampling scheme was employed to train and test the classifier.

To evaluate the improvement in the classifier performance designed by using the temporal change information, an additional classifier was trained using the information extracted from the current images of the temporal pairs. We will refer to these images as current images. Comparison of the two classifiers will reveal the effectiveness of interval change analysis on classification of malignant and benign microcalcification clusters.

3. DATA SET

In this preliminary study, 65 temporal image pairs from 29 patients containing biopsy-proven microcalcification clusters on the current mammograms were chosen from patient files. Eleven of the cases were malignant and 18 were benign. For the 29 patients 102 mammograms were chosen. The mammograms were digitized with a LUMISCAN 85 laser scanner at a pixel resolution of 50 μm $\times$ 50 μm and 4096 gray levels. The digitizer was calibrated so that gray level values were linearly proportional to the optical density (OD) within the range of 0 to 4 OD units, with a slope of 0.001 OD/pixel value. Outside this range, the slope of the calibration curve decreased gradually. The digitizer output was linearly converted so that a large pixel value corresponded to a low optical density. The images were averaged and down-sampled by a factor of 2 resulting in images with a pixel size of 100 μm $\times$ 100 μm for further analysis.

The 102 mammograms contained different mammographic views and multiple years of the microcalcification clusters including the year when the biopsy was performed. By matching microcalcification clusters of the same view from two different exams, a total of 65 temporal pairs were formed, of which 19 were malignant and 46 benign. A malignant temporal pair consisted of a biopsy proven malignant microcalcification cluster or a cluster that was followed up and found to be malignant by biopsy in a future year. Similar definitions were used for the benign temporal pairs. Within the 65 temporal pairs, a total of 56 mammograms were single current mammograms. Of the 56 current mammograms, 16 were malignant and 40 benign. Since all cases in this data set had undergone biopsy, the benign clusters in this set could not be distinguished easily from malignant ones based on current image criteria.

For the malignant microcalcification clusters in this data set, the average cluster size was 8.8 mm on the prior mammograms and 15.1 mm on the current mammograms. The corresponding sizes were 11.4 mm and 11.6 mm, respectively, for the benign microcalcification clusters. The temporal pairs had a time interval of 3 to 32 months. Approximately 50% of the pairs had a time interval of 6 months and more than 30% had a time interval of 12 months.

4. FEATURE EXTRACTION

A rectangular region of interest (ROI) was defined to include the radiologist-identified microcalcification cluster with an additional surrounding breast tissue region of at least 40 pixels wide from any point of the cluster boundary.

The texture features used in this study were calculated from run-length statistics (RLS) matrices[14]. The RLS matrices were computed from the defined ROIs. RLS texture features were extracted from the vertical and horizontal gradient magnitude images, which were obtained by filtering the ROI image with horizontally or vertically oriented Sobel filters and computing the absolute gradient value of the filtered image. Five texture measures, namely, short run emphasis, long run emphasis, gray level nonuniformity, run length nonuniformity, and run percentage were extracted from the vertical and horizontal gradient images in two directions, $\theta = 0^\circ$, and $\theta = 90^\circ$. Therefore, a total of 20 RLS features were calculated for each ROI. The definition of the RLS feature measures can be found in the literature[14].

For the extraction of the morphological features, the locations of the individual microcalcifications in a cluster were identified manually. The true microcalcification were defined as those visible on the film mammograms with a magnifier. The morphological features included features describing the variations of the shape and size of the individual microcalcifications in a cluster such as the area, mean density, eccentricity, moment ratio and axis ratio[11]. To quantify the variation of the visibility and shape descriptors in a cluster, the maximum, the average, the standard deviation and the coefficient of variation were calculated for each feature. The number of microcalcifications in a cluster[11] was also included as a feature.

A total of 41 features (20 RLS and 21 morphological) were extracted from each microcalcification cluster. Additionally, difference features were obtained by subtracting a prior feature from the corresponding current feature. Therefore 20 RLS and 21 morphological difference features were obtained.

5. FEATURE SELECTION

In order to reduce the number of the features and to obtain the best feature subset to design an effective classifier, feature selection with stepwise linear discriminant analysis[15,16] was applied. At each step of the stepwise selection procedure, one feature is entered or removed from the feature pool based on analysis of its effect on the selection criterion. The stepwise selection procedure is controlled by a simplex optimization method[17,18] in such a way that a minimum number of features were selected to achieve a high accuracy of classification by LDA. More details about the stepwise linear discriminant analysis and its application to CAD can be found elsewhere[5].

6. EVALUATION METHODS

To evaluate the classifier performance, the training and test discriminant scores were analyzed using receiver operating characteristic (ROC) methodology[19]. The discriminant scores of the malignant and benign masses were used as decision variables in the LABROC1 program[20], which fits a binormal ROC curve based on maximum likelihood estimation. The classification accuracy was evaluated as the area under the ROC curve, A_z. The performances of the classifiers were also assessed by estimation of the partial area index ($A_z^{(0.9)}$). $A_z^{(0.9)}$ is defined as the area that lies under the ROC curve but above a sensitivity threshold of 0.9 ($TPF_0 = 0.9$) normalized to the total area above TPF_0, ($1-TPF_0$). It indicates the performance of the classifier in the high sensitivity (low false negative) region that is most important for a cancer detection task.

7. CLASSIFICATION RESULTS

For the data set used in this study, an average of 12 features were selected from the 29 training subsets. The most frequently selected features included 3 difference RLS features and 9 morphological features from the current image. Three difference RLSF and 7 morphological features were consistently selected from most of the training subsets. The LDA classifier achieved an average training A_z of 0.98 and a test A_z of 0.87. The LDA classifier using features extracted from the current images of the temporal pairs achieved an average training A_z of 0.88 and a test A_z of 0.81. An average of 4 features were selected from the 29 training subsets. The most frequently selected features were 1 RLS feature and 3 morphological features.

The difference in the test A_z between the two classifiers did not achieve statistical significance. The classifier based on temporal pairs achieved a test partial $A_z^{(0.9)}$ of 0.63 and the classifier based on current images achieved a test $A_z^{(0.9)}$ of 0.43. These results are summarized in Table 1.

Table 1. Classification accuracy for the classifier based on the temporal change information and the classifier based on current single image information.

Classification	Avg. no. Of selected features	Training A_z	Test A_z	Test partial $A_z^{(0.9)}$
Temporal pairs	12	0.98	0.87 ± 0.044	0.63
Current images	4	0.88	0.81 ± 0.059	0.43

8. CONCLUSION

The difference RLS texture features and the current morphological features were useful for identification of malignant microcalcifications in temporal pairs of mammograms. The information on the prior image was important for characterization of the microcalcifications; 3 out of the 12 selected features contained prior information. Morphological features describing the variations of the shape and size of the individual microcalcifications in a cluster were more effective than the features related to the cluster size. This is probably due to the fact that we used biopsy-proven cases in this study and many of the biopsied benign microcalcification clusters also grew over time. Combination of current and temporal change information improved classification accuracy compared to current information alone in terms of the A_z. The increase in A_z (0.06), although large, did not achieve statistical significance due to the small sample size. The partial area under the ROC curve is also improved for the classifier based on current and prior images ($A_z^{(0.9)} = 0.63$) compared to the classifier based only on the current images ($A_z^{(0.9)} = 0.43$). However, the difference did not achieve statistical significance either. Further studies are underway to improve this temporal change classification technique and to evaluate its performance on a larger data set.

ACKNOWLEDGMENTS

This work is supported by a Career Development Award from the USAMRMC (DAMD 17-98-1-8211) (L.H.), a Basic Radiological Science Innovative Research Award, 2001 (L.H.), from the University of Michigan, and a USPHS Grant CA 48129. The content of this publication does not necessarily reflect the position of the funding agency, and no official endorsement of any equipment and product of any companies mentioned in this publication should be inferred.

REFERENCES

1. H. C. Zuckerman, "The role of mammography in the diagnosis of breast cancer," *In: Breast Cancer, Diagnosis and Treatment*, 152-172, Eds. I. M. Ariel and J. B. Cleary, McGraw-Hill, New York, 1987.

2. L. Tabar and P. B. Dean, "The Control of Breast Cancer through Mammography Screening," *Radiologic Clincs of North America* **25**, 961, 1987.

3. L. W. Bassett, B. Shayestehfar, and I. Hirbawi, "Obtaining previous mammograms for comparison: usefullness and costs," *Amer. J. Roentgenology* **163**, 1083-1086, 1994.

4.   E. A. Sickles, "Periodic mammographic follow-up of probably benign lesions: results in 3183 consecutive cases," *Radiology* **179**, 463-468, 1991.

5.   B. Sahiner, H. P. Chan, N. Petrick, M. A. Helvie, and M. M. Goodsitt, "Computerized characterization of masses on mammograms: The rubber band straightening transform and texture analysis," *Medical Physics* **25**, 516-526, 1998.

6.   Z. M. Huo, M. L. Giger, C. J. Vyborny, D. E. Wolverton, R. A. Schmidt, and K. Doi, "Automated computerized classification of malignant and benign masses on digitized mammograms," *Academic Radiology* **5**, 155-168, 1998.

7.   L. M. Hadjiiski, B. Sahiner, H. P. Chan, N. Petrick, and M. A. Helvie, "Classification of malignant and benign masses based on hybrid ART2LDA approach," *IEEE Transactions on Medical Imaging* **18**, 1178-1187, 1999.

8.   H. P. Chan, D. Wei, K. L. Lam, B. Sahiner, M. A. Helvie, D. D. Adler, and M. M. Goodsitt, "Classification of malignant and benign microcalcifications by texture analysis," *Medical Physics* **22**, 938, 1995.

9.   Y. Jiang, R. M. Nishikawa, D. E. Wolverton, C. E. Metz, M. L. Giger, R. A. Schmidt, C. J. Vyborny, and K. Doi, "Malignant and benign clustered microcalcifications: automated feature analysis and classification," *Radiology* **198**, 671-678, 1996.

10. H. P. Chan, B. Sahiner, N. Petrick, M. A. Helvie, K. L. Leung, D. D. Adler, and M. M. Goodsitt, "Computerized classification of malignant and benign microcalcifications on mammograms: texture analysis using an artificial neural network," *Physics in Medicine and Biology* **42**, 549-567, 1997.

11. H. P. Chan, B. Sahiner, K. L. Lam, N. Petrick, M. A. Helvie, M. M. Goodsitt, and D. D. Adler, "Computerized analysis of mammographic microcalcifications in morphological and texture feature space," *Medical Physics* **25**, 2007-2019, 1998.

12. L. M. Hadjiiski, B. Sahiner, H. P. Chan, N. Petrick, M. A. Helvie, and M. Gurcan, "Analysis of temporal change of mammographic features for computer-aided characterization of malignant and benign masses," *Proceedings of the SPIE* **4322**, 661-666, 2001.

13. L. M. Hadjiiski, B. Sahiner, H. P. Chan, N. Petrick, M. A. Helvie, and M. N. Gurcan, "Analysis of Temporal Change of Mammographic Features: Computer-Aided Classification of Malignant and Benign Breast Masses," *Medical Physics* **28**, 2309-2317, 2001.

14. M. M. Galloway, "Texture classification using gray level run lengths," *Computer Graphics and Image Processing* **4**, 172-179, 1975.

15. M. J. Norusis, *SPSS for Windows Release 6 Professional Statistics*, SPSS Inc., Chicago, IL, 1993.

16. M. M. Tatsuoka, *Multivariate Analysis, Techniques for Educational and Psychological Research*, 2nd ed. Macmillan, New York, 1988.

17. S. S. Rao, *Optimization: Theory and Applications*, Wiley Eastern Limited, 1979.

18. F. A. Lootsma, *Numerical methods for non-linear optimization*, Academic Press, New York, 1972.

19. C. E. Metz, "ROC methodology in radiologic imaging," *Investigative Radiology* **21**, 720-733, 1986.

20. C. E. Metz, J. H. Shen, and B. A. Herman, "New methods for estimating a binormal ROC curve from continuously-distributed test results," *Annual Meeting of the American Statistical Association*, Anaheim, CA, 1990.

The use of joint two-view information for computerized lesion detection on mammograms: Improvement of microcalcification detection accuracy

Berkman Sahiner[*], Metin N. Gurcan, Heang-Ping Chan,
Lubomir M. Hadjiiski, Nicholas Petrick, Mark A. Helvie
Department of Radiology, University of Michigan, Ann Arbor

ABSTRACT

We are developing new techniques to improve the accuracy of computerized microcalcification detection by using the joint two-view information on craniocaudal (CC) and mediolateral-oblique (MLO) views. After cluster candidates were detected using a single-view detection technique, candidates on CC and MLO views were paired using their radial distances from the nipple. Object pairs were classified with a joint two-view classifier that used the similarity of objects in a pair. Each cluster candidate was also classified as a true microcalcification cluster or a false-positive (FP) using its single-view features. The outputs of these two classifiers were fused. A data set of 38 pairs of mammograms from our database was used to train the new detection technique. The independent test set consisted of 77 pairs of mammograms from the University of South Florida public database. At a per-film sensitivity of 70%, the FP rates were 0.17 and 0.27 with the fusion and single-view detection methods, respectively. Our results indicate that correspondence of cluster candidates on two different views provides valuable additional information for distinguishing false from true microcalcification clusters.

Keywords: Mammography, Computer-Aided Diagnosis, Microcalcifications, Detection

1. INTRODUCTION

It has been shown that imaging the breast in two views increases the cancer detection sensitivity while decreasing the recall rate[1,2]. The radiologist combines the information from the two views to confirm true positives (TPs) and to reduce false positives (FPs). It is expected that computerized detection could also benefit from the use of the joint two-view information available in a screening study in the form of mediolateral oblique (MLO) and craniocaudal (CC) views. This paper describes our preliminary work on false-positive reduction in computerized microcalcification detection by the use of the joint two-view information.

Analysis of multiple mammograms of the same breast for lesion detection is an active research area. The multiple mammograms can be acquired either at different examination times but using the same geometric orientation (view), or during the same examination but different views. To analyze the information provided by temporal image pairs, Gopal et al.[3] and Hadjiiski et al.[4] developed regional registration methods for identifying corresponding lesions on temporal pairs of mammograms. To identify corresponding regions on two different views, Highnam et al.[5,6] and Kita et al.[5,6] proposed a model for breast deformation under mammographic compression. Chang et al.[7] compared two methods for predicting a search region on the MLO view (or the CC view) for a lesion detected on the CC view (or the MLO view). Good et al.[8] investigated a method for matching computer-detected objects on two views and discriminating a TP-TP pairs from other pairs. Paquerault et al.[9] designed geometric models that can localize corresponding lesions within a search region when two-view or three-view mammograms are available for lesion localization. Paquerault et al.[10,11] and Sahiner et al.[12] recently demonstrated how the geometric, morphological, and texture features from lesion candidates on two different views of the same breast can be combined to increase the accuracy of computerized mass detection on mammograms.

2. METHODS

* berki@umich.edu, phone 734-647-7429, CGC B2102, 1500 E. Medical Center Dr., Ann Arbor, MI 48109-0904

Medical Imaging 2002: Image Processing, Milan Sonka, J. Michael Fitzpatrick,
Editors, Proceedings of SPIE Vol. 4684 (2002) © 2002 SPIE · 1605-7422/02/$15.00

Our joint two-view detection methods is based on the assumption that if a single-view detection algorithm detects a true cluster on the CC and MLO views of the same breast, the detections on the two views will exhibit similarities in their geometric, morphological and textural features. On the other hand, an FP cluster detected on the CC view is expected to exhibit a lesser degree of similarity with the true cluster on the MLO view, and vice-versa. Furthermore, the degree of similarity exhibited by two FP clusters on two different views is expected to be lesser than that between two TPs. Based on this assumption, we performed similarity analysis between cluster candidates detected on the two views and distinguishing true pairs (TP-TP pairs) from false pairs (FP-TP, TP-FP, and FP-FP pairs). The block diagram of the joint two-view detection method is shown in Figure 1. Individual components of this block diagram are explained next.

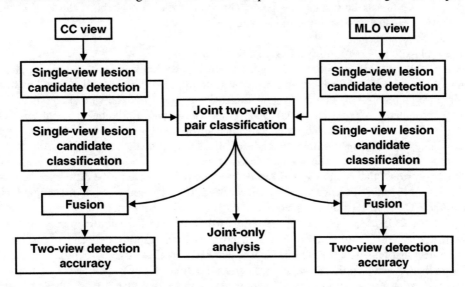

Figure 1:   The block diagram of the computerized two-view microcalcification detection method.

2.1   Single-view lesion candidate detection

The single-view lesion candidate detection technique used in this study includes three major steps as shown in Figure 2.

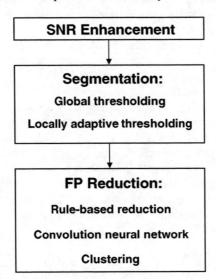

Figure 2:   The block diagram of the single-view microcalcification detection method.

First, the image is processed using a difference-image technique to enhance the signal-to-noise ratio (SNR) of the microcalcifications[13]. Second, potential signals are segmented from the image background using global and locally adaptive segmentation techniques. In the global segmentation stage, potential signal sites are determined using thresholding. A gray level threshold is selected based on the histogram of the preprocessed image, and is iteratively updated until the number of potential signal sites falls within the chosen input maximum and minimum numbers. Locally adaptive segmentation is then applied to each signal site. The threshold in this stage is determined as the product of the local root-mean-square noise and an input SNR threshold. The false-positive reduction step includes three stages, which are rule-based classification, convolution neural network (CNN), and clustering, respectively. In the first stage, upper and/or lower bounds are used on the signal size, contrast and SNR to eliminate false-positives. After rule-based FP reduction, a CNN that has been trained to recognize true microcalcifications is applied to the remaining signals to further reduce FPs[14]. Finally, a regional clustering procedure is used to identify clustered microcalcifications. Signals that are within a neighborhood of other signals are sustained as potential microcalcifications within a cluster. Isolated signals are considered as noise points or isolated calcifications and are excluded.

2.2   Joint two-view classification of true and false pairs

Our joint two-view pair classification algorithm is designed to distinguish between true and false pairs by using the similarities between the two objects on different views that constitute the pair. The initial step in this task is to define the object pairs. From the geometry of the mammographic image acquisition, it is known that an object seen on the CC view can appear only in a limited sub-region in the MLO view, and vice-versa. Radiologists at our institution routinely use the nipple-to-object distance (NOD) on the two views to confirm the correspondence between objects seen on different views of the same breast. Our preliminary studies[9,11] have also shown that the NODs on the two views are highly correlated. Other researchers have considered curved epipolar lines[6] and the Cartesian straight-line distance methods[7]. Based on our previous studies, in this work we defined the pairs based on the difference between the NODs on the CC and MLO views. Figure 3 illustrates our two-view registration procedure. First, the nipple locations N_c and N_m are determined on the CC and MLO views, respectively. Next, the nipple-to-object distance R_c is computed for the cluster candidate C_{C1} on the CC view. To find objects on the MLO view to be paired with C_{C1}, an arc of radius R_c centered at N_m is outlined on the MLO view. Next, two concentric arcs, with radii $R_c + \Delta R$ and $R_c - \Delta R$ are also drawn on the MLO view. Any object that falls with the annular region delineated by these two concentric arcs is paired with the cluster candidate C_{C1} on the CC view. In this example, two pairs are defined: C_{C1}-C_{M1} pair and C_{C1}-C_{M2} pair. Although a third cluster candidate C_{M3} exists on the MLO view, it is not paired with C_{C1} because it falls outside the defined annular region. The width of the annular region, $2\Delta R$, is determined using training data.

A correspondence classifier was used to score the defined pairs as to their likelihood of being a true pair. The correspondence classifier has been designed to use the similarity of a number of features of the suspected clusters in two views. The classifier was designed using stepwise feature selection and linear discriminant analysis (LDA) training on an independent training set. The feature space used in stepwise selection included the similarity measures extracted from texture and morphological features of the microcalcification clusters on the two views, as well as the number of microcalcifications and the CNN scores.

2.3   Single-view lesion candidate classification

Our previous work on the use of joint two-view information for mass detection demonstrated that the two-view pair classification could improve computer detection accuracy. However, the scores resulting from joint two-view pair classification alone (referred to as "joint-only" detection) may not provide adequate sensitivity. We have therefore adopted a strategy in which the two-view pair classification scores supplement the single-view scores. In order to score each lesion candidate based on its single-view features, a classifier was trained using stepwise feature selection and linear discriminant analysis on the training set. The feature space used in stepwise selection included the features that were used to define the similarity measures in the two-view pair classification method. This ensured that the additional information provided by the two-view pair classification method was a result of the use of the similarity information, instead of the application of new or different features.

2.4   Fusion

The correspondence classifier produced a correspondence score for each object pair. These scores were converted into two-view object scores before being combined with the single-view object scores. An object on the CC view can be a member of several object pairs (paired with more than one object on the MLO view), and vice-versa, as illustrated in Figure 3. The two-view object score of an object C_i was defined as the maximum of all correspondence scores for pairs in which C_i is a member. The fusion score for an object was defined as the average of its single- and two-view object scores.

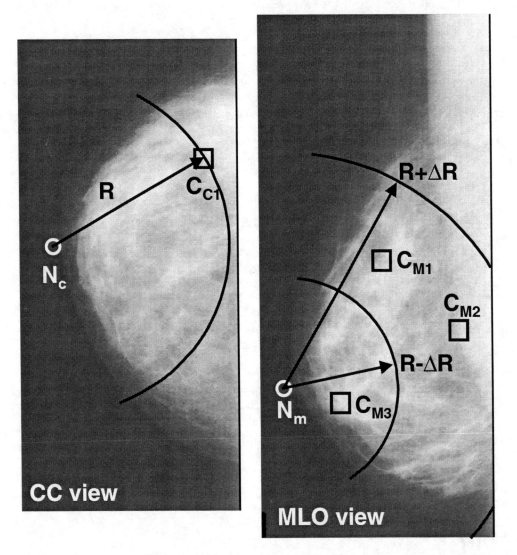

Figure 3: The definition of object pairs based on the nipple-to-object distances on the CC and MLO views in our two-view registration technique.

2.5 Data Set

Our training data set consisted of 38 pairs of biopsy-proven CC and MLO mammograms containing microcalcification clusters, collected with Institutional Review Board approval at the University of Michigan (UM). Ten of the microcalcification pairs were malignant and 28 were benign. The mammograms were digitized with a LUMISYS 85 laser scanner at a pixel size of 50 μm x 50 μm and 4096 gray levels. The digitizer was calibrated so that the gray level values were linearly proportional to the optical density (OD) within the range of 0.1 to 4.0 OD units. The mammograms were filtered with a 2x2 box filter and subsampled by a factor of 2 to produce a 0.1 mm x 0.1 mm images prior to any processing.

Our independent test set consisted of 77 pairs of mammograms, selected from the University of South Florida (USF) public mammogram database[15]. The digitization characteristics of these mammograms were similar to those of the UM database, with the difference that a Lumisys 200 laser scanner with an OD range of 0.1 to 4.0 OD units was used to digitize the USF cases. The test data set contained 175 microcalcification clusters on 154 mammograms, of which 161 were biopsy-proven malignant. Four of the microcalcifications clusters were visible only on one view.

3. RESULTS

The detection accuracy was evaluated using per-film free-response receiver operating characteristic (FROC) curves. In per-film analysis, a microcalcification cluster detected on one view but missed on the other view is considered as one TP and one false-negative (FN). This method provides a more conservative sensitivity estimate than per-case analysis, in which a cluster detected on one view but missed on the other view would be counted as one FP and zero FN.

The single-view lesion candidate detection algorithm correctly detected 83% (146/175) of the microcalcification clusters, at an average FP rate of 1.6 FPs/image. Microcalcification clusters were detected on both views in 71% (55/77) of the mammogram pairs.

Based on the geometric locations of the microcalcification clusters in the training set, a radial width of $2\Delta R=6.0$ cm was used for geometric pair definition. Of a total of 4663 possible pairs in the test set, 2350 object pairs were defined using the two-view registration method described in Section 2.2, while the percentage of mammograms with true pairs was maintained at 71%. The object pairs were classified using the correspondence classifier designed using the training set. The stepwise procedure selected 6 features from the training set, which included the number of microcalcifications, the mean CNN score, two morphological features, and two texture features. The pair scores were converted into object scores as described in Section 2.4. Figure 4 shows the FROC curve resulting from the use of the score from joint-only detection. Also shown in Figure 4 is the FROC curve obtained by the single-view lesion candidate classification. The final FROC curve obtained by the fusion of single-view and two-view scores is compared to the single-view FROC curve in Figure 5 and Table 1.

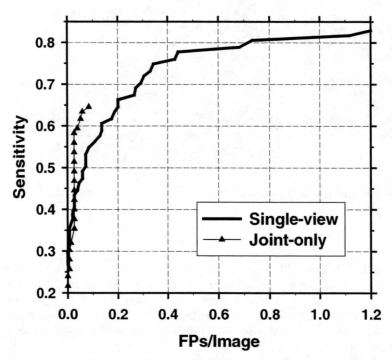

Figure 4: The comparison of the FROC curves obtained by joint two-view detection only and single-view detection.

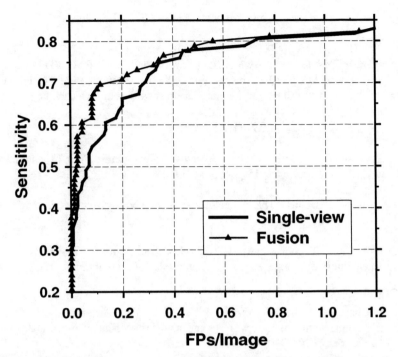

Figure 5:   The comparison of the FROC curves obtained by the fusion and the single-view detection methods.

Sensitivity	False-Positives per Image	
	Fusion	Single-view
70%	0.17	0.27
75%	0.34	0.41
80%	0.55	0.70

Table I.   The comparison of the FP rates generated by the fusion method and the single-view detection method at selected sensitivity levels.

4. CONCLUSION

We have demonstrated the feasibility of improved FP reduction in computerized microcalcification detection by fusing the scores from single-view and joint two-view classifiers designed on a small training set. Joint two-view classification of true and false pairs in this study achieved a very low FP rate at a moderate sensitivity. The fusion of the single-view and two-view scores resulted in a detection algorithm with a reduced number of FPs at comparable sensitivities to single-view detection.

In this study, our objective was to reduce the false-positives produced by our single-view detection technique. As observed from Figure 4, the highest per-film sensitivity achieved by both single-view and two-view techniques was 83%. Another possible application of joint two-view detection is to increase the overall sensitivity. This can be achieved by first relaxing the FP elimination criteria in any of the three stages of FP reduction shown Figure 2, so that a larger number of TPs are detected along with more FPs. One can then investigate whether the redesign of the two–view detection methods will improve the overall sensitivity of computerized detection at FP rates less than 1 FP/image. Our experience with two-view mass detection[11,12] indicates that this is an achievable goal.

Further studies with larger training and test sets are needed to study the generalizability of our approach. Future work also includes the optimization of the similarity measures, improvement of the fusion technique, and the application of two-view detection techniques to improve the overall detection sensitivity.

ACKNOWLEDGMENTS

This work is supported by USPHS Grant CA 48129, USAMRMC grant DAMD 17-96-1-6254, USAMRMC grant DAMD17-01-1-0823, and a Career Development Award (L.H.) from the USAMRMC (DAMD 17-98-1-8211). The content of this publication does not necessarily reflect the position of the government and no official endorsement of any equipment and product of any companies mentioned in the publication should be inferred.

REFERENCES

1. E. Thurfjell, A. Taube, and L. Tabar, "One-view versus 2-view mammography screening - a prospective population-based study," *Acta Radiologica* **35**, 340-344, 1994.

2. R. Warren, S. Duffy, and S. Bashir, "The value of the second view in screening mammography," *British Journal of Radiology* **69**, 105-108, 1996.

3. S. Sanjay-Gopal, H. P. Chan, T. Wilson, M. Helvie, N. Petrick, and B. Sahiner, "A regional registration technique for automated interval change analysis of breast lesions on mammograms," *Medical Physics* **26**, 2669-2679, 1999.

4. L. M. Hadjiiski, H. P. Chan, B. Sahiner, N. Petrick, and M. A. Helvie, "Automated registration of breast lesions in temporal pairs of mammograms for interval change analysis - local affine transformation for improved localization," *Medical Physics* **28**, 1070-1079, 2001.

5. R. P. Highnam, Y. Kita, J. M. Brady, B. J. Shepstone, and R. English, "Determining correspondence between views," *Proc. 4th International Workshop on Digital Mammography*, Nijmegen, Netherlands, 1998.

6. Y. Kita, R. P. Highnam, and J. M. Brady, "Correspondence between different view breast X rays using curved epipolar lines," *Computer Vision and Image Understanding* **83**, 38-56, 2001.

7. Y. H. Chang, W. F. Good, J. H. Sumkin, B. Zheng, and D. Gur, "Computerized localization of breast lesions from two views - An experimental comparison of two methods," *Investigative Radiology* **34**, 585-588, 1999.

8. W. F. Good, B. Zheng, Y. H. Chang, Z. H. Wang, G. S. Maitz, and D. Gur, "Multi-image CAD employing features derived from ipsilateral mammographic views," *Proceedings of the SPIE* **3661**, 474-485, 1999.

9. S. Paquerault, B. Sahiner, N. Petrick, L. M. Hadjiiski, M. N. Gurcan, C. Zhou, and M. A. Helvie, "Prediction of object location in different views using geometrical models," *Proc. 5th International Workshop on Digital Mammography*, 748-755, Toronto, Canada, 2001.

10. S. Paquerault, N. Petrick, H. P. Chan, B. Sahiner, and A. Y. Dolney, "Improvement of mammographic lesion detection by fusion of information from different views," *Proceedings of the SPIE* **4322**, 1883-1889, 2001.

11. S. Paquerault, N. Petrick, H. P. Chan, B. Sahiner, and M. A. Helvie, "Improvement of computerized mass detection on mammograms: Fusion of two-view information," *Medical Physics* **29**, 238-247, 2002.

12. B. Sahiner, N. Petrick, H. P. Chan, S. Paquerault, M. A. Helvie, and L. M. Hadjiiski, "Recognition of lesion correspondence on two mammographic views - A new method of false-positive reduction for computerized mass detection," *Proceedings of the SPIE* **4322**, 649-655, 2001.

13. H. P. Chan, K. Doi, C. J. Vyborny, R. A. Schmidt, C. E. Metz, K. L. Lam, T. Ogura, Y. Wu, and H. MacMahon, "Improvement in radiologists' detection of clustered microcalcifications on mammograms. The potential of computer-aided diagnosis," *Investigative Radiology* **25**, 1102-1110, 1990.

14.   H. P. Chan, S. C. B. Lo, B. Sahiner, K. L. Lam, and M. A. Helvie, "Computer-aided detection of mammographic microcalcifications: Pattern recognition with an artificial neural network," *Medical Physics* **22**, 1555-1567, 1995.

15.   M. Heath, K. Bowyer, D. Kopans, R. Moore, and P. Kegelmeyer, "The digital database for screening mammography," *In: Digital Mammography; IWDM 2000*, 457-460, Eds. M. J. Yaffe, Medical Physics Publishing, Toronto, Canada, 2001.

Effect of Case-Mix on Feature Selection in the Computerized Classification of Mammographic Lesions

Zhimin Huo[a]* and Maryellen L. Giger[b]

[a] Eastman Kodak Company, 1999 Lake Ave., Rochester, USA
[b] The University of Chicago, 5841 S. Maryland Ave., Chicago, USA

ABSTRACT

One potential limitation of computer-aided diagnosis (CAD) studies is that a computerized method may be trained and tested on a database comprised of a limited number of cases. Thus, the performance of the CAD method may depend on the subtlety of the lesions (i.e., the case mix) in the database. The purpose of this study is to evaluate the effect of case-mix on feature selection and the performance of a computerized classification method trained on a limited database.

Keywords: Computer-aided diagnosis, digital mammography, case subtlety, artificial neural network, feature selection

1. INTRODUCTION

Clinically detected breast lesions vary greatly in their appearance with regard to size, density, contrast, shape and margin characteristics [1]. The difficulty to detect breast cancer or to differentiate between benign and malignant breast lesions may depend on the subtlety of these lesions in terms of their appearance. Computer-aided diagnosis in digital mammography has been shown to have potential in improving radiologist s performance in detecting breast cancer and in differentiating between benign and malignant breast lesions [2-4]. However, due to the limited access to clinical cases, performance validation of a computerized method is sometimes performed on the same database on which the training of the algorithm was performed. One common approach to validate the performance of a computer algorithm is to use a leave-one-out method when the number of cases is limited. The leave-one-out approach [5] is usually applied in order to prevent the classifier used in the method (e.g., an artificial neural network) from over-learning due to a limited number of available cases, thus allowing for the classifier to generalize to the cases that are not included in the training database. Note that a computerized method usually includes multiple components such as 1) lesion segmentation, 2) feature extraction, 3) feature selection and 4) classification. The ability of other components to generalize to new cases is not addressed by the leave-one-out approach. Over-learning may occur in the training process of the other components. In this study, we investigated the limitation in the feature selection phase when a small number of cases is used in the training of a computerized classification method and its effect on the performance of the method.

2. METHODS AND MATERIALS

We have developed a computerized method to classify mammographic mass lesions as benign vs. malignant, which is described in detail elsewhere [6]. A schematic overview of the classification method is illustrated in Figure 1. . To characterize a mammographic mass lesion, various features are automatically extracted from an identified mass lesion. We have investigated over 52 features that are similar to features used by radiologists to characterize the margin, shape, density, size, and texture features of a mass lesion [6]. Performance of these individual features in differentiating between benign and malignant mass lesions was analyzed in comparison with the performance of radiologists visually-extracted features (e.g., radiologist s spiculation ratings). Features were selected to quantify the different aspects of a mass lesion, i.e., the margin, shape, density and texture. These features then served as inputs to an artificial neural network (three-layer, feed-forward neural network with a back propagation algorithm) [5]. The selected features are listed in Table 1 along with brief descriptions. Details about these features can be found elsewhere [7,8].

Previously, we showed in an independent evaluation that our computerized classification method is robust to variation in case mix in the task of differentiating between benign and malignant cases [9]. In addition, we have shown

---

* E-mail: zhimin.huo@kodak.com
    m-giger@uchicago.edu

Medical Imaging 2002: Image Processing, Milan Sonka, J. Michael Fitzpatrick, Editors, Proceedings of SPIE Vol. 4684 (2002) © 2002 SPIE · 1605-7422/02/$15.00

that the use of the computerized method improves radiologists performance in the classification of benign and malignant mass lesions [4].

For our current study, we used two independently-collected databases (A and B) for the purpose of development and evaluation of the computerized method. Database A consists of 95 mammographic images (38 benign and 58 malignant) from 65 cases. Database B consists of 212 mammographic images (120 benign and 92 malignant) from 110 cases. The classification method was initially trained on database A. Training includes 1) selection of parameters used in the segmentation phase, 2) selection of the most significant set of features, and 3) determination of the weight table used in the neural net. The features were selected based on their individual performance and their collective performance when merged with an artificial neural network. Receiver operating characteristics (ROC) analysis [10] was used to evaluate the performance of individual features and the ability of the artificial neural network in merging the selected features to differentiate between benign and malignant masses. Both round-robin analysis and independent validation methods were performed to evaluate the performance of the trained classification method.

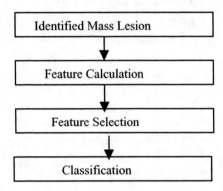

Figure 1. Overview of classification method.

1) Spiculation	Measure (degree) of spiculation along the margin of a mass lesion
2) Margin sharpness	Measure of how well-defined the margin is
3) Avg. gray value	Measure of the density of the mass lesion
4) Texture	Measure of the variation in gradient within the mass lesion
5) Radial gradient	Measure of the margin (spiculation) and shape (irregularity)

Table 1. List of computer-extracted features and brief description.

2.1. Round-Robin Evaluation Using Database A

The performance of the computerized method trained on database A was evaluated on the same database (database A) using the leave-one-out cross-validation method. The leave-one-out method is also called the round-robin method [5]. In this approach, all but one case in the database are used to train the neural network, with the single left-out case used to test the classifier. To avoid bias for cases with images having two views (medio-lateral-oblique and cranio-caudal views) of the breast, both images of a given case were left out in the round-robin training, and the higher of the two values from the round-robin test was reported as the estimated likelihood of malignancy for that case. This procedure was repeated for all the cases so that every case in the database served once as a cross-validation case.

Based on the learning from database A, four features (spiculation, margin sharpness, average gray level and texture) were selected as the inputs to a 4-input artificial neural network. Round-robin analysis was performed to evaluate the 4-input ANN in merging the four features to differentiate between benign and malignant. The area under the ROC curve (A_z) was calculated as an index to indicate the performance of individual features and the performance of the ANN. In addition, we calculated the partial area index $_{0.90}A_z$ to evaluate the performance at high sensitivity levels [11]. The performances of the selected features are listed in Table 2.

2.2. Round-Robin Evaluation Using Database B

To evaluate the effect of differences in case mix on the feature selection, we retrained the computerized method on database B. Note that the training on database B involves feature selecion and the training of an artificial neural. Same criteria for feature selection were applied on databases A and B. The features were selected based on their individual performance and their collective performance in a round-robin evaluation when merged with an ANN classifier, and the number of the features selected was kept at a minimum in order to retain the ability to generalize. Five features were selected based on the analysis of database B and served as inputs to a 5-input ANN. These features are spiculation, margin sharpness, average gray level, texture and radial gradient. Their performances on database B are listed in Table 2. Note that an additional feature was selected when database B was used. Round robin analysis was performed to evaluate the performance of the computerized method on database B.

Table 2. List of performances of individual features in terms of the area under the ROC curve (A_z). Features indicated with an asterisk were selected based on the performance on database A.

Features	Performance on database A	Performance on database B
Spiculation*	0.80	0.77
Margin sharpness*	0.56	0.55
Avg. gray value*	0.54	0.54
Texture*	0.65	0.51
Radial gradient	0.78	0.80

Note that to evaluate the effect of difference in the features selected on the performance of the classification method, we applied both sets of selected features (the 4-feature set and the 5-feature set) to train the ANNs on each database and compared the performances obtained on the same database with different sets of features.

2.3. Independent Evaluation

In a round-robin analysis, the performance of a classifier is evaluated on the same database used in the training. In order to validate the performance of the computerized method, we evaluated it on independent datasets, i.e., database B served as the independent data set to evaluate the computer algorithm trained on database A; and database A served as the independent data set to evaluate the computerized method trained on database B.

3. RESULTS

Listed in Table 3 are the results from the round-robin evaluation of databases A and B using the two sets of selected features. A new feature was included as an additional input feature to the classifier when database B was used for training. In our previous study, this feature was studied along with the spiculation feature to quantitatively assess the spiculation along the margin of a mass [6]. The two features are strongly correlated [7]. Note that the fifth feature was not selected for database A since the performance of the ANN on database A did not improve when the feature was included (an A_z of 0.89 and a $_{0.90}A_z$ of 0.38). However, when we included this feature as an additional feature to the ANN (5 input units, 2 hidden units and one output unit) trained on database B, the performance on database B improved from an A_z of 0.86 and a $_{0.90}A$ of 0.54 to an A_z of 0.91 and a $_{0.90}A'_z$ of 0.77 in a round-robin evaluation. This significant improvement ($\Delta_{0.90}A'_z$ =0.23 with a p-value of 0.004) in $_{0.90}A'_z$ as evaluated using the CLABROC program [12], when the additional feature was included, indicated that case mix in the training database influences the feature selection.

In addition, we found that the variation in case mix may affect the training of an ANN, thus resulting in significant differences in performance. The 4-input ANN trained on database A yielded an A_z of 0.81 and a $_{0.90}A'_z$ of 0.37 on database B (in an independent evaluation). The 4-input ANN trained on database B yielded an A_z of 0.86 and a $_{0.90}A'_z$ of 0.54 on database B (in a round-robin evaluation). The differences in performance (ΔA_z =0.05, p=0.03 and $\Delta_{0.90}A'_z$ =0.17, p=0.04) on database B due to the different learning processes from the two different databases are statistically significant.

Shown in Figure 2 are the distributions of cases in database A and database B based on subtlety in terms of radiologist s ratings of likelihood of malignancy. We have evaluated the effect of difference in case mix, as shown in Figure 2, on feature selection and ANN learning in terms of the performance of the ANNs.

Table 3. Performances from the round-robin analyses and independent evaluations using the two sets of selected features on databases A and B.

Round-Robin Analysis			Independent Evaluation		
Database	A_z	$_{0.90}A'_z$	Database	A_z	$_{0.90}A'_z$
A (4 features)	0.90+/-0.04	0.40+/-0.17	B (4 features)	0.81+/-0.04	0.37+/-0.10
A (5 features)	0.89+/-0.03	0.38+/-0.16	B (5 features)	0.82+/-0.03	0.38+/-0.10
B (4 features)	0.86+/-0.04	0.54+/-0.09	A (4 features)	0.89+/-0.04	0.44+/-0.15
B (5 features)	0.91+/-0.03	0.77+/-0.06	A (5 features)	0.89+/-0.04	0.41+/-0.15

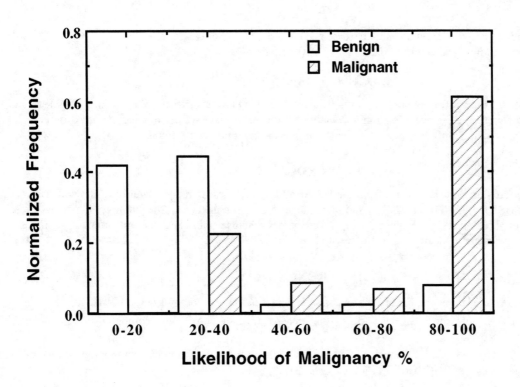

(a)

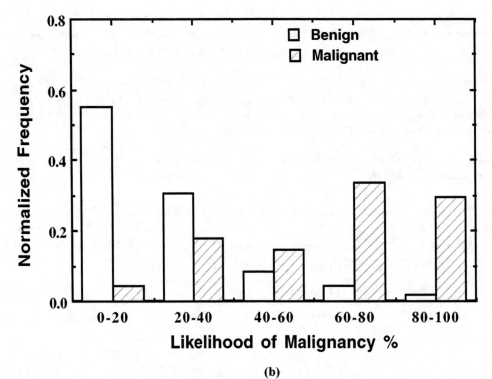

(b)

Figure 2: Distribution of cases based on subtlety (case mix) in terms of radiologist s ratings of likelihood of malignancy for (a) database A and (b) database B.

4. CONCLUSIONS

We have shown that the types of cases in the training database may bias the feature selection and the ANN learning process in the task of differentiating between benign and malignant masses, thus resulting in a significant difference in performance, when a limited number of cases is used in the training of the computerized method.

5. ACKNOWLEDGMENTS

This work was supported in parts by a grant from the US Army Medical Research and Materiel Command (DAMD 17-96-1-6058) and USPHS grant CA89452. Z. Huo and M. L. Giger are shareholders in R2 technology, Inc. (Los Altos, CA). It is the policy of the University of Chicago that investigators disclose publicly actual or potential significant financial interests that may appear to be affected by the research activities.

6. REFERENCES

1. D'Orsi CJ and Kopans DB. Mammographic feature analysis. *Seminars in Roentgenology* 1993; **28**:204-230.

2. Jiang Y, Nishikawa RM, Schmidt RA, et al. Improving breast cancer diagnosis with computer-aided diagnosis. *Academic Radiology* 1999; **6**:22.

3. Chan H-P, Sahiner B, Helvie MA, et al. Improvement of radiologists' characterization of mammographic masses by using computer-aided diagnosis: An ROC study. *Radiology* 1999; **212**:817-827.

4. Huo Z, Giger ML, Vyborny CJ and Metz CE. Effectiveness of CAD in the Diagnosis of Breast Cancer: An Observer Study on an Independent Database of Mammograms. *Radiology* (in press);

5. Haykin S. Neural Networks: A comprehensive foundation. New York, Macmillan College Publishing Company, 1994.

6. Huo Z. Computerized methods for classification of masses and analysis of parenchymal patterns on digitized mammograms. Dissertation. The University of Chicago. 1998.

7. Huo Z, Giger ML, Vyborny CJ, et al. Analysis of spiculation in the computerized classification of mammographic masses. *Med Phys* 1995; **22**:1569-1579.

8. Huo Z, Giger ML, Vyborny CJ, et al. Automated computerized classification of malignant and benign masses on digitized mammograms. *Academic Radiology* 1998; **5**:155-168.

9. Huo Z, Giger ML, Vyborny CJ, Wolverton DE and Metz CE. Computerized classification of benign and malignant masses on digitized mammograms: a study of robustness. *Academic Radiology* 2000; **7**:1077-1084.

10. Metz CE. ROC methodology in radiologic imaging. *Invest Radiol* 1986; **21**:720-733.

11. Jiang Y, Metz CE and Nishikawa RM. A receiver operating characteristics partial area index for highly sensitive diagnostic tests. *Radiology* 1996; **201**:745-750.

12. Metz CE, Herman BA and Roe CA. Statistical comparison of two ROC-curve estimates obtained from partially-paried datasets. *Medical Decision Making* 1998; **18**:110-121.

Intelligent CAD workstation for breast imaging using similarity to known lesions and multiple visual prompt aids

Maryellen L. Giger[*], Zhimin Huo, Carl J. Vyborny, Li Lan, Ioana Bonta,
Karla Horsch, Robert M. Nishikawa, Ingrid Rosenbourgh
Department of Radiology, University of Chicago, Chicago, Illinois 60637, U.S.A.

ABSTRACT

While investigators have been successful in developing methods for the computerized analysis of mammograms and ultrasound images, optimal output strategies for the effective and efficient use of such computer analyses are still undetermined. We have incorporated our computerized mass classification method into an intelligent workstation interface that displays known malignant and benign cases similar to lesions in question using a color-coding scheme that allows instant visual feedback to the radiologist. The probability distributions of the malignant and benign cases in the known database are also graphically displayed along with the graphical "location" of the unknown case relative to these two distributions. The effect of the workstation on radiologists' performance was demonstrated with two preliminary studies. In each study, participants were asked to interpret cases without and with the computer output as an aid for diagnosis. Results from our demonstration studies indicate that radiologists' performance, especially specificity, increases with the use of the aid.

1. INTRODUCTION

Mammography is the most effective method for the early detection of breast cancer, and it has been shown that periodic screening of asymptomatic women does reduce mortality. Many breast cancers are detected and referred for surgical biopsy on the basis of a radiographically detected mass lesion or cluster of microcalcifications. Although general rules for the differentiation between benign and malignant mammographically identified breast lesions exist, considerable misclassification of lesions occurs with human-interpretation methods and variations have also been observed in the positive biopsy rates of individual radiologists [1-6].

Breast sonography is used as an important adjunct to diagnostic mammography and is typically performed to evaluate palpable or mammographically identified masses in order to determine whether they are cystic or solid. Use of ultrasound for the diagnosis of simple benign cysts is accurate. However, many that prove to be indeterminate or solid on sonography are candidates for further intervention.

Various investigators are developing methods for the computerized analysis of lesions on breast images with the computer output serving as an aid to the radiologist. However, optimal output strategies for the effective and efficient use of such computer analyses for computer-aided diagnosis are still undetermined. We have incorporated our computerized mass classification methods into an intelligent workstation interface, which displays similar malignant and benign known cases by use of a color-coding scheme allowing for instant visual feedback to the radiologist.

1.1 Computerized Characterization of Mass Lesions on Mammography

Our mass classification method includes three components: 1) automated segmentation of mass regions, 2) automated feature-extraction, and 3) automated classification [7-9]. The scheme was initially trained with 95 mammograms containing masses occurring in 65 patients. Features related to the margin, shape, and density of each mass are extracted automatically from the image data and merged into an estimate of the likelihood of malignancy using artificial neural networks. In a round-robin analysis, the computer classification scheme yielded an A_z value of 0.94, similar to that of an experienced mammographer ($A_z=0.91$) and statistically significantly higher than the average performance of five

---

[*] m-giger@uchicago.edu

Medical Imaging 2002: Image Processing, Milan Sonka, J. Michael Fitzpatrick,
Editors, Proceedings of SPIE Vol. 4684 (2002) © 2002 SPIE · 1605-7422/02/$15.00

radiologists with less mammographic experience (A_z=0.81). [7-8]. The computerized mass classification method was also independently evaluated on a 110-case clinical database containing 50 malignant and 60 benign mass cases. The effects of variations in both case mix and in film digitization technique on the performance of the method were assessed. In the task of distinguishing between malignant and benign lesions, the computer achieved an A_z value (area under the ROC curve) of 0.90 on the prior training database (Fuji scanner digitization) in a round-robin evaluation, and A_z values of 0.82 and 0.81 on the independent database for Konica and Lumisys digitization formats, respectively. However, in the statistical comparison of these performances, we failed to show a statistical significant difference between the performance on the training database and that on the independent validation database (p-values > 0.10). Thus, our computer-based method for the classification of lesions on mammograms is robust to variations in case mix and film digitization technique [9].

1.2 Computerized Characterization of Mass Lesions on Breast Sonography

We have also developed a computerized method for the automatic classification of breast lesions on ultrasound. The computerized method includes automatic segmentation of the lesion from the ultrasound image background and automatic extraction of four features related to lesion shape, margin, texture, and posterior acoustic behavior [10-11]. Lesion shape is characterized by a depth-to-width ratio and lesion margin is characterized by the normalized radial gradient which yields the average orientation of the gray level gradients along the margin. Lesion texture is characterized an autocorrelation function and the posterior acoustic behavior is characterized by comparing the gray-level values posterior to the lesion to those in adjacent tissue at the same depth. These four features are merged through linear discriminant analysis to yield an estimate of the likelihood of malignancy. The linear discriminant function was determined using 409 cases. In an independent evaluation comprised of eleven jackknife trials, the computerized classification method yielded an average A_z value (area under the ROC curve) of 0.87 in the task of distinguishing between malignant and benign lesions [11].

1.3. Intelligent workstation with multiple visual prompt aids

We previously developed an intelligent workstation based on similarity to a known atlas of breast images [12]. We incorporated the mammographic and sonographic computerized mass classification methods into this workstation. Upon viewing an unknown case, the display shows both the computer classification output as well as images of lesions with known diagnoses (e.g., malignant vs. benign) and similar computer-extracted features. The similarity index used in the search can be selected by the radiologist and can be based on a single feature, multiple features, or on the computer estimate of the likelihood of malignancy. The output of a computer-aided diagnostic scheme can take a variety of forms such as the estimated likelihood that a lesion is malignant either in terms of probabilities or along a standardized rating scale. This information is then available for use by the radiologist when making decisions regarding patient management, as he or she sees fit.

2. PRELIMINARY EVALUATION OF WORKSTATION

In order to assess the potential usefulness of our intelligent workstation interface [12], we demonstrated the workstation at the 2000 and 2001 meetings of the Radiological Society of North America (RSNA) in Chicago, Illinois. The intelligent workstation used in these demonstrations displayed the estimate of the likelihood of malignancy and recalled lesions in the known database atlas based on the computer-estimate of the likelihood of malignancy. The similar lesions were displayed using a color-coding scheme that allowed for instant visual feedback to the radiologist regarding the malignancy of the atlas lesions, with red borders corresponding to malignant lesions and green borders corresponding to benign lesions.

The observer portion of the 2000 demonstration included 20 unknown mammographic cases and 20 unknown sonographic breast cases. The 2001 demonstration study included 20 unknown cases for which both mammograms and ultrasound images were available. Half of the cases were cancerous and the other were benign, with truth obtained from pathology reports. Each participant was asked if they interpreted mammograms or mammograms on a regular basis in their practice.

In the 2000 mammographic study, each participant was presented with a "4 on 1" image collage indicating the location of the lesion in the standard screening mammograms, areas of interest in which the lesions were centered in the standard CC (cranio-caudal) and MLO (medial-lateral-oblique) views and on any available special views. The observer was then asked to indicate his or her likelihood of malignancy on a 0 to 100 scale and his or her patient management decision (whether or not to send the patient to biopsy). Next the computer-determined likelihoods of malignancy was given for the CC and MLO views of the lesion and similar cases from the reference atlas were displayed using the green and red coding as described early. (Figure 1) The known atlas for the mammographic cases included 169 cases (373 images). The observer was then asked to again indicate his or her likelihood of malignancy on a 0 to 100 scale and his or her patient management decision (whether or not to send the woman to biopsy), with the choice of "no change" being available. Windowing and leveling of the images was available.

The 2000 sonographic study was similar to the mammographic one just described except that the participants were given two ultrasound images per case to use in their interpretation. The requested likelihood of malignancy and patient management decision were also asked before and after viewing of the computer aid prompts. The known atlas for the breast sonography cases included 271 cases (488 images).

In the 2001 study, each participant was presented with a more clinically-realistic display in which both the mammograms and the ultrasound images from the case in question were shown. These cases, which were unknown to both the computer and the participant, included the 4-on-1 whole breast mammograms, the regions of interest about the lesion in conventional and special mammographic views as well as the sonograms. The mammographic on-line atlas had 169 cases (373 images) and the sonographic on-line atlas had 438 cases (865 images). The participant was asked to give their BI-RADS recommendation before and after seeing the computer output on both the mammograms and the sonograms. (Figure 2)

As these were demonstration studies, the pathology (i.e., malignant or benign) was given after the second observer interpretation, that is, after presentation of the computer outputs. This method was employed to provide instant feedback in a learning situation and to encourage the RSNA participant to finish the study during the busy meeting.

3. RESULTS

The results in terms of sensitivity and specificity are tabulated below for both the single-modality studies from RSNA 2000 and the multi-modality study from RSNA 2001. All groups of participants for both modalities had equal or improved performance when using the intelligent workstation, although not all increases were statistically significant.

Modality	Participants	Number of Participants	Sensitivity without aid	Sensitivity with aid	p-value	Specificity without aid	Specificity with aid	p-value
Mammography	Radiologists - Mammo*	29	0.81	0.83	0.54	0.62	0.67	0.28
	Others**	13	0.79	0.85	0.34	0.55	0.74	0.0063
Ultrasound	Radiologists - Mammo*	22	0.85	0.85	0.95	0.61	0.63	0.66
	Others**	11	0.84	0.86	0.58	0.34	0.46	0.0058
Multimodality (mammo/US)	Radiologists - Mammo*	48	0.87	0.87	1	0.65	0.70	0.041
	Others**	48	0.66	0.78	0.0004	0.70	0.78	0.0024

* Radiologists who read mammograms as part of their practice.
** All other participants, e.g. other radiologists, medical physicists, technologists.
p-values from two-tail t-test

4. SUMMARY AND CONCLUSION

Results from our demonstration studies indicate that radiologists' performance, especially specificity, increases with the use of the aid. As these were demonstration studies in which feedback was given, one needs to be cautious in extracting definitive conclusions. We are therefore currently conducting a rigorous observer study to show the benefit of the intelligent search workstation.

The intelligent search workstation combines the benefit of computer-aided diagnosis with visual prior knowledge obtained from confirmed clinical cases. It is expected that the display of known lesions with similar features will aid the radiologist in his/her workup of a suspect lesion.

ACKNOWLEDGMENTS

This work was supported in parts by an USPHS grant CA89452 and a grant from the US Army Medical Research and Materiel Command (DAMD 97-2445). M. L. Giger, Z. Huo, R. M. Nishikawa and C. J. Vyborny are shareholders in R2 Technology, Inc. (Los Altos, CA). It is the policy of the University of Chicago that investigators disclose publicly actual or potential significant financial interests that may appear to be affected by the research activities.

REFERENCES

[1]   Bassett LW and Gold RH. *Breast Cancer Detection: Mammography and Other Methods in Breast Imaging*. New York, Grune & Stratton, 1987.

[2]   D'Orsi CJ and Kopans DB. Mammographic feature analysis. *Seminars in Roentgenology* 28:204-230, 1993.

[3]   D'Orsi CJ, Swets JA, Pickett RM, Seltzer SE and McNeil BJ. Reading and decision aids for improved accuracy and standardization of mammographic diagnosis. *Radiology* 184:619-622, 1992.

[4]   Sickles EA. Periodic mammographic follow-up of probably benign lesions: results in 3184 consecutive cases. *Radiology* 179:463-468., 1991

[5]   Kopans DB. *Breast Imaging*. Philadelphia, Lippincott, 1989.

[6]   McKenna RJ: The abnormal mammogram: radiographic findings, diagnostic options, pathology, and stage of cancer diagnosis. *Cancer* 74:244-255, 1994.

[7]   Huo Z, Giger ML, Vyborny CJ, Bick U, Lu P, Wolverton DE and Schmidt RA. Analysis of spiculation in the computerized classification of mammographic masses. *Med Phys* 22:1569-1579, 1995.

[8]   Huo Z, Giger ML, Vyborny CJ, Wolverton DE, Schmidt RA and Doi K. Automated computerized classification of malignant and benign masses on digitized mammograms. *Acad Radiol* 5:155-168, 1998.

[9]   Huo Z, Giger ML, Vyborny CJ, Wolverton DE, Metz CE: Computerized classifications of benign and malignant masses on digitized mammograms: A study of robustness, *Acad Radiol* 7:1077-1084, 2000.

[10].   Horsch K, Giger ML, Venta LA, Vyborny CJ: Automatic segmentation of breast lesions on ultrasound. *Medical Physics* 28: 1652-1659, 2001.

[11]   Horsch K, Giger ML, Venta LA, Vyborny CJ: Computerized diagnosis of breast lesions on ultrasound. *Medical Physics* 29: 157-164, 2002.

[12]   Giger ML, Huo Z, Lan L, Vyborny CJ: Intelligent search workstation for computer-aided diagnosis. *Proc. of Computer Assisted Radiology and Surgery (CARS'2000)*, pp. 822-827, 2000.

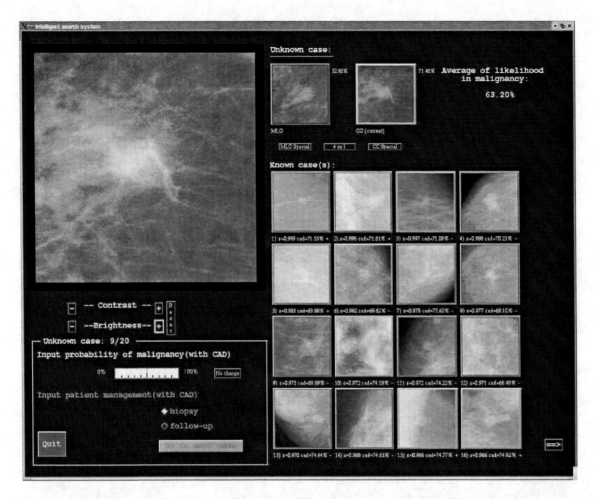

Figure 1. Workstation interface for a malignant case from RSNA 2000. For this malignant case, the computer-estimated likelihood of malignancy was 63%. Both malignant (in red outline but shown as black in the paper) and benign (in green outline but shown as white in the paper) similar images were retrieved automatically by the computer for use by the participant.

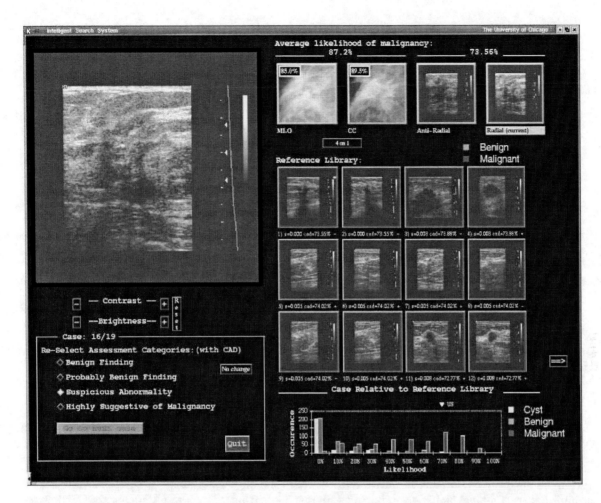

Figure 2. Workstation interface for a malignant case from RSNA 2001. For this malignant case, the computer output estimated an average likelihood of malignancy of 87% and 73% for the mammography and sonography images, respectively. Similar images automatically pulled from the on-line atlas were all malignant.

Image Reconstruction in SPECT with a Half Detector

Xiaochuan Pan, Emil Y. Sidky, and Yu Zou
Department of Radiology,
The University of Chicago, Chicago, IL 60637

Abstract

In parallel beam computed tomography, the measured projections at conjugate views are mathematically identical, and, consequently, this symmetry can be exploited for reducing either the scanning angle or the size of the detector arrays. However, in single-photon emission computed tomography (SPECT), because the gamma-rays in the conjugate views suffer different photon attenuation, the measured projections at conjugate views are generally different. Therefore, it had been widely considered that projections measured data over a full angular range of 360 degrees and over the whole detector face are generally required for exactly reconstructing the distributions of gamma-ray emitters. Recently, it has been revealed that exact image can be reconstructed from projections acquired with a full detector over disjoint angular intervals whose summation is 180 degree when the attenuation medium is uniform. In this work, we show that exact SPECT images can also be reconstructed from projections over 360 degrees, but acquired with a half detector viewing half of the image space. We present an heuristic perspective that supports this claim for SPECT with both uniform and non-uniform attenuation.

1 Introduction

In parallel-beam computed tomography (CT), the sinogram over 2π contains redundant information [1], because the projections from conjugate views are mathematically identical in the absence of noise. It is well known that such redundant information can be exploited for reducing scanning angle from 2π to π in parallel-beam CT. It is also clear that the same redundancy can be made use of to reconstruct the image from a half detector. Namely, as shown in Fig. 1, data from the whole 2π scanning angular range and on one side of the center of rotation are needed to reconstruct a unique image.

In SPECT, the projections from conjugate views generally differ from each other, because the effects of physical factors such as photon attenuation and blurring are distance dependent. Therefore, it is often supposed that accurate image reconstruction (and adequate compensation for the effects of these physical factors) in SPECT requires full knowledge of the data function over 2π radians and the full detector. In SPECT with only

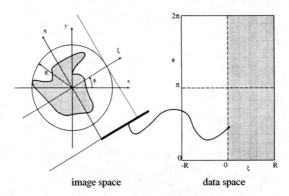

image space   data space

Figure 1: Schematic of scanning configuration. Shaded region is data space indicates data for a half-detector reconstruction.

Medical Imaging 2002: Image Processing, Milan Sonka, J. Michael Fitzpatrick,
Editors, Proceedings of SPIE Vol. 4684 (2002) © 2002 SPIE · 1605-7422/02/$15.00

uniform attenuation (and distance-dependent spatial resolution (DDSR) of certain forms), the data function over 2π and the full detector has been found to contain redundant information [2]. Such information has been exploited for controlling image noise properties [2]. However, only recently has such information been used to reduce the scanning angle [3, 4]. To the best of our knowledge, the connection between the redundant information in the ERT and reconstruction from the half-detector plane has not yet been made.

Recently, we developed a novel, heuristic perspective on redundant information in SPECT for the general case of non-uniform attenuation [5]. In the work reported here, we argue from this new perspective that reconstruction from data acquired from a half detector is sufficient to uniquely reconstruct the activity image for both the ERT case *and* non-uniform attenuation case. Numerical examples of half-detector image reconstructions, using an iterative algorithm, support our claim.

1.1   Half-Detector SPECT with Non-uniform Attenuation

When only the effect of photon attenuation is considered, the attenuated sinogram, $p_\mu(\xi, \phi)$, measured at a view angle ϕ can be written as

$$p_\mu(\xi, \phi) = \int d\eta \; a\left(\xi\hat{\theta}(\phi) + \eta\hat{\theta}^\perp(\phi)\right)$$

$$\times \exp\left[-\int_{D(\xi,\phi)}^{\eta} d\eta' \mu\left(\xi\hat{\theta}(\phi) + \eta'\hat{\theta}^\perp(\phi)\right)\right], \tag{1}$$

where $a(x, y)$ and $\mu(x, y)$ are the image function and the attenuation map, respectively; $(x, y) = (\xi\hat{\theta}(\phi) + \eta\hat{\theta}^\perp(\phi))$; $\hat{\theta}(\phi) = (\cos\phi, \sin\phi)$; $\hat{\theta}^\perp(\phi) = (-\sin\phi, \cos\phi)$; and $D(\xi, \phi)$ characterizes the boundary of the attenuation map. If $\mu(x, y)$ is known, one can readily obtain a modified sinogram [6]:

$$m(\xi, \phi) \;\equiv\; p_\mu(\xi, \phi) \exp\left[\int_{D(\xi,\phi)}^{0} d\eta' \mu\left(\xi\hat{\theta}(\phi) + \eta'\hat{\theta}^\perp(\phi)\right)\right]$$

$$= \int d\eta \; a\left(\xi\hat{\theta}(\phi) + \eta\hat{\theta}^\perp(\phi)\right)$$

$$\times \exp\left[-\int_{0}^{\eta} d\eta' \mu\left(\xi\hat{\theta}(\phi) + \eta'\hat{\theta}^\perp(\phi)\right)\right].$$

$$\tag{2}$$

In half detector SPECT, knowledge of $m(\xi, \phi)$ is available for $0 \leq \phi < 2\pi$ and $0 \leq \xi < \infty$. Below, using an heuristic perspective developed by us previously [5], we argue that the half detector scan contains the information to reconstruct a unique activity image. In the absence of attenuation, the modified sinogram becomes the Radon transform (RT) of the image function:

$$p(\xi, \phi) \;=\; \int d\eta \; a\left(\xi\hat{\theta}(\phi) + \eta\hat{\theta}^\perp(\phi)\right). \tag{3}$$

It is known that the RT is mathematically identical at conjugate views, i.e., $p(\xi, \phi) = p(-\xi, \phi + \pi)$. In SPECT, the presence of attenuation generally spoils this symmetry, i.e., $m(\xi, \phi) \neq m(-\xi, \phi + \pi)$.

For an image function with compact support, however, there is an exception. Points on the outermost edge of the modified sinogram *have* the conjugate view symmetry, i.e., $m(\xi_m, \phi_m) = m(-\xi_m, \phi_m + \pi)$, where (ξ_m, ϕ_m) is a point on the outermost edge in the data space. The reason for the symmetry at this point can be seen in Fig. 2. For any point on the edge of the disk there is a view angle, ϕ_m, for which that point appears at the edge of the modified sinogram. For example, in the figure, point B appears at the edge of the data space, $\xi_m = R$, for the view angle, $\phi_m = \phi_0$. For a point (ξ_m, ϕ_m) at the edge of the modified sinogram space, Eq. (2), simplifies considerably. As $(\xi, \phi) \to (\xi_m, \phi_m)$, η approaches zero, and the modified sinogram, $M(\xi_m, \phi_m)$ in Eq. (2), simplifies to the RT. The fact that the modified sinogram approaches the RT as ξ approaches R is independent of whether or not the attenuation is uniform! This observation leads to the so-called "potato

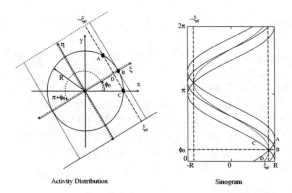

Activity Distribution   Sinogram

Figure 2: Schematic showing opposing views of the activity distribution. Points A, B, C and D in the activity region correspond to the sinusoidal curves with the same labels in the sinogram.

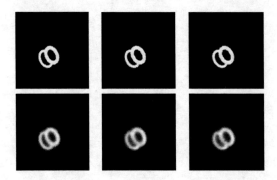

Figure 3: Top row: Reconstruction from a noiseless 2π ERT (left), reconstruction from a noiseless ERT using positive half of the detector (center), and reconstruction from a noiseless ERT using negative half of the detector (right). Bottom row: Same as top row except reconstructions are performed from noisy ERTS. Total number of counts in the data sets is about 1,000,000.

peeler" procedure described in more detail in Ref. [5]. It is clear from Figs. 1 and 2 that every point on the edge of the image support can be determined by the sinogram at $\xi = R$ or $\xi = -R$. Having determined the points on the edge of the support, it can be "peeled" away creating an image with a slightly smaller support. The same argument can be applied for determining the activity at the new edge of the activity image, and so on. The potato peeling stops once R is reduced to zero. Thus, in this way the whole image can be reconstructed from information on a half-detector plane.

2   Numerical Results

We demonstrate reconstruction from half-detector data with the cardiac phantom (the reconstructions are shown in Figs. 3 and 4). To perform the reconstruction, we use the expectation maximization method (EM) iterative approach. The EM algorithm has been shown to be able to invert an integral equation, such as Eq. (2), provided that there exists a unique solution. The potato peeling perspective presented in the previous section argues for the existence and uniqueness of an activity distribution a for sinogram data given on a half-detector plane. Thus, we expect the EM method to converge to the correct activity image from half-detector data. The numerical results on the cardiac phantom support this claim.

We performed simulation studies to investigate and evaluate the numerical and statistical properties of images obtained from projections acquired with a half of the conventional detector in SPECT with either uniform attenuation or non-uniform attenuation. We simulated noisy projections containing Poisson noise. To study the noise properties of the reconstructed images quantitatively, we generated a large number of noisy data sets.

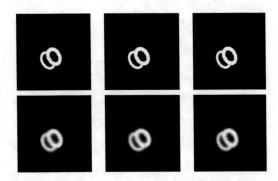

Figure 4: Same as Figure 1 except that the attenuation map is non-uniform.

The matrix size of the reconstructed images is 128x128 pixels. The local statistical properties were calculated empirically from the images reconstructed the simulated noisy data sets. Our simulation studies for uniform and non-uniform attenuation maps clearly show that measurements using only half the detector provide enough information to reconstruct the image.

We demonstrate image reconstruction from the exponential Radon transform (ERT) using data collected on a half detector in Fig. 3 and in general half-detector SPECT with non-uniform attenuation in Fig. 4. The images shown are comprised of 128x128 pixels reconstructed from data over 120 views, covering the full 2π range and 64 bins in the half-detector case or 128 bins in the full detector case. For the images with noisy data, Poisson noise was added to the sinogram prior to reconstruction, where the sinograms were normalized to 1,000,000 total counts. In both figures the images, going from left to right, represent reconstructions using the full, positive half, and negative half of the detector. The top row in both figures show reconstructions from noiseless data, and the bottom row gives results from noisy sinogram. All the images shown support the claim that information from either half of the detector is enough to provide an accurate image reconstruction even for the case of SPECT with non-uniform attenuation.

3   Conclusion

In this work, SPECT with a half detector is proposed. We developed the algorithm for image reconstruction from the data. Numerical results confirm that exact images can be obtained from data in SPECT with a half detector. The implication of this work is significant theoretically as well as practically. It suggests that redundant information exist in projections in SPECT with either uniform attenuation or non-uniform attenuation. Such redundant information can be used for reducing either the scanning angle or the detector size.

4   Acknowledgement

This work was supported in part by National Cancer Institute Grants CA70449 and CA85593. Its contents are solely the responsibility of the authors and do not necessarily represent the official views of the National Cancer Institute.

References

[1] F. Natterer. *The Radon Transform*. Wiley and Sons, New York, 1986.

[2] C. E. Metz and X. Pan. A unified analysis of exact methods of inverting the 2-D exponential Radon transform, with implications for noise control in SPECT. *IEEE Trans. Med. Imaging*, 14:643–658, 1995.

[3] F. Noo and J.-M. Wagner. Image reconstruction in 2D SPECT with 180-degree acquisition. *Inverse Problems*, 17:1357–1372, 2001.

[4] X. Pan, C.-M. Kao, and C. Metz. A family of pi-scheme exponential Radon transforms and the uniqueness of their inverses. *Inverse Problems*, (submitted), 2001.

[5] X. Pan, E. Y. Sidky, C.-M. Kao, Y. Zou, and C. Metz. Image reconstruction in pi-scheme short-scan SPECT with non-uniform attenuation. *IEEE Trans. Nucl. Sci.*, (submitted), 2001.

[6] O. J. Tretiak and C. E. Metz. The exponential Radon transform. *SIAM J. Appl. Math.*, 39:341–354, 1980.

CARDIAC STATE DRIVEN CT IMAGE RECONSTRUCTION ALGORITHM FOR CARDIAC IMAGING

Erdogan Cesmeli[1], Peter M. Edic[1], Maria Iatrou[1], Jiang Hsieh[2], Rajiv Gupta[1] and Armin H. Pfoh[1]

[1]GE Corporate Research and Development, Niskayuna, NY 12309
[2]GE Medical Systems, Milwaukee, WI 53201

ABSTRACT

Multi-slice CT scanners use EKG gating to predict the cardiac phase during slice reconstruction from projection data. Cardiac phase is generally defined with respect to the RR interval. The implicit assumption made is that the duration of events in a RR interval scales linearly when the heart rate changes. Using a more detailed EKG analysis, we evaluate the impact of relaxing this assumption on image quality. We developed a reconstruction algorithm that analyzes the associated EKG waveform to extract the natural cardiac states. A wavelet transform was used to decompose each RR-interval into P, QRS, and T waves. Subsequently, cardiac phase was defined with respect to these waves instead of a percentage or time delay from the beginning or the end of RR intervals. The projection data was then tagged with the cardiac phase and processed using temporal weights that are function of their cardiac phases. Finally, the tagged projection data were combined from multiple cardiac cycles using a multi-sector algorithm to reconstruct images. The new algorithm was applied to clinical data, collected on a 4-slice (GE LightSpeed Qx/i) and 8-slice CT scanner (GE LightSpeed Plus), with heart rates of 40 to 80 bpm. The quality of reconstruction is assessed by the visualization of the major arteries, e.g. RCA, LAD, LC in the reformat 3D images. Preliminary results indicate that Cardiac State Driven reconstruction algorithm offers better image quality than their RR-based counterparts.

Keywords: multi-slice computed tomography; cardiac imaging; multiphasic image reconstruction, adaptive sector selection

1. INTRODUCTION

The goal of the CT cardiac reconstruction algorithms is to obtain a 3D image of the heart at a given cardiac phase. However, the coverage of the entire heart is still not possible in a single gantry rotation with the current multi-slice detector technology. As a result, it is required that multiple cardiac cycles and gantry rotations be combined to reconstruct 3D volume. Since helical scan provides more axial coverage for a given breath-hold time, algorithms, in general, are based on a protocol employing a helical scan mode.

The first challenge of the cardiac reconstruction algorithms is common to all algorithms using helical scan data. In an ideal reconstruction space, projections lying on the plane of reconstruction are needed to form the image. In contrast, helical projections that are assumed to belong to the same plane cover a finite slice thickness due to the cone angle of the projections. As a result, the reconstruction at a desired z-location has to be created using z-interpolation with a compromise in the axial resolution.

In cardiac CT imaging, the additional challenge of the reconstruction process is due to the motion of the heart. To minimize the motion induced artifacts, clinical protocols include the acquisition of EKG during the scans to obtain cardiac phase information. During the rotations of the gantry, the heart continues its motion and makes a limited set of projections available for a given cardiac phase. In an ideal CT system, where the entire 3D volume of the heart could be scanned instantaneously relative to length of the cardiac period, the cardiac imaging would not be different from that of a stationary body part. In reality, however, projections cannot be acquired instantaneously, compelling algorithms to combine projections belonging to different cardiac phases using temporal interpolation.

Existent algorithms assume that cardiac phases occur at a fixed delay with respect to the preceding or the succeeding R peak of any RR interval regardless of the heart rate. However, cardiac physiology suggests that the diastole phase get longer with decreased heart rate while the systole almost stays the same [1]. Motivated by this observation, we propose a novel algorithm, namely, the Cardiac State Driven Algorithm, which tracks cardiac phases using the characteristic waves of the EKG. The purpose of this paper is to describe the Cardiac State Driven Algorithm and how it generates 3D cardiac volume by reconstructing a set of 2D axial images of the heart for a given cardiac phase. It assumes helical scan data, however, the principles of the algorithm are general enough to make it applicable to cine scan data. The proposed algorithm distinguishes itself from others in the selection of projections and their temporal interpolation.

2. PROJECTION DOMAIN

2.1 Spatial Domain

Projections can be visualized in z-t domain as shown in Figure 1, where a horizontal group of four rectangles represents the z-locations of four rows of detectors, or equivalently those of their projections, across time. Starting from the beginning of the scan, projections in each detector row have linearly increasing z-heights, resulting in slanted trajectories. In contrast, if the projections were from a cine scan mode, rectangles would line up vertically. One of the goals in the helical reconstruction algorithms is to form a vertical line in z-t domain by interpolation.

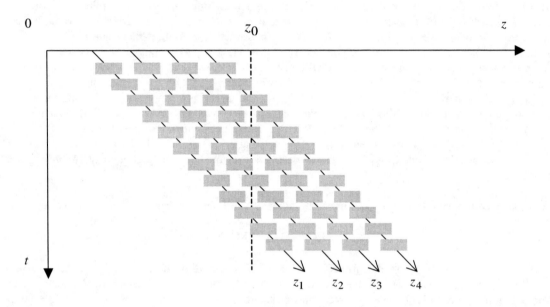

Figure 1. Interpolation in z takes place across multiple rows of detectors, namely slices. For a particular location, z_0, different rows, shown as filled rectangles, provide the z-coverage at different time intervals. Dark rectangles indicate the rows and the instances at which their projections contribute to the interpolation.

2.2 Temporal domain

The behavior of projections in $6 - \phi$ [1] is shown in Figure 2. In the representation, for simplicity, it was assumed that $T_g \leq T_c$ where T_g and T_c are the periods of gantry and a cardiac cycle, respectively. In the figure where one common trajectory for all rows is shown for simplicity, projections form linear trajectories covering different $6 - \phi$ combinations. The trajectory of the projections starts from the origin at the upper-left corner and proceeds towards right. Each time the trajectory reaches the end of the cardiac cycle, $\phi = T_c$, it wraps back to $\phi = 0.0$ horizontally (6 is continuous). Similarly, when the trajectory reaches $6 = 360°$, it wraps back to $6 = 0°$ vertically. Here, for the simplicity of the illustration, the heart rate is assumed to be constant and as a result, the trajectories in the phase domain all have the same slope.

1. _____

[1] Note that ϕ is equivalent to time, t; here, a different symbol is used to emphasize the periodicity of the heart motion.

Each line segment is labeled with a subscripted number, i_j, where i and j are the cardiac cycle and gantry rotations of the projections forming that line segment. For instance, 1_2 shows that the corresponding line segment is the set of projections belonging to the first cardiac cycle that are acquired during the second rotation of the gantry.

The difference between the projections of a beating heart and those of a stationary body part can also be visualized using the representation in Figure 2. In the former, lines are slanted because projections for different angles are acquired at different cardiac phases. In the latter, however, the segments would be vertical, like the vertical dashed line at ϕ_0, since projections would not have distinguishable phases. In the dynamic case, however, only a pseudo vertical line can be obtained, usually by combining projections from different cardiac phases. This process entails a temporal interpolation method, which inherently tends to introduce errors. A specific goal of the cardiac reconstruction algorithms is to minimize the temporal interpolation errors.

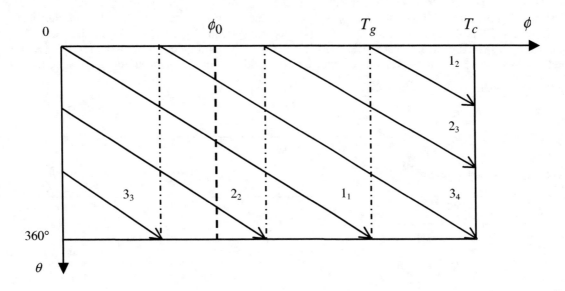

Figure 2. The trajectories of the projections in $\theta - \phi$ are composed on slanted line segments.

3. METHOD

There are four major steps in the Cardiac State Driven Algorithm. First, the projections are tagged with z-location and phase information using EKG data. Next, projections are interpolated in z to obtain pseudo-cine projections for a given z-height. In order to reconstruct the image of the heart at a desired cardiac phase ϕ, a set of z-interpolated projections is selected based on a temporal distance objective function. Finally, selected projections are combined using temporal interpolation and an axial image is obtained using a reconstruction angle of $\Theta_r < 360°$. The last three steps are repeated for different z-heights to cover the entire heart.

3.1 Tagging projections with phase and z information

The projections in the scan data do not have their phase information available explicitly. As a result, a simultaneously collected EKG waveform is used to extract this information. Thus, the goal of the first step is to tag each projection, $P_{ijk}(\theta)$, with a cardiac phase, $\Phi_{ijk}(\theta)$, extracted from the EKG data and z-location information, $Z_{ijk}(\theta)$, calculated based on the speeds of the gantry and the table.

The goal of the phase tagging step is to enable the temporal interpolation process to combine the projections belonging to approximately the same desired phase after relative weighting. The step starts with processing EKG signal by a dyadic quadratic spline wavelet transformation [2]. The wavelet transformation generates a filtered output, W_λ, for different scales, $\lambda = 1 \ldots \Omega$. In our analysis, we found $\lambda = 6$ as the characteristic scale to do the analysis. In order to determine the peaks in the original EKG signal, zero crossings in W_λ are detected. First, the most prominent peaks in W_λ are detected by finding modulus maximum line. A modulus maximum at a zero crossing is the product of the minimum and the maximum values that sandwich the zero crossing. After finding the global maximum of the moduli, a threshold set to 40% of the global maximum is selected for the detection of R-peaks. Temporal locations with moduli larger than the threshold are included in the R-peak candidate list. To avoid false positives, maximum moduli from consecutive R-peaks are compared. When the difference was larger than the global average maximum modulus, R-peak with the smaller value is deleted from the list. Remaining list members are identified as the R-peaks.

Next, preceding each R-peak a search window for P-peaks is considered. The size of the window is set adaptively to 50% of the RR interval containing the target P-peak. The location with the largest maximum modulus in this window is identified as the P-peak. Similarly, T-peak is determined in a window succeeding each R-peak. The size of this window, too, is set according to the corresponding RR interval (25%). Finally, the first maximum modulus locations just before and after each R-peak are taken as Q- and S-peaks, respectively. A typical result similar to the one shown in Figure 3 is produced.

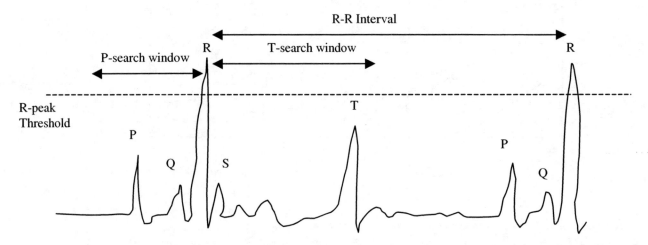

Figure 3. Characteristic points of EKG signal are identified using a dyadic quadratic spline wavelet transformation.

Having identified the characteristic points, a piecewise linear phase map between two consecutive R-peaks is defined where the phase is increased from 0.0 to 1.0 as time traces the interval from the first R-peak to the second (Fig. 4). By mapping these phases to the temporal locations of the projections, each projection is assigned with a cardiac phase, $\Phi_{ijk}(\theta)$ where i, j, and k correspond to cardiac cycle, gantry rotation, and detector row, respectively. Repeating this procedure for all consecutive R-peak pairs, all views in the scan data are marked with their associated cardiac phases, $\Phi_{ijk}(\theta)$.

Like phase information, the z-locations of projections are not available in the scan data but can be calculated from the gantry and the table motions. Knowing the starting z-location of the detector rows, the gantry period, and the table speed, z-locations, $Z_{ijk}(\theta)$, of all projections, $P_{ijk}(\theta)$, are determined and recorded.

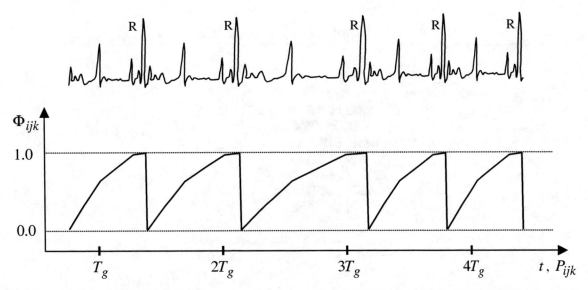

Figure 4. Projections are tagged with phase information, based on the characteristic peaks of EKG signal. Phase is assumed to be piecewise linear between two consecutive R-peaks, which are assigned the phases of 1.0.

3.2 Z- interpolation

Recall that if the projections were from a cine scan mode, rectangles in Figure 1 would line up vertically. The goal in the first step of the algorithm is to obtain pseudo cine projections, namely a vertical line at z_0 in Figure 1, from helical projections.

The Cardiac State Driven Algorithm utilizes the advantage of having multi-slice data to achieve this goal. It combines the projections from different detector rows using interpolation. According to the detector geometry, rows pass through z_0 as the table moves forward and hence, provide projections whose z-locations, Z_{ijk}, are in the neighborhood of z_0. In Figure 5, rows contributing to the interpolation are colored darker than the others are. As depicted in the figure, for any horizontal group of four rows, there are at most two rows that are included in the interpolation. For certain instances, only one row contributes to the interpolation, as indicated by a single dark colored rectangle in a horizontal group of four rectangles. A pseudo cine projection at z_0, $P_{ij}(\theta, z_0)$, can be obtained from the helical projections $P_{ijk}(\theta)$ where i, j, and k correspond to cardiac cycle, gantry rotation, and detector row, respectively:

$$P_{ij}(\theta, z_0) = \sum_{\substack{k \in \{1,2,3,4\} \\ ijk \ni |Z_{ijk}(\theta) - z_0| \leq d_z}} \omega_k(z_0) \cdot P_{ijk}(\theta) \tag{1a}$$

$$\omega_k(z_0) = |Z_{ijk}(\theta) - z_0| / d_z \tag{1b}$$

where $Z_{ijk}(\theta)$ is the z-location of projection $P_{ijk}(\theta)$ and d_z is the collimation, namely, the inter-row distance. Note that the phase of the projection $P_{ij}(\theta)$, $\Phi_{ij}(\theta)$, is the same as that of $P_{ijk}(\theta)$'s, $\Phi_{ijk}(\theta) = \Phi_{ij}(\theta)$, since it is obtained using the projections collected at the same time instance.

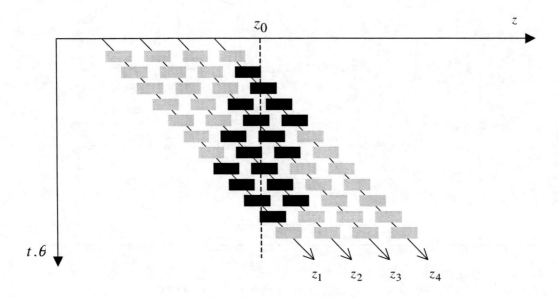

Figure 5. Interpolation in z takes place across multiple rows of detectors, namely slices. For a particular location, z_0, different rows, shown as filled rectangles, provide the z-coverage at different time intervals. Dark rectangles indicate the rows and the instances at which their projections contribute to the interpolation.

3.3 Determination of θ_s and θ_e

Imagine an ideal CT machine that can instantaneously obtain the set of projections necessary for a reconstruction. Acquired projections would have had exactly the same phase, eliminating the necessity to perform an interpolation in phase. Since this is not the case in reality, the Cardiac State Driven Algorithm has to combine projections having different phases to form a set of projections of a common phase, ϕ, as if they were obtained from an ideal CT machine. Hence, the goal of this step of the algorithm is to form this set from projections with phases in the neighborhood of the reconstruction phase ϕ.

As seen in Figures 2 and 5, at different projection angles, θ, $P_{ij}(\theta)$'s have different cardiac phases, $\Phi_{ij}(\theta)$. When $T_g \neq T_c$, for the same angle, θ, $P_{ij}(\theta)$'s from different gantry rotations have different phases. In forming the reconstruction set, the Cardiac State Driven Algorithm assumes that the heart motion is stationary and thus, combines $P_{ij}(\theta)$'s from cardiac cycles to obtain an interpolated projection at ϕ. This assumption is consistent with the one stated in [3].

When the reconstruction is limited to use $\theta_r < 360°$, only a subset of projection angles is needed for reconstruction. This implies that the algorithm has the flexibility to avoid certain projection angles, at which the projections have phases that are not close to the reconstruction phase, ϕ. Exploiting this fact, the Cardiac State Driven Algorithm selects an angular range defined by a starting and an ending angle, θ_s and θ_e, such that the $P_{ij}(\theta)$'s in the selected range have the minimum total temporal distance to ϕ. Let us define the total phase (temporal) distance for projections whose projection angles are between θ_1 and θ_2 as:

$$D(\theta_1, \theta_2, \phi) = \sum_{\theta \in [\theta_1, \theta_2]} d(\theta, \phi) \qquad (2a)$$

$$d(\theta, \phi) = \mathop{\arg\min}_{i,j} \left| \Phi_{ij}(\theta) - \phi \right| \qquad (2b)$$

Here, $\Phi_{ij}(\theta)$ is the cardiac phase of projection $P_{ij}(\theta)$. Equation (2b) finds the minimum temporal distance achieved for the angle θ by searching projections from multiple cardiac gantry rotations/cardiac cycles for the same angle. Equation (2a) simply adds up these temporal distances for the angles in the angular range defined by $[\theta_1, \theta_2]^2$.

The algorithm calculates $D(\theta_1, \theta_2, \phi)$ for all possible $[\theta_1, \theta_2]$ where the reconstruction angle is $\Theta_r = |\theta_2 - \theta_1|$. By selecting θ_s and θ_e such that $D(\theta_s, \theta_e, \phi)$ is the minimum, the Cardiac State Driven Algorithm assures that the included $P_{ij}(\theta)$'s forms a projection set whose members are the closest to ϕ in the temporal space. It is important to note that the Cardiac State Driven Algorithm is not limited by the particular distance function implemented in (2). Its flexibility lies in its generality allowing other forms of functions used in the selection of projections for reconstruction and its capability to capture other multi-sector algorithms within the same framework.

3.4 Temporal interpolation

The goal of the temporal interpolation is to obtain a set of interpolated projections that forms a vertical line at ϕ (Fig. 5). Let $P_{ij}(\theta)$ represent the z-interpolated projection from i^{th} cardiac cycle and j^{th} gantry rotation corresponding to angle θ. The temporally interpolated projection at phase ϕ, $P_\phi(\theta)$, can be expressed as:

$$P_\phi(\theta) = \sum_{ij} w_{ij}(\theta, \phi) \cdot P_{ij}(\theta) \qquad (3)$$

Here, $\theta \in [\theta_s, \theta_e]$, $\Theta_r = |\theta_e - \theta_s|$, and $w_{ij}(\theta)$ is the associated interpolation weight.

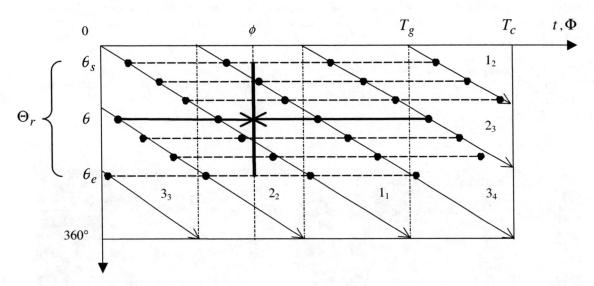

Figure 6. Forming the temporally interpolated projections from z-interpolated projections. Each horizontal dashed line represents one such interpolation.

In Figure 6, the temporal interpolations for projection angles θ are shown as horizontal dashed line segments. Black dots along these lines correspond to the z-interpolated projections obtained in equation (1). For angle θ, two converging arrows are drawn to show the resulting position of the temporally interpolated projections. Temporally interpolated projections form a reconstruction set indicated as a solid vertical line segment at ϕ.

The idea of combining projections from multiple cardiac cycles, which is the backbone of all multi-sector algorithms, heavily relies on the assumption that the heart motion is stationary in consecutive cardiac cycles. However, it is believed this

1. ───────────────────────────

[2] Note that, in general θ_2 could also be less than θ_1 whereby $[\theta_1, \theta_2] = [\theta_1, 2\pi] \cup [0, \theta_2]$.

assumption is more likely to be valid when the set of cardiac cycles used in (3) are close in time. This condition implies that the interpolation of projections should include a minimum number of temporally close cardiac cycles. One way of satisfying this condition is to have interpolation weights as a fast decaying function of temporal distances. In current implementation, the Cardiac State Driven Algorithm employs:

$$w_{ij}(\theta,\phi) = \frac{w'_{ij}(\theta,\phi)}{\sum w'_{ij}(\theta,\phi)} \text{ where } w'_{ij}(\theta,\phi) = (\Phi_{ij}(\theta) - \phi)^{-p} \tag{4}$$

Here $p = 2$ to achieve a fast decay. Note that other possibilities include assigning non-zero weights to either a single projection whose phase is the closest to ϕ (nearest neighborhood) or to a pair of projections whose phases sandwich ϕ.

A unique feature of the Cardiac State Algorithm is that depending on the heart rate it varies the number of sectors it includes in the reconstruction. This feature is a data driven process unlike some other algorithms where the number of sectors is provided externally by an expert user. The Cardiac State Algorithm, however, adapts to the heart rate changes. It selects more sectors when the heart rate increases and fewer sectors when the rate decreases.

4. RESULTS

In order to test the performance of the algorithm, we applied it to clinical studies collected on a 4-slice (GE LightSpeed Qx/i) and 8-slice CT scanners (GE LightSpeed Plus), where the mean patient heart rates were between 40 to 80 bpm. The quality of reconstructions was assessed by the visualization of the major arteries, e.g. RCA, LAD, LC in the reformat 3D images.

In the first study where the subject had a mean heart rate 80 bpm (Fig. 7), we also applied a generic multisector algorithm to scan data collected using GE LightSpeed Qx/i, a 4-slice CT scanner. As compared to the multi-sector algorithm, the Cardiac State Driven Algorithm provides smoother edges along the surface of the heart and its inner structures such as its chambers, an important image quality feature for the clinical cardiac functional evaluations. The Cardiac State Algorithm utilized 3-4 sectors in this study.

In another study with a mean heart rate of 44 bpm, the scan data was collected using 8-slice CT scanner, GE LightSpeed Plus. The Cardiac State Algorithm generated images by utilizing 1-2 sectors (Fig. 8). Both RCA and left coronary arteries were reconstructed quite successfully as shown in Figures 8-9. Curved reformat images in Figure 9 attest to the performance of the algorithm, which provided contiguous arteries along the surface of the heart.

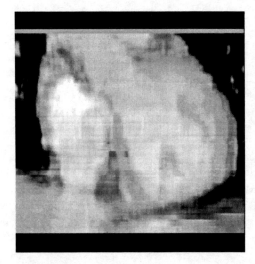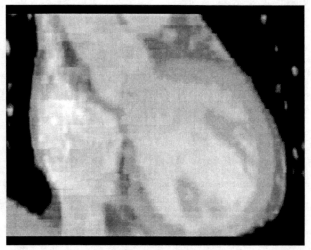

Figure 7. Coronal views from the reconstruction of an in-vivo beating heart. The images are obtained using the generic multisector (left) and Cardiac State Driven (right) algorithms. Note that the cardiac surface near the right edge of the view and those of the neighboring chambers are smoother and continuous with the Cardiac State Driven Algorithm.

In a study where the heart rate variation was the main challenge (mean: 70 bpm std: 6.5 bpm), 3D volume of the heart is reconstructed using three different approaches including a generic multisector and a half-scan, and the Cardiac State algorithms (Fig. 10). As the figure suggests, the Cardiac State Algorithm performs at least as well as the half scan reconstruction does and quite better than the multisector counterpart does. The Cardiac State achieves this by adaptively selecting sectors, which is mostly one in this study, as opposed the preset selection in the other two algorithms.

5. CONCLUSIONS

We have proposed a novel reconstruction method, namely the Cardiac State Driven Algorithm, for cardiac CT imaging. It provides a flexible way of combining projections from multiple cardiac cycles with an objective function optimizing the temporal interpolation. We observed that the Cardiac State Driven Algorithm offers improved results with clinical studies.

As part of our future studies, we are planning to include additional classes of heart rate variations and a complete set of phases covering the entire cardiac cycle in our analysis.

ACKNOWLEDGMENT

Authors would like to thank Harvey E. Cline for his valuable discussions and his help in the preparation of the visualization of clinical results.

REFERENCES:

1. R. M. Berne and M. N. Levy, *Physiology*, Mosby Year Book: St. Louis, MI, 1993.
2. C. Li, C. Zheng, and C. Tai, "Detection of ECG Characteristic Points Using Wavelet Transforms," IEEE Trans. Biomed. Eng., vol. 42(1):21-28, Jan. 1995.
3. G. C. Mc Kinnon and R. H. T. Bates, "Towards imaging the bating heart usefully with a conventional CT scanner," *IEEE Trans. Biomed. Eng.*, vol. 28 (2), pp. 123-127, 1981.

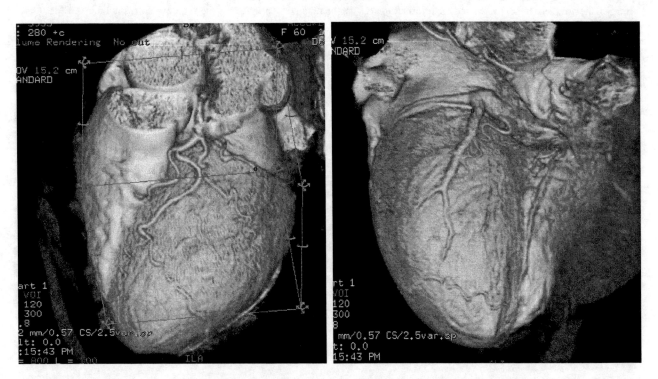

Figure 8. The Cardiac State Algorithm reconstructs the stack of images to cover the entire 3D volume of the heart by adaptively changing the number of sectors utilized. As shown in the front and the back views of the heart, the right and left coronary arteries are reconstructed contiguously.

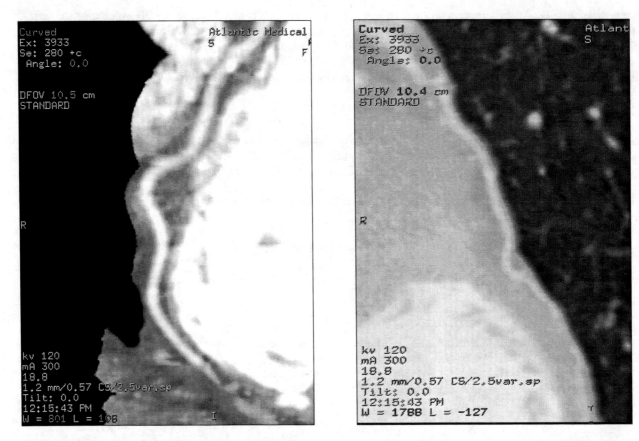

Figure 9. The curved reformat images of the right and the left coronary arteries are shown. By dropping seed points in the axial images, the arteries can be tracked and the reformat images can be obtained using Advantage Window Workstation by GEMS.

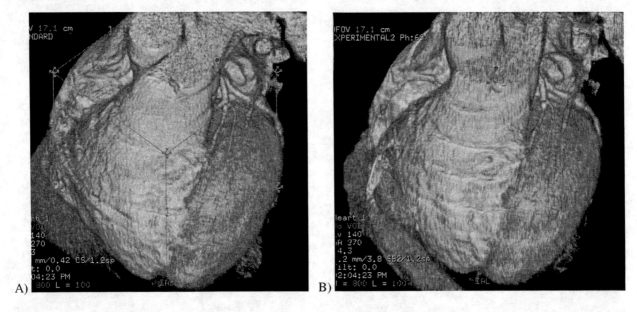

Figure 10. (Continued)

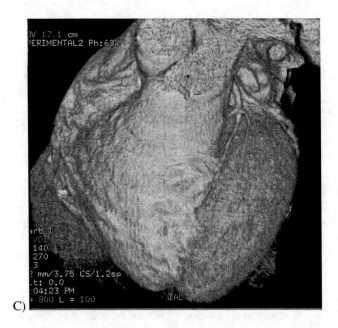

C)

Figure 10. A study with a heart rate variation. Results from A) Cardiac State, b) A Generic Multisector, and C) Half-scan Reconstruction Algorithms. The Cardiac State Algorithm performs better since it can adaptively select number of sectors depending on the data availability.

Noise Properties of the Inverse π-Scheme Exponential Radon Transform

Emil Y. Sidky, Chien-Min Kao, Patrick J. LaRiviere,
and Xiaochuan Pan
Department of Radiology,
The University of Chicago, Chicago, IL 60637

Abstract

Because the effects of physical factors such as photon attenuation and spatial resolution are distance-dependent in single-photon emission computed tomography (SPECT), it has been widely assumed that accurate image reconstruction requires knowledge of the data function over 2π. In SPECT with uniform attenuation, Noo and Wagner recently showed that an accurate image can be reconstructed from knowledge of the data function over a contiguous π-segment. More generally, we proposed π-scheme SPECT that entails data acquisition over disjoint angular intervals without conjugate views, totalling to π radians, thereby allowing flexibility in choosing projection views at which the emitted gamma-rays may undergo the least attenuation and blurring. In this work, we study the general properties of the π-scheme inverse exponential Radon Transform, and discuss how to take advantage of the π-scheme flexibility to improve noise properties of short-scan SPECT.

1 Introduction

In parallel-beam computed tomography (CT), the sinogram over 2π contains redundant information, because the projections from conjugate views are mathematically identical in the absence of noise. It is well known that such redundant information can be exploited to reduce the scanning angle from 2π to π. It was also observed previously that, in some other tomographic imaging modalities such as fan-beam CT [1] and diffraction tomography (DT) [2], the data functions over 2π contain redundant information and that this redundancy can be used to reduce the scanning angles in these imaging systems [3].

In SPECT with uniform attenuation, the projection data can be transformed into a modified sinogram which is the exponential Radon transform (ERT) of the activity distribution:

$$m(\xi, \phi) = \int_{-\infty}^{\infty} f(\xi\hat{\theta}(\phi) + \eta\hat{\theta}^{\perp}(\phi))e^{-\mu_0\eta}d\eta, \tag{1}$$

where f is the activity image function; μ_0 is the constant linear attenuation coefficient; ξ and η are detector frame coordinates; ξ measures distance along the detector and η indicates distance away from the detector. The projections from conjugate views generally differ from each other, $m(\xi, \phi) \neq m(-\xi, \phi + \pi)$, because the effects of physical factors such as photon attenuation and blurring are distance dependent. Therefore, it has often been assumed that accurate image reconstruction (and adequate compensation for the effects of these physical factors) in SPECT requires full knowledge of the data function over 2π.

In SPECT with only uniform attenuation, the data function over 2π has been found to contain redundant information [4]. Such information has been exploited for controlling image noise properties [4]. However, it remained unclear whether such information can be used to reduce the scanning angle until recent work by Noo and Wagner [5] demonstrated that the redundant information inherent in the data function in uniform-attenuation SPECT can be employed to reduce the scanning angle from 2π to π.

In the work reported here, we discuss so-called π-scheme SPECT [6] and investigate the problem of accurate image reconstruction in this context. As shown in Fig. 1, the full angular range $[0, 2\pi)$ is divided into $4n + 2$

Medical Imaging 2002: Image Processing, Milan Sonka, J. Michael Fitzpatrick,
Editors, Proceedings of SPIE Vol. 4684 (2002) © 2002 SPIE · 1605-7422/02/$15.00

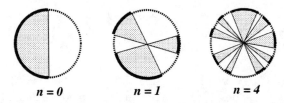

Figure 1: π-scheme scanning configurations. Data are acquired in the intervals indicated by the shaded areas.

angular intervals, where n is a non-negative integer, and the data in the π-scheme SPECT are acquired only over disjoint angular intervals whose summation without conjugate views is larger than or equal to π. For example, with $n = 1$, as displayed in Fig. 1, the full angular range 2π is divided into six angular intervals, and the data are acquired over the shaded angular intervals depicted with solid curves. Obviously, the short-scan SPECT described above in which the data are acquired at scanning angles from 0 to π can be interpreted as a special ($n = 0$) case of the π-scheme SPECT, i.e., the situation in which the 2π angular interval is divided evenly into two regions, and the data are acquired only over one of the two regions. In this article, we present two principal results about the properties of the inverse π-scheme ERT: (1) from a general, image-independent analysis we show that the noise properties of the inverse π-scheme ERT approach that of the full-scan ERT in the limit of an infinite number of scanning segments and (2) from a practical, image-dependent point of view we demonstrate by example that the π-scheme ERT allows the flexibility to choose angular views with the highest integrated intensity, which provides the short-scan with the lowest global image variance.

2 π-Scheme ERT

Using a method similar to that developed by Noo and Wagner [5], we have shown analytically [6] that accurate images can be reconstructed from data in π-scheme SPECT with uniform attenuation. In the π-scheme ERT the activity distribution satisfies the following Fredholm integral equation:

$$f(x,y) = \chi(x,y)H^{(n)}(x,y) + \chi(x,y)K^{(n)} \otimes f(x,y), \qquad (2)$$

where

$$K^{(n)} = \sum_{i=0}^{2n} h_i,$$

where χ is the characteristic function enforcing the compact support of the image f. The first term on the right-hand side is a sum of Tretiak-Metz (TM) reconstructions

$$H^{(n)} = \sum_{i=0}^{2n} TM\left[\phi_{2i}, \phi_{2i+1}\right] \qquad (3)$$

with,

$$TM\left[\phi_1, \phi_2\right] = \int_{\phi_1}^{\phi_2} d\phi\, e^{\mu_0\, \vec{r}\cdot\hat{\theta}^\perp(\phi)} \int_{\mu_0 \le |\nu_m|} d\nu_m |\nu_m| e^{j2\pi\nu_m\, \vec{r}\cdot\hat{\theta}(\phi)} M(\nu_m, \phi).$$

The second term (the convolution term) involves a convolution of the activity distribution with the sum $K^{(n)}$ over h_i. $M(\nu_m, \phi)$ is the one dimensional Fourier Transform of the ERT, $m(\xi, \phi)$, of f. The function h_i is simply the function h_0 rotated in the xy-plane by the angle ϕ_{2i}, and the expression for h_0, which we will study in greater detail, is:

$$h_0(x,y) = j\nu_0 \int_{-1}^{1} dp\, e^{\mu_0 py} \int_{|\nu_m| \ge \nu_0 |p|} d\nu_m sign(\nu_m) e^{j2\pi x\nu_m}, \qquad (4)$$

where the frequency ν_0 is $\mu_0/(2\pi)$. The sequence of angles ϕ_{2i} specify the angular intervals of the π-scheme, where data is available on the intervals:

$$[\phi_{2i}, \phi_{2i+1}), \quad i = 0, 1, 2, \ldots, 2n + 1, \tag{5}$$

where n characterizes the number of non-overlapping angular intervals. The $n = 0$ case is the short-scan ERT of Noo and Wagner [5]. The noise properties of the TM term are already well understood; thus we focus on characterizing the convolution term.

2.1 Convolution Term

The integrals in Eq. (4) can be carried out analytically:

$$
\begin{aligned}
h_0(x, y) &= \frac{\sinh \mu_0 y}{\pi y} g(x) \\
&+ \frac{\nu_0}{\pi x} \left[\frac{2 \sinh \mu_0 y}{\mu_0 y} - \frac{\sinh \mu_0 (y + ix)}{\mu_0 (y + ix)} - \frac{\sinh \mu_0 (y - ix)}{\mu_0 (y - ix)} \right],
\end{aligned} \tag{6}
$$

where

$$g(x) = \frac{1}{\pi x} = \int_{-\infty}^{\infty} dp \; i \, \text{sign}(p) \, e^{i 2 \pi x p}. \tag{7}$$

From Eq. (6) a few properties are evident: h_0 is real since the last two terms are the sum of complex conjugates; $h_0(x, y) = h_0(-x, y)$; $h_0(x, y) = -h_0(x, -y)$; and $h_0(x, y) = -h_0(-x, -y)$. All other $h_i's$ are also odd functions, because h_i is simply a rotation of the h_0 by the angle ϕ_{2i}. As a result the convolver $K^{(n)}$ is always an odd function, which, like the derivative operator, tends to amplify noise. Moreover, the first term in Eq. (6) is singular because of the function $g(x)$. In practice, this singularity can be controlled by redefining $g(x)$ through its Fourier Transform in Eq. (7) setting the frequency limits to the Nyquist frequency of the image [5].

2.2 Limit as $n \to \infty$

The π-scheme ERT allows the flexibility to scan over a homogeneously distributed set of angular segments that total to π, which intuitively should improve the noise properties of the inverse short-scan ERT. We show here that indeed the importance of the convolution term is reduced in the limit that $n \to \infty$ for equal size intervals. We write h_0 in polar form, since the other $h_i's$ are simply $h_i^{(\text{pol})}(r, \phi) = h_0^{(\text{pol})}(r, \phi + \phi_{2i})$. We rearrange the sum in Eq. (2):

$$
\begin{aligned}
K^{(n)} = \sum_{i=0}^{2n} h_i &= \sum_{i=0}^{2n} h_0^{\text{pol}}(r, \phi + \phi_{2i}) \\
&= \sum_{i=0}^{n-1} h_0^{\text{pol}}(r, \phi + \phi_{2i}) - h_0^{\text{pol}}(r, \phi + \phi_{2i+1}) + \\
&\quad h_0^{\text{pol}}(r, \phi + \phi_{2n}).
\end{aligned} \tag{8}
$$

In the first line of Eq. (8), the sum over $h's$ is performed at the angles corresponding to the beginning of all the angular segments of the π-scheme; hence the $2i$ index on the angular interval. In the second line of Eq (8), we use the fact that shifting the angular index in the π-scheme sequence by $2n + 1$ shifts the angle itself by π; the minus sign comes about because h is an odd function. In words, a particular angle at the beginning of an angular segment necessarily corresponds to the end of an angular segment at π plus the same angle; such an arrangement of the angular segments prevents the inclusion of conjugate rays.

Consider the case that a number of equally spaced angles are placed between ϕ_a and ϕ_b, where both angles coincide with even numbered angles in the sum over h_i:

$$K_{ab}^{(\text{lim})} = \lim_{M \to \infty} \sum_{j=1}^{M/2} \left[h_0^{(\text{pol})}(r, \phi + \phi_a + 2\phi') - h_0^{(\text{pol})}(r, \phi + \phi_a + 2\phi' + \Delta) \right]$$

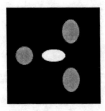

Figure 2: White, central ellipse represents the activity image, which is taken to be constant inside the ellipse. Gray ellipses represent the attenuation map, where the attenuation in those regions is 0.15 cm^{-1}.

$$
\begin{aligned}
\phi' &= (j-1)\Delta \\
\Delta &= (\phi_b - \phi_a)/M.
\end{aligned}
$$

Rearranging $K_{ab}^{(\text{lim})}$ yields:

$$
K_{ab}^{(\text{lim})} = -\frac{1}{2} \lim_{M \to \infty} \sum_{j=1}^{M/2} \frac{h_0^{(\text{pol})}(r, \phi + \phi_a + 2\phi' + \Delta) - h_0^{(\text{pol})}(r, \phi + \phi_a + 2\phi')}{\Delta} 2\Delta
$$

Taking the limit, one has:

$$
\begin{aligned}
K_{ab}^{\text{lim}} &= -\frac{1}{2} \int_{\phi_a}^{\phi_b} \frac{dh_0^{\text{pol}}(r, \phi + x)}{dx} dx \\
&= -\frac{1}{2} \left[h_0^{\text{pol}}(r, \phi + \phi_b) - h_0^{\text{pol}}(r, \phi + \phi_a) \right].
\end{aligned} \tag{9}
$$

From Eq. (9) evaluating various limiting cases is straightforward.

We are specifically interested in the case with N equally spaced angular intervals of size ϵ and $N \to \infty$; $\epsilon = \pi/N$. Since Eq. (9) only applies to even numbers of intervals the sum over h_i is written as follows:

$$
\begin{aligned}
K_\epsilon^{\text{lin}} &= K_{0,\pi-2\epsilon}^{\text{lim}} + h_0^{\text{pol}}(r, \phi + \pi - \epsilon) \\
&= -\frac{1}{2} \left[h_0^{\text{pol}}(r, \phi + \pi - 2\epsilon) - h_0^{\text{pol}}(r, \phi) \right] + h_0^{\text{pol}}(r, \phi + \pi - \epsilon) \\
&= \frac{1}{2} h_0^{\text{pol}}(r, \phi) + \frac{1}{2} h_0^{\text{pol}}(r, \phi + 2\epsilon) - h_0^{\text{pol}}(r, \phi + \epsilon) \\
&\to 0.
\end{aligned} \tag{10}
$$

Thus, the convolution term tends to cancel out as n gets large for equally spaced intervals.

3 Using the π-Scheme to Choose Maximum Intensity Views

From a practical point of view the primary advantage of the π-scheme is that a reconstruction can be performed from a short-scan using the appropriate subset of views where the intensity is expected to be highest. In Fig. 2 we show a model phantom for which it is obvious that an $n = 1$ π-scheme scan is most desirable. In this example, a center region of activity is surrounded by three distinct regions where the outgoing gamma rays undergo attenuation. Intuitively, the π-scheme should use the angular intervals that avoid the views that are obstructed by the attenuators. Figure 3 shows the total intensity, integrated over the detector and normalized to the maximum value, as a function of the view angle. From Figs. 2 and 3, it is clear that the π-scheme that maximizes the number of counts in equal collection times is the one that covers the angular intervals $[60° - 120°]$, $[180° - 240°]$, and $[300° - 360°]$, which avoid the regions of attenuation. We perform a quantitative study with the phantom in Fig. 2, comparing the noise properties of various equal-time scanning configurations and show that indeed this $n = 1$ π-scheme minimizes the bias and variance of the reconstructed image compared to other scanning configurations.

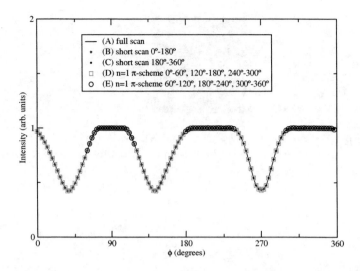

Figure 3: The intensity from the activity image in Fig. 2 integrated over the detector as a function of scanning angle. Intensities normalized to the maximum value. The various scanning configurations are indicated in the legend.

In the study, five equal time scanning configurations were simulated ; their angular ranges are shown graphically in the intensity graph in Fig. 3. In study A, a full 2π scan was performed, and Poisson noise was added to the sinogram, which was normalized to a count total of 500,000. The sinogram data include 120 view angles and 128 detector bins. In studies $B - E$, of which all include only π-data, the full sinograms were normalized to 1,000,000 counts from which only half the number of views were taken. As a result, all five scanning configurations studied here represent scans that are performed over equal times. Note, however, that this does *not* mean the π-schemes in $B - E$ have total counts of 500,000, because the intensity is not uniform as a function of scanning angle. Indeed, we are exploiting this non-uniformity to come up with the optimal scanning configuration. To perform the reconstruction, we employ a variation on the expectation maximization method (EM) using ordered subsets (OSEM), which speed up the convergence of the EM iterative approach. The EM algorithm has been shown to converge to the solution of equations like the Fredholm integral equation, Eq. (2); indeed, in this case it has been proven that there exists a unique solution [6]. Now, the image function f has been shown to satisfy the Fredholm equation shown in Eq. (2) only for the case of *uniform* attenuation. The example illustrated by Fig. 2 clearly violates the assumption of uniform attenuation. However, in order to use the OSEM method we need only to demonstrate the existence of a unique inverse of Eq. (1) when $m(\xi, \phi)$ is known only over π-data. While we have not yet proved this rigorously, we have presented an heuristic argument that demonstrates that there is such a unique inverse [7].

3.1 Results

To compare the noise properties of the various, equal-time scanning schemes, we show the normalized bias and standard deviation of each of the reconstructions in Table 1. All reconstructions were performed with 10 OSEM iterations using 10 ordered subsets. The subsets were divided by interlacing the view angle. In the table the relative intensities are shown by taking the total number of counts, from the part of the sinogram used for construction, and dividing that number by 1,000,000 counts. From the true activity map, f, the fractional bias b and the fractional standard deviation s were calculated from a set of reconstructed images of N random realizations of noisy SPECT sinograms, $\{f_i, i = 1, \ldots, N\}$, by

$$b = |\overline{f} - f|/|f|, \tag{11}$$

$$s = \left(\sqrt{\frac{1}{N} \sum_{i=1}^{N} |f_i - \overline{f}|^2} \right) /|f|, \tag{12}$$

Table 1: Statistical properties of five equal scanning time reconstructions, where A is a full-scan and $B - E$ are various π-scheme reconstructions. The scanning configurations are shown in Fig. 3. The sinogram for the full-scan study was normalized to 500,000 counts and the π-scheme studies were normalized to 1,000,000 total counts. The "intensity" column shows the fraction of counts, compared to 1,000,000, detected in the simulation of each scanning configuration. The fractional bias and standard deviation are shown in the last two columns.

scan	intensity	bias	standard deviation
A	50.0%	1.07%	0.72%
B	45.7%	0.97%	0.75%
C	54.4%	1.37%	0.69%
D	40.4%	1.21%	0.79%
E	59.6%	1.07%	0.66%

where $\overline{f} = N^{-1} \sum_{i=1}^{N} f_i$ and $N = 800$. As expected the fractional standard deviation reflects the total number of counts collected in each simulation. Scanning configuration E, which represents an $n = 1$ π-scheme reconstruction that makes use of angular views that are nearly unobstructed, collects 60% of the total available counts in the full 2π sinogram. As a result study E's standard deviation is the lowest at 0.66%. Interestingly, the fractional bias does not have a clear correlation with the intensity. In particular, study C that represents a short-scan over the left side of the phantom in Fig. 2 shows a worse bias than the short-scan, B, on the right side of the phantom even though the intensity argument should favor the left side scan. The behavior of the image bias for different π-schemes needs to be explored in more detail to see what aspect of the reconstruction the image bias is sensitive to and if general, image independent conclusions can be made. In any case, the scanning configuration E that collects the most counts in equal total scanning time and that, of all the π-schemes, utilizes data the most uniformly distributed about the image appears to have lowest standard deviation and at the same time a low bias compared to the other studies.

4 Conclusions

We have explored the novel π-scheme reconstruction of SPECT data, seeking to determine the noise properties of various scanning configurations. We have detailed a general argument showing that the properties of the π-scheme reconstruction approaches the full-scan reconstruction in the limit that the scanning configuration consists of an increasing large number of equally spaced and equally sized angular intervals. Our numerical example indicates that the π-scheme that maximizes the total collected counts also minimizes the global variance of the reconstructed image. However, the image bias seems to be more sensitive to the mathematical properties of the various π-scheme reconstructions, and further work is necessary to understand the connection between the π-scheme scanning configuration and the image bias.

5 Acknowledgement

This work was supported in part by National Cancer Institute Grants CA70449 and CA85593. Its contents are solely the responsibility of the authors and do not necessarily represent the official views of the National Cancer Institute.

References

[1] D. L. Parker. Optimal short scan convolution reconstruction for fan-beam CT. *Med. Phys.*, 9:245–257, 1982.

[2] X. Pan. A unified reconstruction theory for diffraction tomography with considerations of noise control. *J. Opt. Soc. Am.*, 15:2312–2326, 1998.

[3] X. Pan and M. Anastasio. Minimum-scan filtered backpropagation algorithms in diffraction tomography. *J. Opt. Soc. Am.*, 16:2896–2903, 1999.

[4] C. E. Metz and X. Pan. A unified analysis of exact methods of inverting the 2-D exponential Radon transform, with implications for noise control in SPECT. *IEEE Trans. Med. Imaging*, 14:643–658, 1995.

[5] F. Noo and J.-M. Wagner. Image reconstruction in 2D SPECT with 180-degree acquisition. *Inverse Problems*, 17:1357–1372, 2001.

[6] X. Pan, C.-M. Kao, and C. Metz. A family of pi-scheme exponential Radon transforms and the uniqueness of their inverses. *Inverse Problems*, (submitted), 2001.

[7] X. Pan, E. Y. Sidky, C.-M. Kao, Y. Zou, and C. Metz. Image reconstruction in pi-scheme short-scan SPECT with non-uniform attenuation. *IEEE Trans. Nucl. Sci.*, (submitted), 2001.

Full non-linear inversion of microwave biomedical data

Aria Abubakar[a], Peter M van den Berg[a] and Jordi J Mallorqui[b]

[a]Laboratory of Electromagnetic Research, Delft University of Technology
Mekelweg 4, 2628 CD, Delft, The Netherlands
[b]Department of Signal Theory and Communications, Universitat Politecnica de Catalunya
D3-Campus Nord-UPC, 08034, Barcelona, Spain

ABSTRACT

In this paper the contrast source inversion method using a multiplicative weighted L^2-norm total variation regularizer is applied to image reconstructions from electromagnetic microwave tomography experiments. This iterative method avoids solving a full forward problem in each iteration which makes the method suitable to handle a large scale computational problem. The numerical results from experimental data with high contrast biological phantom are presented and discussed.

Keywords: medical imaging, nonlinear inversion, optimization, microwave tomography

1. INTRODUCTION

Image reconstruction is a complicated nonlinear problem in microwave tomography because both the material parameters and the field distribution in the investigation domain are unknowns. If the unknown object has small contrast of dielectric properties, a linearization procedure like the Born approximations[1] can be used to provide images with spatial resolution of a fraction of the wavelength. Computer codes based on these Born approximations demonstrate a high speed and can be used for almost real time imaging. Iterative procedures for the Born approximation have been used for intermediate contrast objects.[4] More complicated mathematical reconstruction algorithms have been developed for reconstruction objects with high contrast in dielectric properties.[3, 5–8, 10] These algorithms require large computer resources, but nevertheless theoretically provide a resolution with a sufficiently high signal-to-noise ratio. The Newton method[12] has been successfully applied to high contrast objects. The main bottlenecks of this Newton approach are the multiple forward solutions needed to construct the Hessian matrix. Other methods which avoid solving any forward problem in each iterative step are the Modified Gradient (MG) method[9] and the Contrast Source Inversion (CSI) method.[13] These last two approaches can solve the nonlinear inverse problem without dealing with a high-dimensional linear equation system but it requires a larger number of iterations.

Recently, due to the simplicity of the CSI method, this method has been armed with a Total Variation (TV) regularizer in order to handle high contrast objects.[14] Although the addition of the TV to the cost functional has a very positive effect on the quality of the reconstructions for both 'blocky' and smooth profiles, a drawback is the presence of an artificial weighting parameter in the cost functional, which can only be determined through considerable numerical experimentation and a priori information of the desired reconstruction. It was suggested to include the TV as a multiplicative constraint,[14] with the result that the original cost functional is the weighting parameter of the regularizer, so that this parameter is determined by the inversion procedure itself. This eliminates the choice of the artificial regularization parameters completely. The multiplicative type of regularization seems to handle noisy as well as limited data in a robust way without the usually necessary a priori information. In this paper the latter method using the new weighted L^2-norm total variation regularizer[15] is applied to handle more complicated biological objects embedded in a lossy medium. Numerical examples using experimental data collected by a circular microwave scanner operating at 2.33 Ghz demonstrate the ability of the CSI method using the weighted L_2-norm TV regularizor. Furthermore, some comparisons with other nonlinear inversion methods will also be presented and discussed.

Send correspondence to Aria Abubakar, E-mail: abubakar@its.tudelft.nl, Telephone: 31 15 2784429, Address: Laboratory of Electromagnetic Research, Delft University of Technology, Mekelweg 4, 2628 CD, Delft, The Netherlands

2. PROBLEM STATEMENT

We consider an object, B, of arbitrary bounded cross section with complex dielectric permittivity $\varepsilon(\boldsymbol{x})$ and arbitrary shape. The complex permittivity and the shape of this object B are unknown, but they are known to lie within a bounded simply connected object domain D. This object domain D is assumed to be embedded in the background medium, the immersion liquid, with permittivity ε_{b}. We assume a time harmonic dependence $\exp(\mathrm{j}\omega t)$, where $\mathrm{j}^2 = -1$, ω is angular frequency, and t is time. We also assume that the object is irradiated successively by a number of known incident electric fields due to line source with polarization in the vertical direction parallel to the cylindrical objects. Then, we have only one non-zero componenent of the electric field, namely the vertical component of the electric field. The problem associated with this polarization is known as the two-dimensional TM electromagnetic scattering problem. The line sources are located in a data domain S surrounding the object domain D, where the measurements are made as well. The two-dimensional position vector is denoted by $\boldsymbol{x} = (x_1, x_2)$.

For each incident field u_s^{inc} with (for $s = 1, 2, \cdots$), the total electric field will be denoted by u_s. Nowadays, it is well-known that the total field u_s and the scattered field u_s^{sct} satisfy the following domain integral representations:

$$u_s(\boldsymbol{x}) = u_s^{\mathrm{inc}}(\boldsymbol{x}) + k_{\mathrm{b}}^2 \int_D g(\boldsymbol{x}-\boldsymbol{x}')\chi(\boldsymbol{x}')u_s(\boldsymbol{x}')\,\mathrm{d}v(\boldsymbol{x}')\,, \quad \boldsymbol{x} \in D\,, \tag{1}$$

$$u_s^{\mathrm{sct}}(\boldsymbol{x}) = k_{\mathrm{b}}^2 \int_D g(\boldsymbol{x}-\boldsymbol{x}')\chi(\boldsymbol{x}')u_s(\boldsymbol{x}')\,\mathrm{d}v(\boldsymbol{x}')\,, \quad \boldsymbol{x} \in S\,, \tag{2}$$

where

$$\chi(\boldsymbol{x}) = \frac{\varepsilon(\boldsymbol{x})}{\varepsilon_{\mathrm{b}}} - 1 \quad \text{and} \quad g(\boldsymbol{x}) = \frac{\mathrm{j}}{4}H_0^{(2)}(k_{\mathrm{b}}|\boldsymbol{x}|)\,, \tag{3}$$

in which $k_{\mathrm{b}} = \omega\left(\varepsilon_{\mathrm{b}}\mu_0\right)^{1/2}$ denotes the wavenumber in the embedding.

In the inverse scattering problem u_s^{sct} will be measured on some domain S outside D, so the integral representation in (2) for points exterior to D is written symbolically as the *data equation*,

$$u_s^{\mathrm{sct}} = G_S\chi u_s\,, \quad \boldsymbol{x} \in S\,, \tag{4}$$

while the integral equation in (1) is written symbolically as the *object equation*,

$$u_s^{\mathrm{inc}} = u_s - G_D\chi u_s\,, \quad \boldsymbol{x} \in D\,, \tag{5}$$

where the operator G_S is an operator mapping from $L^2(D)$ into $L^2(S)$ and the operator G_D is an operator mapping $L^2(D)$ into itself.

The inverse scattering problem consists of determining χ from a knowledge of the incident fields, u_s^{inc}, on D and the scattered fields, u_s^{sct}, on S. Because the total fields u_s on D are also unknown, this problem is non-linear.

3. INVERSION ALGORITHM

In the CSI method, one chooses to reconstruct the material contrast χ and the contrast sources w_s instead of the fields u_s. The contrast sources are defined by

$$w_s(\boldsymbol{x}) = \chi(\boldsymbol{x})u_s(\boldsymbol{x})\,. \tag{6}$$

Using (6) in (4), the data equation becomes

$$u_s^{\mathrm{sct}} = G_S w_s\,, \quad \boldsymbol{x} \in S\,, \tag{7}$$

while the object equation becomes

$$u_s = u_s^{\mathrm{inc}} + G_D w_s\,, \quad \boldsymbol{x} \in D\,. \tag{8}$$

Substituting (8) into (6), we obtain an object equation for w_s

$$\chi u_s^{\mathrm{inc}} = w_s - \chi G_D w_s\,, \quad \boldsymbol{x} \in D\,. \tag{9}$$

3.1. Contrast source inversion method

In the CSI method, the sequences of the contrast sources $w_{s,n}$ and the contrast χ_n (for $n = 1, 2, \cdots, n_{max}$), are iteratively found by minimizing a cost functional,

$$F_n(w_s, \chi) = F^S(w_s) + F_n^D(w_s, \chi), \tag{10}$$

where

$$F^S(w_s) = \frac{\sum_s \|u_s^{sct} - G_S w_s\|_S^2}{\sum_s \|u_s^{sct}\|_S^2} \qquad \text{and} \qquad F_n^D(w_s, \chi) = \frac{\sum_s \|\chi u_s^{inc} - w_s + \chi G^D w_s\|_D^2}{\sum_s \|\chi_{n-1} u_s^{inc}\|_D^2}, \tag{11}$$

where $\|\cdot\|_{S,D}^2 = <\cdot, \cdot>_{S,D}$ denotes the squared norm on S or D. This CSI method starts with backpropagation as the initial estimates for the contrast sources and the contrast. In each iteration, we first update the contrast sources $w_{s,n}$ using a conjugate gradient step. Note that the functional is a quadratic function in terms of the contrast sources, and only one minimizer is arrived at. Subsequently, we compute the field using (8), after which an updated approximation of the contrast χ_n is found as

$$\chi_n = \arg \min\nolimits_{\text{complex } \chi} \left\{ \sum_j \|\chi u_{j,n} - w_{j,n}\|_D^2 \right\} \tag{12}$$

and its solution can be found in closed-form. In this way the total computational complexity of the CSI method is approximately equal to the complexity of solving two linear forward problems using Conjugate Gradient (CG) method. The details of the CSI algorithm is summarized in Table 1.

3.2. Multiplicative regularized contrast source inversion method

Although the inclusion of the object equation in the second term of (10) can be considered as a physical regularization of the ill-posed data equation in the first term of (10), the inversion results may be improved by taking into account *a priori* information about the contrast profile. The standard way to include this *a priori* information is to modify the functional by introducing an extra penalty function, viz.,

$$C_n(w_s, \chi) = F^S(w_s) + F_n^D(w_s, \chi) + \gamma^2 F_n^R(\chi). \tag{13}$$

As known in the literature the addition of the regularization term F_n^R to the cost functional has a very positive effect on the quality of the reconstruction. The drawback is the presence of the positive weighting parameter γ^2 in the cost functional, which, with the present knowledge, can only be determined through considerable numerical experimentation and *a priori* information of the desired reconstruction. Further, numerical experiments have shown that the results improve when we let the parameter γ^2 decrease with increasing number of iterations. In fact, a good choice seems to take this parameter proportional to the value of the cost functional F_{n-1} of the previous iteration. This numerical experimentation has led us to the idea of multiplicative regularization technique,[14] viz.

$$C_n(w_s, \chi) = [F_S(w_s) + F_n^D(w_s, \chi)] F_n^R(\chi). \tag{14}$$

As the regularization factor we choose the one introduced in.[15] This so-called weighted L_2-norm TV regularizer is given by

$$F_n^R(\chi) = \frac{1}{V} \int_D \frac{|\boldsymbol{\nabla}\chi(\boldsymbol{x})|^2 + \delta_n^2}{|\boldsymbol{\nabla}\chi_n(\boldsymbol{x})|^2 + \delta_n^2} \, dv(\boldsymbol{x}), \tag{15}$$

where $\boldsymbol{\nabla}$ denotes the spatial differentiation with respect to $\boldsymbol{x}$ and $V = \int_D dv(\boldsymbol{x})$ denotes the area of the test domain D. Although this regularizer is a L_2-norm regularizer, it has all the benefits of the original L_1-norm TV regularizer.[11] The constant parameter δ_n^2 is originally introduced for restoring differentiability of the TV regularizator, it also controls the influence of the regularization. We therefore have chosen to increase the regularization as a function of the number of iterations by decreasing this parameter δ_n^2. Since the object error term will decrease as a function of the number of iterations, we choose

$$\delta_n^2 = F_n^D(w_{j,n}, \chi_n) \tilde{\Delta}^2, \tag{16}$$

Table 1: The algorithm of the Contrast Source Inversion (CSI) method.

Initializing contrast sources:

$\alpha_0 = \sum_s \|G_S^* u_s^{\text{sct}}\|_D^2 / \sum_s \|G_S G_S^* u_s^{\text{sct}}\|_S^2$

$w_{s,0} = \alpha_0 G_S^* u_s^{\text{sct}}$

Initializing contrast:

$u_{s,0} = u_s^{\text{inc}} + G_D w_{s,0}$

$\chi_0 = \sum_s w_{s,0} \overline{u}_{s,0} / \sum_s |u_{s,0}|^2$

Initializing residuals and CG search directions:

$\rho_{s,0} = u_s^{\text{sct}} - G_S w_{s,0}$ % residual in data equation

$r_{s,0} = \chi_0 u_{s,0} - w_{s,0}$ % residual in object equation

$\eta_0^D = \sum_s \|\chi_0 u_s^{\text{inc}}\|_D^2$

$F_0^D = \eta_0^D \sum_s \|r_{s,0}\|_D^2$

$F^S = \eta^S \sum_s \|\rho_{s,0}\|_S^2$

$v_{s,0} = 0$ % search direction for contrast sources

For $n = 1$ to $n = n_{\max}$

    Updating contrast sources:

      $g_{s,n}^w = -\eta^S G_S^* \rho_{s,n-1} - \eta_{n-1}^D (I - G_D^* \overline{\chi}_{n-1}) r_{s,n-1}$ % gradient

      $v_{s,n} = g_{s,n}^w + \sum_s < g_{s,n}^w, g_{s,n}^w - g_{s,n-1}^w >_D / \sum_s \|g_{s,n-1}^w\|_D^2 \, v_{s,n-1}$ % CG direction

      $\alpha_n = \text{argmin}_{\text{real}\alpha} \{F_n(w_{s,n-1} + \alpha v_{s,n}, \chi_{n-1})\}$ % CG weight

      $w_{s,n} = w_{s,n-1} + \alpha_n v_{s,n}$

    Updating contrast:

      $u_{s,n} = u_{s,n-1} + \alpha_n G_D v_{s,n}$

      $\chi_n = \sum_s w_{s,n} \overline{u}_{s,n} / \sum_s |u_{s,n}|^2$

    Updating residuals:

      $\rho_{s,n} = \rho_{s,n-1} - \alpha_n G_S v_{s,n}$

      $r_{s,n} = \chi_n u_{s,n} - w_{s,n}$

      $\eta_n^D = \sum_s \|\chi_n u_s^{\text{inc}}\|_D^2$

      $F_n^D = \eta_n^D \sum_s \|r_{s,n}\|_D^2$

      $F^S = \eta^S \sum_s \|\rho_{s,n}\|_S^2$

    If $F^S(w_{s,n}) <$ error criterium then

      stop

    end If

    $n = n + 1$

end For

---

where $\tilde{\Delta}$ denotes the reciprocal mesh size of the discretized domain D, and F_n^D is the normalized norm of the error in the object equation, before the extra regularization. Its choice is inspired by the idea that in the first few iterations, we do not need the minimization of the TV regularizator and as the iterations proceed we want to increase the effect of the TV regularizator.

Minimization of this cost functional C_n with respect to changes in the contrast will change the minimizer χ_n given in (12) to χ_n^R. Our aim is not to change the updating procedure of the contrast sources $w_{s,n}$. At the beginning of each iteration we have to replace the quantity χ_{n-1} by χ_{n-1}^R, but the remainder of the contrast source updating procedure is not changed, when we keep the regularization factor to be equal to one during this part of the iteration. Then, only the updating of the contrast for given $w_{s,n}$ has to be modified. Instead of taking the previous iterate of the contrast as done in,[15] we now take the analytic value of (12) as starting value. From this point we make an additional minimization step,

$$\chi_n^R = \chi_n + \beta_n d_n, \tag{17}$$

where χ_n is given by (12) and d_n is the Polak-Ribière CG direction. We remark that we prefer now a line minimization around the minimum of the cost functional F_n^D (physical cost criterion). In view of (12) we take

g_n^R as

$$g_n^R = \frac{\left[\partial F_n^R(\chi)/\partial\chi\right]_{\chi=\chi_n}}{\sum_s |u_{s,n}|^2}, \tag{18}$$

being a preconditioned gradient of the regularization factor F_n^R with respect to changes in the contrast around the point $\chi = \chi_n$. In view of the previous minimization step, the gradient of F_n^D with respect to changes in the contrast around the point χ_n vanishes. Hence, the gradient with respect to the contrast, in contrary to the previous approaches of the CSI method with regularizator,[14,15] contains only a contribution of the regularization additionally imposed. This simplifies the algorithm. For the weighted L_2-norm TV regularizator in (15), the real parameter β_n is found from a closed-form line minimization as the minimizer of

$$\beta_n = \arg\min_{\text{real }\beta} \left\{C_n(w_{s,n}, \chi_n + \beta d_n)\right\}. \tag{19}$$

The structure of this minimization procedure is such that it will minimize the regularization factor with a large weighting parameter in the beginning of the optimization process, because the value of F_n is still large, and that it will gradually minimize more and more the error in the data and object equations when the regularization factor F_n^R remains a nearly constant value close to one. If noise is present in the data, the data error term F_S will remain at a large value during the optimization and therefore, the weight of the regularization factor will be more significant. Hence, the noise will, at all times, be suppressed in the reconstruction process and we automatically fulfill the need of a larger regularization when the data contains noise. After we have obtained a new estimate χ_n^R for the contrast, we update the contrast sources starting with $\chi_{n-1} = \chi_{n-1}^R$ of the previous iteration. This CSI method using TV regularizator is denoted as the Multiplicative Regularized CSI (MR-CSI) method. The algorithm is summarized in Table 2.

4. NUMERICAL EXAMPLES

We consider inversion from the two-dimensional TM polarization measurement. For this measurement there are experimental data available which have been measured using a circular microwave scanner operating at 2.33GHz. The scanner consists of a 12.5cm radius circular array of 64 water-immersed horn antennas.[2] The measurement procedure records the total electric field values at the receiving antennas. If one antenna is transmitting, the fields are measured only with the 33 antennas located in front of the active source. The scattered fields are deduced from the total field by subtracting the incident field, measured in the absence of any targets. Further, the measured scattered fields have been calibrated so that a directed unit line source can be used as the model for the incident fields, viz.,

$$u_s^{\text{inc}}(\boldsymbol{x}) = -\frac{\omega\mu_0}{4} H_0^{(2)}(k_b|\boldsymbol{x} - \boldsymbol{x}_s^{\text{S}}|), \tag{20}$$

where $\mu_0 = 4\pi \times 10^{-7}$ is the permeability in vacuum.

In the inversion of experimental data we assumed that the unknown object is entirely located within a test domain D with dimension of 6.3λ by 6.3λ where λ is the wavelength in water. The permittivity of water is approximately $\epsilon_b/\epsilon_0 = 77.3 - j\,8.66$ at frequency $f = 2.33$ GHz. Hence, the wavelength $\lambda = 14.6$ mm. The discrete form of the algorithm is obtained by dividing the test domain D into 63 by 63 subsquares. The discrete spatial convolutions are efficiently computed using Fast Fourier Transform routines. The lower and upper bounds of the reconstructed complex permittivity in the inversion algorithm are enforced as follows:

$$0 \leq \text{Re}[\varepsilon(\boldsymbol{x})]/\varepsilon_0 \leq 80 \quad \text{and} \quad 0 \leq -\text{Im}[\varepsilon(\boldsymbol{x})]/\varepsilon_0 \leq 20. \tag{21}$$

The first experimental data were obtained from a human arm phantom. The external layer (supposed to model the skin) and bones of the human arm phantom were made with PVC with complex permittivity $\varepsilon/\varepsilon_0 = 2.73 - j\,0.01$ and the muscle was $\varepsilon/\varepsilon_0 = 54.5 - j\,17.2$. We show first the results obtained using the so-called Modified Gradient (MG) method[9] after 1024 iterations, see Figure 1a. The results of the CSI and MR-CSI method after 1024 iterations are given in Figures 1b and 1c. Note that for all three methods, although the total number of iterations is large, the total computation time is very limited. Note that we do not solve any forward problem at each iteration of the algorithm. The computational time of the CSI and MR-CSI method

Table 2: The algorithm of the Multiplicative Regularized CSI (MR-CSI) method.

Initializing contrast sources:

$$\alpha_0 = \sum_s \|G_S^* u_s^{\text{sct}}\|_D^2 / \sum_s \|G_S G_S^* u_s^{\text{sct}}\|_S^2$$

$$w_{s,0} = \alpha_0 G_S^* u_s^{\text{sct}}$$

Initializing contrast:

$$u_{s,0} = u_s^{\text{inc}} + G_D w_{s,0}$$

$$\chi_0 = \sum_s w_{s,0} \overline{u}_{s,0} / \sum_s |u_{s,0}|^2$$

Initializing residuals and CG search directions:

$$\rho_{s,0} = u_s^{\text{sct}} - G_S w_{s,0} \quad \text{\% residual in data equation}$$

$$r_{s,0} = \chi_0 u_{s,0} - w_{s,0} \quad \text{\% residual in object equation}$$

$$\eta_0^D = \sum_s \|\chi_0 u_s^{\text{inc}}\|_D^2$$

$$F_0^D = \eta_0^D \sum_s \|r_{s,0}\|_D^2$$

$$F^S = \eta^S \sum_s \|\rho_{s,0}\|_S^2$$

$$v_{s,0} = 0 \quad \text{\% search direction for contrast sources}$$

$$d_0 = 0 \quad \text{\% search direction for contrast}$$

For $n = 1$ to $n = n_{\max}$

　Updating contrast sources:

$$g_{s,n}^w = -\eta^S G_S^* \rho_{s,n-1} - \eta_{n-1}^D (I - G_D^* \overline{\chi}_{n-1}) r_{s,n-1} \quad \text{\% gradient}$$

$$v_{s,n} = g_{s,n}^w + \sum_s < g_{s,n}^w, g_{s,n}^w - g_{s,n-1}^w >_D / \sum_s \|g_{s,n-1}^w\|_D^2 \, v_{s,n-1} \quad \text{\% CG direction}$$

$$\alpha_n = \text{argmin}_{\text{real} \alpha} \{F_n(w_{s,n-1} + \alpha v_{s,n}, \chi_{n-1})\} \quad \text{\% CG weight}$$

$$w_{s,n} = w_{s,n-1} + \alpha_n v_{s,n}$$

　Updating contrast:

$$\rho_{s,n} = \rho_{s,n-1} - \alpha_n G_S v_{s,n}$$

$$r_{s,n} = r_{s,n-1} - \alpha_n (I - \chi_{n-1} G_D) v_{s,n}$$

$$u_{s,n} = u_{s,n-1} + \alpha_n G_D v_{s,n}$$

$$\chi_n = \sum_s w_{s,n} \overline{u}_{s,n} / \sum_s |u_{s,n}|^2$$

$$r_{s,n} = \chi_n u_{s,n} - w_{s,n}$$

$$\eta_n^D = \sum_s \|\chi_n u_s^{\text{inc}}\|_D^2$$

$$F_n(w_{s,n}, \chi_n) = \eta_n^D \sum_s \|r_{s,n}\|_D^2 + \eta^S \sum_s \|\rho_{s,n}\|_S^2$$

$$g_n^R = -F_n(w_{s,n}, \chi_n) \boldsymbol{\nabla} \cdot (b_n \boldsymbol{\nabla} \chi_n) / \sum_s |u_{s,n}|^2 \quad \text{\% gradient}$$

$$d_n = g_n^R + \langle g_n^R, g_n^R - g_{n-1}^R \rangle_D \, d_{n-1} / |g_{n-1}^R|_D^2 \quad \text{\% CG direction}$$

$$\beta_n = \text{argmin}_{\text{real} \beta} \{C_n(w_{s,n}, \chi_n + \beta d_n)\} \quad \text{\% CG weight}$$

$$\chi_n^R = \chi_n + \beta_n d_n$$

$$\chi_n = \chi_n^R \quad \text{\% contrast to be used in next iteration}$$

　Updating residuals:

$$r_{s,n} = \chi_n u_{s,n} - w_{s,n}$$

$$\eta_n^D = \sum_s \|\chi_n u_s^{\text{inc}}\|_D^2$$

$$F_n^D = \eta_n^D \sum_s \|r_{s,n}\|_D^2$$

$$F^S = \eta^S \sum_s \|\rho_{s,n}\|_S^2$$

　If $F^S(w_{s,n}) <$ error criterium then

　　stop

　end If

　$n = n + 1$

end For

---

is almost equal and they are approximately three times more faster than the MG method. From the results, it is obvious that the CSI method outperforms the MG method and the MR-CSI produces the best reconstructed images. Further we observe that the bones are clear and sharp. The only drawback is that the reconstructed imaginary part of the complex permittivity for one of the bones is completely wrong. This can be caused by the presence of the noise in the experimental data.

For the second experiment we consider data that were taken from a human forearm. The MG method reconstructions after 1024 iterations are given in the Figure 2a. The results of the CSI and the MR-CSI method

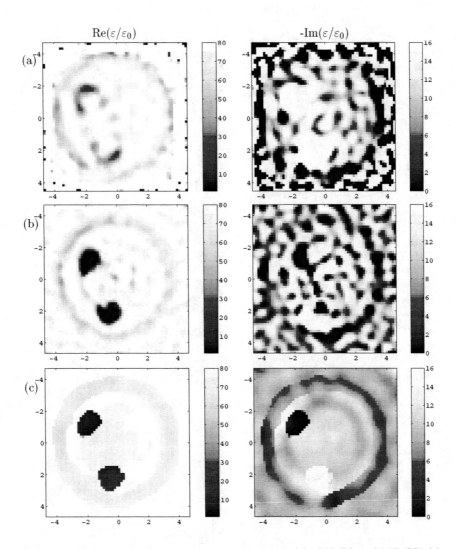

Figure 1: Human arm phantom images: using MG (a), CSI (b) and MR-CSI (c).

after 1024 iterations are given in Figures 2b and 2c. Again, the MR-CSI method provides us with the best reconstructed results. The reconstructed images from the MR-CSI method show the positions of the two bones and the correct value of the muscle (approximately $54.5 - j\,17.2$). Conversely, due to the water and tissue attenuation and the reduced dynamic range of the available data, the complex permittivity values of the bones are higher than the real ones (it should approximately be $5.5 - j\,0.59$ at the present frequency of operation).

5. CONCLUSIONS

The presented results for biomedical data, using a two-dimensional TM polarization measurement, show that the Contrast Source Inversion method using multiplicative weighted L_2-norm Total Variation regularization leads to an effective inversion technique. The algorithm is fully iterative and does not solve any forward problem in each iteration. This makes the method suitable for large-scale computations. Furthermore, the artificial tuning process with a weighting parameter of the regularization to obtain the "cosmetically best" results seems superfluous.

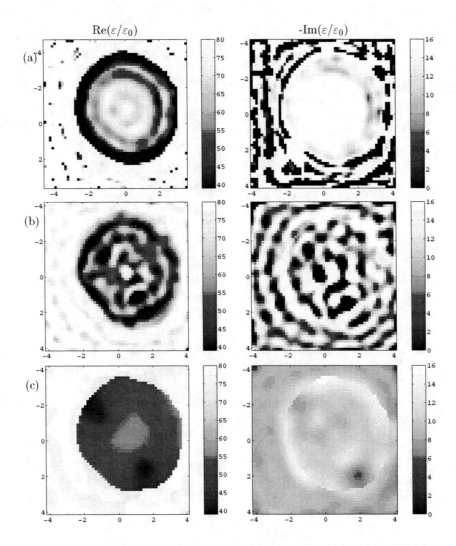

Figure 2: Human forearm images: using MG (a), CSI (b) and MR-CSI (c).

REFERENCES

1. Bolomey, J., Pichot, C.: Some applications of diffraction tomography to electromagnetics - the particular case of microwaves in: Inverse Problems in Scattering and Imaging, M. Bertero and E.R. Pike, Eds., London, U.K.: Adam Hilger (1982) 319–344

2. Broquetas, A., Romeu, J., Rius, J.M., Elias-Fuste, A.R., Cardama, A., Jofre, L.: Cylindrical geometry: A further step in active microwave tomography. IEEE Trans. Microwave Theory Tech. **39** (1991) 836–844

3. Bulyshev, A.E., Souvorov, A.E., Semenov, S.Y., Svenson, R.H., Nazarov, A.G., Sizov, Y.E., Tatsis, G.P.: Three-dimensional microwave tomography. Theory and computer experiments in scalar approximation. Inverse Probl. **16** (2000) 863-875

4. Chew, W.C., Wang, Y.M.: An iterative solution of two-dimensional electromagnetic inverse scattering problem. Int. J. Imag. Syst. Technol. **1** (1989) 100–108

5. Chew, W.C., Wang, Y.M.: Reconstruction of 2D permittivity distribution using the distorted Born iterative method. IEEE Trans. Med. Imag. **9** (1990) 218–225

6. Franchois A., Pichot, C.: Microwave imaging - complex permittivity reconstruction with a Levenberg-Marquadt method. IEEE Trans. Microwave Theory Tech. **46** (1997) 133–141

7. Harada, H., Wall, D., Takenaka, T., Tanaka, T.: Conjugate gradient method applied to inverse scattering problem. IEEE Trans. Antennas Propagat. **43** (1995) 784–792

8. Joachimowicz, N., Mallorqui, J.J., Bolomey, J.Ch., Broquetas, A.: Convergence and stability assessment of Newton-Kantorovich reconstruction algorithms for microwave tomography. IEEE Trans. Med. Imag. **17** (1998) 562–569

9. Kleinman, R.E., van den Berg, P.M.: An extended range modified gradient technique for profile inversion, Radio Sci. **28** (1993), 877–884

10. Meaney, P.M., Paulsen, K.D., Hartov, A., Crane, R.K.: Microwave imaging for tissue assessment: Initial evaluation in multitarget tissue equivalent phantoms. IEEE Trans. Biomed. Enq. **43** (1996) 878–890

11. Rudin, L., Osher, S., Fatemi, C.: Nonlinear total variation based noise removal algorithm. Physica. **60D**, (1992) 259–268.

12. Souvorov, A.E., Bulyshev, A.E., Semenov, S.Y., Svenson, R.H., Nazarov, A.G., Sizov, Y.E., Tatsis, G.P.: Microwave tomography: A two-dimensional Newton iterative scheme. IEEE Trans. Microwave Theory Tech. **46** (1998) 1654–1659

13. van den Berg, P.M., Kleinman, R.E.: A contrast source inversion method. Inverse Probl. **13** (1997) 1607–1620

14. van den Berg, P.M., van Broekhoven, A.L., Abubakar, A.: Extended contrast source inversion. Inverse Probl. **15** (1999) 1325–1344

15. van den Berg P.M., Abubakar, A.: Contrast source inversion method: State of art. Prog. in Electromag. Research **34** (2001) 189–218

Filter design for filtered back-projection guided by the interpolation model

Stefan Horbelt, Michael Liebling, and Michael Unser

Biomedical Imaging Group, Swiss Federal Institute of Technology, CH-1015 Lausanne EPFL

ABSTRACT

We consider using spline interpolation to improve the standard filtered back-projection (FBP) tomographic reconstruction algorithm. In particular, we propose to link the design of the filtering operator with the interpolation model that is applied to the sinogram. The key idea is to combine the ramp filtering and the spline fitting process into a single filtering operation. We consider three different approaches. In the first, we simply adapt the standard FBP for spline interpolation. In the second approach, we replace the interpolation by an oblique projection onto the same spline space; this increases the peak signal-noise ratio by up to 2.5 dB. In the third approach, we perform an explicit discretization by observing that the ramp filter is equivalent to a fractional derivative operator that can be evaluated analytically for splines. This allows for an exact implementation of the ramp filter and improves the image quality by an additional 0.2 dB. This comparison is unique as the first method has been published only for degree n=0, whereas the two other methods are novel. We stress that the modification of the filter improve the reconstruction quality especially at low (faster) interpolation degrees ($n = 1$); the difference between the methods becomes marginal for cubic or higher degrees ($n \geq 3$).

Keywords: tomographic reconstruction, filtered back-projection, ramp filter, fractional splines, oblique projection, spline interpolation

1. INTRODUCTION

Mathematically, the measurement process in X-ray tomography is conveniently described by the Radon transform[1]. An attractive feature of this transform is that it has an exact inversion formula. The digital implementation of this analytical formula leads to the standard filtered back-projection (FBP) algorithm, which goes back to the early 70s[2]. Despite the considerable research efforts devoted to alternative reconstruction techniques (in particular, algebraic or statistical ones), the FBP is still the method of choice used in commercial CT scanners. It owes its success to the fact that it is direct, fast and reasonably simple to implement. Even though the standard implementation uses a rather rudimentary discretization—at least by modern standards, it has not been much improved over the years, except for the aspect of filter design[3]. The filtering part of the algorithm is essential to avoid excessive smoothing and to suppress aliasing; in practice, the design is mostly guided by practical considerations, such as noise reduction.

An important aspect of FBP is the interpolation step that takes place during the back-projection part of the algorithm. Most practical implementations use linear interpolation to minimize computations, but there is also evidence that the performance can be improved be using higher order models. In this paper, we are especially interested in the interpolation aspect of the problem and we want to determine the extent to which high quality methods can make a difference. As a novelty, we are proposing to modify the filtering step of the algorithm so that it is best matched to the interpolation that is applied to the sinogram. We have chosen here to concentrate on B-splines since these functions were found to offer the best cost-performance tradeoff for the interpolation of medical images[4,5]. The quality of the polynomial spline model is determined by its degree; for $n = 1$, it is equivalent to linear interpolation and it gets closer and closer to the band-limited model (sinc interpolation) as n increases. Another advantage of splines is that the effect of ramp filtering can be determined analytically; a property that will be exploited in the third method that is considered in this paper. We will essentially compare three methods—all based on spline interpolation; practically, they will differ only by the type of filter being used. Interestingly, we will see that we can outperform the standard approach by selecting a filter that is different from the traditional Ram-Lak (or ramp) filter.

Medical Imaging 2002: Image Processing, Milan Sonka, J. Michael Fitzpatrick, Editors, Proceedings of SPIE Vol. 4684 (2002) © 2002 SPIE · 1605-7422/02/$15.00

2. STANDARD FBP

We recall the standard filtered back-projection (FBP), which is based on the inverse of the Radon transform[1].

The Radon transform $R_\theta f$ of an image $f(\vec{x})$, $\vec{x} \in R^2$, is the set of line integrals along the direction $\vec{\theta}$ at the distance t from the origin

$$R_\theta\{f(\vec{x})\} = R_\theta f(t) = \int_{\vec{x} \in \mathbb{R}^2} f(\vec{x})\delta(t - \vec{x}^\top \cdot \vec{\theta})d\vec{x}, \tag{1}$$

where $\delta(t)$ is the Dirac impulse and $\vec{\theta} = (\cos\theta, \sin\theta)^\top$ specifies the direction of integration.

The basis for the inverse Radon transform is the well-known identity

$$f(\vec{x}) = R^*(q * R_\theta\{f(\vec{x})\}), \tag{2}$$

where q denotes the 1D ramp filter whose Fourier transform is $\hat{q}(\omega) = |\frac{\omega}{2\pi}|$; R^*, the adjoint of R, is the back-projection operator:

$$(R^*p)(\vec{x}) = \int_0^\pi p(\vec{x}^\top \cdot \vec{\theta}, \theta)d\theta,$$

The widely used FBP algorithm corresponds to the direct discretization of the right-hand side of (2). However, instead of the infinite ramp filter q, one usually uses an attenuated version $\hat{h}(\omega) = |\frac{\omega}{2\pi}|\widehat{\Omega}(\omega)$, where $\widehat{\Omega}(\omega)$ is a suitable spectral window (e.g. Shepp-Logan filter).

3. FRACTIONAL B-SPLINES AND THEIR DERIVATIVES

The basic building blocks for spline interpolation are the B-spline basis functions. Here, we describe an extension for fractional degree α; not necessarily integer[6]. The symmetric B-spline of degree α is defined in the Fourier domain by

$$\hat{\beta}_*^\alpha(\omega) = \frac{\left|1 - e^{j\omega}\right|^{\alpha+1}}{|j\omega|^{\alpha+1}}. \tag{3}$$

This definition is essentially the same as the one for the classical B-splines of integer degree n[7]. The difference is that $\alpha = n$ is allowed to be fractional; i.e., non integer. Here, we are especially interested in the fractional derivative properties of these B-splines.

The n-th derivative of the function $f(x)$ can be defined in the Fourier domain as $D^n f(x) \leftrightarrow (j\omega)^n \hat{f}(\omega)$, where $\hat{f}(\omega) = \int_{-\infty}^{+\infty} f(x)e^{-j\omega x}dx$ denotes the Fourier transform of $f(x)$. By extension, we define a symmetric version of fractional derivatives $D_*^\gamma f(x) \leftrightarrow |\omega|^\gamma \hat{f}(\omega)$, where γ is any fractional number. Note that this derivative only corresponds to the usual one when γ is even.

The relevance for our purpose of the D_* operator is that it is a scaled version of the ramp filter $\hat{q}(\omega) = |\frac{\omega}{2\pi}|$. The key property is that we have a simple analytical formula for the fractional derivative of a fractional B-spline

$$D_*^\gamma \beta_*(x) = \Delta_*^\gamma \beta_*^{\alpha-\gamma}(x), \tag{4}$$

where Δ_*^γ is the fractional finite difference operator

$$\Delta_*^\gamma \leftrightarrow |1 - e^{-j\omega}|^\gamma.$$

The argument for the proof is as follows

$$D_*^\gamma \beta_*(x) \leftrightarrow |j\omega|^\gamma \left|\frac{1 - e^{j\omega}}{j\omega}\right|^{\alpha+1} = \left|1 - e^{-j\omega}\right|^\gamma \left|\frac{1 - e^{j\omega}}{j\omega}\right|^{\alpha+1-\gamma}.$$

Spline interpolation amounts to fitting a sequence $f(k)$ with a spline of the form

$$f(x) = \sum_{k \in Z} c(k) \beta_*^\alpha (x - k).$$

The $c(k)$'s are determined by inverse filtering[9]:

$$c(k) = \left((b_*^\alpha)^{-1} * f \right) (k), \tag{5}$$

where

$$(b_*^\alpha)^{-1}(k) \leftrightarrow \frac{1}{\sum_k \beta_*^\alpha(k) e^{-j\omega k}} = \frac{1}{\sum_{l \in Z} |\mathrm{sinc}(\frac{\omega}{2\pi} + l)|^{\alpha+1}}.$$

4. SPLINE FBP

Next, we show how to modify the standard FBP so that the filtered sinogram can be fitted using splines. We will first describe the general principle of the method and then derive the filters that combine the spline fitting process (e.g. interpolation) and the ramp filter in one step. We will consider three different approaches.

4.1. Spline-based FBP: general principle

Here, we assume that the projection data $p_\theta(x)$ is known in a continuous fashion for $x \in R$, but for a discrete set of N equidistant angles $\theta_i = i \cdot \pi / N$.

The first step is to filter the sinogram $\hat{p}_\theta(\omega)$ in the Fourier domain with the ideal ramp filter (see Section 2):

$$\hat{g}_\theta(\omega) = \hat{p}_\theta(\omega) \cdot \hat{q}(\omega).$$

The second step is to fit the sinogram with a model that is represented as a linear combination of shifted basis functions $\varphi(t - k)$ (e.g. B-splines):

$$\tilde{g}_\theta(t) = \sum_{k \in Z} c_\theta(k) \cdot \varphi(t - k). \tag{6}$$

Typically, we have that $c_\theta(k) = \langle \tilde{\varphi}(t - k), g_\theta(t) \rangle$, where $\tilde{\varphi}$ is a suitable analysis function that is biorthogonal to $\varphi = \beta^n$ as described elsewhere[7]. In our implementation, the $c_\theta(k)$'s will be computed from the $p_\theta(k)$'s by filtering in the Fourier domain using FFTs:

$$c_\theta(k) = (h * p_\theta)(k) \leftrightarrow H(e^{j\omega}) \cdot P_\theta(e^{j\omega}).$$

What will make the difference between the three methods below is the choice of the filter $h \leftrightarrow H(e^{j\omega})$.

The last step is to calculate the back-projection $R^*\{\tilde{g}_\theta(t)\}$ at the pixel location (x, y)

$$\tilde{f}(x, y) = \int_0^\pi \tilde{g}_\theta((x, y) \cdot \vec{\theta}) d\theta \cong \frac{\pi}{N} \sum_{i=1}^N \tilde{g}_{\theta_i}(x \cos \theta_i + y \sin \theta_i),$$

where the right-hand side is the Riemann-sum approximation of the back-projection integral. This approximation is justifiable as long as the number N of projections is sufficiently large (typ., twice the size of the image). The arguments of the sum are computed using the 1D spline interpolation model (6).

4.2. Ramp filter with B-spline prefilter

In the first method, we compute the B-spline coefficients $c_{\theta_i}(k)$ such that the function $\tilde{g}_\theta(t)$ interpolates the integer samples of the filtered sinogram. This involves the application of the digital interpolation filter (5), which can be merged with the ramp-filtering step of the algorithm.

Here, the basic assumption is that the sinogram is band-limited; in this case, the ramp-filtered sinogram is band-limited as well, and represented by its samples. Thus, to get the B-spline coefficients of the filtered sinogram, these samples needs to be filtered with the prefilter $\widehat{\Omega}_1(\omega)$:

$$\widehat{\Omega}_1(\omega) = 1/B^n(e^{j\omega}) = 1/\sum_{l \in Z} \left(\text{sinc}(\frac{\omega}{2\pi} + l) \right)^{n+1}. \tag{7}$$

We combine the prefilter $\widehat{\Omega}_1(\omega)$ with the ramp filter, and get the B-spline interpolating ramp filter

$$H_1(e^{j\omega}) = |\frac{\omega}{2\pi}| \widehat{\Omega}_1(\omega).$$

4.3. Ramp filter with oblique projection

Again, we assume that the sinogram is band-limited, which implies that the filtered sinogram is band-limited as well. Instead of B-spline interpolation, we use an oblique projection to get a continuous spline approximation of the sinogram. Because the computation needs to be performed in Fourier space, the projection is chosen to be perpendicular to the subspace of band-limited functions.

This projection can be derived as a direct application of Theorem 2 in the work of Unser and Aldroubi[8]. Specifically, the oblique projection of the filtered sinogram $g_\theta(t)$ is given by

$$\text{Proj}\{g_\theta(t)\} = \sum_{k \in Z} \underbrace{c_1 * (a_{12})^{-1}(k)}_{=c_\theta(k)} \cdot \beta^n(x - k),$$

where $c_1(k) = \langle g_\theta(t), \text{sinc}(t - k) \rangle \leftrightarrow |\frac{\omega}{2\pi}| P_\theta(e^{j\omega})$, and where a_{12} (the cross-correlation between the analysis and synthesis functions) is

$$a_{12}(k) = \langle \text{sinc}(x), \beta^n(x - k) \rangle$$

$$\leftrightarrow A_{12}(e^{j\omega}) = \sum_{k \in Z} \text{rect}(\omega + 2\pi l) \cdot \hat{\beta}^n(\omega + 2\pi k).$$

The effect of the rect function is to suppress aliasing so that we have

$$A_{12}(e^{j\omega}) = \hat{\beta}^n(\omega) \text{ for } -\pi \leq \omega \leq \pi.$$

Combining the ramp filter and the projection filter $A_{12}^{-1}(e^{j\omega})$ in the Fourier domain, we get the oblique B-spline ramp-filter

$$H_2(e^{j\omega}) = |\frac{\omega}{2\pi}|/\hat{\beta}^n(\omega) = |\frac{\omega}{2\pi}|/\text{sinc}^{n+1}(\frac{\omega}{2\pi}).$$

We can already predict that this projection approach will be better than the more standard interpolation described in Section 4.2. It is essentially equivalent to the least-squares solution: first, because it is guaranteed to be asymptotically optimal; and second, because the angle between the spline and the Sinc spaces is small, especially for higher degrees n.

Filters	Frequency response $H(e^{j\omega})$ for $0 \le \omega \le 2\pi$
Shepp–Logan[3]	$h_0(k) \leftrightarrow \lvert\omega/(2\pi)\rvert\mathrm{sinc}(\omega)$
Inter–polation	$h_1(k) \leftrightarrow \dfrac{\lvert\omega/(2\pi)\rvert}{B^n(e^{j\omega})} = \dfrac{\lvert\omega/(2\pi)\rvert}{\sum_{l\in Z}\mathrm{sinc}^{n+1}(\frac{\omega}{2\pi}+l)}$
Oblique	$h_2(k) \leftrightarrow \dfrac{\lvert\omega/(2\pi)\rvert}{\mathrm{sinc}^{n+1}(\frac{\omega}{2\pi})}$
Fractional	$h_3(k) \leftrightarrow \dfrac{\lvert 1-e^{j\omega}\rvert/(2\pi)}{B_*^\alpha(e^{j\omega})} = \dfrac{\lvert\sin(\omega/2)\rvert/\pi}{\sum_{l\in Z}\lvert\mathrm{sinc}(\frac{\omega}{2\pi}+l)\rvert^{\alpha+1}}$

Table 1: Modified ramp filters for splines. These filters project onto the B-spline space of degree n or $\alpha - 1$.

4.4. Ramp filter with fractional B-splines

In the two cases before (4.2 and 4.3), the band limitation assumption was necessary to justify the multiplication with the theoretical ramp filter $\lvert\frac{\omega}{2\pi}\rvert$ in the FFT domain. We now consider a third approach which does not require this hypothesis. The idea is to fit the sinogram with a fractional spline, and then determine the effect of the ramp filter analytically.

First, the unfiltered sinogram $p_\theta(t)$ is fitted using fractional B-splines of degree α:

$$p_\theta(t) = \sum_{k\in Z} d_\theta(k)\beta_*^\alpha(t-k). \tag{8}$$

This is achieved with the digital prefiltering technique described by (5).

Since the ramp filter corresponds to the fractional derivative operator D_*, we can use our theoretical formula (4) to differentiate (8) analytically. This allows to apply the ramp filtering step directly onto the fitted sinogram (8):

$$g_\theta(t) = D_*\{p_\theta(t)\}/(2\pi) = \sum_{k\in Z} c_\theta(k)\beta_*^{\alpha-1}(t-k), \tag{9}$$

which reduces the spline degree by one. We can obtain the spline coefficients $c_\theta(k)$ of the filtered sinogram in one step by applying a single digital filter which combines the fitting and finite differences operations:

$$c_\theta(k) = (h_3 * p_\theta)(k).$$

$$H_3(e^{j\omega}) = \frac{\lvert 1-e^{j\omega}\rvert/(2\pi)}{B_*^\alpha(e^{j\omega})} = \frac{\lvert\sin(\omega/2)\rvert/\pi}{\sum_{l\in Z}\lvert\mathrm{sinc}(\frac{\omega}{2\pi}+l)\rvert^{\alpha+1}}.$$

If the fractional spline degree α is even ($\alpha = 2, 4, \ldots$), then the B-spline in (9) will be of odd degree $\alpha - 1 = n = 1, 3, \ldots$, and the basis functions is compactly supported. This means that the same back-projection method as before is applicable.

5. RESULTS

The Shepp-Logan phantom[3] of size 128×128 was used as our test image. Its Radon transform was computed over $K = 256$ equidistant angles. Figures 1 and 2 display the reconstructed images (with details) and the errors for the three methods for linear and cubic degrees, respectively. The FBP reconstruction error with the Shepp-Logan filter and linear interpolation is 29.16 dB. With linear splines ($n = 1$), the FBP reconstruction errors are 30.98 dB (interpolation filter), 32.91 dB (oblique projection filter), and 33.10 dB (fractional derivative filter).

Filter type \ degree	$n = 1$	$n = 3$
Shepp-Logan	29.16	32.49
B-spline interpolation	30.98	34.69
Oblique projection	32.91	34.80
Fractional derivative	33.10	34.90

Table 2. FBP reconstruction error (PSNR given in dB) for different spline interpolating ramp filters with various interpolation degrees n. The image size is $N = 128$, the angular resolution is $K = 256$ and the sampling step on the sinogram is 1.

Note that the first case here also corresponds to the standard approach: Ram-Lak filter with linear interpolation since $B^1(e^{j\omega}) = 1$. With cubic splines ($n = 3$), the corresponding results are 32.49 dB (Shepp-Logan filter), 34.69 dB (interpolation filter), 34.80 dB (oblique projection filter), and 34.90 dB (fractional derivative filter). See Table 2.

When looking at the error images, the edges are sharper for the interpolation filter and more diffuse for the oblique projection. Remember that the less visible the error, the better the result. The fractional derivative filter is slightly better than the two others. These results demonstrate that there is a clear improvement when using ramp filters that adapt to the interpolation method. Further, it appears that the optimization of the filter is especially useful when the interpolation model is low. This is especially interesting for applications where computational speed is a key issue.

6. CONCLUSION

We compared three different versions of the filtered back-projection based on spline interpolation. The first approach uses interpolation combining the ramp and direct B-spline filter in to a single FFT filtering operation. The second implements an oblique projection of the sinogram into a spline space. It outperforms the first by up to 2 dB, because it better takes into account the band-limited nature of the sinogram. The third filter is based on an explicit discretization using fractional splines. The advantage is that the ramp-filtering of the sinogram produces a spline of reduced degree, which leads to an implementation perfectly coherent with the underlying model. This yields another gain in quality for the same computational cost.

In conclusion, for low interpolation degrees ($n = 1$) we recommend to use either the method based on the oblique projection or fractional splines in order to achieve a quality improvement of up to 2.5 dB. Switching to higher degree—cubic instead of linear—pays off by an additional 2-4 dB in all three cases, but the quality differences between the methods are less significant.

A software demo (JAVA applet) of the methods developed in this paper is available at:
`http://bigwww.epfl.ch/demo/jtomography/`

REFERENCES

1. D. Ludwig, "The Radon transform on Euclidean space," *Comm. Pure and Appl. Math.*, vol.19, pp.49-81, 1966.
2. G. N. Ramachandran and A. V. Lakshminarayanan, "3D reconstructions from radiographs and electron micrographs: Appl. of convolution instead of Fourier trans.," *Proc. Nat. Acad. Sci.*, vol.68, pp.2236-40, 1971.
3. L. A. Shepp and B. F. Logan, "The Fourier reconstruction of a head section," *IEEE Trans. Nucl. Sci.*, vol.21, pp.21-43, 1974.
4. E. H. W. Meijering, "Spline Interpolation in Medical Imaging: Comparison with other convolution-based approaches," *EUSIPCO*, vol. 4, pp. 1989-1996, 2000.
5. P. Thévenaz, T. Blu, M. Unser, "Interpolation revisited," *IEEE Trans. MI*, vol. 9, no. 17, pp. 739-758, 2000.
6. M. Unser, T. Blu, "Fractional Splines and Wavelets," *SIAM Review*, vol. 42, no. 1, pp. 43-67, March 2000.
7. M. Unser, "Sampling—50 Years After Shannon," *Proceedings of the IEEE*, vol. 88, no. 4, pp. 569-587, 2000.
8. M. Unser, A. Aldroubi, "A general sampling theory for nonideal acquisition devices", Signal Processing, IEEE Trans. on Signal Processing, vol. 42, no. 11 , pp. 2915-2925, Nov. 1994.
9. M. Unser, "Splines: A Perfect Fit for Signal and Image Processing," *IEEE Signal Processing Magazine*, vol. 16, no. 6, pp. 22-38, Nov. 1999.

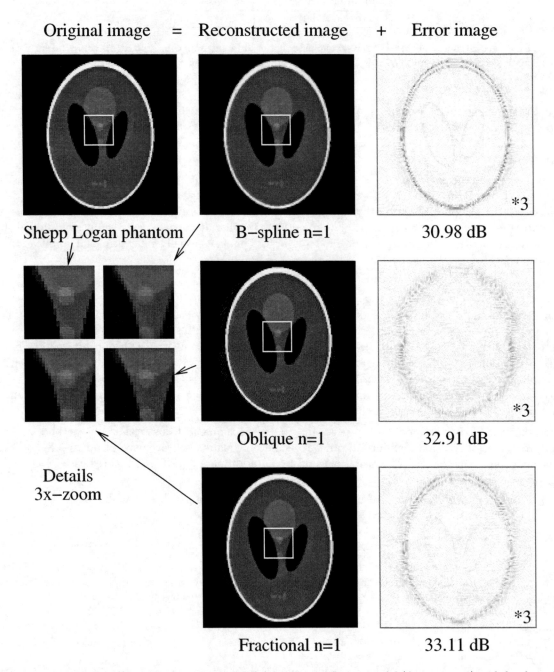

Original image = Reconstructed image + Error image

Shepp Logan phantom

B–spline n=1

30.98 dB

Details
3x–zoom

Oblique n=1

32.91 dB

Fractional n=1

33.11 dB

Figure 1. Results of Spline-filtered back-projection with linear interpolation model (degree $n = 1$) and the three different ramp filters. To highlight differences, the absolute error images have been amplified by a factor of 3.

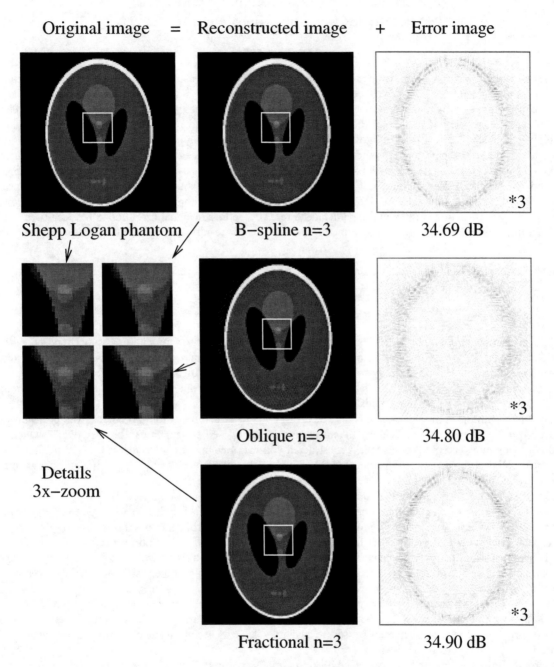

Figure 2. Results of Spline-filtered back-projection with cubic interpolation model (degree $n = 3$) and three different ramp filters. To highlight differences, the absolute error images have been amplified by a factor of 3.

A new method for 3D reconstruction in digital tomosynthesis

Bernhard E.H. Claus[*], Jeffrey W. Eberhard
General Electric Company, Global Research Center

ABSTRACT

Digital tomosynthesis mammography is an advanced x-ray application that can provide detailed 3D information about the imaged breast. We introduce a novel reconstruction method based on simple backprojection, which yields high contrast reconstructions with reduced artifacts at a relatively low computational complexity. The first step in the proposed reconstruction method is a simple backprojection with an order statistics-based operator (e.g., minimum) used for combining the backprojected images into a reconstructed slice. Accordingly, a given pixel value does generally not contribute to all slices. The percentage of slices where a given pixel value does not contribute, as well as the associated reconstructed values, are collected. Using a form of re-projection consistency constraint, one now updates the projection images, and repeats the order statistics backprojection reconstruction step, but now using the "enhanced" projection images calculated in the first step. In our digital mammography application, this new approach enhances the contrast of structures in the reconstruction, and allows in particular to recover the loss in signal level due to reduced tissue thickness near the skinline, while keeping artifacts to a minimum. We present results obtained with the algorithm for phantom images.

Keywords: Tomosynthesis, 3D reconstruction, order statistics, contrast enhancement, artifact reduction, mammography

1. INTRODUCTION

In standard projection radiography one sees in a single image the "structures of interest" superimposed with other, "interfering" structures that are located at a different height within the imaged object. Depending on the particular structure of the object, this problem may represent a significant obstacle in obtaining a clear interpretation of x-ray radiographs, and potentially prevents the detection of lesions, etc. This problem of superimposed (or encompassing) tissue is the main reason why cancers are missed in mammography[1].

The aim of tomosynthesis is the three-dimensional reconstruction of structures within an object from projection images acquired from different viewpoints. Thereby the interfering superimposed structures can be "removed", which enables easy and non-ambiguous interpretation of the reconstructed volume, thus making it easy to identify structures within the imaged object. Digital tomosynthesis mammography addresses the problem of overlying tissue, and has therefore the potential to significantly improve sensitivity and specificity in mammography.

In digital tomosynthesis, generally only a small number of digital projection radiographs are acquired, typically with a relatively small angular range. Therefore, image reconstruction represents a difficult limited-angle tomography problem. One of the most frequently used reconstruction methods is the simple backprojection (or shift-and-add) algorithm, which is the digital equivalent to the image formation process in conventional motion tomography[2,3]. The simple backprojection algorithm is popular because it is computationally fast and straightforward to implement. To reconstruct a single horizontal slice (parallel to the detector plane) one just needs to appropriately shift and add (or average) the set of projection images.

However, simple backprojection reconstructions exhibit "streak artifacts", that are generated when a high-contrast structure in a projection image is backprojected (i.e., "smeared" across) the imaged volume, thereby creating a "streak" in the reconstruction. These artifacts can be severe and may lead to a significant reduction in the quality and the diagnostic value of the reconstructed images.

Furthermore, if some structure within the imaged object is relatively small, then this structure suffers from a significant loss in contrast (compared to its "true" 3D contrast) in both the projection images and the reconstruction. This effect also manifests itself when a non-constant pathlength through the imaged object leads to a variation in gray-level, which does not correspond to varying object composition, but only to varying object shape or geometry. In mammography, the

---

[*] claus@crd.ge.com; phone 1 518 387 6260; fax 1 518 387 5975; General Electric – Global Research Center, One Research Circle, Niskayuna, NY 12309

Medical Imaging 2002: Image Processing, Milan Sonka, J. Michael Fitzpatrick, Editors, Proceedings of SPIE Vol. 4684 (2002) © 2002 SPIE · 1605-7422/02/$15.00

compressed breast is essentially of constant thickness, but we have a substantial variation in thickness near the skinline of the breast which leads to a significant variation in signal level which is not due to varying composition of the breast. The corresponding decrease in gray level cannot be recovered by simple backprojection reconstruction.

In this paper, we introduce a new reconstruction algorithm, which has the simple backprojection at its basis, but addresses both problems of the simple backprojection reconstruction: artifacts and loss of contrast.

The new reconstruction technique is based on the observation that simple backprojection with an order statistics-based operator (e.g., minimum) used for combining the backprojected images can significantly reduce streak artifacts. This approach represents the initial step in our new reconstruction algorithm, and is discussed in Section 3, after introducing mammographic tomosynthesis in Section 2. This first reconstruction step alone, however, does not enhance the contrast in the reconstructed volume. In a second step, which is introduced in Section 4, one uses information collected during the first step to "enhance" the projection images, and then repeat the order statistics based reconstruction using the enhanced images as input. We demonstrate the applicability of the presented approach to reconstruction of breast phantoms from limited-angle tomosynthesis projection data, and present results in Section 5.

In mammography, the breast can be viewed as consisting of high contrast structures embedded in a low-contrast "background". The order statistics operator used in this framework is essentially a minimum operator, and is therefore efficient in eliminating streak artifacts caused by calcifications, or radiographically dense glandular tissue. For other applications, other order statistics operators (e.g., median) may be more suitable. In our digital mammography application, this new approach allows in particular to recover the loss in contrast due to reduced tissue thickness near the skinline, while keeping skinline and other artifacts to a minimum. It also exhibits relatively low computational cost and memory requirements.

2. DIGITAL MAMMOGRAPHIC TOMOSYNTHESIS

In our experiments, a number of projection radiographs of the imaged object were acquired for different projection angles within a relatively narrow angular range of about 30 degrees.

In mammography, the breast is generally compressed between a radiolucent compression paddle and the detector cover, i.e., the volume of interest is the volume between the compression paddle and the detector cover, and the thickness of imaged tissue can be assumed to be constant in a significant portion of the projection image, with the exception of the regions close to the skinline (in the projection images). The compressed thickness (i.e., the height of the compression paddle above the detector cover) is assumed to be known. Typical values for breast imaging lie in the range of 4-7 cm. The x-ray dose in our acquisition protocol was set to be about 1.5 times the standard dose for a digital mammogram.

A digital projection radiograph represents essentially at each pixel the value $I \cdot e^{-\int \mu(s)ds}$, where I denotes the signal level observed with no imaged object being present, and the integral is the line-integral of the local linear attenuation value of the tissue along the path of the corresponding ray through the imaged object. The value I is systematically varying as a function of the location on the detector as well as the tube position, due to effects like varying distance to the x-ray source, and incident angle of the x-rays at detector. We performed a preprocessing of each image, including correction for these geometric effects, taking the log, and correcting for varying pathlength through an object of constant thickness, such that in the corrected images each pixel value corresponds to the average attenuation along the path of the ray. After the pre-processing step, the signal values at any given pixel in the resulting images correspond to the average linear attenuation value along the corresponding ray path for an assumed object of known, fixed, thickness. See Figure 1 for an illustration. Scatter can represent a significant fraction of the signal, and should ideally also be removed from the signal[4], but we did not perform this correction here.

Once the volume of interest is reconstructed, the dataset is usually displayed either slice by slice, by volume rendering[5], or using other display techniques. In this paper we present the results as images of reconstructed slices.

When reconstructing a single slice through the imaged volume, which is here always assumed to be parallel to the detector, the simple backprojection translates into a shift, scale (to counteract magnification in cone beam imaging) and add/average operation. I.e., by appropriately shifting and scaling the different projection images, the features corresponding to structures located at a given height above the detector can be aligned, and subsequent averaging yields an image where the features of that slice appear with the same contrast as they appear in the projection images, while features corresponding to structures from slices at other heights are decreased in contrast (as their backprojections don't line up). This is illustrated in Figure 2(a). Obviously, the above-mentioned streak artifacts caused by high contrast structures in the projection images manifest themselves in a reconstructed slice as several repeated low contrast copies of that structure, the so-called out-of-plane artifacts. If the volume of interest (VOI) is partitioned into a set of N equally spaced slices, then we can denote by

$$P^{(j)}(\bar{x}) = \frac{1}{N} \cdot \sum_{i=1}^{N} O(x_i^{(j)}) \tag{1}$$

the projection image (after preprocessing) of imaged object O at detector location $\bar{x}$, where $j \in \{1,...,M\}$ denotes the respective tube position, and x_i denotes the location of the intersection of the corresponding ray-path j with slice i (recall that the projections were normalized to reflect the average linear attenuation along the ray). The simple backprojection reconstruction now reads

$$\tilde{S}(x) = \frac{1}{M} \cdot \sum_{j=1}^{M} P^{(j)}(\bar{x}^{(j)}) . \tag{2}$$

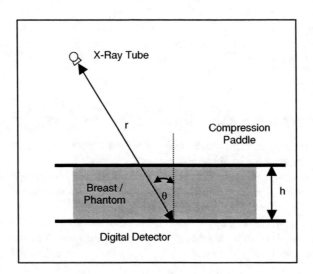

Figure 1: The signal at the detector is of the form $I_0 \cdot \frac{1}{r^2} \cdot \cos\theta \cdot e^{-\bar{\mu}\frac{h}{\cos\theta}}$, where r denotes the distance from the tube, h denotes the height of the imaged object, and θ denotes the incident angle. The value $\bar{\mu}$ denotes the average linear attenuation along the ray-path. After preprocessing, the projection image values reflect this average attenuation coefficient $\bar{\mu}$ at each pixel.

3. ORDER STATISTICS BASED BACKPROJECTION

To minimize streak artifacts caused by high intensity (high attenuation) structures one can replace the averaging operator, used in simple backprojection to combine pixel values in backprojected images, by a minimum operator. Intuitively, the motivation for using this order statistics operator can be illustrated by the following "voting" interpretation of the reconstruction of "structures" embedded in a transparent background. Here every pixel value of a backprojected image represents a vote for "structure present" or "no structure present". Obviously, even if at a given location only a single backprojection clearly indicates "no structure present", then the reconstruction should be "no structure present", in spite of the fact that all other backprojections may indicate "structure present". Correspondingly, by using the minimum operator instead of the averaging operator, one can minimize the effect of high contrast structures "bleeding" into their respective background. Examples of this type of artifact in mammographic tomosynthesis include streak artifacts from calcifications, or artifacts at the air/tissue interface (i.e., tissue "bleeding" into the background/air) near the skinline. The effect of using the minimum operator instead of the averaging operator is illustrated in Figure 2 (b).

There is, however, a tradeoff between the number of backprojected images contributing to the reconstructed slice, and the noise characteristics of the reconstruction. In order to retain some of the noise minimizing effects of the averaging operator, it may be advantageous to average all but the K largest values at any given pixel. Also, to eliminate a strong impact by small signal value outliers that are caused by noise, the minimum itself (or even the L smallest values) may also not be taken into account, which now leads us to the general order statistic filters (OS filters, or L-filters[6,7]). Obviously, these modifications due to noise management requirements may increase the level of artifacts somewhat over the achievable optimum. Using the same notation as in (2), the order statistics-based reconstruction can be written

$$\tilde{S}(x) = \frac{1}{(M-L-K)} \cdot \sum_{j=L+1}^{M-K} P^{(\tilde{j})}(\overline{x}^{(\tilde{j})}) \,, \qquad (3)$$

where $\tilde{j}$ denotes a permutation of j such that $P^{(\tilde{j})}(\overline{x}^{(\tilde{j})}) \le P^{(\tilde{j}+1)}(\overline{x}^{(\tilde{j}+1)})$.

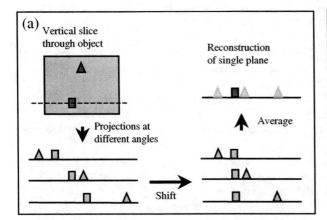 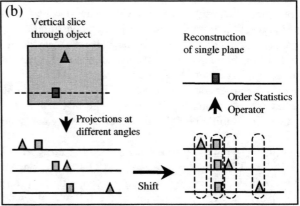

Figure 2: (a) Illustration of simple backprojection, or "shift-and-add" reconstruction of the horizontal slice containing the structure indicated by the square. One can see how the structure indicated by the square appears with the same contrast as it appears in the projection images, while the triangle appears as three low-contrast copies, although this structure is in fact not present in this slice. (b) Use of a suitable order statistics operator eliminates in this example the out-of-plane artifacts, i.e., the low-contrast copies of the structure represented by the triangle.

This order statistics-based backprojection reconstruction approach is especially well-suited for mammography. The breast consists essentially of high-attenuation structures, e.g., calcifications, which are typically very small, with a very high attenuation value, and non-fatty tissue (which includes glandular tissue as well as cancerous tissue), embedded in a low-attenuation background consisting of fatty tissue. Furthermore, the breast itself can be viewed as a high-attenuating object, embedded in a low-attenuating background, namely air. Due to this specific structure, some "minimum-type" operator as defined in (3) is ideally suited to combine backprojected mammographic projection images. For other applications[8], other operators from order statistics (maximum, median, different L-filters, etc.) may be more appropriate.

The order statistics-based reconstruction approach presented in this section prevents high contrast structures from bleeding into the background, but it does not recover a loss in contrast, which will be addressed in the next section.

4. NEW METHOD FOR 3D RECONSTRUCTION

3.1 Motivation

A projection image (after preprocessing) is essentially the average of (scaled and shifted copies of) horizontal slices through the object. Assuming only a small high contrast structure located within an otherwise homogeneous object, most of these slices have an essentially constant profile, with only few slices showing the high contrast structure. Therefore, already the projection image exhibits a potentially significant relative reduction in the contrast of the imaged high contrast structure, because the relative contrast of the structure in the projection is the average of the contrast in all contributing slices. For example, for an imaged object composed of N thin slices containing a high-contrast structure at only one slice, the contrast of that structure in the projection is 1/N of the true 3D contrast.

The simple backprojection reconstruction does not recover this loss in contrast, because it consists essentially of taking the average of the (scaled and shifted) projection images, thereby not increasing the contrast. The re-projection consistency constraint states that the gray-value at any given pixel of a projection image is equal to the average of gray-values along the path of the corresponding ray through the reconstructed volume. Simple backprojection from a single image satisfies this constraint by distributing the pixel values and the contrast of a structure equally across the reconstructed slices (note that this is generally only true for backprojection reconstruction from a single image).

The order statistics-based reconstruction method also does not enhance the contrast of reconstructed structures when compared to the projection images, but it does eliminate artifacts created by out-of-plane structures. Here, however, pixel values are not equally distributed across reconstructed slices. This applies in particular to pixels corresponding to high-contrast structures, the values of which are either relatively large (or relatively small), and therefore contribute only to a fraction of reconstructed slices. Consequently, the contrast of structures in the reconstruction needs to be enhanced in order to meet the re-projection consistency constraint.

The idea to accomplish this is to replace all values in the projection images that correspond to (small) structures in the object, by "suitably enhanced" values, and then performing an order statistics-based reconstruction. In one example, one may replace a large value with an even larger value. This will not have an impact on the reconstruction at "background locations": the order statistics operator, which ignored the initial value, will also ignore the new value. However, because all values corresponding to a given structure in the object underwent a similar enhancement, the reconstruction of the structure will exhibit an enhanced contrast – even when some of the enhanced values are ignored by the order statistics operator.

How do we determine the "suitably enhanced" values? If we assume that the initial reconstruction of the "background" is already good, but that now the contrast of structures needs to be enhanced, one can use the following strategy. Note that we consider for this argument only a single pixel corresponding to some structure in the imaged object. The initial order statistics-based reconstruction of the full volume will give us as a by-product a partition of the slices into a set where a structure was present (on the ray-path corresponding to the considered pixel) defined by the set of slices where the considered pixel-value was taken into account, and a set where no structure was present. The reconstruction of the background in slices where "no structure was present" gives us an estimate of a partial ray-sum, which, together with the partial ray-sum of the "structure present" slices must add up to the corresponding value in the projection image, i.e., must satisfy the re-projection consistency constraint. This condition allows us to determine an estimate of what the value in the "structure present" locations should be. This is exactly the value that we choose as our "suitably enhanced" value. In the subsequent reconstruction step, due to the order statistics operator, this enhanced value is not taken into account when reconstructing "background", but potentially enters in the reconstruction of structures, which now exhibit a higher contrast.

Note that this approach does not rely on a pre-determined classification of "structure" and "no structure" pixels in the projection images, but can be applied directly using only information on the location of slices where a pixel value was not taken into account in the first reconstruction, as well as the associated partial ray-sum.

3.2 Overview of the method

We give here a more formal presentation of the reconstruction strategy. Let us denote by

$$P(\overline{x}) = \frac{1}{N} \cdot \sum_{i=1}^{N} O(x_i)$$

the projection image of imaged object O at detector location $\overline{x}$, where x_i denotes the location of the intersection of the corresponding ray-path with slice i. Note that this notation does not reflect that fact that we have set of several projection images. The VOI (defined by the maximum thickness of the imaged object, given by the height of the compression paddle) is partitioned into a set of N equally spaced slices. Let $S(x_i)$ and $R(x_i)$ denote the initial order statistics-based, and the final reconstruction, respectively.

The present algorithm consists of a sequential processing of the data, where in a first step an order statistics-based reconstruction of the full volume of interest (VOI) is performed, according to equation (3). In this first step, at each location in the volume, the backprojected values of some projection images are ignored, while the others are taken into account. For every given location $\overline{x}$ in a projection image, with associated value $P(\overline{x})$, one collects now the set of slices where that value did not contribute, $\kappa \subset \{1, \dots, N\}$. The re-projection consistency constraint for the ray-sum of the final reconstruction can now be written

$$P(\overline{x}) = \frac{1}{N} \cdot \sum_i R(x_i) = \frac{1}{N} \cdot \sum_{i \in \kappa} R(x_i) + \frac{1}{N} \cdot \sum_{i \notin \kappa} R(x_i). \tag{4}$$

Obviously, one can view this expression as the sum of a partial ray-sum across the slices where a structure associated with the current pixel $\overline{x}$ is assumed to be present, and a partial ray-sum over the "background" (i.e., the slices in κ). Now, according to the argument that the order-statistics based reconstruction minimizes artifacts due to high-contrast structures bleeding into the background, the order statistics-based reconstruction of the background can be assumed to represent a good estimate of the 3D structure of the background, i.e., we have the approximation

$$\sum_{i \in \kappa} R(x_i) \approx \sum_{i \in \kappa} S(x_i). \tag{5}$$

That is, an estimate of the partial ray-sum corresponding to background is already available after the order statistics-based reconstruction step. Based on the pixel value $P(\overline{x})$ (which is given by the projection image), and the partial ray-sum (5), which can be determined from the first reconstruction step, one can derive from the re-projection consistency constraint (4) what the value of the partial ray-sum $\sum_{i \notin \kappa} R(x_i)$ should be. This value, which we denote by $\widetilde{P}(\overline{x})$, then replaces the original value $P(\overline{x})$ in the projection image. In particular, from (4), (5) it follows that

$$\widetilde{P}(\overline{x}) = \frac{N}{\text{card}(\kappa)} \cdot \left(P(\overline{x}) - \frac{1}{N} \sum_{i \in \kappa} S(x_i) \right), \tag{6}$$

where card(κ) is the cardinality of the set κ (i.e., the number of elements in the set κ). Using the enhanced projection images $\widetilde{P}(\overline{x})$ as input, the order statistics-based reconstruction is repeated, yielding a reconstruction with enhanced contrast.

In summary, one performs an initial order statistics-based reconstruction of the full VOI, and then generates the enhanced projection images $\widetilde{P}(\overline{x})$ using equation (6), followed by a repeat of the order statistics-based reconstruction process, using the enhanced images $\widetilde{P}(\overline{x})$ as input.

If some value which is due to noise or some other spurious effect (and not due to a high contrast structure within the imaged volume) has been enhanced in the first part of the previously described process, then this value will not be taken into account in the subsequent reconstruction, as a consequence of the order statistics characteristic of the nonlinear reconstruction algorithm, which minimizes the occurrence of high contrast artifacts.

The initial nonlinear reconstruction process followed by the update of the projection images leads to modified versions $\widetilde{P}(\overline{x})$ of the projection images where the contrast of structures has been enhanced to a value which corresponds to the estimated actual contrast of that structure within the imaged volume. As such, the modified projection images can already be considered to be "enhanced" projection images, where for example the contrast of small structures within the imaged object is enhanced, and signal level variations due to the varying thickness of the imaged tissue at the skinline are reduced significantly.

3.3 Practical considerations in the implementation of the algorithm
In practice, the initial reconstruction of the volume is performed slice by slice, and no reconstructed slice needs to be stored in memory. For every projection image one uses two auxiliary images of the same size, one of which is used to

incrementally generate the partial ray-sum corresponding to background (i.e., the sum $\sum_{i \in \kappa} S(x_i)$), while the other tracks the number of slices where each pixel did not contribute (i.e., the expression card(κ)). These images can then be used to compute the enhanced projection images $\tilde{P}(\overline{x})$ using equation (6).

Note that, unlike iterative approaches like ART, for example, at no time in the reconstruction procedure do we need to store the full reconstructed volume. In addition, although our approach involves two reconstruction steps, we don't need to compute the re-projection of the initially reconstructed volume.

Furthermore, for the initial reconstruction of the volume the reconstructed slices do not necessarily need to be spaced such that any small structure will in fact be reconstructed. The contrast enhancement of small structures hinges on the fact that these structures are identified as "artifacts" in a significant fraction of the reconstructed slices, and therefore this enhancement will be effective through the fact that the small structures are identified as artifacts in most (or even all) slices, even when these slices are widely spaced.

Due to the noise propagation properties of the present algorithm, and also the computational effort and memory requirements, it may be advantageous to separate each of the projection images into a coarse scale image (which can be downsampled) and a detail image. Then the present reconstruction method can be applied to the coarse scale and the detail images separately, and the results can then be combined in an appropriate fashion. Alternatively, the coarse scale image can be enhanced according to our strategy, and then the detail image (multiplied with an appropriate constant factor) can be added to the enhanced coarse scale image. The resulting enhanced projection images are then used as input for the final order statistics-based reconstruction step. The results in this paper have been generated using this strategy.

Furthermore, although the previous discussion may suggest that the enhancement of contrast is effective for structures that have a higher signal level than the background, it is of course also effective for the enhancement of structures with a lower signal level than the background. A slightly different behavior of the present algorithm with respect to these different scenarios can be achieved by choosing the order statistics operator in the reconstruction process accordingly.

5. RESULTS

In our experiments we used a CIRS breast phantom[9] containing a number of structures at a fixed height. The structures include line pair targets, hemispheric masses, small calcium carbonate grains simulating calicifications, and fibers, all in varying sizes or diameters. In addition, the phantom contains a ring structure, and a step wedge. The phantom has a thickness of 4.5 cm, and has rounded edges. All attenuation parameters are in the range that can be expected in mammographic imaging. A simple backprojection reconstruction of the center slice of the phantom is shown in Figure 3, together with an indication of the respective positions of different embedded structures.

A tomosynthesis projection dataset was acquired, consisting of 11 projection radiographs. After pre-processing of the 11 projections, a reconstruction of the imaged volume was performed. With a total number of 11 projections, we used here $K = 4$ and $L = 2$ (see equation (3)), i.e., the 4 largest and the 2 smallest values were ignored when combining the backprojected images. In the initial order-statistics based reconstruction a total of 5 slices was reconstructed, with a slice separation of 10mm.

The results are shown in Figures 4 and 5. In particular, the reconstructions shown in Figure 4 correspond to the center slice of the phantom, while the reconstructions shown in Figure 5 correspond to a slice close to the compression paddle, about 22 mm above the center slice. In each Figure the top-left image shows the result of the initial order statistics-based reconstruction, the bottom left image shows the final, contrast-enhanced reconstruction result. These reconstruction images are all displayed with the same gray-scale setting, for easy comparison. In addition, the top-right image shows the difference between simple backprojection reconstruction, and order statistics-based reconstruction. It is obvious from this difference image in Figure 4, that for example the ring structure loses some of its contrast in the order statistics-based reconstruction, when compared to the simple backprojection. This effect is due to the nonlinear operator. However, the positive effect of that operator with respect to streak artifact suppression is obvious in Figure 5, where it is clearly visible in the top-right image how the "bleeding" of the ring structure into the background is efficiently suppressed, as is the bleeding of the phantom into the background (visible here as the dark region at the skinline of the phantom). The bottom-right image in both Figure 4 and Figure 5 shows the difference between the final "contrast enhanced" reconstruction result and the result of the order statistics-based reconstruction. In Figure 4 it is obvious how the contrast of many structures in the phantom was enhanced, including the ring structure, the masses, fibers, and the step-wedge. It is also obvious here, and even more so in Figure 5, how the signal level inside the phantom, near the skinline, was enhanced. The present algorithm is thus efficient in enhancing the contrast of reconstruction images, while suppressing some of the artifacts (note, for example, that there are no noticeable streak artifacts due to the ring structure in the final reconstruction, as can be seen in Figure 5). However, some of the artifacts from the line pair target seem to be more pronounced in the final reconstruction, than, for example, in the order statistics-based reconstruction.

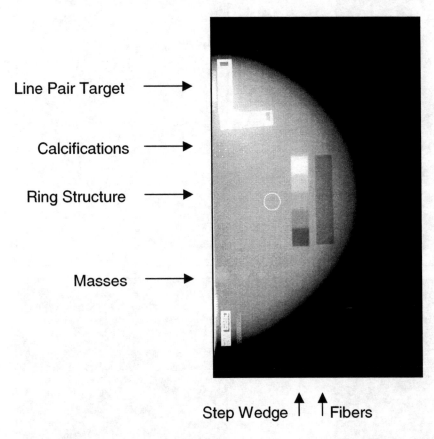

Figure 3: Simple backprojection reconstruction of the central slice of the breast phantom, and illustration of the position of the embedded structures. Due to the gray-scale settings for optimal display of the structures within the phantom, and the reduced thickness of the phantom near the "skinline", the region near the skinline is not visible here.

6. CONCLUSIONS

The present algorithm is efficient in enhancing the contrast of reconstruction images, while suppressing some of the artifacts due to high contrast structures in the imaged object. However, more work is needed to optimize the image quality of the reconstructions.
Although a two-step approach, the algorithm does not require re-projection of the reconstructed volume, or even storing the full reconstructed dataset, and is thus computationally efficient.

ACKNOWLEDGMENTS

This work was supported by the Office of Naval Research under Grant Number MDA905-00-1-0041.

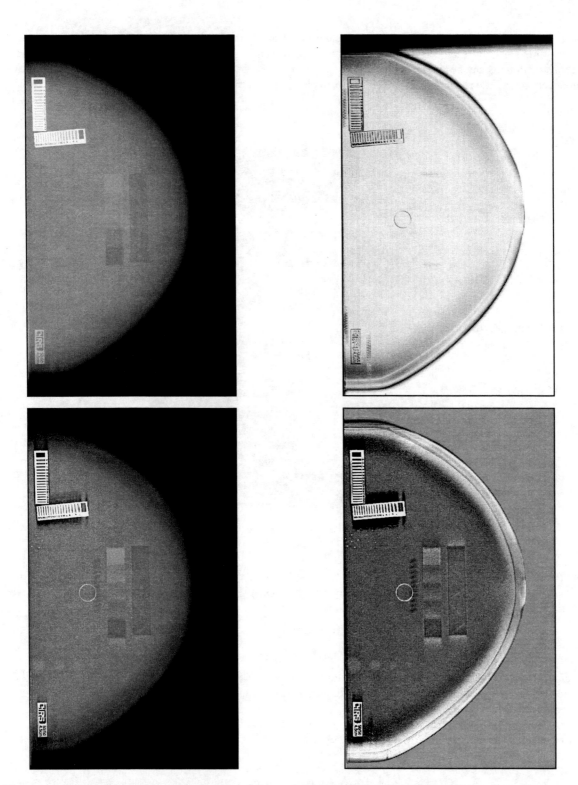

Figure 4: Order-statistics based reconstruction of central slice of phantom (top-left), and reconstruction from enhanced projection images (bottom-left). The top-right image shows the difference between simple backprojection and order statistics-based reconstruction, the bottom-right image shows the difference between order statistics-based and final reconstruction. The removal of artifacts, and the enhanced contrast in the reconstruction are clearly visible.

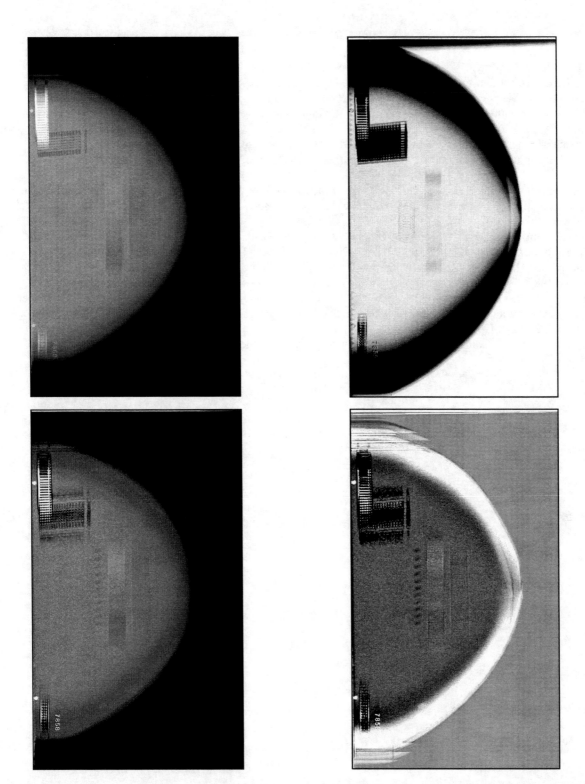

Figure 5: Order-statistics based reconstruction of slice about 22mm above center slice (top-left), and reconstruction from enhanced projection images (bottom-left). The top-right image shows the difference between simple backprojection and order statistics-based reconstruction, the bottom-right image shows the difference between order statistics-based and final reconstruction. The removal of artifacts, and the enhanced contrast in the reconstruction are clearly visible.

REFERENCES

1. L. Ma, E. Fishell, B. Wright, W. Hanna, S. Allan, N.F. Boyd: "Case-Control Study of Factors Associated with Failure to Detect Breast Cancer by Mammography", J. Natl. Cancer Inst., 1992; 84:81-785.

2. W.J. Meredith, J.B. Massey, *Fundamental Physics of Radiology*, John Wright & Sons, Bristol, England, 1977.

3. D.G. Grant, "Tomosynthesis: A Three-Dimensional Radiographic Imaging Technique", *IEEE Trans. on Biomed. Eng.*, **BME-19**, no.1, 20-28, 1972.

4. D.E. Gonzalez-Trotter, J.E. Tkaczyk, B.Claus, J. Kaufhold, J.W.Eberhard, "Thickness_dependent Scatter Correction Algorithm for Digital Mammography", *Medical Imaging 2002: Physics of Medical Imaging*, Proc. SPIE **4682**, 2002.

5. A.M. Alyassin, "Automatic Transfer Function Generation for Volume Rendering of High Resolution X-Ray 3D Digital Mammography", *Medical Imaging 2002: Visualization, Image-Guided Procedures, and Display*, Proc. SPIE **4681**, 2002.

6. H.G. Longbotham, A.C. Bovik, "Theory of Order Statistic Filters and Their Relationship to Linear FIR Filters", *IEEE Trans. Acoust. Speech, Signal Proc.*, **37**, no. 2, 275-287, February 1989.

7. S.A. Kassam, and H.V. Poor, "Robust Techniques for Signal Processing: A Survey", *Proceedings of the IEEE*, **73**, no. 3, March 1985.

8. U. Ewert, V.A. Baranov, and K. Borchardt: "Cross-Sectional Imaging of Building Elements by new Non-Linear Tomosynthesis Techniques Using Imaging Plates and ^{60}Co-Radiation", NDT&E International (Elsevier Science Ltd.), **30**, no.4, 243-248,1997.

9. CIRS-Breast Phantom – Computerized Imaging Reference Systems, Inc., 2428 Almeda Ave., Suite 212, Norfolk, VA 23513, USA.

Image reconstruction using shift-variant resampling kernel for magnetic resonance imaging

Ahmed S. Fahmy, Bassel S. Tawfik, Yasser M. Kadah[*]

Biomedical Engineering Department, Cairo University, Giza, Egypt

ABSTRACT

Nonrectilinear k-space trajectories are often used in MRI applications due to their inherent fast acquisition and immunity to motion and flow artifacts. In this work, we develop a more general formulation for the problem of resampling under the same assumptions as previous techniques. The new formulation allows the new technique to overcome the present problems with these techniques while maintaining a reasonable computational complexity. The image space is decomposed into a complete set of orthogonal basis functions. Each function is sampled twice, once with a rectilinear trajectory and the other with a nonrectilinear trajectory resulting in two vectors of samples. The mapping matrix that relates the two sets of vectors is obtained by solving the set of linear equations obtained using the training basis set. In order to reduce the computational burden at the reconstruction time, only a few nonrectilinear samples in the neighborhood of the point of interest are used. The proposed technique is applied to simulated data and the results show a superior performance of the proposed technique in both accuracy and noise resistance and demonstrate the usefulness of the new technique in the clinical practice.

Keywords: Resampling, image reconstruction, magnetic resonance imaging, least-squares problems.

1. INTRODUCTION

In Magnetic Resonance Imaging (MRI), data is collected in the k-space which represents the Fourier transform of the imaged slice. The sampling trajectory along the k-space is determined by the shape of the waveform of the applied magnetic gradients. On-Off gradient waveforms result in evenly spaced k-space samples which can be easily transformed into the image domain using the fast Fourier transform (FFT). Unfortunately, generation of fast switching gradients is not easily accomplished. Thereby smoothly varying gradient waveforms are usually implemented in fast MRI acquisition techniques. However, this results in non-rectilinear sampling trajectories with a multitude of loop-like patterns such as spiral[1,2], radial sampling[2], Rossettes[3], or Lissajous[4]. Such data points must be resampled onto a rectilinear grid in order to take advantage of the speed of the FFT.

Ideal reconstruction is theoretically guaranteed by the sampling theory as long as the Nyquist criterion is satisfied [5,6]. That is, if $f(k)$ is the continuos k-space representation of the imaged slice at a spatial frequency coordinate k, and $S(k-k^r)$ is a sampling function consisting of 2-dimensional evenly spaced impulse functions located at the rectilinear k-space points, k^r, the sampling theory guarantees that $f(k)$ can be completely recovered from its sampled version $f_s(k) = f(k).S(k-k^r)$ as follows[5],

$$f(k) = f_s(k) * C(k) \quad , \tag{1}$$

where $C(k)$ is an infinite Sinc function, and $*$ is the convolution operator. Since working with an infinite sinc function is not feasible in practice, truncating the Sinc function is necessary. Substituting $k=k^{nr}$, where k^{nr} is the non-rectilinear k-space grid coordinates and assuming (without loss of generality) that both the rectilinear and the non-rectilinear grids carry the same number of points ($=N$), then equation (1) can be written in vector form as follows:

$$f^{nr}_{Nx1} = C_{NxN} f^r_{Nx1} \quad , \tag{2}$$

where f^r, and f^{nr} are vectors containing the rectilinear and the non-rectilinear samples, respectively, while C is a matrix whose entries are $Sinc(k^r-k^{nr})$. In the Uniform Re-Sample algorithm (URS)[4], f^r is directly obtained from f^{nr} by inverting

---

[*] E-mail: ymk@ieee.org

the matrix C in equation (2). While such matrix inversion can be directly achieved for one-dimensional signals, the URS algorithm becomes impractical in the 2-dimensional signals due to the huge size of the matrix C in this case.

The Block Uniform Re-Sampling algorithm (BURS)[7,8] was introduced by way of approximation to the URS method in order to reduce the computational effort. The BURS algorithm is in essence a numerical method for obtaining the inverse of a large sparse matrix. It is based on isolating a small block, C^b_{mxq}, of the matrix C centered at entries (i,j), where j represents an unknown point in f^r, which is to be estimated from m measured non-rectilinear samples centered around the entry i in f^{nr}. The block is assumed to reasonably approximate the entire mapping (2) for the unknown point j. Next, the inverse of the matrix C is obtained, namely C^{b-1}, of which one row corresponding to the sample j is kept. This row is used later, during image reconstruction, to estimate the rectilinear sample j from the selected few measured samples. This process is repeated for the entire points in f^r. This method does not guarantee the best available estimate of the resampling process. Moreover, unreasonable estimates of the rectilinear points may be obtained when Lissajous trajectories are used to acquire the k-space as pointed out by Moriguchi, et al [4].

In the conventional gridding algorithm[5,6], the measured samples are convolved with a small shift-invariant interpolation kernel, usually a Kaiser-Bessel function, to estimate the rectilinear k-space grid. Steps of pre and post compensation of the data are required to reduce certain artifacts inherent to the technique such as cupping or wings[7]. But the main concern in conventional gridding is that the Kaiser-Bessel function is not optimal in the least squares sense, which was shown by Sedarat, et al.[9]. In an attempt to overcome this problem, a methodology was devised to obtain the optimal kernel and showed that it can be shift-variant. However, this method is not readily applicable to high-resolution images because of the associated intensive calculations.

In this paper, we present a new method for estimating of shift-variant resampling kernels that map the non-rectilinear samples to their rectilinear counterparts. Each sample on the rectilinear grid is estimated from its neighboring sampling on the non-rectilinear grid using a least squares criterion. We present the mathematical formulation of the proposed method as well as the results of the implementing the proposed technique compared to those of URS and BURS techniques.

2. THEORY

Estimating a point, p, on the rectilinear grid from m sampled (non-rectilinear) points can be represented as

$$p = a_{1xm} \cdot p_{mx1} \quad , \tag{3}$$

where p is a vector containing the m neighboring samples of the point p. For this equation to correctly represent the required mapping from the nonrectilinear grid to the rectilinear one, it should be valid for the k-space of any given image. In other words, if $\Phi = \{ \phi_i, i=1:L \}$ represents a basis (continuous) functions for the imaged field of view (FOV), then equation (1) should be valid for every ϕ_i. Rewriting (1) for the given set of the basis functions yields the following set of linear overdetermined system of equations,

$$\varphi = a \cdot \phi_i \qquad , i=1:L \quad , \tag{4}$$

where φ_i is a sample on the rectilinear grid representation of the basis function ϕ_i, and ϕ_i is a k-space vector of m neighboring samples on the non-rectilinear grid. In vector form, the equations in (2) can be written as

$$\varphi_{1xL} = a_{1xm} \cdot \Phi_{mxL} \qquad , \tag{5.a}$$

or,

$$a = \varphi \cdot \Phi^{\dagger} \qquad , \tag{5.b}$$

where Φ is a matrix whose columns are the vectors ϕ_i, and $\Phi^{\dagger}$ is its pseudo-inverse given by $\Phi^T \cdot (\Phi \cdot \Phi^T)^{-1}$. The matrix inverse involved in this pseudo-inverse does not represent a computation burden since $(\Phi \cdot \Phi^T)$ is an mxm matrix (usually $m=9$ to 25). A mapping vector a is calculated for every point on the rectilinear grid. That is, equation (5.b) is solved N^2

times for image size of $N \times N$. We will call this least-squares resampling based on spatially variant kernel *LR-based* sampling throughout this paper.

3. RESULTS AND DISCUSSION

3.1   One Dimensional Results

The LR-based estimate of the gridding kernel is used to reconstruct 1-dimension signals of finite extent. The functions, ϕ_i, are complex exponentials representing the Fourier transform of spatial domain impulses spanning the entire field of view (fig. 1). In our 1-dimensional simulations, a sampling scheme of the k-space is used such that the sampling density is an integral multiple, referred to as the *density factor* hereon, of the Nyquist sampling rate. The locations of the measured samples, x_i, are given by $x_i = i + r$, where i is a location in the rectilinear grid, and r is a random number such that $|r| < 0.5$. The case where the entire set of non-rectilinear samples is used to estimate each rectilinear point ($m = L$) is considered first followed by the case where ($m << L$).

In the first case ($m = L$), It was found that both the LR-based and the URS techniques give the same results (error below 0.5%), which means that the LR-technique reaches the optimal solution in this case. Interesting results are obtained when the same simulation settings is used but with the sampling trajectory misses one sample. Figures 2.a,b show the reconstruction of the two techniques when the sample at spatial frequency $k = 0.7\pi$ is missed (entry 16 in f^{nr}). In Figure 2.a, the signal reconstructed by the LR-based technique overlaps the true signal. At the same time, the URS result suffers artifacts due to the violation of the sampling theorem at certain region in the k-space. These results were obtained without introducing any regularization techniques when obtaining the URS or the LR-based mapping matrices. It was found that truncation of some singular values of the Sinc interpolation matrix used in the URS technique improves the reconstruction yet the LR-based technique is still better (see Figure 2.b). The mapping matrices for both techniques in this case are shown in Figure 3. The effect of varying the location of the missed sample is shown in Figure 4, where the reconstruction error is plotted for both BURS and LR-based algorithms when the location of the missed sample varies from $\pi/16$ to π.

The second case ($m << L$), is practically a typical case since the target is to reduce the reconstruction time. In the BURS algorithm, the block matrix C^b, of dimension $m \times q$, represents a k-space region of size $\delta k \times \Delta k$. This means that m varies from place to another inside the k-space according to the sampling density. In our simulation, m is fixed and the sampling density is made variable. This means that the reconstruction time, which depends on m rather than δk, is fixed allover the k-space regardless what the sampling density is. Moreover, all of the BURS simulations given below use a value of Δk equal ∞ to obtain the best results for BURS.

Table 1 shows the reconstruction error of both the BURS and LR-based techniques at different sampling densities and different values for δk. The reconstruction error of both techniques in the presence of noise is shown in Figure 5.

3.2.   Two Dimensional Results

In this section, the LR-based technique is used to reconstruct images acquired using polar trajectories. The images are for numerical phantom and each is of resolution 128×128. For each sampling trajectory, a number of sample locations, $m = 16$, nearest to each rectilinear point is calculated and stored in a look-up table. The table is used first to construct the required optimal mapping, which is stored also in another table to be used in the resampling process. The number of basis functions used to construct the mapping is taken to be 128^2 thereby, cover the entire FOV with the specified spatial resolution. Calculating the mapping matrix takes about 3.5 hours on a personal computer with PII 400MHz processore and 192 Mbytes of RAM. Image reconstruction takes about 2 seconds on the same workstation (resampling process plus Fourier transformation). Figure 6 shows the LR-based reconstruction in case of polar acquisition of a numerical phantom (Figure 6.b) compared with Fourier reconstruction when rectilinear acquisition is used (Figure 6.a). Cross sectional profiles in the images in Figure 6 are plotted in Figure 7, where we observe that the results from the new method and that of the true almost match each other.

Although the URS algorithm was usually thought of as the perfect resampling algorithm, the results in the previous section indicate that this is not true for all sampling schemes. To demonstrate this, consider the trivial case of resampling data points from a rectilinear grid to the same rectilinear grid. In this case, the samples of the Sinc function used in the URS algorithm, i.e. the rows of the C matrix in (2), will take unity value at one location corresponding to the row index and zeros in the rest. Therefore, C is an identity matrix of size NxN. If one sample is missing from the measurements, the corresponding column in the C matrix is also missed turning the problem into an underdetermined system of equations. Therefore, the obtained solution is the minimum norm solution, and in the above case the missing sample will be substituted for by zero. On the other hand, the proposed method still provides the least squares solution for the same problem. That is, when the mapping is being established by equation (5), the problem is still over-determined because the basis vectors outnumber the grid points, i.e. the number of columns in matrix Φ is larger than the number of rows. This conclusion can also be illustrated by examining the mapping matrices in Figure 3, where the mapping matrices are shown to be band-limited in general. Nonetheless, when a sample is missing, the URS matrix ignores its absence while the proposed method matrix tries to estimate it based on the larger set of the non-rectilinear samples. Moreover, regularization techniques should be used for the URS algorithm to give acceptable reconstruction results. It was found that the regularization depends on the location where the sample is missing and since many samples are expected to be missing in practical situations, it might be difficult to achieve reasonable regularization.

As mentioned earlier, the main concern in any resampling or gridding algorithm is to reach optimal reconstruction meanwhile maintain the reconstruction time at low limit. The proposed method in this work establishes a mapping between each rectilinear point and a given finite number of neighboring points on the non-rectilinear grid. For each rectilinear point, the mapping is not restricted to certain functional form, instead, it is determined through an optimization process based on a least squares error criterion. Consequently, the obtained mapping is shift-variant which is apparent clearly in Figure 3. This result contradicts with the thoughts involved in the current resampling algorithms, which rely mainly on the convolution with a shift-invariant kernel (e.g., Sinc, Kaiser-Bessel, etc.). However, a work of Sedarat et al.[9] showed that the optimal mapping can be shift-variant but the methodology used to obtain such mapping requires intensive computations and thus not readily applicable to high-resolution images. Moreover, although our simulations show that the mapping is complex, we can observe that the reconstruction error when ignoring the imaginary part is almost the same. This approximately halves the computational time of the resampling process and reduces the memory size required for storing the mapping matrix.

From Table 1, it is obvious that the reconstruction error of the LR-based technique is lower than that of the BURS technique especially at small values of δk (the smaller the values of δk, the lower the reconstruction time and memory requirements). At large values of δk, e.g. 2.5, the performance of both techniques is nearly the same. Unexpectedly, there is a rise in the reconstruction error at $\delta k = 1.5$ this is because this result is given by using only three non-rectilinear samples to estimate each rectilinear point.

Finally, although the described LR-based algorithm is applied to resample the data from a non-rectilinear grid to rectilinear one, it can be used to establish mapping between arbitrary grids by changing the locations of the samples in the two vectors f^r, and f^{nr} in equation (2). The proposed LR-algorithm achieves the required mapping on one step only. This is faster than the method proposed by Rasche et al.[10], which requires a two-step convolution interpolation.

4. CONCLUSIONS

In this work, a least squares error solution is developed to resample data points from a non-rectilinear grid into a rectilinear grid. The results of this work show that the URS algorithm is not the optimal method in the least squares sense when the sampling density decreases below the Nyquist limit. The proposed technique, on the other hand, is superior in the least squares sense regardless of the sampling pattern. Moreover, the proposed algorithm does not restrict the mapping to be shift-invariant or real valued which allows more freedom to achieve optimality. Future work includes the potential of the new method to be extended for use in extrapolation besides interpolation or resampling.

REFERENCES

1. E. Haacke, R. W. Brown, M. R. Thompson, and R. Venkatesan, *Magnetic Resonance Imaging: Physical Principles and Sequence Design*, John Wiley & Sons, New York, 1999.
2. C. H. Meyer, B. S. Hu, D. G. Nishimura, and A. Macovski, "Fast spiral coronary artery imaging," *Magnetic Resonance in Medicine*, vol. 28, pp 202-213, 1992.
3. D. C. Noll, S. J. Peltier, and F. E. Boada, "Simultaneous Multislice Acquisition Using Rosette Trajectories (SMART): A New Imaging Method for Functional MRI," *Magnetic Resonance in Medicine*, vol. 39, pp. 709-716, 1998.

4. H. Moriguchi, M. Wendt, and J. L. Duerk, "Applying the Uniform Resampling (URS) algorithm to Lissajous trajectory: Fast image reconstruction with optimal gridding," *Magnetic Resonance in Medicine*, vol. 44, pp 766-781, 2000.

5. J. I. Jackson, C. H. Meyer, D. G. Nishimura, and A. Macovski, "Selection of a convolution function for Fourier inversion using gridding," *IEEE Trans. Medical Imaging*, vol. 10, no.3, pp. 473-478, Sept. 1991.

6. J. D. O'Sullivan, "A fast sinc function gridding algorithm for Fourier inversion in computer tomography," *IEEE Trans. Medical Imaging*, vol. 4, no. 4, pp. 200-207, 1985.

7. D. Rosenfeld, "An optimal and efficient new gridding algorithm using singular value decomposition," *Magnetic Resonance in Medicine,* vol. 40, pp 14-23, 1998.

8. H. Moriguchi, and J. L. Duerk, "A modified block uniform resampling (BURS) algorithm using truncated singular value decomposition: fast gridding with noise reduction," *Proc. International Society of Magnetic Resonance in Medicine*, Glasgow, 2001.

9. H. Sedrat, and D. G. Nishimura, "On the optimality of the gridding reconstruction algorithm," *IEEE Trans. Medical Imaging*, vol. 19, no.4, pp. 306-317, April 2000.

10. V. Rasche, R. Proska, R. Sinkus, P. Bornert, and H. Eggers, "Resampling of data between arbitrary grids using convolution interpolation, *IEEE Trans. Medical Imaging*, vol. 18, no. 5, pp. 385-392, May 1999.

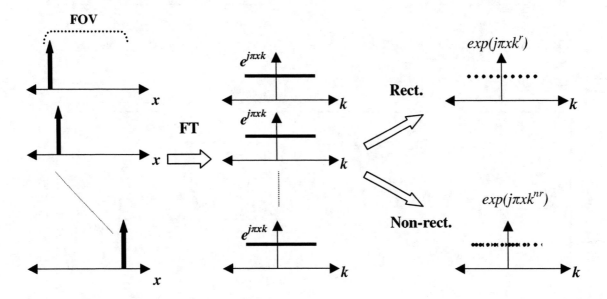

Figure 1. The basis set used in the LR equations are the Fourier transforms of impulse functions spanning the field of view. Note that the magnitude of the functions φ_i are the same and equal to unity while the phase (not shown) depends on the location of each impulse, x.

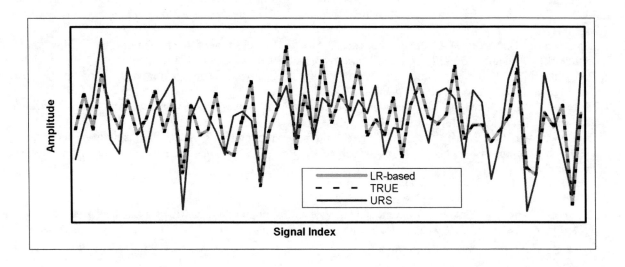

Figure 2.a Reconstruction using URS versus LR-based technique, both are without regularization.

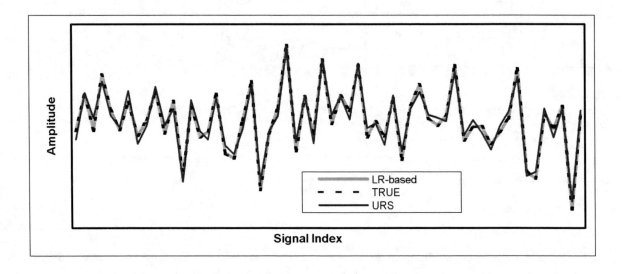

Figure 2.b Reconstruction using URS (with regularization) versus LR-based technique.

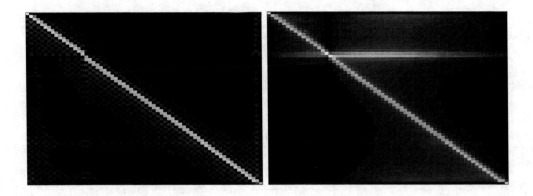

Figure 3. The mapping matrix of the URS (left) and LR-based technique (right). Note the difference at row number 16, where the trajectory has missed a k-space sample.

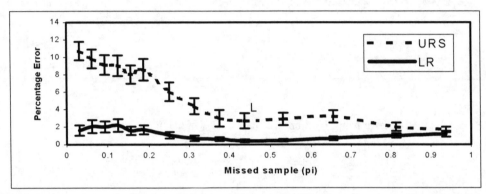

Figure 4. Reconstruction error using URS and LR-based algorithms when the missed sample varies from $\pi/16$ to π.

Density Factor	8	8	10	8	6	4	2	8	2
# Points, m	5	7	11	9	7	5	3	13	5
Corresponding δk	.625	.875	1.1	1.125	1.167	1.25	1.5	1.625	2.5
LR-based	3.5%	3%	0.6%	.56%	.47%	0.78%	9.5%	0.23%	0.6%
BURS (Δk=∞)	17.5%	14.1%	11.9%	11.8%	9.7%	3.3%	10.2%	2%	0.8%

Table 1. Reconstruction error of both LR-based and BURS techniques at different sampling densities and different values for *m*.

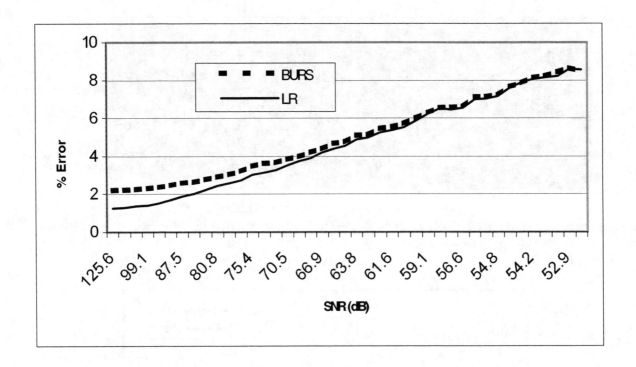

Figure 5. Reconstruction error using URS and LR-based algorithms in presence of noise.

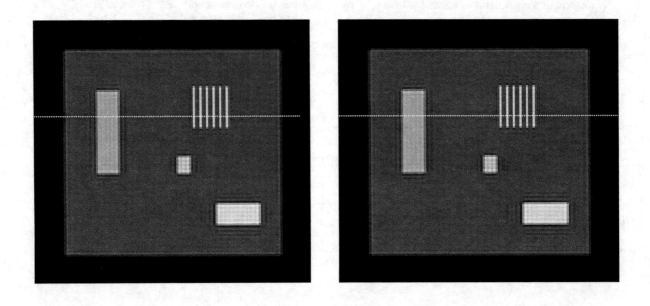

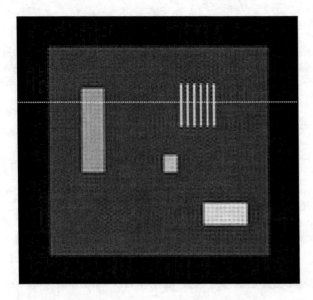

Figure 6. Phantom image when acquired using rectilinear trajectory (a), and when acquired using polar trajectories and reconstructed using LR-based and BURS algorithms in (b), and (c) respectively.

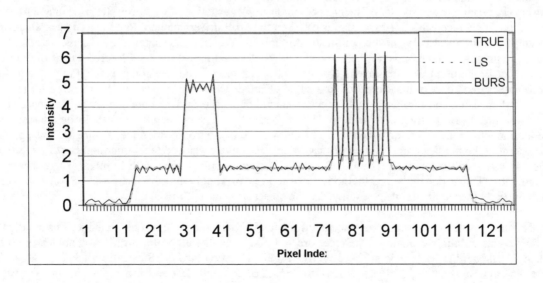

Figure 7. Cross-sectional profiles of the images in Figure 6 at the level of the dotted white line. It is shown that the LR-based reconstructed image coincides with the true one.

A study of the effect of reconstruction parameters on defect detection in fan-beam SPECT

George K. Gregoriou

Department of Computer and Electronics Engineering, Intercollege, CYPRUS

ABSTRACT

The effect of reconstruction parameters on the fan-beam filtered backprojection method in myocardial defect detection was investigated using an observer performance study and receiver operating characteristics (ROC) analysis. A mathematical phantom of the human torso was used to model the anatomy and Thallium-201 (Tl-201) uptake in humans. Half-scan fan-beam realistic projections were simulated using a low-energy high resolution (LEHR) collimator that incorporated the effects of photon attenuation, spatially varying detector response, scatter, and Poison noise. A focal length of 55 cm and a radius of rotation of 25 cm were used, which resulted to a magnification of two at the center of rotation and a maximum magnification of three in the reconstructed region of interest. By changing the reconstruction pixel size, five different projection bin width to reconstruction pixel size (PBWRPS) ratios were obtained which resulted in five classes of reconstructed images. Myocardial defects were simulated as Gaussian-shaped decreases in Tl-201 uptake distribution. The total projection count per 3 mm image slice was 44,000. A total of 96 reconstructed transaxial images from each one of the five classes were shown to eight observers for evaluation. The results indicate that the reconstruction pixel size has a significant effect on the quality of fan-beam SPECT images. Moreover, the study indicated that in order to ensure best image quality the PBWRPS ratio should be at least as large as the maximum possible magnification inside the reconstructed image array.

Keywords: single photon emission computed tomography, fan-beam filtered backprojection, reconstruction pixel size, myocardial defect detection, observer performance study

1. INTRODUCTION

Converging-hole collimators, enhance the trade-off between spatial resolution and detection efficiency that limits the single photon emission computed tomography (SPECT) images. Data obtained from such collimators have to be reconstructed using converging backprojectors. The most common implementation of backprojector used in a fan-beam filtered backprojection (FBP) reconstruction algorithm is based on the pixel-driven method. Pixel-driven backprojectors trace a ray passing from the focal point of the collimator through the center of the pixel to be reconstructed to the projection plane. The pixel is assigned a value that is obtained by interpolating between the filtered values of the two projection bins nearest to the point of intersection. This type of backprojectors must include a weighting factor for each pixel to account for the effect of magnification and angle of incidence of the converging beam geometry [1, 2]. More importantly, when using the fan-beam backprojectors one should take into account the magnification of the system when determining the reconstruction pixel size. The convergent projections magnify objects by an amount that depends on the focal length of the collimator, the radius of rotation, and the source location (see Figure 1). Thus, pixels close to the focal point of the fan-beam undergo larger magnifications and are mapped to a larger number of projection bins than pixels close to the collimator face. The use of a large reconstructed pixel size results in images of low contrast and signal to noise ratio. This is due to the fact that in reconstructing a pixel only information from two projection bins is used, although the pixel (depending on its position inside the object) may have contributed to a larger number of bins.

The work described in [3] evaluates the statistical uncertainties (standard deviations) in reconstructed regions of interest directly from the projection data. By changing the reconstructed pixel size, the algorithm in [3] was implemented in order to calculate the standard deviations in a 20x20 cm (see Figure 1) region for PBWRPS ratios of 1, 2, 3, 4, and 5. The reconstructed arrays were 64x64, 128x128, 192x192, 256x256, and 320x320 and the regions of interest were adjacent square arrays of dimensions 1x1, 2x2, 3x3, 4x4, and 5x5 for the ratios of 1, 2, 3, 4, and 5, respectively. This way, 64x64 standard deviation images resulted for each one of the five ratios. Figure 2 shows these images together with a reconstructed image of the actual activity distribution for comparison. Notice the resemblance of the standard deviation images to the actual reconstructed image slice. The standard deviation images (b-f) look like blurred versions

Medical Imaging 2002: Image Processing, Milan Sonka, J. Michael Fitzpatrick,
Editors, Proceedings of SPIE Vol. 4684 (2002) © 2002 SPIE · 1605-7422/02/$15.00

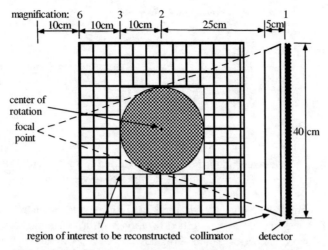

Figure 1. The fan-beam geometry used in the experiment.

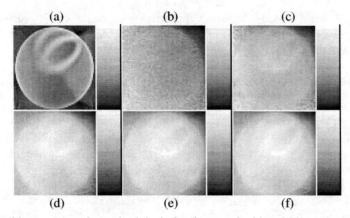

Figure 2. The reconstructed image (a) and standard deviation images for bin width to pixel size ratios of 1 (b), 2 (c), 3 (d) , 4 (e), and 5 (f). Each image from (b) to (f) has been individually scaled in order to show the resemblance to (a).

of the reconstructed image slice (a). The same behavior was also observed in a study reported in [4] where noise properties of filtered backprojection reconstructed images were investigated. Bear in mind, though, that each picture in Figure 2 was individually scaled in order to emphasize the correlation of the images to the object. In absolute terms, the variation in the standard deviation throughout each one of the images is small. The standard deviation is in the order of ~8 % higher in the myocardium than in the background. In order to make a quantitative assessment of the errors associated with reconstructed images of different PBWRPS ratios, average standard deviations were calculated from pixels in a disk of radius 25 pixels (surrounding the myocardium) for each one of the images shown in Figure 2 (b) - (f). The resulting average standard deviations are shown in Figure 3. The average standard deviation falls dramatically as the pixel size decreases (or as the PBWRPS ratio increases), followed by a less significant decrease and finally it falls asymptotically to a minimum. In other words, the signal to noise ratio increases asymptotically as the pixel size decreases. This interesting result motivated me to perform an observer performance study to test whether this trend in the signal to noise ratio results in a similar trend in the observer performance study.

The goal of this work was to study the effect of the reconstruction pixel size in the pixel-driven fan-beam FBP method through the use of a human observer performance study and ROC analysis. Specifically, for a simple detection task the specificity and sensitivity of SPECT images obtained with different reconstruction pixel sizes was evaluated. In order to obtain images necessary for the observer performance study, a three-dimensional (3D) mathematical phantom that realistically models the anatomy and uptake of Tl-201 in the myocardium and other organs was used. Computer-generated projection data, which included the effects of photon attenuation, spatially-varying system geometric response, photon scatter, and Poisson distributed random noise were simulated and reconstructed with five different

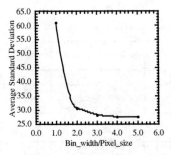

Figure 3. The average standard deviation obtained from a circular disk
with a radius of 25 pixels for the different PBWRPS ratios.

reconstruction pixel sizes. The reconstructed images were used in observer studies where the observers specified their degree of confidence that a defect was present at a specified location within the myocardium. Since the presence or absence of a defect was known a-priori, the performance of the observers was evaluated by an ROC methodology [5, 6].

2.   METHOD

In this section the mathematical phantom used in the study is described, the method with which realistic projection data were obtained is explained, the way in which the SPECT images were reconstructed and prepared for display is shown, and the design and conduction of the observer experiments and ROC analysis are discussed.

2.1 The mathematical cardiac torso (MCAT) phantom

The 3D MCAT phantom [7] was modified and used to define the Tl-201 uptake distribution and photon attenuation in the different organs. Both the Tl-201 activity distribution and the linear attenuation coefficients were digitized into 128x128x128 matrices with $3.1x3.1x3.1 \ mm^3$ cubic voxels. For this study four transaxial slices, spaced 12.5 mm apart, were selected in the myocardium. In each slice a total of eight possible defect sites were chosen, avoiding the area where the two ventricles meet. Eight different defect sets have been used in this study, resulting in as many phantoms with defects. On a specific phantom only a set of four defects was placed, one on each slice, and at such positions so as to avoid crosstalk between defects [7]. The defects were modeled as 3D Gaussian-shaped decreases in myocardial uptake of activity distribution. The standard deviation of a defect was 0.65 cm. A phantom with no defects was also generated to simulate a defect-free situation.

2.2 Simulating realistic SPECT projection data

Projection data which included the effects of photon attenuation, 3D spatially-varying geometric response, scatter and Poisson noise were simulated. A LEHR collimator was used which had a spatial resolution of 14 mm at 25 cm from its face. A 40 cm large-field-of-view (LFOV) scintillation camera with 4 mm intrinsic resolution was simulated. Half-scan projections were obtained over 180° plus the fan angle with the center-of-rotation (COR) and the focal point at 25 cm and 55 cm from the collimator face, respectively (see Figure 1). Thus, a total of 78 projection views were simulated, from 52° right anterior oblique (RAO) to 75° left posterior oblique (LPO). The projection bin size for the 40 cm camera was 3.1 mm.

Using the 3D MCAT phantom, noise-free projections were simulated that included the effects of attenuation and detector response. Projection data of the myocardium without defects, the defects, and the other organs in the torso were obtained separately. The projection data obtained from the defects and the heart were then combined, as shown in Figure 4 (left). In order to obtain areas under the ROC curves in the desirable range of 0.75 - 0.85 [6], a contrast of 80% was used in this study. The defect contrast was adjusted by varying the magnitude of the Gaussian distribution. The effects of scatter response function were incorporated by convolving each one of the 2D projection views by a series equivalent scatter response function (SRF). The SRF for each angle was calculated separately for the heart and the torso at the water equivalent depth of their center of mass [7]. The projection data for the heart and the torso were then combined and scaled so that the total number of counts over all projection views in a 3 mm slice resembled clinically obtained counts of 44,000. Lastly, Poisson noise was added to the projections in order to simulate experimentally obtained data (Figure 4 (right)).

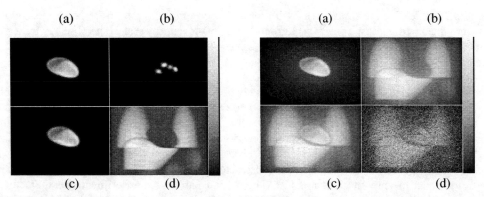

Figure 4. Left: Anterior projection view which includes the effect of 3D detector response and attenuation: heart (a), defects (b), heart and defects with a contrast of 0.8 (c), and torso (d). Right: Anterior projection view which includes photon scatter: heart with defects (a), torso (b), heart with defects and torso combined (c), and with simulated Poisson noise added (d).

For each one of the eight different phantoms that included defects in four slices, two noisy sets of 78 projections were generated in 128x128 matrices. Thus, a total of sixteen projection data sets were simulated with defects. Similarly, sixteen noisy projection sets were obtained for the defect-free phantom. The same projection data sets were reconstructed using five different PBWRPS ratios. This resulted in five different classes of images. The projection data sets provided a total of 128 noisy reconstructed images for each class, half of which contained a defect and half of which did not. Furthermore, the noise-free projection data (eight with defects and one without) were reconstructed using a PBWRPS ratio of 3 and were used in training the observers.

2.3 Obtaining the reconstructed SPECT images

Whereas the geometry used resulted in a magnification at the COR of two, the reconstructed region of interest (ROI) (a 20x20 cm square including the myocardium as shown in Figure 1) had a maximum magnification of three along its side closest to the focal point. Five different PBWRPS ratios were used: 1, 2, 3, 4 and 5. In order to accomplish this, the same projection data were reconstructed by the pixel-driven FBP algorithm [8] with pixel sizes of 1, 1/2, 1/3, 1/4, and 1/5 times the bin width. The corresponding array sizes were 64x64, 128x128, 192x192, 256x256, and 320x320, respectively. The reconstructed slices were then collapsed into 64x64 arrays by summation, post-filtered with a 2D Butterworth filter of order 8 and a cut-off frequency of 0.4 cycles/cm in order to suppress high frequency noise, and masked to remove the ring artifact in the reconstructed image due to the truncated projections. Subsequently, the individual slices were extracted from the reconstructed phantoms and extrapolated to 256x256 arrays. With this array size, the images occupied about 8x8 cm^2 on the display monitor. Before the reconstructed images were displayed for the observer study, the pixel values were normalized and converted to displayed intensities. The normalization was important in order to control the effects of noise fluctuations on observer performance.

2.4 Observer experiment and ROC analysis

For the observer performance experiment, the observers were shown transaxial reconstructed image slices from the five classes of images obtained with the five different reconstructed pixel sizes shown in Table 1. Half of the images contained a myocardial defect and half were defect-free. The task of the observer was to indicate his/her confidence in

Table 1. The five classes of images used in the observer study.

Class #	PBWRPS ratio	Reconstructed array size	Reconstructed pixel size (cm)
1	1	64x64	0.3125
2	2	128x128	0.1562
3	3	192x192	0.1042
4	4	256x256	0.0781
5	5	320x320	0.0625

detecting a defect in a specified location indicated by a cross. The observer sessions were performed in a darkened room. The images were displayed against a black background in a 256-level gray scale. The observer indicated his/her confidence level by the position selected on a continuous scale. The area under the ROC curves (A_z) was used for comparing the five classes of images.

A total of 128 reconstructed images from each class were evaluated half of which contained a defect. A subset of 32 images from each class was used for training the observers. The remaining 96 images were split into two blocks of 48 images (resulting to ten blocks) for the observer study. The observer session consisted of two parts. During the first part, 16 training images from each class were shown to the observers to familiarize them with the characteristics of the images and also the experimental procedure [6]. After the observers had indicated their certainty with which they detected a defect at a specified location, the noise-free reconstructed image corresponding to that slice was presented, together with the truth about the presence of a defect. The second part of the experiment was the actual observer performance test. The ten blocks of images from the different classes and the ordering of images within each block were randomized for different observers. This was done to eliminate any reading order effect [6]. This way, each observer viewed a different mix of image blocks and a different ordering of images. A smaller training set consisting of eight images was shown before each test block of images.

Eight observers participated in this study: 5 medical imaging scientists experienced in observer experiments and three graduate students in biomedical engineering. A total of 640 images had to be evaluated - 128 for each class. On the average, the study required about two 50-minute sessions. The software package described in [9] was used for the ROC analysis of the experimentally obtained data. Statistical tests were performed to evaluate the differences between the average ROC curves obtained from all eight observers. The null hypothesis (H_0) that the average areas under two ROC curves (A_z) were the same was tested against the alternative hypothesis (H_a) that they were different. Specifically, a two-tailed paired Student's t-test was used to test the null hypothesis that the difference in the average areas under the ROC curves obtained from two different classes was zero, against the alternative hypothesis that this difference was non-zero. Since the average areas were calculated from all observers, seven degrees of freedom (df) resulted for the t-test. The test was applied pairwise on the five different classes of images, i.e. a total of 10 comparisons were performed. In addition, 95% confidence intervals around the sample mean differences were also calculated. Finally, the associated P-values for each possible comparison were calculated.

3. RESULTS

The areas under the ROC curves along with the averages over the observers and the associated standard deviations are shown in Table 2. Figure 5 shows the ROC curves averaged over all observers. The areas under the average ROC curves are 0.5899, 0.8011, 0.8421, 0.8540, and 0.8487 for ratios of 1, 2, 3, 4, and 5, respectively. Thus, a large improvement is seen in going from a ratio of 1 to a ratio of 2 and a smaller one in going from 2 to 3. An insignificant improvement is seen in going from 3 to 4. Finally, an insignificant deterioration can be seen in further decreasing the pixel size from a ratio of 4 to a ratio of 5. Table 3 shows the Student's t-statistic obtained from a paired two-tailed t-test where the null hypothesis is that the difference in the area is zero. The corresponding P-value and the associated 95% confidence interval around the difference is also shown for each pair of classes being compared. The null hypothesis that the area under the curve is the same (i. e. the difference is zero) can be rejected at the levels of significance of less than 0.001 for the image class pairs (1,2), (1,3), (1,4), (1,5), (2,3), (2,4), (2,5), 0.085 for (3,4), 0.058 for (3,5) and 0.262 for (4,5). Thus, at the 0.01 significance level the defect detectability improves by decreasing the pixel size from a ratio of 1 to 2 and from 2 to 3, but doesn't significantly change by a further decrease.

Table 2 . Area under the ROC curves for the observers.

Class #	Observer # :								Average A_z index	Standard deviation
	1	2	3	4	5	6	7	8		
1	0.5565	0.5941	0.5750	0.5903	0.5994	0.6056	0.5823	0.6159	0.5899	0.0066
2	0.7930	0.8045	0.8080	0.8196	0.7975	0.8055	0.7870	0.7936	0.8011	0.0037
3	0.8349	0.8414	0.8499	0.8452	0.8285	0.8602	0.8417	0.8219	0.8421	0.0048
4	0.8418	0.8364	0.8644	0.8587	0.8364	0.9042	0.8382	0.8650	0.8540	0.0083
5	0.8262	0.8425	0.8548	0.8763	0.8393	0.8631	0.8446	0.8427	0.8487	0.0055

Table 3. Two-tailed t-test of observer data.

Classes being compared	Difference in the average A_z	Standard deviation of the difference	t-statistic (7 df)	P-value (7 df)	95 % confidence interval
1 Vs 2	- 0.2112	0.0204	- 29.3120	< 0.0010	(- 0.22826, - 0.19414)
1 Vs 3	- 0.2523	0.0245	- 29.0810	< 0.0010	(- 0.27278, - 0.23180)
1 Vs 4	- 0.2641	0.0235	- 31.7800	< 0.0010	(- 0.28375, - 0.24445)
1 Vs 5	- 0.2588	0.0200	- 36.5810	< 0.0010	(- 0.27552, - 0.24208)
2 Vs 3	- 0.0411	0.0097	- 11.9730	< 0.0010	(- 0.04921, - 0.03299)
2 Vs 4	- 0.0529	0.0235	- 6.3720	< 0.0010	(- 0.07255, - 0.03325)
2 Vs 5	- 0.0476	0.0094	- 14.3190	< 0.0010	(- 0.05546, - 0.03974)
3 Vs 4	- 0.0118	0.0214	- 1.5563	0.0853	(- 0.02969, - 0.00609)
3 Vs 5	- 0.0065	0.0095	- 1.9416	0.0578	(- 0.01444, - 0.00143)
4 Vs 5	0.0053	0.0219	0.6800	0.2622	(- 0.01301, 0.02361)

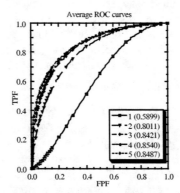

Figure 5. The average ROC curves.

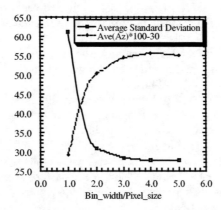

Figure 6. The average standard deviation in the circular region of Figure 1 (solid line) and the linearly scaled average area under the ROC curves (dashed line) as a function of the ratio of the bin width to the reconstructed pixel size.

Recall that in this study five different reconstructed pixel sizes which resulted in reconstructed images of different sizes (64x64, 128x128, 192x192, 256x256, and 320x320) that were subsequently collapsed into 64x64 were used. The program that was used to obtain the reconstructions [8], also calculates the standard deviations associated with each reconstructed pixel. The problem is that, whilst the reconstructed images of different array sizes can all be collapsed to 64x64 arrays by summation, the same cannot be done with the corresponding reconstruction variance images because the covariances among pixels to be collapsed are not known. In order to overcome this problem, the algorithm in [3] was implemented to calculate the standard deviation images. Figure 6 shows the average standard deviation obtained in a disk with a radius of 25 pixels (solid line) together with the average area under the ROC curve (dashed line) as a function of the PBWRPS ratio. Note that the trend of the two curves is similar, with both curves reaching a maximum or minimum at the same PBWRPS ratio of 3, which is the maximum magnification in the reconstructed region of interest.

Therefore, the noise being higher for larger reconstructed pixel sizes results in reduced defect detectability as verified by the results of the observer performance study.

4. DISCUSSION

The results of the study indicate that the proper choice of the pixel size in fan-beam reconstruction when using the pixel-driven algorithm is indeed a very important issue. In fan-beam geometries, depending on their position in the object and the associated magnification, voxels may get projected to a large number of projection bins. Because of the nature of pixel-driven backprojectors, reconstruction pixel sizes that are too large result in reconstructed images of low contrast and signal to noise ratio. Reconstructing a larger number of smaller pixels and then collapsing (summing up) the data is effectively equivalent to pixel-driven backprojection using more than two projection bins. The theoretical results in [3] were verified by the observer study which showed that when the pixel size is larger than the proper size, the images are of lower contrast, the noise level is higher, and the detectability of defects deteriorates. The reconstructed images improve (in terms of myocardial defect detection) as the pixel size decreases and as the bin width to pixel size ratio approaches the highest magnification in the reconstructed region of interest. Images of adequate qualitative and quantitative accuracy are obtained when the PBWRPS ratio is equal to the highest magnification in the ROI. Further decreasing the pixel size, the gain in defect detectability is not significant, while the time required for the reconstruction and the memory requirements are increased. Therefore, as a rule of thumb, the pixel size should be chosen so that the ratio of the projection bin size to the reconstruction pixel size is at least as large as the maximum possible magnification within the reconstruction space.

5. REFERENCES

1. G. T. Herman and A. Naparstek, "Fast image reconstruction based on a Radon inversion formula appropriate for rapidly collected data," *SIAM J. Appl. Math.*, vol. 33, pp. 511-533, Nov. 1977.
2. C. R. Crawford, G.T. Gullberg, and B.M.W. Tsui, "Reconstruction for fan beam with an angular-dependent displaced center-of-rotation," *Medical Physics*, 5 (1), Jan.1988.
3. R. H. Huesman, "A new fast algorithm for the evaluation of regions of interest and statistical uncertainty in computed tomography", *Physics in Medicine and Biology*, vol. 29, no. 5, pp. 543-552, May 1984.
4. D. W. Wilson and B. M. W. Tsui,"Noise properties of filtered-backprojection and ML-EM reconstructed emission tomographic images", *IEEE Transactions on Nuclear Science*, vol. 40, no. 4, pp. 1198-1203, August 1993.
5. C. E. Metz, "ROC methodology in radiologic imaging", *Investigative Radiology*, 1986;21, pp. 720-733.
6. C. E. Metz, "Some practical issues of experimental design and data analysis in radiological ROC studies", *Investigative Radiology*, 1989:24, pp. 234-245.
7. B. M. W. Tsui, J. A. Terry, and G. T. Gullberg, "Evaluation of cardiac cone-beam Single Photon Emission Computed Tomography using observer performance experiments and receiver operating characteristic analysis," *Investigative Radiology*, vol. 28, no. 12, pp. 1101-1112, Dec. 1993.
8. R. H. Huesman, G. T. Gullberg, W. L. Greenburg, T. F. Budinger, *RECLBL Library: Donner algorithms for reconstructed tomography*, Berkley, CA: Lawrence Berkley Laboratory, 1977.
9. C. E. Metz, J. H. Shen, and B. A. Herman, "New methods for estimating a binormal ROC curve from continuously-distributed test results", presented at the1990 Annual Meeting of the Americal Statistical Association, Anaheim, CA, August, 1990.
10. G. K. Gregoriou, B. M. W. Tsui, and G. T. Gullberg, "Effect of truncated projections on defect detection in attenuation-compensated fan-beam cardiac SPECT", the Journal of Nuclear Medicine, vol. 39, no. 1, pp. 166 – 175, January, 1998.

A novel method for reducing high attenuation object artifacts in CT reconstructions

Laigao Chen,[a] Yun Liang,[b*] George A Sandison,[a] Jonas Rydberg[b]

[a]School of Health Sciences, Purdue University, West Lafayette, IN 47907
[b]Department of Radiology, Indiana University Medical School,
541 Clinical Drive, RM 157, Indianapolis, IN 46202

ABSTRACT

A new method to reduce the streak artifacts caused by high attenuation objects in CT images has been developed. The key part of this approach is a preprocessing procedure based on the raw projection data using an adaptive scaling-plus-filtering method. The procedure is followed by the conventional filtered-back projection to reconstruct artifact-reduced images. Phantom and clinical studies have demonstrated that the proposed method can effectively reduce the streak artifacts caused by high attenuation objects for different anatomical structures and metal materials while still faithfully reproduce the positions and dimensions of the metal objects. The visualization of tissue features adjacent to metal objects is greatly improved. The proposed method is computational efficient and can be easily adapted to the current commercial CT scanners.

Keywords: computed tomography (CT), high attenuation object artifacts, metal artifact reduction, beam hardening correction

1. INTRODUCTION

High attenuation objects cause streak artifacts in CT images that may overlap with the images of surrounding tissues and thereby cause misdiagnosis.[1-6] Such high attenuation objects include surgical clips, metal prosthesis and implants, dental fillings and cryotherapy probes. Since most of them are various types of metal materials, the streak artifacts caused by these objects are typically termed "metal artifacts".

One major source of metal artifacts in CT images is the inaccurate beam hardening correction for high attenuation objects. CT reconstruction theory assumes that the incident x-ray beam is monoenergetic. Only under this assumption, the linear attenuation coefficient for a given tissue material is uniquely defined and the relationship between measured attenuation data (after logarithm operation) and the thickness of a given material is linear. Unfortunately in practice the x-ray beam in commercial CT scanners is polyenergetic which typically contains a energy spectrum from 20keV to 120keV or 140keV. Because low energy x-rays are attenuated more than high energy x-rays by a given tissue material, the x-ray beam spectrum changes (hardens) when it travels through an object. This leads to a nonlinear relationship between the measured attenuation data and the thickness of a given material and hence creates so-called beam hardening artifacts in the reconstructed images. To remedy this problem, CT manufacturers typically apply a polynomial correction function to the measured attenuation data to estimate the idea attenuation data for a monoenergetic x-ray beam.[7] This beam hardening correction function is usually derived and calibrated for normal tissues and not accurate enough for high attenuation objects. To demonstrate this inaccuracy in beam hardening correction for metal objects, we simulated the attenuation data of a typical polyenergetic x-ray beam in CT scanners for different thickness of iron (Fig. 1). The x-ray spectrum was generated using a C program written by John M. Boone[8] (http://www.aip.org/epaps/epaps.html). In this simulation we set the

---

* Correspondence: Email:yliang1@iupui.edu; telephone:317-274-1843; Fax: 317-274-4074

peak voltage as 120 kVp with 5mm added Aluminum filtration and 3.5% KV ripples. The x-ray attenuation coefficients of iron for different energy of x-ray beams are taken from the well-known web site (http://physics.nist.gov/). As shown by the simulation results, there are huge deficiencies between the idea monoenergetic attenuation data and the corrected attenuation data using the polynomial correction formula optimized for water. Typically this results in broad dark streaks emanating from the high attenuation object in the reconstructed CT image.

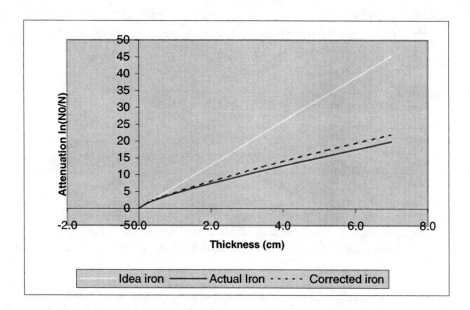

Figure 1. Attenuation of iron as a function of object thickness calculated for a typical CT scanner. Both idea (without beam-hardening) and actual cases are plotted. The dashed line corresponds to the corrected attenuation data of iron using the polynomial correction formula optimized for water.

Another important source of the metal streak artifacts stems from the poor signal-to-noise ratio due to photon starvations in the projection rays passing through the high attenuation object. This high fluctuations in the projection data of corresponding rays will lead to thin streaks (alternately dark and bright) along radial directions in the reconstructed image. Other possible sources of metal artifacts include scattering, exponential edge-gradient effect, relative motion between metal objects and patient tissues, etc. [9]

Many methods have been proposed to suppress metal artifacts in CT images.[1-6] Basically they can be classified into two categories: projection interpolation methods and iterative reconstruction methods. In the projection interpolation methods, [1-3;5] projection data passing through metal objects are replaced by data interpolated from adjacent non-metal projections. The interpolation methods can be either a very simple two-point linear interpolation[2] or other sophisticated interpolation methods in spatial domain[1] or frequency domain.[3] The corrected projections are then fed into normal filtered backprojection reconstruction to get the artifacts reduced image. This type of metal artifacts reduction algorithms is typically fast and easy to implement. However, they also have certain disadvantages. One disadvantage is that metal objects are totally removed from the corrected images and hence the position and dimension information of the metal objects are lost after correction. This is not desired by many clinical applications. More importantly, extra artifacts will be created when there are bony structures existing in the imaging field of view because the interpolated data typically cannot represent surrounding bony structures correctly. [2]

Iterative metal artifacts reduction methods treat the projection rays passing through metal objects as "missing projection data" and reconstruct the image using iterative reconstruction algorithms such as algebraic reconstruction technique (ART) or maximum likelihood expectation maximization algorithm.[4;10] This category of algorithms achieves relative better image quality than interpolation methods. However they are computationally expensive and cannot make use of the reconstruction hardware in current commercial CT scanners. In other words, it is difficult to implement them in current stage.

In this article, we present a new method to reduce the streak artifacts caused by high attenuation objects in CT images. This method significantly reduces the metal artifacts from both beam hardening and photon starvations while still faithfully reproduces the positions and dimensions of the metal objects. Furthermore, it is computationally efficient and can be easily adapted to commercial CT systems. In the following sections, the principle and implementation details of our method will be discussed. Both phantom and clinical cases will be used to testify the effectiveness of our method. Finally, a discussion of the proposed algorithm and conclusions will be stated.

2. METHODS

The framework of our metal artifacts reduction algorithm is similar to the projection interpolation methods discussed in last section. In both algorithms, the first step is to extract the metal objects with a suitable threshold from an initial image reconstructed without metal artifact correction. For each viewing angle, the metal parts are then reprojected to form clear delineation of their corresponding projection channels. The second step is to modify the projection data passing through the metal objects to correct for possible sources that can introduce steak artifacts. Finally the modified projection data are fed into a conventional filtered backprojection routine to reconstruct the artifacts-reduced image.

The main difference between our new approach and the projection interpolation methods lies in the second step of this framework. In the projection interpolation methods, any projections passing through metal objects are considered to contain two parts. One part is contributed by attenuation of tissues, which can be estimated by the interpolation from projections outside of the metal regions. Another part is contributed by metal objects. This part of projection data is typically considered "corrupted" and removed from the original projection data. By doing this, the metal artifacts are largely reduced in the reconstructed image. However, the removed metal projection data contain all the attenuation information from the metal objects as well as some information of bony structures in the imaging field because the interpolation from adjacent non-metal regions cannot separate the projection data purely contributed by the metal parts. This results in the loss of metal object positions and blurred bony structures in the reconstructed image after correction. Since the removed projection data contain important information, we try to keep this part of projection data in our new approach. Instead of totally removing them, an adaptive scaling-plus-filtering technique is used to partly correct the attenuation inaccuracies associated with this part of projection data and also reduce the relative contributions of these projections to other surrounding tissues during filtered backprojection. Specifically, the "corrupted" metal projection part is adaptively scaled to compensate for the inaccurate beam hardening corrections and also the amplitude of the metal projection profile is lowered down to be between 5% and 30% of the original amplitude. This lowered amplitude helps to reduce the effect of any errors within the metal projections when backprojecting them to other tissue positions in the reconstructed image. An adaptive filtering is applied to the scaled metal projection part to further reduce the streak artifacts due to photon starvation noises. The scaled and filtered metal profile is then added to the interpolated tissue baseline to form a new projection profile for each view. Reconstruction of the image from the processed projection data then proceeds as usual to generate corrected images.

In the following sections, we discuss in detail all the processing steps involved in our new metal artifacts reduction algorithm.

2.1 Step 1 - Find Metal Projection Regions

Our algorithm starts from the measured parallel beam projection data P(m,n), m=1,...M, n=1,...N. Here M is the total number of detectors and N is the total number of projection views. If the original scanning geometry is in fan beam format, we assume it has already been rebinned to parallel beam format. A standard filtered backprojection algorithm is applied to reconstruct an initial image from P(m,n). Metal objects are extracted with a suitable threshold, say, 2000 HU, from the initial image. For each view, the metal parts are reprojected to form clear delineation of their corresponding projection channels. Unlike the typical projection ray driven reprojection technique,[11] pixel driven reprojection technique is used in our approach. Specifically, each pixel corresponding to the metal objects is reprojected onto all view angles. Linear interpolation is performed to distribute the pixel value onto corresponding detector channels under each view. This pixel-by-pixel reprojection method is very computational efficient in this particular application due to the fact that the total number of metal pixels only occupy a very small portion of the whole image matrix. After doing this, the regions corresponding to the metal objects under each projection view can be determined:

$$R(n) = \{[s(i,n),e(i,n)]\}, \qquad i=1,\ldots I(n) \tag{1}$$

where $I(n)$ is the total number of metal regions under view n and $s(i,n)$, $e(i,n)$ are the starting and ending channels of region i under view n respectively.

When only single metal object exists in the imaging field, it is not necessary to perform the segmentation and reprojection of the metal object from the first initial reconstructed image. It is possible to directly detect the boundary of the metal object from the measured projection data. However, the reprojection method is still the most robust approach to find the regions corresponding to metal objects in measured projection data.

2.2 Step 2 - Adaptive Scaling

A baseline profile $b(m,n)$ is formed for all $m \in R(n)$ by performing a linear or polynomial fit to the projection data on both side of the metal region $[s(i,n),e(i,n)]$. This baseline is subtracted from the measured projection yielding a measured profile of the metal objects in this view (Fig. 2b):

$$P_m(m,n) = [P(m,n)-b(m,n)], \quad m \in R(n) \tag{2}$$

This metal profile is adaptively scaled using following formula:

$$P_1(m,n) = W_c W_b(m,n) P_m(m,n), \quad m \in R(n) \tag{3}$$

where $W_b(m,n)$ is a scaling factor adaptively calculated from the amplitude of the metal projection $P_m(m,n)$ to compensate for the inaccurate beam hardening correction to metal objects (Fig. 1). This can be determined from the x-ray beam spectrum and the material of the metal objects. W_c is a constant scaling factor which is less than unity for all metal regions to lower the amplitude of the metal projection profile (Fig. 2). This lowered amplitude helps to reduce the effect of any errors within the metal projections when backprojecting them to other tissue positions in the reconstructed image. A typical value of W_c is between 0.5 and 0.3. Actually the scaling factor W_c can be used as a parameter to control a trade-off between reducing streak artifacts and keeping bony structures in the final reconstructed image. A larger W_c creates an image with less bony structure distortion but more streak artifacts, while a smaller W_c creates an image with less streak artifacts but more bony structure distortions. When W_c is equal to zero, our method becomes equivalent to those interpolation methods. When W_c is equal to one, it restores the original measured projection data.

In many practical cases, the x-ray spectrum or the metal material information is not available. Then we can simply set $W_b(m,n)=1$ and only apply one single scaling factor W_c for all metal projection data. We will show in the following sections that even the constant scaling factor generates very good metal artifacts reduction effects for many applications.

2.3 Step 3 - Adaptive Filtering

Adaptive filtering is widely used in commercial CT scanners for reducing streak artifacts caused by projection data fluctuations.[12;13] Here we apply adaptive filtering specifically to the scaled metal projection data $P_1(m,n)$ to further reduce the noises within the projection data of the metal objects. This filtering procedure can be represented as:

$$P_2(m,n) = P_1(m,n) \otimes G(m), \quad m \in R(n) \tag{4}$$

where G is a filter function which can be different types such as running mean filters, boxcar filters, median filters, trimmed mean filters, etc. According to our experience, the trimmed mean filters[12] work very well for reducing the streak artifacts caused by photon starvation noises.

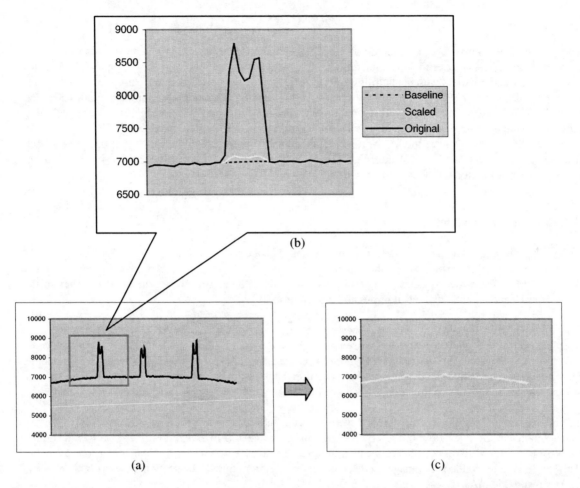

(b)

(a)   (c)

Figure 2. Schematic illustration of the scaling factor W_c applied to the metal projection profiles to lower the amplitude of the metal peaks. (a) Original projection data at one viewing angle. Three peaks correspond to enhanced attenuation by metal objects; (b) Scaling of one metal peak. First a baseline is formed by performing a polynomial fit to the projection data adjacent but not including the metal parts. This baseline is subtracted from the measured projection yielding a profile of the metal objects in this view. The metal projection profile is scaled down to 5% of the original amplitude (W_c =0.05) and then added back onto the baseline to form the scaled projection data; (c) projection data after all three metal peaks are scaled. Only 5% of the metal peak amplitude is preserved.

2.4 Step 4 - Filtered Backprojection

After the metal projection profiles are adaptively scaled and filtered, they are added back to the baseline to form the corrected projection data:

$$P_3(m,n) = P_2(m,n) + b(m,n), \quad m \in R(n), \tag{5}$$

All projection data outside of the metal regions are kept unchanged as the original measured values. That is:

$$P_3(m,n) = P(m,n), \quad m \notin R(n) \tag{6}$$

The new projection data $P_3(m,n)$ are fed into a filtered backprojection procedure as usual to reconstructed the artifacts reduced image.

3. RESULTS

The proposed metal artifacts reduction algorithm has been applied to several application cases to evaluate its performance. These cases include a gelatin phantom with five metallic cryoprobes, a patient elbow with a metal screw and a patient with dental fillings. All the CT scans are performed in a Philips MX8000 quad-slice spiral CT scanner (Philips Medical Systems). After scanning, the raw projection data are downloaded from the scanner to a HP Unix workstation in our lab. All following processing procedures including rebinning, filtered backprojection and metal artifacts reduction are implemented on the HP workstation using IDL (Research Systems, Inc.). The reconstructed image sets before and after correction are sent back to a dedicated view workstation of the MX8000 CT scanner (Philips Medical Systems) for 3D rendering, multi-planar reformation (MPR) and maximum intensity projection (MIP).

3.1 Metallic Cryoprobes

Cryotherapy is a therapeutic procedure to use freezing damage to kill tumors.[14] This involves the direct contact application of cryoprobes to the desired tumor tissues. Typically the probes are hollow metallic tubes within which a gas or liquid cryogen is caused to flow. After certain period of time, water in the tissue freezes and an ablating iceball grows about each probe.

Image guidance in cryotherapy is usually performed using ultrasound. However, x-ray CT imaging is an alternate means of guidance which has several advantages over ultrasound including displaying 3D structures of the iceballs and quantitatively monitoring the growth of iceballs by CT number measurements. Unfortunately the CT images during cryotherapy suffer badly by metal artifacts from metallic cryoprobes. It is highly desired to reduce the metal artifacts while still keeping the probes in the reconstructed images.

In our experiment set-up, five cryoprobes were inserted into a homogeneous gelatin phantom to form a pentagon shape. Cryogen flow in the cryoprobes causes the gelatin to freeze and form an iceball around each probe. After all five iceballs are formed, an axial CT scan is performed to cover the whole phantom. The whole volume contains 32 images and each of them is 2.5mm thick. The scanning parameters are set as 120 kVp and 250 mAs.

As shown in Fig. 3(a), there are severe streak artifacts in the CT images caused by the cryoprobes if no corrections are applied. Fig. 3(b) is the corrected image using our metal artifacts reduction approach (W_c=0.05, $W_b(m,n)$=1). The streak artifacts are largely reduced while the positions of the five probes are well preserved. The contrast between the cryoprobes and the iceballs are also enhanced. Fig. 3(c) and 3(d) are 3D renderings of the cryoprobes and iceballs. Before correction, the iceballs are rendered in irregular shapes because of the streak artifacts while after correction the five iceballs are clearly rendered around each cryoprobe.

The line profiles of the 256th row in the reconstructed axial images before and after metal artifacts correction are also plotted. From the line profile of the corrected image, we can see nicely a drop in the middle of the profile which corresponds to the region of iceballs. But in the profile before correction, this region is much more noisy because of the streak artifacts. Apparently the image before correction cannot be used for quantitatively monitoring the growth of iceballs.

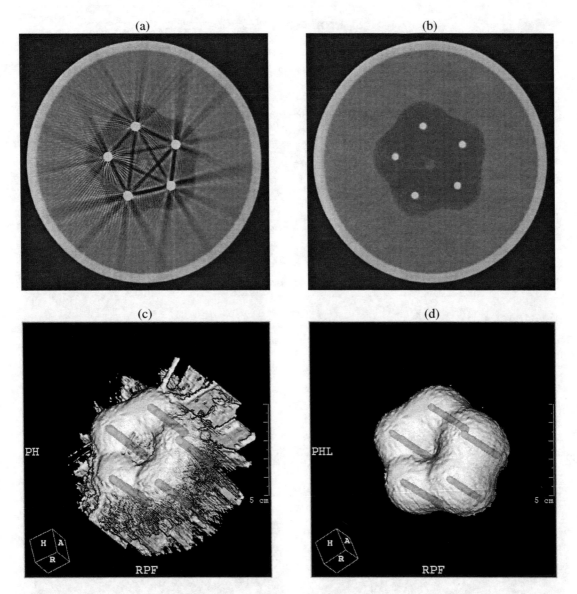

Figure 3. Comparison of CT images of cryoprobes and iceballs before and after metal artifacts reduction: (a) axial image before correction; (b) axial image after correction; (c) 3D rendering before correction; (d) 3D rendering after correction.

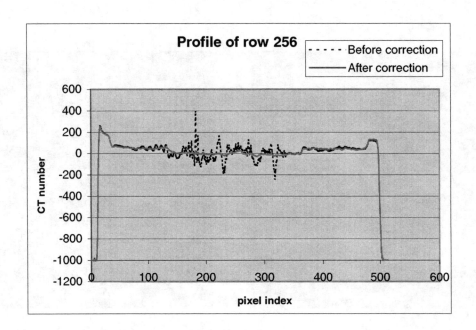

Figure 4. Comparison of line profiles in CT images of cryoprobes and iceballs before and after metal artifacts reduction.

3.2 A metal Screw in the Elbow

Fig. 5(a) shows the metal streak artifacts caused by a metal screw in the patient's elbow. This case is a spiral scan with a scanning pitch 0.625x4 and 1mm slice thickness. The tube voltage and current are 140kVp and 175 mAs respectively.

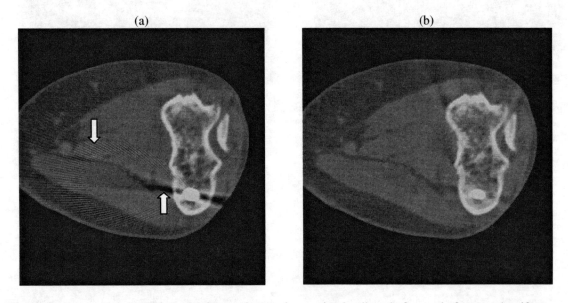

Figure 5. Comparison of CT images of a metal screw in a patient's elbow before and after metal artifacts reduction: (a) axial image before correction; (b) axial image after correction.

Both broad dark streaks caused by inaccurate beam-hardening correction (pointed by the upper arrow) and thin bright-dark streaks (pointed by the down arrow) caused by projection noises can be observed. After correction using the proposed algorithm (W_c=0.20, W_b(m,n)=1), both broad dark streaks and thin bright-dark streaks are significantly removed (Fig 5b). The surrounding bone structures are also well preserved.

3.3 Dental Filling and Carotid Artery Case

Fig. 6(a) shows the metal streak artifacts caused by dental fillings in a patient's teeth. This case is a spiral scan with a scanning pitch 0.875x4 and 1mm slice thickness. The tube voltage and current are 120kVp and 210 mAs respectively.

The streak artifacts are so severe that they obscure the carotid arteries, which are the region of interest for physicians in this case. After correction using the proposed algorithm (W_c=0.25, W_b(m,n)=1), the streak artifacts are significantly reduced (Fig 6b), especially around the carotid artery region. As a result, the maximum intensity projection (MIP) image in Fig 6(c) nicely depicts the carotid artery.

(a)   (b)   (c)

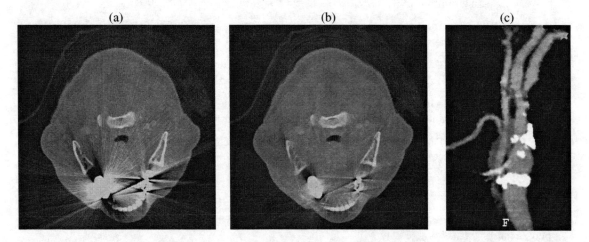

Figure 6. Comparison of CT images of a patient with dental fillings before and after metal artifacts reduction: (a) axial image before correction; (b) axial image after correction; (c) MIP of the carotid artery after correction.

4. CONCLUSIONS AND DISCUSSIONS

The proposed method is a very promising algorithm for reducing high attenuation object artifacts in medical CT systems because of the following advantages: (1) robust metal artifacts reduction ability. Phantom and clinical studies have demonstrated that the proposed method can effectively remove the streak artifacts caused by high attenuation objects for different anatomical structures and metal objects; (2) the metal objects can be preserved and differentiated from other tissues after the metal artifact reduction procedure; (3) the scaling factor W_c can be used as a parameter to control a trade-off between reducing streak artifacts and keeping bony structures. (4) all the procedures in our method can be automated and the algorithm can be easily implemented in current commercial CT scanners.

Currently all the examples presented in the article have not incorporated the x-ray spectrum information and the attenuation property of the metal objects. The optimal scaling strategy with consideration of these information is still under investigation. It involves the measurement of the effective spectrum of CT scanners.

REFERENCES

1. Glover GH, Pelc NJ. "An algorithm for the reduction of metal clip artifacts in CT reconstructions." *Med.Phys.* **8**: 799-807, 1981.

2. Kalender WA, Hebel R, Ebersberger J. "Reduction of CT Artifacts Caused by Metallic Implants." *Radiology* **164**: 576-577, 1987.

3. Zhao S, Robertson DD, Wang G, Whiting B, Bae KT. "X-ray CT metal artifact reduction using wavelets: an application for imaging total hip prostheses." *IEEE Trans.Med.Imaging* **19**: 1238-1247, 2000.

4. Wang G, Snyder DL, OSullivan JA, Vannier MW. "Iterative deblurring for CT metal artifact reduction." *IEEE Transactions on Medical Imaging*, **15**: 657-664, 1996.

5. Tuy H K. "A post-processing algorithm to reduce metallic clip artifacts in CT images." *European Radiology* **3**: 129-134, 1993.

6. De Man B, Nuyts J, Dupont P, Marchal G, Suetens P. "An iterative maximum-likelihood polychromatic algorithm for CT." *IEEE Trans.Med.Imaging* **20**: 999-1008, 2001.

7. Herman GT. "Correction for beam hardening in computed tomography." *Phys.Med.Biol.* **24**: 81-106, 1979.

8. Boone JM, Seibert J A. "An accurate method for computer-generating tungsten anode x-ray spectra from 30 to 140KV." *Med.Phys.* **24**: 1661-1670, 1997.

9. De Man B, Nuyts J, Dupont P, Marchal G, Suetens P. "Metal streak artifacts in X-ray computed tomography: A simulation study." *IEEE Transactions on Nuclear Science* **46**: 691-696, 1999.

10. De Man B, Nuyts J, Dupont P, Marchal G, Suetens P. "Reduction of metal streak artifacts in x-ray computed tomography using a transmission maximum a posteriori algorithm." *IEEE Transactions on Nuclear Science* **47**: 977-981,2000.

11. Crawford CR. Reprojection using a parallel backprojector. *Med.Phys.* **13**: 480-483, 1986.

12. Hsieh J. "Adaptive streak artifact reduction in computed tomography resulting from excessive x-ray photon noise." *Med.Phys.* **25**: 2139-2147, 1998.

13. Kachelriess M, Watzke O, Kalender WA. "Generalized multi-dimensional adaptive filtering for conventional and spiral single-slice, multi-slice, and cone- beam CT." *Medical Physics* **28**: 475-490, 2001.

14. Baissalov R, Sandison G A, Donnelly B J. "Suppression of high-density artefacts in x-ray CT images using temporal digital subtraction with application to cryotherapy." *Phys.Med.Biol.* **45**: N53-N59, 2000.

Sensitivity analysis of textural parameters for vertebroplasty

Gye Rae Tack[*], Seung Yong Lee[*], Kyu Chul Shin[**], and Sung Jae Lee[***]

[*]Dept. of Biomedical Eng., Konkuk Univ./Chungju, Korea
[**]Dept. of Orthopedics, Hanyang Univ./Seoul, Korea
[***]Dept. of Biomedical Eng., Inje Univ./Kimhae, Korea

ABSTRACT

Vertebroplasty is one of the newest surgical approaches for the treatment of the osteoporotic spine. Recent studies have shown that it is a minimally invasive, safe, promising procedure for patients with osteoporotic fractures while providing structural reinforcement of the osteoporotic vertebrae as well as immediate pain relief. However, treatment failures due to excessive bone cement injection have been reported as one of complications. It is believed that control of bone cement volume seems to be one of the most critical factors in preventing complications. We believed that an optimal bone cement volume could be assessed based on CT data of a patient. Gray-level run length analysis was used to extract textural information of the trabecular. At initial stage of the project, four indices were used to represent the textural information: mean width of intertrabecular space, mean width of trabecular, area of intertrabecular space, and area of trabecular. Finally, the area of intertrabecular space was selected as a parameter to estimate an optimal bone cement volume and it was found that there was a strong linear relationship between these 2 variables (correlation coefficient = 0.9433, standard deviation = 0.0246). In this study, we examined several factors affecting overall procedures. The threshold level, the radius of rolling ball and the size of region of interest were selected for the sensitivity analysis. As the level of threshold varied with 9, 10, and 11, the correlation coefficient varied from 0.9123 to 0.9534. As the radius of rolling ball varied with 45, 50, and 55, the correlation coefficient varied from 0.9265 to 0.9730. As the size of region of interest varied with 58 x 58, 64 x 64, and 70 x 70, the correlation coefficient varied from 0.9685 to 0.9468. Finally, we found that strong correlation between actual bone cement volume (Y) and the area (X) of the intertrabecular space calculated from the binary image and the linear equation $Y = 0.001722 X - 2.10922$. We could see that this equation slightly overestimated bone cement volume and those amounts would not make any serious complications. We hope this will help to control a proper amount of bone cement volume injection during vertebroplasty.

Keywords: sensitivity analysis, vertebroplasty, bone cement, texture analysis, osteoporosis

1. INTRODUCTION

In the United States, 25% of women over the age of 70 and 50 % of women over the age of 80 show the evidence of vertebral fractures[1]. The majority of those fractures occur in midthoracic region and thoracolumbar junction that results in increasing morbidity. Percutaneous vertebroplasty is an effective surgical procedure that was introduced to treat hemangiomas in the spine in late 1980's in France[2], and still regarded as a relatively new procedure considering the fact that it was not introduced in the United States until 1994. It includes puncturing vertebrae and injecting polymethylmethacrylate(PMMA) into the vertebrae.

Recent studies have shown that it is a minimally invasive and safe procedure that can reinforce the structural integrity of the weakened vertebrae with immediate pain relief. It is also known to be very effective for the patients suffering from osteoporotic fractures or selected vertebral column neoplasms. However, there exist several limitations: They include

---

[*]grtack@kku.ac.kr; phone 82 43 840 3762; fax 82 43 851 0620; http://bsl.kku.ac.kr; Biomedical Eng., Konkuk Univ., 322 Danwall-dong, Chungju, Chungbuk, Korea 380-701; [**]shinkcos@netsgo.com; phone 82 2 501 6868; fax 82 2 501 6898; Dept. of Orthopedics, Hanyang Univ., Hangdang-dong, Seongdong-gu, Seoul, Korea 130-100; [***]sjl@bme.inje.ac.kr; phone 82 55 320 3452; fax 82 55 337 1303; http://www.inje.ac.kr; Biomedical Eng., Inje Univ., Kimhae, Kyongnam, Korea 621-749

the inability to restore the original height of the vertebrae, lack of clinical reports on its use on younger people, insufficient data on long-term effects, and thermal damage by the polymerization of bone cement after injection. There are many possible complications[3-7]. Bleeding at the puncture site, bone infection or fracture, damage to the nerve roots or spinal cord, extravasation of material into the venous system with embolization to the pulmonary vasculature or compression of neural tissue is possible. Dysphagia or radiculopathy, presumably due to extravasation of PMMA into nerve root or esophageal compression, and decreased pulmonary function may occur. But life-threatening complications have not been reported in vertebroplasty.

Thus we believed that disproportionate volume of PMMA injection is one of the most common causes of complications. Therefore, clinical success of vertebroplasty can be dependent on the injected PMMA volume for a given patient. Since the level of the osteoporosis can influence the porosity of the cancellous bone in the vertebral body, the injection volume can be different from patient to patient. Gray-level run length analysis was used to extract textural information of the trabecular. At initial stage of the project[8], four indices were used to represent the textural information: mean width of intertrabecular space, mean width of trabecular, area of intertrabecular space, and area of trabecular. Finally, the area of intertrabecular space was selected as a parameter to estimate an optimal bone cement volume. In this study, we examined several factors affecting overall procedures to derive the relationship between area of the intertrabecular space and an optimal bone cement volume during vertebroplasty.

2. METHOD

2.1 TEXTURE ANALYSIS

Vertebroplasty was performed after patient was sedated with intravenous fentanyl (Sublimase, Abott Labs; Chicago, IL) and midazolam (Versed, Roche; Manati, Puerto Rico). Blood pressure, electrocardiographic readings, and oxygen saturation were monitored continuously. Patient was given 1 gm of cefazolin intravenously immediately prior to the procedure. Patient was placed in a prone position on high-resolution-angiographic-table capable of biplane imaging. Local anesthesia was applied to the skin and deep structures, including the periosteum of the bone at the intended site of entry by the bone needle. Biplane fluoroscopic guidance allowed the placement of an 11-gauge Jamshidi bone biopsy needle (Manan Medical; Northbrook, IL) via a transpedicular approach to approximately the junction of the anterior and middle thirds of the vertebral body. Intraosseous venography was performed through the 11 gauge needle, using 5cc of nonionic x-ray contrast medium (Omnipaque 300, Nycomed; Princeton, NJ) to assess the flow characteristics within the vertebral body and to determine if there was abnormally large or dangerous communication with the epidural space. Methacrylate (Codman cranioplastic, CMN Laboratories; Blackpool, England) was prepared by adding the sterile opacification agent barium sulfate (E-Z-EM; Westbury, NY), which allowed better visualization during fluoroscopy. Careful monitoring of the PMMA during injection is required in order to recognize any flow into an undesirable location such as the epidural space or inferior vena cava. Approximately 2-5cc of PMMA was injected into each half of the vertebral body via separate, bihemisheric injections. At the termination of each procedure, the patient was transferred to holding area and monitored for 2-3 hours before discharge.

Fifteen female patients (age, 57-78 years) underwent this procedure. A total of 26 vertebrae in which osteoporosis was assessed were involved. Xpeed Unit (Toshiba, 120kvp, 170 mA, 2.7sec) was used for CT measurement (512 x 512). Table 1 shows patient's data such as fracture location, bone mineral density, T-score, and Z-score. Vertebrae in Table 1 were scanned with 1 mm thickness before and after operation.

In previous study[8], the gray level run length analysis was used to extract textural features of the trabecular bone. Four indices - the width of trabecular, the width of intertrabecular spaces, the area of intertrabecular space, and the area of trabecular - were calculated. Brief explanation is as follows: Preoperative CT images (512 x 512, 12 bits) of patients were converted into binary images to obtain textural features of each image. The CT values of each image were converted in a linear fashion into 256 gray levels. The rolling ball subtraction algorithm was used to remove the smooth, continuous background of the gray level image before making a binary image. After removal of background, the images were converted into binary images with two gray levels (0 and 1). The same threshold was used for all series and was applied to the ROI (64 x 64) within an image. The ROI was selected manually within the trabecular. The bound of the run length was set to 64, and the spatial frequency of the run length in the binary image was calculated.

Table 1: Patient's data

Patient Number	Fracture Location	BMD (mg/cc)	T-score	Z-score
1	T11, T12	20.5	-6.3	-3.2
2	T8	-0.1	-0.7	-3.2
3	T7, T11, T12	0.8	-7.1	-3.2
4	T7, T8, T10, T12	18.1	-6.4	-2.7
5	T8, L1	20.4	-6.3	-3.2
6	T11	11.2	-6.7	-2.7
7	L1	30.8	-5.9	NA
8	L1	49.1	-5.2	NA
9	L3	NA	NA	NA
10	L2	36	-5.7	NA
11	L1	9.7	-6.7	NA
12	T8, T12, L1	NA	-6.9	-3.1
13	L1	NA	-6.0	-3.4
14	T10, L2, L3	NA	-7.0	-3.4
15	T12	NA	-4.6	-3.0

2.2 SENSITIVITY ANALYSIS

A total of 26 vertebrae of fifteen patients were used to do texture analysis and sensitivity analysis. Each vertebrae has the average of 8 slices of CT images, thus a total of approximately 200 images were used for this study. Since CT was taken before and after vertebroplasty, the number of the preoperative images and that of the postoperative images are approximately 200, respectively. The preoperative images were used for texture analysis and sensitivity analysis whereas the postoperative images were used for comparison between actually injected bone cement volume and calculated bone cement volume.

Previous results[8-9] showed that among four indices the area of intertrabecular space was selected as a parameter to estimate an optimal bone cement volume since the area of intertrabecular space showed very strong linear relationship with actually injected PMMA volume (correlation coefficient = 0.9433, standard deviation = 0.0246). From previous studies, more in-depth tests on the factors affecting this procedure need to be followed. They include the threshold level for segmentation of trabecular and intertrabecular spaces, the size of region of interest in CT images, and the radius of rolling ball[10-11] during image processing of CT images that were the important factors in this study. From several trial-and-error approaches, we found that the texture analysis showed good results when threshold level was 10, the size of region of interest was 64 x 64, and the radius of rolling ball was 50.

In order to investigate the effects of these parameters during overall procedure, with fixed two parameters the value of one parameter was changed as follows: The level of threshold varied with 9, 10, and 11. The radius of rolling ball varied with 45, 50, and 55. The size of region of interest varied with 58 x 58, 64 x 64, and 70 x 70. In order to do quantitative analysis, the correlation coefficient(r) was calculated. The equation for estimating an optimal bone cement volume for vertebroplasty was derived based on these results by using least square estimation.

3. RESULTS

Figure 1 showed the typical results of the preoperative (before vertebroplasty) and postoperative (after vertebroplasty) images. The radiopaque region of the image is the actual PMMA injected area. Distribution patterns of PMMA were different from patient to patient and from vertebral body to vertebral body. Figure 2 showed the relationship between injected PMMA volume and the area of trabecular and that of intertrabecular space. The injected PMMA volume increased as the area of the intertrabecular space increased. It increased also with decreases in the area of trabecular. Figure 3 showed typical results of binary images after image processing by changing the radius of rolling ball and the level of threshold with fixed size of region of interest. White region is the intertrabecular space whereas black region is the trabecular. As the radius of rolling ball increases and the level of threshold decreases, segmented intertrabecular space increases. Table 2 showed the correlation coefficients between injected PMMA volume during vertebroplasty and the area of intertrabecular space by changing size of region of interest, level of threshold, and radius of rolling ball. In case that the size of region of interest is 64 x 64 (Table 2-b), as the radius of rolling ball increased and the level of threshold increased, the correlation coefficient between injected PMMA volume and the area of intertrabecular space increased, which means that there exists very strong linear relationship between them. But in case that the size of region of interest is 58 x 58 and 70 x 70, there did not show any trends in the variation of correlation coefficient.

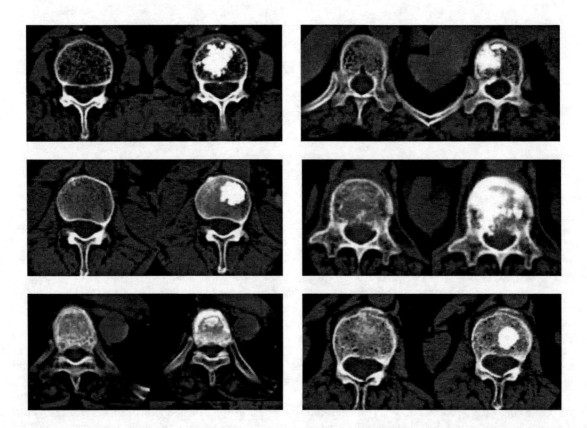

Figure 1: Typical results of the preoperative and postoperative images. The radiopaque region of the images is the actual PMMA injected area. Distribution patterns of PMMA were different from patient to patient and from vertebral body to vertebral body.

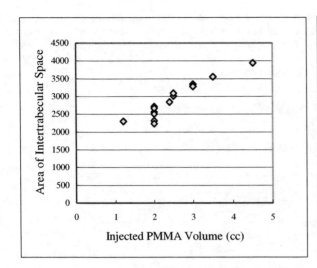 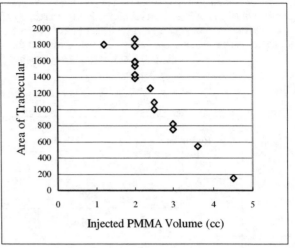

Figure 2: Relationship between actually injected PMMA volume and the area of intertrabecular space and that of trabecular. As the area of the intertrabecular space increased and that of trabecular decreased, the injected PMMA volume increased.

		Level of Threshold		
		9	10	11
Radius of Rolling ball	45			
	50			
	55			

Figure 3: Typical results of binary images after image processing due to the changes of the radius of rolling ball and the level of threshold (the region of interest is 70 x 70, pixel size = 0.234mm). White region is the intertrabecular space whereas black region is the trabecular. As the radius of rolling ball increases and the level of threshold decreases, segmented intertrabecular space increases.

Table 2: Correlation coefficients between injected PMMA volume during vertebroplasty and the area of intertrabecular space by changing size of region of interest, level of threshold, and radius of rolling ball. In case that the size of region of interest is 64 x 64, as the radius of rolling ball increased and the level of threshold increased, the correlation coefficient between injected PMMA volume and the are of intertrabecular space increased. But in case that the size of region of interest is 58 x 58 and 70 x 70, there did not show any trends in the variation of correlation coefficient.

(a) Size of the region of interest = 58 x 58

Radius of Rolling ball	Level of Threshold		
	9	10	11
45	0.9367	0.9873	0.9919
50	0.9840	0.9685	0.9769
55	0.9579	0.9594	0.9653

(b) Size of the region of interest = 64 x 64

Radius of Rolling ball	Level of Threshold		
	9	10	11
45	0.9078	0.9265	0.9457
50	0.9123	0.9428	0.9534
55	0.9458	0.9730	0.9809

(c) Size of the region of interest = 70 x 70

Radius of Rolling ball	Level of Threshold		
	9	10	11
45	0.9822	0.9798	0.9882
50	0.9459	0.9468	0.9698
55	0.9491	0.9595	0.9716

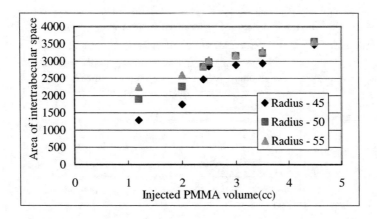

(a) Level of threshold = 10 and Size of ROI = 64

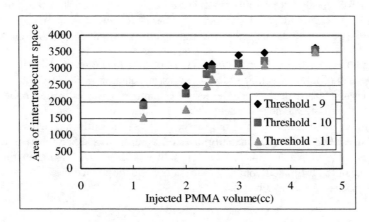

(b) Radius of rolling ball = 50 and Size of ROI = 64

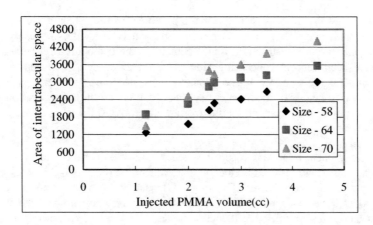

(c) Radius of rolling ball = 50 and Level of threshold = 10

Figure 4: Relationship between the area of interbecular space and injected PMMA volume by changing the radius of rolling ball, level of threshold, and the size of region of interest. In all cases, as the area of the intertrabecular space increased, the injected PMMA volume increased.

Table 3: Comparison between actually injected bone cement volume and estimated bone cement volume based on the derived equation, $Y = 0.001722 X - 2.10922$, where X is the area of intertrabecular space and Y is an estimated bone cement volume.

Patient Number	Estimated bone cement volume (cc)	Injected bone cement volume (cc)
12	2.66 (2.42~2.78)	2.5
13	2.68 (2.46~2.78)	2.5
14	3.25 (2.81~3.68)	3.0
15	3.07 (2.51~3.18)	3.0

Figure 4 showed that the relationship between the area of intertrabecular space and injected PMMA volume by changing the radius of rolling ball, level of threshold, and the size of region of interest. Like figure 2, as the area of the intertrabecular space increased, the injected PMMA volume increased. Changes in the radius of rolling ball, level of threshold, and the size of region of interest did not show any significant variations in overall trends.

Using least square estimation, the best linear fitting was carried out to find the relationship between actually injected bone cement volume and the area of intertrabecular space. The linear equation $Y = 0.001722 X - 2.10922$, where X is the average area of intertrabecular space in the same series of CT and Y is an estimated bone cement volume, was selected for the estimation of an optimal bone cement volume. Based on this equation, four patients underwent vertebroplasty. Table 4 showed the results of the comparison between actually injected bone cement volume and estimated bone cement volume. For patient 12, actually injected volume was 2.5cc whereas estimated volume was 2.66cc. For patient 13, 2.5/2.68, for patient 14, 3/3.25, for patient 15, 3/3.07. Value in the parenthesis was the minimum and maximum value of the estimated volume based on the equation since the image in the same series of CT had different intertrabecular space in the axial direction.

4. CONCLUSIONS AND DISCUSSION

Vertebroplasty is one of the newest surgical approaches for the treatment of the osteoporotic spine. It is very efficient for treatment of pain. Recent studies have shown that it is a minimally invasive, safe, promising procedure for patients with osteoporotic fractures while providing structural reinforcement of the osteoporotic vertebrae and immediate pain relief. However, there have been reports concerning side effects and complications during procedure. Certain complications are linked with leakage of PMMA into adjacent structures during vertebroplasty. It is believed that control of PMMA volume seems to be one of the most critical factors in preventing complications. Thus, we examined whether we could estimate an optimal bone cement volume from preoperative CT images and investigate several factors affecting this procedure.

We found that there was a strong linear relationship between actually injected bone cement volume and the area of the intertrabecular space. Through this relationship, the linear equation $Y = 0.001722 X - 2.10922$, where X is the average area of the intertrabecular space in the same series of vertebral CT scan and Y is an optimally estimated bone cement volume, was derived and applied to vertebroplasty. For the sensitivity analysis, in case that the size of region of interest is 64 x 64 (Table 2-b), as the radius of rolling ball increased and the level of threshold increased, the correlation coefficient between injected PMMA volume and the area of intertrabecular space increased. But in case that the size of region of interest is 58 x 58 and 70 x 70, there did not show any trends in the variation of correlation coefficient. This is due to the fact that each patient has different osteoporotic level. The sensitivity analysis of textural parameters such as level of threshold, size of region of interest, radius of rolling ball showed that those parameters did not show much significant effect on the procedure. We believed that the value of each parameter was well selected and an estimated bone cement volume was good agreement with the actually injected bone cement volume. Thus we can rely on the equation to estimate a bone cement volume even though the equation slightly overestimates the bone cement volume. Those amounts will not make any serious complications.

For further studies, it is necessary that the volume of isolated intertrabecular spaces be considered, since the calculated PMMA volume was found to be slightly more than actually injected PMMA volume. It is also necessary to collect more data on this procedure, to analyze the distribution patterns (see Figure 1) of PMMA during procedure and the relationship between bone mineral density (BMD) and the amount of injected PMMA volume, since our unpublished data showed that the amount of injected PMMA volume did not have much effect on the augmented strength of the vertebrae. In conclusion, we were able to demonstrate that proper amount of PMMA volume injection could be predicted based on the results from this study and could be used for better clinical outcome in percutaneous vertebroplasty.

ACKNOWLEDGMENTS

This study was supported by a grant (HMP-98-G-1-010) of the HAN (Highly Advanced National) Project, Ministry of Heath & Welfare, R.O.K.

REFERENCES

1. J. A. Kanis, E. V. Closkey, "The epidemiology of vertebral osteoporosis," *Bone*, **13**, pp. S1-S10, 1992
2. H. Deramond, C. Depriester, P. Galibert, and D. Le Gars, "Percutaneous vertebroplasty with PMMA polymethylmethacrylate – technique, indications and results," *Radiol. Clinics of N. America*, **36**, No. 3, pp. 533-546, 1998
3. J. B. Martin, B. Jean, D. S. Ruiz, M. Piotin, K. Murphy, B. Rufenacht, M. Muster, and D. A. Rufenacht, "Vertebroplasty: clinical experience and follow-up results," *Bone*, **25**, No. 2, Supplement, pp. S11-S15, 1999
4. J. D. Barr, M. S. Barr, T. J. Lemley, and R. M. McCann, "Percutaneous vertebroplasty for pain relief and spinal stabilization," *Spine*, **25**, No. 8, pp. 923-928, 2000
5. M. E. Jensen, A. J. Evans, J. H. Mathis, D. F. Kallmes, H. J. Cloft, and J. E. Dion, "Percutaneous polymethylmethacrylate Vertebroplasty in the Treatment of Osteoporotic Vertebral Body Compression Fractures: Technical Aspects," *Am. J. Neuroradiol.*, **18**, pp. 1897-1904, 1997
6. A. Weil, J. Chiras, and J. Simon, "Spinal metastases: indications for and results of percutaneous injection of acrylic surgical cement," *Radiology*, **199**, pp. 241-247, 1996
7. H. Deramond, N. T. Wright, and S. M. Belkoff, "Temperature elevation caused by bone cement polymerization during vertebroplasty," *Bone*, **25**, No. 2, Supplement, pp. 17S-21S, 1999
8. G. R. Tack, H. G. Choi, K. C. Shin, and S. J. Lee, "Relationship between trabecular texture features of CT images and an amount of bone cement volume injection in percutaneous vertebroplasty," *Proc. SPIE*, Vol. **4324**, pp. 227-233, 2001
9. G. R. Tack, S. Y. Lee, K. C. Shin, S. J. Lee, B. J. Chon, K. K. Kim, S. S. Kim, and J. B. Choi, "Estimation of PMMA volume for vertebroplasty," *Proc. METMBS'01*, pp. 382-388, 2001
10. S. R. Sternberg, "Biomedical image processing," *IEEE Computer*, pp. 22-34, 1983
11. M. Ito, M. Ohki, K. Hayashi, M. Yamada, M. Uetani, and T. Nakamura, "Trabecular texture analysis of CT images in the relationship with spinal fracture," *Radiology*, **194**, pp. 55-59, 1995

Investigation of Using Bone Texture Analysis on Bone Densitometry Images

Michael R. Chinander, Maryellen L. Giger, Ruchi D. Shah, Tamara J. Vokes

The University of Chicago, 5841 S. Maryland Avenue, MC2026, Chicago, IL, USA

ABSTRACT

We previously developed bone texture analysis methods to assess bone strength on digitized radiographs. Here, we compare the analyses performed on digitized screen-film to those obtained on peripheral bone densitometry images. A leg phantom was imaged with both a PIXI (GE Medical Systems; Milwaukee, WI) bone densitometer (0.200-mm pixel size) and a screen-film system, with the films being subsequently digitized by a laser film digitizer (0.100-mm pixel size). The phantom was radiographically scanned multiple times with the densitometer at the default parameters and for increasing exposure times. Fourier-based texture features were calculated from regions of interest from images from both modalities. The bone densitometry images contained more quantum noise than the radiographs resulting in increased values for the first moment of the power spectrum texture feature (1.22 times higher than from the standard radiograph). Presence of such noise may adversely affect the texture feature's ability to distinguish between strong and weak bone. By either increasing the exposure time or averaging multiple scans in the spatial frequency domain, we showed a reduction in the effect of the quantum mottle on the first moment of the power spectrum.

Keywords: bone densitometry, texture analysis, computer vision, computer-aided diagnosis, radiographic skeletal imaging

1. INTRODUCTION

Osteoporosis reduces the quality of life of the millions of people it afflicts. Osteoporosis has been defined as "a systemic skeletal disease characterized by low bone mass and microarchitectural deterioration of bone tissue, with a consequent increase in bone fragility and susceptibility to fracture".[1] Although there are many factors that affect bone quality, two primary determinants of bone mechanical properties are bone mass and bone structure. Currently, the the most common method to assess osteoporosis status is bone densitometry which only measures bone mass. The ability to characterize both bone structure and bone mass has the potential to better assess bone strength than bone mass alone.

In previous work, we investigated the use of texture analysis of the bone trabecular pattern on digitized radiographs to assess bone structure.[2, 3] In that work, we radiographed excised femoral neck specimens obtained from total hip arthroplasties. Stress to failure values from mechanical strength testing of the specimens was used as our 'gold standard' with which to compare the texture features and BMD measurements abilities in distinguishing between strong and weak bone. When using linear discriminant analysis to combine BMD and a texture feature, the combined feature was able to better distinguish between strong and weak bone compared to BMD alone; areas under the ROC curves (A_z) were 0.85 and 0.75 respectively.[3]

Ideally, bone mass and bone structure information would be obtained from a single diagnostic exam, which could be used for the effective and efficient screening for osteoporosis. Current bone densitometers may provide adequate image quality to characterize bone structure as well as measure bone mineral densitometry. In this study we investigate the use of a peripheral bone densitometer for bone texture analysis and compare it to digitized screen-film texture analysis measurements.

Further author information: (Send correspondence to M.R.C.)

M.R.C.: E-mail: m-chinander@uchicago.edu, Telephone: 1 773-834-5101

Medical Imaging 2002: Image Processing, Milan Sonka, J. Michael Fitzpatrick, Editors, Proceedings of SPIE Vol. 4684 (2002) © 2002 SPIE · 1605-7422/02/$15.00

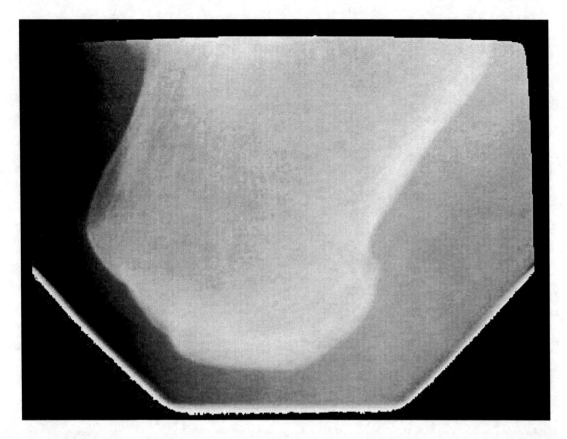

Figure 1: Example of an image of the calcaneous obtained from the PIXI peripheral bone densitometer.

2. MATERIALS AND METHODS

Images of the heel of a leg phantom were acquired using both a screen-film system and a heel bone densitometer. The leg phantom was an Alderson phantom which consisted of real human bone encased in tissue-equivalent plastic. We used a Lanex medium/TMG (Eastman Kodak; Rochester, NY) screen-film system which is typically used for bone radiography. The phantom was radiographed five times with standard exposure parameters so that the resulting radiograph had an optical density of approximately 1.0 in the calcaneous. The radiograph was then digitized to 100 micron pixel size using an Abe Sekkei laser film scanner.

The phantom was also scanned with a PIXI peripheral bone densitometer (GE-Lunar Corp.; Madison, WI). The PIXI is a CCD-based imaging system with a GdO_2S screen and 200 micron pixel size. The phantom was scanned eight times using the default clinical settings. To investigate the effect of exposure time, the phantom was scanned an additional ten times at increasing exposure times up to 2.5 times the standard clinical exposure time. Figure 1 shows an example of an image acquired from the PIXI.

In order to characterize the bone structure, a Fourier-based texture feature was calculated from regions of interest (ROIs) selected in the central part of the calcaneous. Since the two imaging systems differed in pixel size by a factor of two, the screen-film ROIs were taken as twice as large as those from the bone densitometer (128×128 vs. 64×64) so that the ROIs contained the same region of the bone in both imaging systems. A background trend correction using a second-order polynomial fit was performed on the ROIs prior to texture analysis. The first moment of the power spectrum was calculated as show below.

$$\text{First moment of the power spectrum} = \frac{\sum_m \sum_n \sqrt{m^2 + n^2}\, |F_{m,n}|^2}{\sum_m \sum_n |F_{m,n}|^2} \tag{1}$$

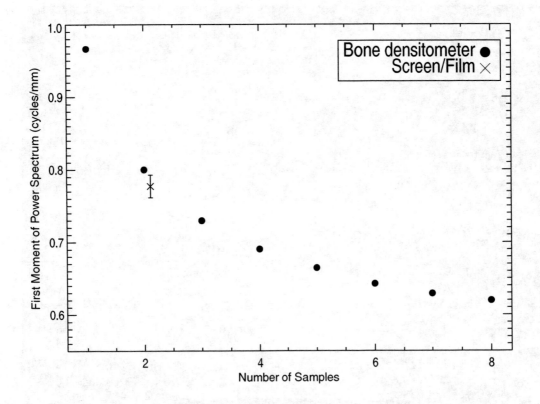

Figure 2. Effect of averaging multiple ROIs from different bone densitometry images on the first moment of the power spectrum texture feature.

In this equation F is the Fourier transform of the background corrected ROI. For the reduction of noise in the bone densitometry images, ROIs extracted at the same location from multiple scans were averaged. The number of ROIs that were averaged ranged from two to eight. In order to avoid blurring of the bone structure due to motion between the scans, the averaging was performed in the spatial-frequency domain rather than in the spatial domain.

3. RESULTS

The effect of averaging ROIs from multiple bone densitometry images of the heel phantom is shown in Figure 2. The data point for the screen-film system is the average value of the first moment obtained from the five screen-film images with the error bar indicating $+/-$ one standard deviation. Figure 3 shows the effect of increasing the exposure time on the first moment of the power spectrum. Exposure values are given relative to the initial exposure of the bone densitometer. The relative exposure of the screen-film imaging system was estimated from measurement of the entrance exposure with a dosimeter and relating that to the dose quoted for the PIXI bone densitometer in GE-Lunar's product literature.

4. SUMMARY

By either averaging multiple ROIs in the spatial frequency domain or increasing the exposure time, it was possible to decrease the contribution of quantum noise to the first moment of the power spectrum texture feature. The value of the first moment of the power spectrum from a single bone densitometry image was higher than from a digitized screen-film image largely due to more noise. Using two exposures or doubling the exposure time had a similar decrease in the first moment of the power spectrum texture features and resulted in similar values as those from digitized screen-film images. We are currently investigating whether these methods to

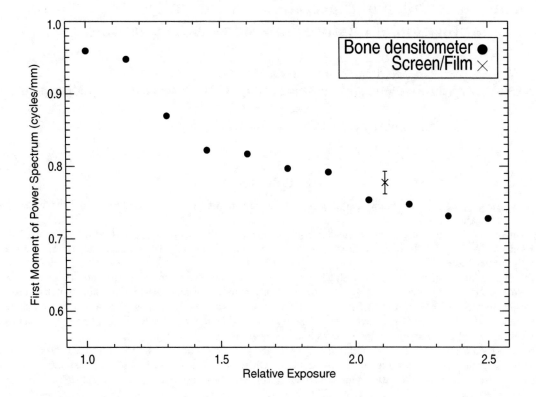

Figure 3. Effect of increasing the exposure time on the first moment of the power spectrum texture feature from images acquired from the PIXI peripheral bone densitometer.

improve the characterization of bone structure from bone densitometry images improves the texture feature's ability to distinguish between normal and osteoporotic bone.

ACKNOWLEDGMENTS

This work has been supported in part by USPHS Grants RO1 AR42739, RR11459, and T32 CA09649.

M.L. Giger is a shareholder in R2 Technology, Inc. (Los Altos, CA). It is The University of Chicago Conflict of Interest Policy that investigators disclose publicly actual or potential significant financial interest which would reasonable appear to be directly and significantly affected by the research activities.

REFERENCES

1. W. Peck, P. Burckhardt, C. Christiansen, and et al., "Consensus development conference: diagnosis, prophylaxis, and treatment of osteoporosis," *American Journal of Medicine* **94**(6), pp. 646–650, 1993.

2. M. R. Chinander, M. L. Giger, J. M. Martell, C. Jiang, and M. J. Favus, "Computerized radiographic texture measures for characterizing bone strength: A simulated clinical setup using femoral neck specimens," *Medical Physics* **26**(11), pp. 2295–2300, 1999.

3. M. R. Chinander, M. L. Giger, J. M. Martell, and M. J. Favus, "Computerized analysis of radiographic bone patterns: Effect of imaging conditions on performance," *Medical Physics* **27**(1), pp. 75–85, 2000.

Genetic algorithm and expectation maximization for parameter estimation of mixture Gaussian model phantom

Nariman Majdi Nasab, Mostafa Analoui

Indiana University School of Dentistry, Imaging Facility, 1121 W. Michigan St., Indianapolis, IN 46202.

nmajdina@ecn.purdue.edu, manaloui@iupui.edu

ABSTRACT

We present a new approach for estimating parameters of Gaussian mixture model by Genetic Algorithms (GAs) and Expectation Maximization (EM).

It has been shown that GAs is independent of initialization parameters. In this work we propose combination of GAs and EM algorithms (GA-EM) for learning Gaussian mixture components to achieve accurate parameter estimation independent of initial values.

To assess the performance of the proposed method, a series of Gaussian phantoms, based on modified Shepp-Logan method, were created. In this phantom, each tissue segment presents a Gaussian density function that its mean and variance can be controlled. EM, GAs and GA-EM were employed to estimate the tissue parameters in each phantom. The results indicate that EM algorithm, as expected, is heavily impacted by the initial values. Coupling GAs with EM not only improves the overall accuracy, it also provides estimates that are independent of initial seed values.

The proposed method offers a solution for accurate and stable solution for parameter estimation in for Gaussian mixture models, with higher likelihood of achieving global optimal. Obtaining such accurate parameter estimation is a key requirement for several image segmentation approaches, which rely on *a priori* knowledge of tissue distribution.

Key words: Expectation Maximization, Mixture Gaussian Model, and Genetic Algorithms.

1. INTRODUCTION

Decomposing a finite mixture of distributions is very difficult problem. The likelihood approach to fitting of mixture models has since been utilized by several authors [1-3]. Finite mixture distributions provide a simple framework for modeling population heterogeneity. Multivariate observations on a set of n entities forming an array can be represented as $x_1,\ldots,x_n$, where each x_j is a vector of p-dimensions. Under the finite mixture models to be fitted here, each x_j can be viewed as arising from a super population G, which is a mixture of a finite number of populations $G_1,\ldots,G_g$ in some proportions $\pi_1,\ldots,\pi_g$, respectively, where

$$\sum_{i=1}^{g}\pi_i = 1 \quad and \quad \pi_i \geq 0 \quad (i=1,\ldots,g). \tag{1}$$

The probability density function (p.d.f.) of an observation x in G can therefore be represented in the finite mixture form,

$$f(x;\phi) = \sum_{i=1}^{g}\pi_i p_i(x,\theta), \tag{2}$$

where $p_i(x;\theta)$ is the p.d.f. corresponding to G_i, and θ denotes the vector of all unknown parameters associated with the parametric forms adopted these g component densities. In particular case, especially in this paper, of multivariate normal component densities consists of the elements of the mean vectors μ_i and the distinct elements of the covariance matrices Σ_i for $i=1,\ldots,g$ are used.

The vector, ϕ,:

$$\phi = (\pi,\theta)^T \tag{3}$$

of all unknown parameters belongs to some parameters space Ω; "T" denotes vector transpose.

Medical Imaging 2002: Image Processing, Milan Sonka, J. Michael Fitzpatrick, Editors, Proceedings of SPIE Vol. 4684 (2002) © 2002 SPIE · 1605-7422/02/$15.00

Learning the mixture, namely, estimating the weights π_i and the parameters θ_i of each component, is often carried out through likelihood maximization using the EM algorithm [2]. However, known limitations of EM are:

(*i*) It assumes that the number *g* of mixing components is known,

(*ii*) There is no widely accepted 'good' method for initialization the parameters, and

(*iii*) The algorithm is of local nature and thus can get stuck in local maxima of the likelihood function.

Good abilities of GAs, Escaping from local minima, and finding global minima and no dependency of GAs to initial values are important advantage of GAs in comparing with EM algorithm.

GAs is adaptive search techniques designed to find out near optimal solutions of large-scale optimization problem with multiple local maxima.

2. GENETIC ALGORITHMS

GAs are an efficient technique to optimize difficult functions in large search spaces. By testing populations of solutions represented as strings of bits (called chromosomes) in an iterative process, a genetic algorithm is able to find a near-optimal solution in robust manner, with the ability to produce a best 'guess' from incomplete or noisy data [5].

GAs tackle the problem of minimizing a function, objective function, of the vector $x_i^j = (x_i^l, ..., x_i^l)$. It is standard practice to formulate problems so that each x_i^j, $j=1, ...,l$, is binary, taking the value 0 or 1; the basic GAs starts by randomly generating an even number *n* of binary strings of length *l* to form an initial population. Rules are then applied to create successive generations in turn.

These parents are considered in pairs and, for each pair, a crossover operation is performed with a pre-selected probability p_c. If the crossover occurs, an integer *k* is generated from the uniform distribution on $\{1,...,l-1\}$ and the last *l-k* elements of each parent are exchanged to create two new strings, thus, one string takes values $x_i^l,...,x_i^l$ from the first parent and $x_i^{k+l},...,x_i^l$ from the second while the other takes values $x_i^l,...,x_i^l$ from second parent and $x_i^{k+l},...,x_i^l$ from the first. If crossover does not occur, the parent the parent is copied unaltered into new strings. Finally, the mutation operator switches the value at each string position from 0 to 1 or vice versa with probability p_m, mutation occurring independently at each element of each string. The algorithm is allowed to continue for a certain number of generations. On termination, the string in the final population with the highest value of *F* can be returned as the solution to the optimization problem. However, since a good solution may be lost by algorithm, a more efficient strategy is to note the best solution seen at any stage and return this as the solution.

A positive fitness *F* is calculated as a monotone decreasing function of objective function, Λ, for each individual in the current generation and *m* parents for the next generation are selected with replacement, the probability F_n of choosing *n*-th individual in the current population being proportional to its fitness Λ_n, i.e.

$$F_n = \frac{\Lambda_n}{\sum_{i=1}^{m} \Lambda_n} \tag{4}$$

The population size *m*, probabilies of crossover, mutation and fitness function *F* must be specified before the algorithm is applied, although trial runs may hopeful in choosing appropriate values.

The sensivity of the algorithm to the choice of p_m is evident. If p_m is too small the algorithm can become trapped in a local minimum at an early age, but if p_m is too high random mutations disrupt what would otherwise be good solutions and the algorithm struggles to create the very best solutions.

A simple genetic algorithm is given below, where $p(t)$ is a population of candidate solutions to a given problem at generation *t*.

```
t=0;
    Initialize p(t) ;
        Evaluate p(t) ;
            While not <termination condition>
            Begin
                t=t+1;
                Reproduce p(t) from p(t-1) ;
                Recombine p(t) ;
```

Evaluate p(t) ;

End

3. GENETIC ALGORITHMS AND EXPECTATION MAXIMIZATION (GA-EM)

Any image processing task needs correct and appreciate a *priori* information. The main difficulty is that the model and its parameters are unknown and need to be computed from the given before any image processing. In practice one does not have any knowledge to those parameters. An alternative approach to this problem is to have a two step process, first estimating the parameters by GAs and getting crude a *priori* information. Then the *priori* information is used as initial guess for EM algorithm to find out the final parameters. So the problem of parameters can be solved using both GAs and EM (GA-EM) algorithm.

In our previous work [6], we have showed that using EM algorithm could not be successful always because of the true number of mixing component is unknown and algorithm can get stuck in one of the many local maxima of the likelihood function and specially there is not generally accepted method for parameter initialization. In that, we presented a new method to find out Gaussian mixture model parameters by Genetic Algorithms. GAs is adaptive search techniques designed to find out near optimal solutions of large-scale optimization problem with multiple local maxima.

It is shown that using GAs can find fast and accurate, proportionally, mixture model components, weights for noisy and noiseless normal mixture model.

4. SIMULATION AND RESULTS

4.1. GAs simulation

Implementation of GAs requires a positive valued fitness function F, monotically decreasing in the objective function $\Lambda(x)$ where,

$$\Lambda_n(x) = \left| 1 - \sum_{i=1}^{g} \hat{\pi}_i \right| + \left| f(x;\phi) - \hat{f}_n(x;\phi) \right| \tag{5}$$

The hat sign, ^, demonstrates the values which were generated by GAs for *n*-th individual, *n=1, ..., m,* in the current population. This function must provide sufficient selectivity to ensure that the algorithm performs superior solutions to the extent that it eventually produces an optimal or near-optimal answer.

In this work, population size $m = 500$ was selected. Mutation is randomly applied with low probability, typically in the range 0.001 and 0.01, and modifies elements in the chromosomes. Usually considered as a background operator, the role of mutation is often seen as providing a guarantee that the probability of searching any given string will never be zero and acting as a safety net to recover good genetic material that may be lost through the action of selection and crossover.

The value for, mutation, $p_m = \dfrac{0.7}{Lind}$ is selected, where *Lind* is the chromosome length. Chromosome length is bit value for each individual, which is number of bits for ϕ in Eq. 3. The basic operator for producing new chromosomes in the GA is that of crossover. Like in counterpart in the nature, crossover produces new individuals that have some parts of both parent's genetic material. Normally probability of crossover is selected between 0.6 - 0.9 and in this work we have selected, p_c, 0.8.

Objective function plays important rule to find out ϕ parameters. The objective function is used to provide a measure of how individuals have performed in the problem domain. In this work, minimization problem, the most fit individuals will have the lowest numerical value of the associated objective function. In this way, we have examined different type of objective functions and eventually the best of them, Eq. 5, is used for simulation our data. We have done simulation for a six-component normal mixture function.

The first term of Eq. 10 constrains the probability summation of mixture and the second term tries to fit the best parameters, ϕ, to original mixture model.

GAs are iteration programs and we have set number of iteration, based on experiment, to 300. Once the program finishes, the GAs results are used as initial value for EM algorithm.

The following table is used as distribution of bits for ϕ. These values are selected based on 8 bits per pixel on 'Modified Shepp-Logan' phantom [7].

Table 1. Bits values for estimation ϕ_i in 'Modified Shepp-Logan' phantom, total length of ϕ_i is 18 bits.

ϕ_i ; $i=1,...,6$	π_i	μ_i	Σ_i
Bits	6	8	4

4.2. EM simulation

The probability density function (p.d.f) of an observation x is defined in the finite mixture form for Guassian model as:

$$f(x;\phi) = \sum_{i=1}^{g} \pi_i \cdot p_i(x;\theta) = \sum_{i=1}^{g} \pi_i \cdot \frac{1}{(2\pi)^{1/2}|\Sigma_i|^{\frac{1}{2}}} \exp{-\frac{1}{2}(x-\mu_i)^T \Sigma_i^{-1}(x-\mu_i)} \tag{6}$$

where π_i is the mixing parameter, $p_i(x;\theta)$ is the p.d.f. corresponding to G_i, and θ denotes the vector of all unknown parameters associated with parametric forms adopted for these g component densities. For the case of multivariate Guassian components, θ consists of the elements of the mean vectors μ_i, and the distinct elements of the covariance matrices Σ_i for $i=1, ..., g$. The vector $\phi = (\pi^T, \theta^T)^T$ of all unknown parameters is estimated using EM algorithm.

We have obtained the following update equations for the parameters of mixture model [2]:

$$\mu_i^{t+1} = \frac{\sum_{j=1}^{n} p'(i|x_j)x_j}{\sum_{j=1}^{n} p'(i|x_j)} \tag{7}$$

$$\Sigma_i^{t+1} = \frac{\sum_{j=1}^{n} p'(i|x_j)(x_j - \mu_i^t)^T(x_j - \mu_i^t)}{\sum_{j=1}^{n} p'(i|x_j)} \tag{8}$$

$$\pi_i^{t+1} = \frac{1}{n}\sum_{j=1}^{n} p'(i|x_j) \tag{9}$$

where

$$p'(i|x_j) = \frac{p'(x_j|i)\pi'(i)}{p'(x_j)} \tag{10}$$

4.3. Results

In this work, we show performance of three algorithm, EM, GAs, and GA-EM, for three set, image 1, image2, and image 3, of 'Modified Shepp-Logan' phantoms. For each of them ϕ is different than others. The purpose of selecting various ϕ is to evaluate performance of algorithms in different ϕ.

4.3.1. Image 1

We constructed a 'Modified Shepp-Logan' phantom, image 1, based on following parameters from table 2.

Table 2. ϕ values for image 1

π	0.5818	0.0014	0.3293	0.0434	0.0008	0.0434
μ	60	91	122	153	184	220
Σ	14	15	8	6	10	10
Model simulation error = 0.0778						

There is always an error between phantom and values on each image, this error was shown on table 2, and we so-called it Model simulation error. This error exists because of limitation of generation Guassian model data to construct the image. In figure 1, we show image, its histogram and constructed histogram based on ϕ values.

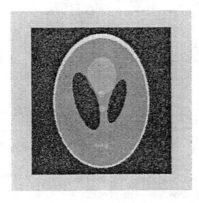 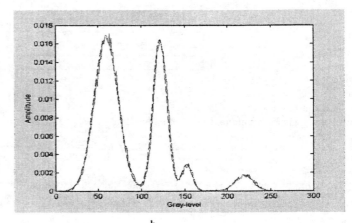

a.   b.

Figure 1. a) Constructed image, image 1 b) Comparison between histogram of image 1 vs. its mixture model Parameters, solid line is image histogram and '-' line is mixture model.

Model simulation error can calculate between image histogram and mixture model is calculates as follows:

$$Error_{model} = \left| Hist_{image\#} - f_{image\#}(x;\phi) \right| \quad (11)$$

where $Hist_{image\#}$ is histogram of image number image and $f_{image\#}(x;\phi)$ is mixture model based on their values, *e.g.* image 1 is on table 2. This error was calculated for image 1 and we got 0.0778.

To measure performance of each algorithm error of each algorithm is calculated as follow:

$$Error = \left| f_{image\#}(x;\phi) - \hat{f}_{algorithm}(x;\phi) \right| \quad (12)$$

where $\hat{f}_{algorithm}(x;\phi)$ is mixture model as result of EM, GAs, and GA-EM.

Table 3. Result of there algorithms to find out ϕ values for image 1 and corresponds error. The original values of ϕ are in table 2. The table consists three connected blocks showing its error algorithm based on Eq. 12.

EM	π	μ	Σ	Error=0.077659
	0.3334	58.8089	13.4930	
	0.2494	61.6118	14.6530	
Image 1	0.3300	122.0843	8.0102	
	0.0430	152.9463	6.0467	
	0.0013	189.8242	13.3320	
	0.0430	220.0953	10.0869	
GAs	π	μ	Σ	Error=0.043931
	0.2381	61	14	
	0.3333	61	14	
Image 1	0.2063	123	8	
	0.1270	123	8	
	0.0476	154	6	
	0.0476	221	11	
GA-EM	π	μ	Σ	Error=0.077806
	0.3398	59.9912	14.0448	
	0.2427	59.9912	14.0448	
Image 1	0.2042	122.0594	8.0099	
	0.1257	122.0594	8.0099	
	0.0434	152.9567	6.2423	
	0.0441	219.4660	10.8739	

The same technique was used to calculate errors for image 2 and the image 3. The original values and result for image 2 is appeared on figure 2, table 4 and 5.

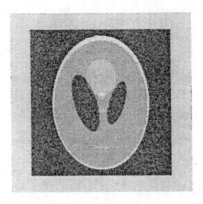
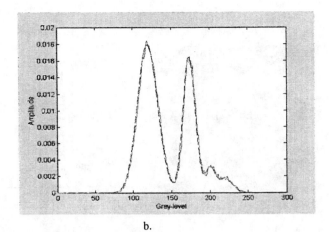

a.   b.

Figure 2. a) Constructed image, image 2 b) Comparison between histogram of image 2 vs. its mixture model Parameters, solid line is image histogram and '-' line is mixture model.

Table 4. ϕ values for image 2

π	0.5818	0.0014	0.3293	0.0434	0.0434	0.0008
μ	120	147	174	201	220	228
Σ	13	15	8	6	10	5
Model simulation error = 0.0735						

Table 5. Result of there algorithms to find out ϕ values for image 2 and corresponds error. The original values of ϕ are in table 4.

EM	π	μ	Σ	Error=0.073101
	0.0001	66.3399	1.4239	
	0.1494	117.7900	12.2838	
Image 2	0.4336	120.8733	13.1791	
	0.3279	173.9489	7.9048	
	0.0496	201.4160	6.6086	
	0.0395	221.6849	9.3253	
GAs	π	μ	Σ	Error=0.063871
	0.0794	120	12	
	0.4127	120	13	
Image 2	0.0794	126	11	
	0.3492	175	9	
	0.0635	208	10	
	0.0159	228	6	
GA-EM	π	μ	Σ	Error=0.072877
	0.0816	118.7489	11.8259	
	0.4233	119.2581	13.0396	
Image 2	0.0780	125.8640	12.6687	
	0.3287	173.9755	7.9369	
	0.0463	201.1930	6.2403	
	0.0421	220.8628	9.7119	

Image 3 is shown in the figure 3, table 6 and 7, again the same technique was used to calculate errors. It is shown that for this image EM algorithm could not find any solution for mixture model and EM algorithm over flew for image 3 to find ϕ values.

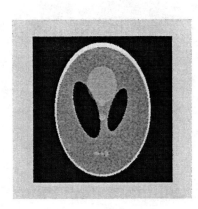

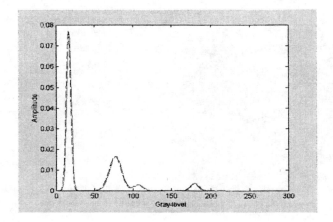

a.   b.

Figure 3. a) Constructed image, image 3 b) Comparison between histogram of image 3 vs. its mixture model Parameters, solid line is image histogram and '-' line is mixture model.

Table 6. ϕ values for image 3

π	0.5818	0.0014	0.3293	0.0434	0.0008	0.0434
μ	17	47	77	107	137	180
Σ	3	10	8	6	2	5
Model simulation error = 0.1972						

Table 7. Result of there algorithms to find out ϕ values for image 3 and corresponds error. The original values of ϕ are in table 5.

EM	π	μ	Σ	Error=Not Defined
	NaN	NaN	NaN	
	NaN	NaN	NaN	
Image 3	NaN	NaN	NaN	
	NaN	NaN	NaN	
	NaN	NaN	NaN	
	NaN	NaN	NaN	
GAs	π	μ	Σ	Error=0.088913
	0.2381	16	2	
	0.0952	18	4	
Image 3	0.2381	20	2	
	0.2381	77	7	
	0.1429	89	16	
	0.0476	181	5	
GA-EM	π	μ	Σ	Error=0.2188
	0.2911	15.8476	2.5772	
	0.1118	17.0783	3.5104	
Image 3	0.1789	18.7917	2.3955	
	0.2688	75.9938	7.1013	
	0.1059	91.7424	16.4299	
	0.0434	180.1618	5.0417	

5. CONCLUSION

In this work the GAs is used to estimate six-component normal mixture function as initial step for EM algorithm. One of the great advantages of GAs in this case is that the algorithm does not depend of initial condition, which is one of the limitations of EM algorithm to find mixture model parameters.

The performance of GAs is highly depending of how Objective function defines. We tested several type of objective function and in this paper we presented the best of them. In this work we propose combination of GA and EM algorithms (GA-EM) for learning Gaussian mixture components to achieve accurate parameter estimation independent of initial values.

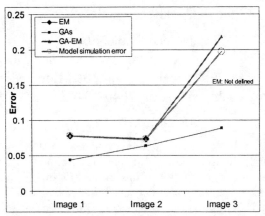

Figure 4. Error of EM, GAs, and GA-EM algorithms for three set of 'Modified Shepp-Logan' phantom.

To assess the performance of the proposed method, a series of Gaussian phantoms, based on modified Shepp-Logan method, were created. EM, GAs and GA-EM were employed to estimate the tissue parameters in three phantoms and relative error of them were calculated. The results indicate that EM algorithm, as expected, is heavily impacted by the initial values and for the image 3 it failed to calculate ϕ values. Coupling GA with EM not only improves the overall accuracy, it also provides estimates that are independent of initial seed values.

Error of GA-EM is very close to error model for all three images, Fig. 4, however the minimum error was obtained by GAs and error for EM in image 3 was undefined.

The proposed method offers a solution for accurate and stable solution for parameter estimation in for Gaussian mixture models, with higher likelihood of achieving global optimal. Obtaining such accurate parameter estimation is a key requirement for several image and signal processing approaches.

6. REFERENCE

1. Geoffrey J. McLachlan, Kaye E. Basford, *Mixture Model Inference and Application to Clustering*, Marcel Dekker, Inc. 1988.
2. Richard A. Render and Homer F. Walker, "Mixture densities, maximum likelihood and the EM algorithm", SIAM review, **26**, No. 2, April 1984.
3. N. A. Vlassis, G. Papakonstantinou, and P. Tsanakas, "Mixture Density Estimation Based on Maximum Likelihood and Test Statistics" *Neural Processing Letters Journal,* 1998.
4. A. P. Dempster, N. M. Laird, and D. B. Rubin, "Maximum likelihood from incomplete data via the EM algorithm," *J. Roy. Statist. Soc. B,* **39**, pp. 1-38, 1977.
5. D. E. Goldberg, *Genetic Algorithms in Search Optimization and Machine Learning*, Addison Wesley Publishing Company, January1989.
6. N. Majdi Nasab and M. Analoui "Mixture conditional estimation using genetic algorithms", IEEE ISSPA 2001: Statistical Signal Processing, Kuala-Lampur, Malaysia, 13-16 August 2001.
7. A. Jain, *Fundamental of Digital Image Processing*, Prentice Hall, NJ, 1989.

Optimized statistical modeling of MS lesions as MRI voxel outliers for monitoring the effect of drug therapy

Zhanyu Ge, and Sunanda Mitra

Texas Tech University
Computer Vision and Image Analysis Laboratory
Department of Electrical and Computer Engineering
Lubbock, Texas 79409-3102

ABSTRACT

This paper presents the results of applying the modified deterministic annealing (DA) algorithm to simulated and clinical magnetic resonance (MR) brain data with multiple sclerosis (MS) lesions. Modified deterministic annealing algorithm is a very efficient segmentation algorithm for isolating MS lesions in the MR images when utilizing all the information contained in all modalities. To fully utilize the information contained in all the modalities, vector segmentation is carried out instead of unimodal segmentation. The vectors to be clustered are formed by multi-modal MR brain data. Through some arithmetic manipulations synthesized image data can be obtained which greatly alleviate the effect of noise and intensity inhomogeneity. Isolated multiple sclerosis lesions are outliers to the brain tissues. Even with noise level up to 7% the MS MR brain data can still be satisfactorily segmented. This method does not need a prior model, and is conceptually very simple. It delineates not only large lesions but small ones as well. The whole process is completely automated without any intervention by an operator, which can be a very promising tool for MS follow-up studies. Comparison between the segmentation results from the simulated MS brain data and from the clinical MS brain data shows that with the current high quality MRI facilities, images with noise above 3% and intensity inhomogeneity above 20% will usually not be produced. Segmentation results for the clinical data are much better and easier to obtain than the simulated noisy data. To get even better results for the MS lesions, inverse problem techniques have to be applied. Noise model and intensity inhomogeneity model have to be established and improved using the given MRI data during iteration.

Keywords: Multiple sclerosis, deterministic annealing, clustering, vector segmentation, magnetic resonance imaging.

1. INTRODUCTION

Multiple sclerosis is a disease of young adults, especially females. It is not curable yet, but can only be controlled through drug therapy. The magnetic resonance imaging scan is a diagnostic tool that currently offers the most effective non-invasive way of imaging the brain. MRI is very useful in detecting central nervous system demyelination, and thus a powerful tool in helping to establish the diagnosis of MS. Demyelination or the destruction of myelin (the fatty sheath that surrounds and protects nerve fibers) causes nerve impulses to be slowed or halted and produces the symptoms of MS. Lesions in MR images of confirmed Multiple Sclerosis patients vary in size, number, and location during follow-up periods and therefore precise assessment by human experts is extremely time consuming and prone to intra- and inter-observer variability. The evaluation of the effect of drug therapy over a period of time for a large number of patients becomes complicated because of the above factors. Recent studies have emphasized the role of post processing and automated analysis of MR images in order to develop a reproducible methodology for identification of MS lesions in multi-spectral MR images based on models [1][2]. We present an optimized and automated statistical clustering procedure for isolating MS lesions from multi-modal (or multi-spectral) MR intensity images with potential of an automated tool for follow-up studies.

Based on a statistical classification technique known as the deterministic annealing (DA) [5], we modified and applied it to volumetric segmentation of simulated normal brain [3] tissues into white matter, gray matter, and cerebrospinal fluid by clustering the intensity values in unimodal MR images. Isolation of MS lesions is, however, is a challenging task since the intensity of the lesions could overlap with the intensities of the other tissues. Deterministic annealing minimizes the expected distortion subject to two constraints: a specified level of randomness (by incorporating the system entropy) and the constraint for the *a priori* probabilities. The methodology used in this work is based on obtaining an efficient and accurate global solution of non-convex optimization problems by including a structural constraint of *a posteriori* probabilities in a deterministic annealing schedule. Location of the lesions in MRI of confirmed MS patients are identified either as outliers or presence of dark spots in the segmented tissues.

Medical Imaging 2002: Image Processing, Milan Sonka, J. Michael Fitzpatrick, Editors, Proceedings of SPIE Vol. 4684 (2002) © 2002 SPIE · 1605-7422/02/$15.00

Segmentation of an image is to separate an image into regions or parts of common attributes (such as proximity, similarity, and continuity), while image segmentation itself belongs to the category of clustering. Clustering is partitioning the given data set into optimal groups, which correspond to an optimal minimum of a cost function of some form. Development of a global optimization technique for 3-D medical image segmentation is a difficult task and is currently being investigated for diagnostic and research applications by researchers throughout the world. Image segmentation is to find two basic kind of segments: boundaries and regions, which may be achieved by object classification and recognition techniques, like AFLC, AFCM, EM, DA, etc. [11, 12, 13, 14, 7, 5]. Here the modified DA algorithm will focus only on local pixel values and globally optimize the segmentation solution.

Leemput et al. [1] developed an automated algorithm for segmenting MS lesions from multispectral (T1-weighted, T2-weighted, and PD-weighted) MR images. The segmentation is an iterative process. The prior classification (probability) that prescribes a voxel to belong to a brain tissue is first obtained from a digital normal brain atlas that contains information about the expected locations of the white matter (WM), gray matter (GM), and cerebrospinal fluid (CSF). Then intensity constraints (thresholding of the T2- and PD-weighted images) and contextual constraints (an application of Markov random theory) are applied to make the M-estimator (a modified EM algorithm) perform satisfactorily. There is still a parameter, k, needing to be experimentally determined. The posteriori probability for each of the voxels is a Gibbs distribution. The tissue model excludes extraneous tissues and only includes WM, GM, and CSF and outliers (within WM and CSF). The intensity inhomogeneity is approximated by a fourth-order polynomial. This method heavily relies on a well-trained normal brain atlas, errors may occur when the patients brains are of different size and different gesture, and when the patients' tissue volumes are different from those in the atlas. Besides accurate registration and correspondence would be a tough problem before segmentation can take place. The whole process is very complicated and may be very time-consuming.

Johnston et al. [2] segments MS lesions in a multi-step way using T2- and PD-weighted MR images. The acquired T2 and PD images are first masked to get rid of the non-brain tissues. Then the data are homomorphically filtered (a form of high pass filtering) to make an RF-correction of the intensity inhomogeneities. The filtered T2 and PD brain data are then separately and softly segmented into 4 clusters using their modified iterated conditional modes algorithm (using histogram profiles). This method also needs a truth model trained by samples. Segmentation results of the T2 and PD data are then combined by multiplying their probabilities and normalized to make the total probability for any voxel add to unity. White matter and lesion segmentations are then extracted and summed to get a WM/lesion mask. This WM/lesion mask is then segmented using the above segmentation algorithm once again and thresholded to separate the lesions from the white matter. Small size lesions will be eliminated. This method also appears to be complicated and inaccurate.

Udupa et al. [4] used fuzzy-connectedness principle to find potential MS lesions as an outlier of the brain tissues. But the brain tissue seeds have to be manually and accurately labeled by an operator. The final decision is made by the operator through a mouse button. Pham and Prince [7] used adaptive fuzzy C-means algorithm to segment brain tissues and model the intensity inhomogeneity with a gain field model. There are other techniques used for segmenting MS lesions, but some post-processing (morphologic operation, connectivity manipulation, or thresholding) must be used and decision parameters are experimentally determined, as in [8].

In this paper we present our approach to segment MS lesions by first semi-automatically removing the non-brain tissues from the T1-, T2-, PD-weighted MR images, then arithmetically manipulating the brain data of different modalities to get synthesized brain data, and finally applying the modified deterministic annealing algorithm to segment the MS lesions and brain tissues through multidimensional vectors formed from the synthesized data and the above multi-modal brain data. The obtained results are satisfactory for simulated brain data of various levels of noise and intensity inhomogeneity and for clinical brain data downloaded from the internet.

2. THEORETICAL BACKGROUND

Deterministic annealing algorithm is a clustering technique derived from an optimization criterion. Based on [5 and 3], a brief description of DA is provided. The cost function to be minimized is

$$F = D - T\left[H + \left(\sum_j p(y_j) - 1\right)\right] \tag{1}$$

where, D = expected distortion $= \sum_i \sum_j p(x_i, y_j) d(x_i, y_j) = \sum_i p(x_i) \sum_j p(y_j \mid x_i) d(x_i, y_j)$;

H = Shannon Entropy $= -\sum_i \sum_j p(x_i, y_j) \log p(x_i, y_j)$;

T = a Lagrangian multiplier, called the pseudo-temperature variable;

x_i = source vector;

y_j = reproduction vector;

$p(x_i, y_j)$ = probability of assigning x_i to the cluster represented by y_j;

$p(x_i)$ = source vector probability distribution;

$p(y_j \mid x_i)$ = the *a posteriori* probability;

$d(x_i, y_j)$ = distortion measure between x_i and y_j;

$p(y_j)$ = the *a priori* probability of the class represented by y_j.

Minimizing F with respect to $p(y_j \mid x_i)$, considering the constraints $\sum_j p(y_j \mid x_i) = 1$ and let $p(y_j \mid x_i) \propto p(y_j)$, we

obtain the following distribution of the *a posteriori* probability

$$p(y_j \mid x_i) = \frac{p(y_j) e^{-\frac{d(x_i, y_j)}{T}}}{\sum_k p(y_k) e^{-\frac{d(x_i, y_k)}{T}}}. \tag{2}$$

By taking partial derivative of F with respect to vector y_j, centroid condition is obtained,

$$\sum_i p(x_i, y_j) \frac{d}{dy_j} d(x_i, y_j) = 0, \quad \forall j. \tag{3}$$

For squared error distortion, (3) becomes

$$y_j = \sum_i x_i p(x_i \mid y_j) \quad \forall j \tag{3a}$$

Minimization of F with respect to $p(y_j)$ gives

$$\sum_i p(x_i) \frac{e^{-\frac{d(x_i, y_j)}{T}}}{\sum_k p(y_k) e^{-\frac{d(x_i, y_k)}{T}}} = 1 \quad \forall j. \tag{4}$$

or $\quad p(y_j) = \sum_i p(x_i) \dfrac{p(y_j) e^{-\frac{d(x_i, y_j)}{T}}}{\sum_k p(y_k) e^{-\frac{d(x_i, y_k)}{T}}} = \sum_i p(x_i) p(y_j \mid x_i) \quad \forall j \tag{4a}$

If ω_j denotes the jth cluster, represented by y_j, the decision rule is

$$x_i \in \omega_j, \quad \text{if } p(y_j \mid x_i) > p(y_k \mid x_i) \quad \forall k \neq j \tag{5}$$

Cluster splits or phase transition occurs when $T = T_c = 2\lambda_{max}$, λ_{max} is the maximum eigenvalue of the covariance matrix, $C_{x\mid y}$, formed by the state-conditional probability distribution $p(x_i \mid y_j)$,

$$C_{x\mid y} = \sum_i p(x_i \mid y_j)(x_i - y_j)(x_i - y_j)^t. \tag{6}$$

where t means "transpose".

3. DETERMINISTIC ANNEALING ALGORITHM

The flowchart of the DA algorithm is shown in Figure 1. Nomenclature used in the figure and later on is listed below:

K = the number of clusters during iteration;
$Kmax$ = the desired number of clusters;
T = pseudotemperature;
Tc_i = critical temperature for the ith cluster;
y_i = centroid of the ith cluster;
$p(y_i)$ = a priori probability of the ith cluster;
α = cooling schedule coefficient, $0 < \alpha < 1$;
δ = perturbation factor during phase transition;
Δ = stopping criterion for updating centroids.

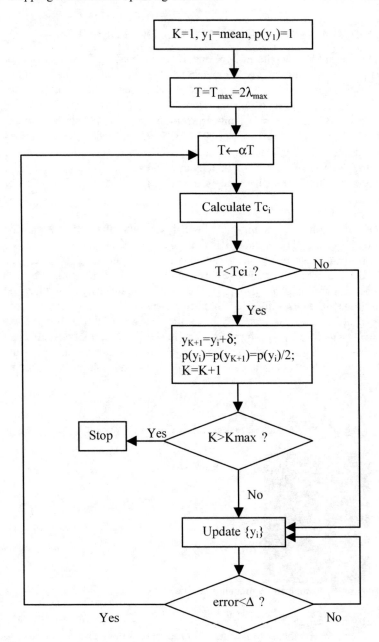

Fig. 1: Flowchart of the deterministic annealing algorithm

The deterministic annealing algorithm adapted to the MRI brain data segmentation is as follows:

(1) Input patterns (source vectors) and iteration and initialization parameters;
(2) Initialize cluster number K=1, y_1 = mean of all the input data, $p(y_1) = 1.0$;
(3) Find initial critical temperature;
(4) Cool the system: $T \leftarrow \alpha T$ ($0 < \alpha < 1$);
(5) Check condition for phase transition. If $Tc_i > T$, cluster splits, K=K+1;
(6) Update cluster centroids till convergence;
(7) Eliminate repeated centroids;
(8) Check the cluster number, if necessary go to (4);
(9) Assign patterns to clusters according to maximum $p(y_j|x_i)$;
(10) Output patterns with their cluster centroids;
(11) Determine misclassification (for labeled training patterns);
(12) Stop.

4. SIMULATED MS MRI BRAIN DATA SETS AND SEGMENTATION RESULTS

The simulated MS MR brain data were downloaded from the web-site of McConnell Brain Imaging Center, Montréal Neurological Institute, McGill University, Canada [9]. Each database is a 3-dimensional MR data set simulated using 3 sequences (3 modalities, namely, T1-, T2-, and PD-weighted or SD-weighted), 5 slice thicknesses (1 mm, 3 mm, 5 mm, 7 mm, and 9 mm), 6 noise levels (0, 1, 3, 5, 7, and 9%), and 3 levels of intensity non-uniformity (0, 20, and 40%). The data set is composed of voxels of 181×217×181 (X×Y×Z) when it is at a 1 mm isotropic voxel grid in Talairach space. The 3-D MS MR brain data sets of modalities T1, T2, and PD, of noise levels 0, 1, 3, 5, 7, 9%, and of intensity non-uniformity levels 0, 20, and 40%, were downloaded and analyzed. The slice thickness is 1 mm. The truth MS model brain data were also downloaded and used to do the comparison. The 2-D images are slices (perpendicular to Z-axis) from the 3-D data sets. 2-D segmentation is the segmentation of the slice images, 3-D segmentation is the clustering of the whole 3-D data sets.

Because the intensity overlapping of the MS lesions with brain tissues, uni-modal MR brain data usually do not provide good lesion segmentation results. Using all the T1-, T2-, and PD-weighted MR data, we may obtain more information about the MS lesions and each of the brain tissues. Adverse effects of noise and intensity inhomogeneity can be compromised through arithmetic manipulations of the brain data in the above three modalities, as demonstrated below. The synthesized brain data come from the arithmetic manipulations of data of the three modalities. The synthesized image data combined with the data of the above three modalities are used to form vectors, which are clustered into groups. Because the brain data of different levels of noise and inhomogeneity have different intensity distributions, we could not fix the number of clusters to be segmented, which means we have to segment the data into bigger number of clusters than the number of tissues plus background and lesions (outliers). Because the lesions are within the white matter and close to the CFS areas, lesions can be easily recognized, and the segmented and split tissues can be recombined.

4.1 Truth MS brain model
Figure 2 shows the truth model for the MS lesions for Slice No. 90. These lesions are located in areas within the white matter, and close the cerebrospinal fluid.

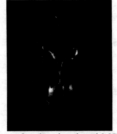

Fig. 2: Truth model image for the simulated MS brain image, Slice #90

4.2 MS brain data with 0% noise and 0% intensity inhomogeneity
Figure 3 shows the original MS brain images, Slice #90 in the z-direction, of three modalities. The image size is 217x181. Images in Figure 4 were obtained automatically by masking out the extraneous tissues. The mask was made

manually. Because the lesions are inside the CSF, minor errors of the mask will not affect the segmented lesions. All the following slice images are masked first before synthesized images are formed in the same way. Figure 5 shows the synthesized image for Slice #90. It is obtained by first subtracting T2-weighted images from PD-weighted images, and then subtracting the difference images from the T1-weihgted images, expressed by T1 - (PD - T2). Two-dimensional vectors (2xtotal number of voxels) are formed using the PD-weighted data set and this synthesized data set. These vectors are clustered into 6 instead of 5 groups because the partial volume effects. The extra cluster was added to the gray matter, as shown in Figure 6. Segmented tissues and lesions in Figure 6 are obtained by hard clustering using the *a posteriori* probability. It can be seen that the isolated lesions are almost identical to the truth model (after thresholding), which demonstrated the power of the modified DA algorithm in he detection of MS lesions.

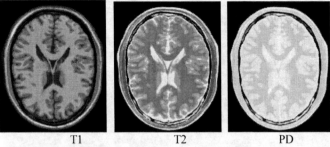

T1   T2   PD

Fig. 3: Original images (Slice #90), 0% noise and 0% intensity inhomogeneity

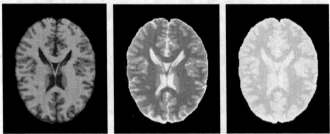

Fig. 4: Removal of the Extraneous Tissues

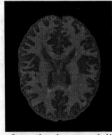

Fig. 5: Synthesized image from the three modalities in Fig. 4, T1-(PD-T2)

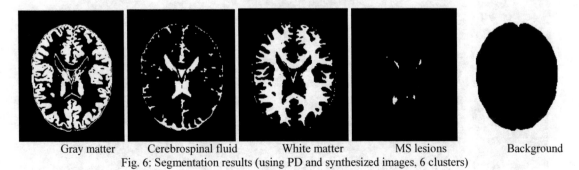

Gray matter   Cerebrospinal fluid   White matter   MS lesions   Background

Fig. 6: Segmentation results (using PD and synthesized images, 6 clusters)

4.3 MS brain data with 3% noise and 0% intensity inhomogeneity

Figure 7 shows the original images of Slice #90. Figure 8 are the brain data after removal of extraneous tissues and median filtering to reduce spike noise. Figure 9 are two synthesized images by arithmetic manipulations of the three modalities. PD - T1 means that the synthesized data are obtained by subtracting T1-weighted data from the PD-weighted data, and T1 - (PD - T2) is similar to that in Figure 5. Segmentation is carried out based on vectors formed from these two synthesized data sets. Because the noise and partial volume effects, the vectors are grouped into 12 clusters. The original segmentation results are shown in Figure 10 (a). The split brain tissues are recombined and shown in Figure 10 (b). It can be seen that because of the added noise some of the MS lesions are misclassified into the white matter, but the segmentation results are still satisfactory.

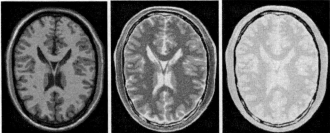

Fig. 7: Original images, 3% noise and 0% intensity inhomogeneity

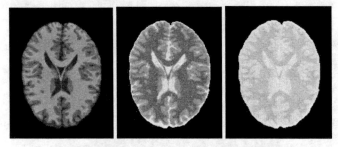

Fig. 8: Removal of extraneous tissues for images in Fig. 7

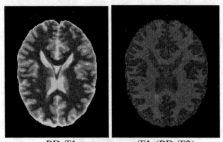

PD-T1   T1-(PD-T2)

Fig. 9: Synthesized images

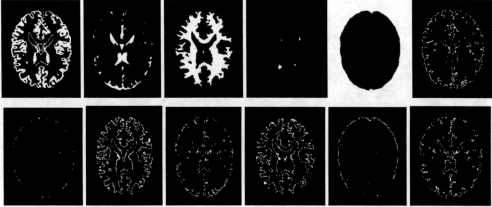

Fig. 10: (a) Original segmentation results (using 2 synthesized images in Fig.9, 12 clusters)

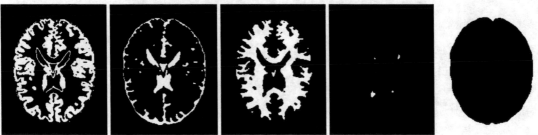

Fig. 10: (b) Segmentation results after recombining the split tissues

4.4 MS brain data with 3% noise and 20% intensity inhomogeneity

Figure 11 are the original images and Figure 12 are the images after removal of non-brain tissues and median filtering. Synthesized images in Figure 13 are similar to those in Figure 9. Figure 14 shows the segmented lesions and tissues, which shows that the segmentation results are even better than those in Figure 10 without intensity inhomogeneity. This is because of the larger number of clusters used and the recombination of the split tissues.

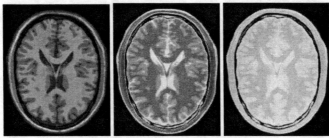

Fig. 11: Original images, 3% noise and 20% intensity inhomogeneity

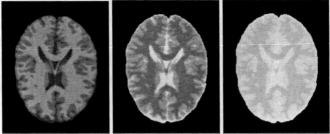

Fig. 12: Removal of extraneous tissues for images in Fig. 11 (after median filtering)

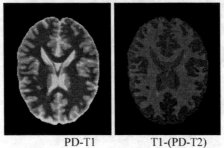

PD-T1   T1-(PD-T2)
Fig. 13: Synthesized images

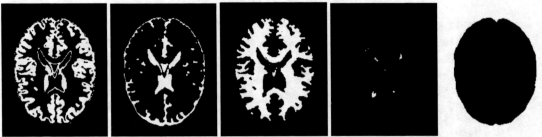

Fig. 14: Segmentation results (using 2 synthesized images in Fig.13, 12 clusters)

4.5 MS brain data with 7% noise and 0% intensity inhomogeneity

Figure 15 are the original images of Slice #90. Figure 16 shows the images after non-brain tissues are removed and median filtered. Synthesized images in Figure 17 are similar to those in Figure 9 and 13. Figure 17 are the segmented lesions and brain tissues. Segmentation results up to this noise level are still pretty good. As far as the literature is searched we have not see similar results.

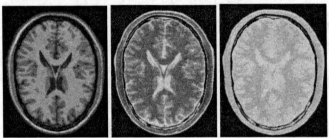

Fig. 15: Original images, 7% noise and 0% intensity inhomogeneity

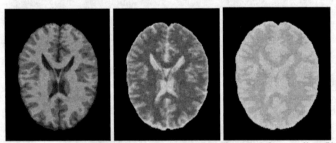

Fig. 16: Removal of extraneous tissues for images in Fig. 15 (after median filtering)

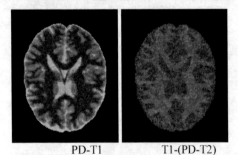

PD-T1   T1-(PD-T2)
Fig. 17: Synthesized images

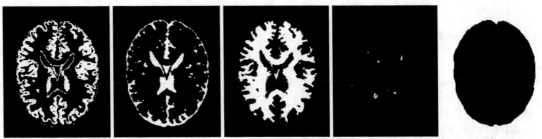

Fig. 18: Segmentation results (using 2 synthesized images in Fig.17, 12 clusters)

5. CLINICAL MS MRI BRAIN DATA SETS AND SEGMENTATION RESULTS

The clinical MS MR brain data were downloaded from Harvard university[10]. On the Harvard web-site there are 58 cases of various brain diseases with Case 5 and Case 38 being multiple sclerosis patients. Case 5 only has T2 images, taken at 23 discrete times with 53 slices each time. Case 38 consists of images of 4 modalities (T1, T2, PD, and Gad) and 23 pictures for each modality taken at one time. There is no truth models for the MS lesions, only some simple symptom descriptions. We can not assess our results according to some known standard for these clinical data. Compared with the simulated MS brain data, clinical data are much easier to manipulate. There is no needs to median filter these data. It is not clear whether these clinical data have already been preprocessed or denoised. Figure 19 shows the MS brain images of four modalities of the Slice #15. Figure 20 are the two synthesized images used for segmentation, and Figure 21 presents the segmentation results after recombining the split tissue segments.

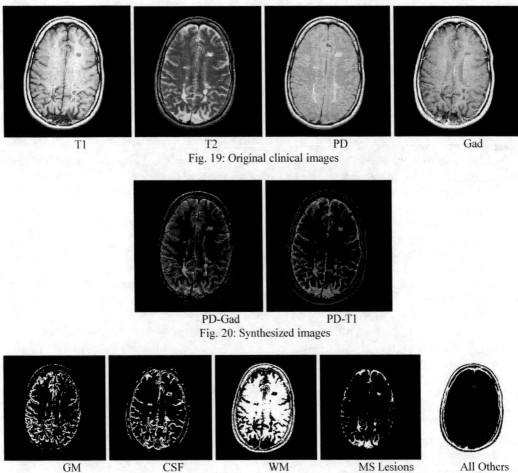

T1   T2   PD   Gad

Fig. 19: Original clinical images

PD-Gad   PD-T1

Fig. 20: Synthesized images

GM   CSF   WM   MS Lesions   All Others

Fig. 21: Segmentation results (using 2 synthesized images in Fig.20, 10 clusters)

6. CONCLUSIONS AND SUGGESTIONS

Modified deterministic annealing algorithm is a very efficient segmentation algorithm for isolating MS lesions in the MR volumes when utilizing all the information contained in all the modalities. Through some arithmetic manipulations we can obtain synthesized image data which greatly alleviate the effect of noise and intensity inhomogeneity. Isolated multiple sclerosis lesions are outliers to the brain tissues. Even with noise level up to 7% the MS MR brain data can still be satisfactorily segmented. This method does not need a prior model, and is conceptually very simple. It segments not only large lesions but small ones as well. The whole process is completely automated without any intervention by an operator, which can be a very promising tool for MS follow-up studies. Comparison between the segmentation results from the simulated MS brain data and from the clinical MS brain data shows that with the modern high quality MRI equipment images with noise above 3% and intensity inhomogeneity above 20% may not be produced. Segmentation results for the clinical data are much better and easier to obtain than the simulated noisy data. So modeling images with noise above 3% and inhomogeneity above 20% may not be very necessary. To get even better results for the MS lesions, inverse problem techniques have to be applied. Noise and intensity inhomogeneity models have to be used and improved during iteration using the provided MRI data.

ACKNOWLEDGEMENT

This research has been partially supported by funds from the Advanced Research Program (ARP) (Grant No. 003644-176-ARP), the Advanced Technology Program (ATP) (Grant # 003644-0280-ATP) of the state of Texas and NSF Grant # EIA-9980296.

REFERENCES

1. Koen Van Leemput, et al., "Automated segmentation of multiple sclerosis lesions by model outlier detection", *IEEE Trans. on Medical Imaging*, **20**, No. 8, pp. 677-688, 2001.
2. B. Johnston, et al., "Segmentation of multiple sclerosis lesions in intensity corrected multispectral MRI", *IEEE Trans. on Medical Imaging*, **15**, No. 2, pp. 154-169, 1996.
3. Zhanyu Ge, and Sunanda Mitra, "Efficient 3D volume segmentation of MR images by a modified deterministic annealing approach", *SPIE Proceedings, Image Processing*, Vol. **4322**, 2001.
4. J. K. Udupa, et at., "Multiple sclerosis lesion quantification using fuzzy-connectedness principles", *IEEE Trans. on Medical Imaging*, **16**, No. 5, pp. 598-609, 1997.
5. Kenneth Rose, "Deterministic annealing for clustering, compression, classification, regression, and related optimization problems", *Proc. of the IEEE*, **86**, No.11, pp. 2210-2239, 1998.
6. Sunanda Mitra and Sujit Joshi, "Generalized nonconvex optimization for medical image segmentation", *SPIE Proc., Image Processing*, **3979**, Part I, pp160-168.
7. Dzung Pham and Jerry Prince, "Adaptive fuzzy segmentation of magnetic resonance images", *IEEE Trans. on Medical Imaging*, **18**, No.9, pp.737-752, 1999.
8. R. Kikinis et al., "Quantitative follow-up of patients with multiple sclerosis using MRI: technical aspects", *J. Magnetic Resonance Imaging*, **9**, No. 4, pp. 519-530, 1999.
9. Remi Kwan, et al., "An extensible MRI simulator for post-processing evaluation", BrainWeb: Simulated Brain Database, http://www.bic.mni.mcgill.ca/brainweb/.
10. Keith Johnson, and Alex Becker, "The whole brain atlas", http://www.med.harvard.edu/AANLIB/home.html
11. Scott Newton, Surya Pemmaraju and Sunanda Mitra, "Adaptive fuzzy leader clustering of complex data sets in pattern recognition", *IEEE Trans. on Neural Networks*, **3**, No.5, pp. 794-780, 1992.
12. S. K. Lee and M. W. Vannier, "Post-acquisition correction of MR inhomogeneities", *Magnetic Resonance Imaging*, **36**, pp. 276-286, 1996.
13. J. C. Bezdek, "A convergence theorem for the fuzzy ISODATA clustering algorithms", *IEEE Trans. Pattern Anal. Machine Intell.*, **PAMI-2**, pp. 1-8, 1980.
14. Z. Liang et al., "Parameter estimation of finite mixtures using the EM algorithm and information criteria with application to medical image processing", *IEEE Trans. Nucl. Sci.*, **39**, pp. 1126-1133, 1992.

Determination of biplane geometry and centerline curvature in vascular imaging

Daryl P. Nazareth[c], Kenneth R. Hoffmann[abcd], Alan Walczak[e], Jacek Dmochowski[f], Lee Guterman[b], Stephen Rudin[abcd], Daniel R. Bednarek[abcd]

Toshiba Stroke Research Center, University at Buffalo (SUNY), [a]Dept. of Radiology, [b]Dept. of Neurosurgery, [c]Dept. of Physics, [d]Dept. of Physiology and Biophysics, [e]Dept. of Computer Science and Engineering, [f]Div. of Biostatistics SPM

ABSTRACT

Three-dimensional (3-D) vessel trees can provide useful visual and quantitative information during interventional procedures. To calculate the 3-D vasculature from biplane images, the transformation relating the imaging systems (i.e., the rotation matrix $\mathbf{R}$ and the translation vector $\mathbf{t}$) must be determined. We have developed a technique to calculate these parameters, which requires only the identification of approximately corresponding vessel regions in the two images. Initial estimates of $\mathbf{R}$ and $\mathbf{t}$ are generated based on the gantry angles, and then refined using an optimization technique. The objective function to be minimized is determined as follows. For each endpoint of each vessel in the first image, an epipolar line in the second image is generated. The intersection points between these two epipolar lines and the corresponding vessel centerline in the second image are determined. The vessel arclength between these intersection points is calculated as a fraction of the entire vessel region length in the image. This procedure is repeated for every vessel in each image. The value of the objective function is calculated from the sum of these fractions, and is smallest when the total fractional arclength is greatest. The 3-D vasculature is obtained from the optimal $\mathbf{R}$ and $\mathbf{t}$ using triangulation, and vessel curvature is then determined. This technique was evaluated using simulated curves and vessel centerlines obtained from clinical images, and provided rotational, magnification and relative curvature errors of 1°, 1% and 14% respectively. Accurate 3-D and curvature measures may be useful in clinical decision making, such as in assessing vessel tortuousity and access, during interventional procedures.

Keywords: biplane, 3D, imaging, neurovascular, optimization, downhill simplex

1. INTRODUCTION

Determination of the three-dimensional (3-D) configuration of blood vessel networks may be useful for interventional procedures[1-4], where there is limited visibility and restricted access to the patient. A single x-ray image does not contain the depth information required for network reconstruction. However, a second image of the vessel network may be acquired using an image plane that is rotated and translated with respect to the original imaging system. The 3-D information can then be recovered from the two images[5,6].

Methods exist for determining the geometry when a calibration object is used[3,4]. Investigators have also proposed self-calibration techniques which do not require calibration objects[2,7-10]. Instead, corresponding vessel bifurcation points in the two images are employed. The geometry is then determined using epipolar constraints[3,4]. However, these techniques rely on the bifurcation points being visible in both views, which is often not the case with vascular images, due to vessel overlap in the bifurcation regions.

Zhang *et al.* have developed a method[11] for determining biplane geometry which was applied to objects consisting of straight line segments. This method requires the identification of corresponding line segments, not points, in the two views. Epipolar constraints are then employed to evaluate an objective function. The geometry is determined by minimizing this function. Our technique is a generalization of Zhang's, applied to a set of curves, such as a network of vessels.

2. METHODS

2.1 Biplane geometry

The biplane geometry configuration is shown in Figure 1. In each coordinate system, the focal spot is the origin, and the positive z-axis (or z'-axis) points in the direction of and perpendicular to the image plane. The source-to-image distances are denoted D and D', respectively. The primed coordinate system is obtained from the unprimed system by a 3-D rigid rotation followed by a translation. Therefore, if $\mathbf{x}$ represents the coordinates of a 3-D point in the unprimed system, then

$$\mathbf{x'} = \mathbf{R}(\mathbf{x}-\mathbf{t}) \tag{1}$$

represents the coordinates of the same point in the primed system, where $\mathbf{R}$ and $\mathbf{t}$ are respectively the rotation and translation relating the two systems. In the unprimed image plane, the u-axis and v-axis are parallel to the x- and y-axes, respectively. Therefore, the image point (u,v) corresponding to the 3-D point (x,y,z) is given by

$$u = x\, D/z \tag{2}$$

and

$$v = y\, D/z, \tag{3}$$

and similarly for the primed system.

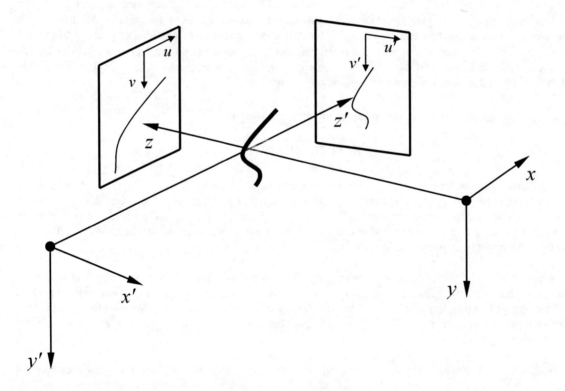

Figure 1: Biplane geometry and images of a curve.

For a given point P in the unprimed image, there is a corresponding epipolar line in the primed image, as shown in Figure 2. The epipolar line is the projection in the primed image of the line between P in the unprimed image and the source O. Generation of the epipolar line requires knowledge or an estimate of $\mathbf{R}$ and $\mathbf{t}$. The point P', corresponding to P, will lie on this epipolar line in the primed image if the geometry (i.e., $\mathbf{R}$ and t) is correct. P' can be determined by finding the intersection point of this epipolar line and the appropriate curve in the primed image. The corresponding 3-D point $\mathbf{P}$ can then be recovered by triangulation, that is, by finding the intersection of the lines OP and $O'P'$.

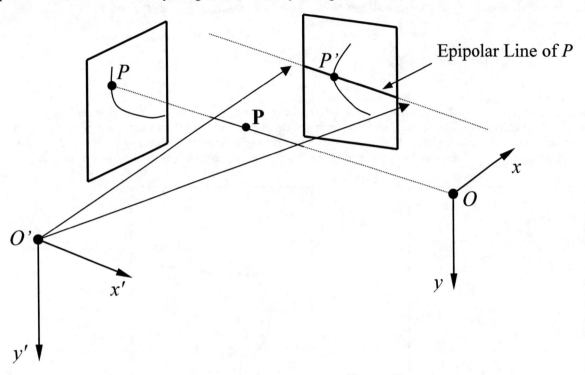

Figure 2: 3-D point $\mathbf{P}$, point P in unprimed frame and corresponding epipolar line and point P' in primed frame.

2.2 Indication and initial estimates

The 3-D vessel tree reconstruction proceeds as follows. Two images of the 3-D vessel tree are acquired. The user indicates approximately-corresponding vessel regions in the two views, by indicating the two endpoints of each vessel region. Correspondence can be estimated using local vessel features (e.g., visible bifurcation points, vessel size, relative contrast or calibration objects). A vessel centerline tracking technique[12] is employed to provide centerlines in each image. Initial values of the transformation relating the imaging systems, i.e., the rotation matrix $\mathbf{R}$ and the translation vector $\mathbf{t}$, are generated based on the gantry information, i.e., the gantry angles, magnification and source-to-image distance (SID) for each view. Since $\mathbf{t}$ can only be determined up to a scale factor, we assume that its magnitude is known.

2.3 Optimization

The initial $\mathbf{R}$ and $\mathbf{t}$ are then refined using an optimization technique based on the downhill simplex method[13]. The objective function F to be minimized is a function of $\mathbf{R}$ and $\mathbf{t}$, and its value is determined as follows.

For each endpoint of the ith vessel region in the unprimed image, an epipolar line is generated in the primed image. The intersection point between each of these two epipolar lines and the ith vessel centerline in the primed image is determined, as shown in Figure 3. The vessel arclength, L'_i, between these intersection points in the primed image is calculated. This arclength corresponds to the amount of overlap of the indicated vessel regions in the two views, for a given imaging geometry. If there is no intersection because the epipolar lines lie outside the vessel region in the primed image, the entire vessel region is considered to be overlapped. If no section of the vessel region in the second image lies between the epipolar lines, then L'_i is defined as the negative distance from the vessel region endpoint to the nearer epipolar line. L'_i is then divided by l'_i (the length of the vessel region in the primed image) to yield the fractional overlap in the primed image for vessel region i.

The fractional overlaps, L'_i/l'_i, are recalculated for every vessel in the unprimed image, and likewise for the primed image. Their deviations from one are squared and then summed over all vessels to provide the value of the objective function:

$$F(\mathbf{R},\mathbf{t}) = \sum_{i=1}^{n}\left[\left(1-\frac{L_i}{l_i}\right)^2 + \left(1-\frac{L'_i}{l'_i}\right)^2\right]. \qquad (4)$$

The objective function is smallest when the total fractional overlap is greatest. Note that if a region defined by epipolar lines is larger than the vessel segment in one view, the epipolar region will be smaller than the corresponding vessel segment in the other view. Thus, only when both views are optimally overlapped is the objective function minimized. The $\mathbf{R}$ and $\mathbf{t}$ which provide the minimal objective function value are taken as the best estimate of the biplane geometry.

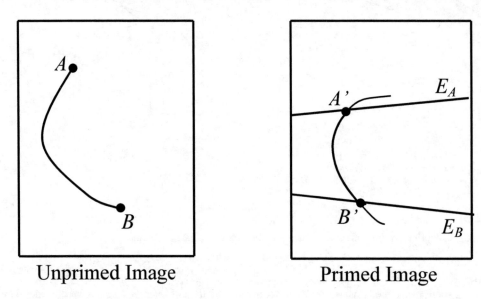

Figure 3: The endpoints A and B of a vessel region in the unprimed image are used to generate epipolar lines E_A and E_B which intersect the corresponding vessel in the primed image at A' and B', respectively. The vessel arclength between A' and B' is taken as the overlap between the vessel region in the two views.

The 3-D vasculature is then reconstructed for each point along each vessel centerline in the first image, by using the optimal $\mathbf{R}$ and $\mathbf{t}$ to generate the corresponding epipolar line in the second image. The intersection point between this epipolar line and the corresponding centerline in the second image is determined. The corresponding 3-D point is then calculated using these two image points and triangulating.

2.4 Calculating curvature
The curvature of the 3-D at each point of the vessel tree can be calculated once the tree has been reconstructed. Curvature is determined in the following way. For each point along the centerline, a 1-cm segment of the centerline is generated centered on that point, yielding a 3-D curve approximately 1 cm long. The coordinates of the points along this segment are fit with polynomials. Coordinates x, y and z are fitted independently as functions of arclength. The polynomial with the smallest residual is used as the best fit polynomial for that x, y, z coordinate of the curve. The second derivatives of the x, y and z polynomials are obtained and the curvature is then calculated as

$$K = | \, \mathrm{d}^2\mathbf{r}/\mathrm{d}s^2 \, |, \tag{5}$$

where $\mathbf{r}$ is the 3-D position vector, and s is the arclength along the centerline.

2.5 Evaluations

Simulations were performed in order to evaluate our technique's ability to improve the initial gantry information. A rotation matrix corresponding to a 90° rotation about the y-axis, and a translation vector of (-50 cm, 0, 50 cm) were selected. The SID in each imaging system was 100 cm, and the pixel size was 0.1 mm. Simulated projected 2-D vascular trees were generated as follows. Clinical biplane images of a five-vessel network were acquired, from which the 3-D centerline was generated using imaging geometry determined by the Enhanced Metz-Fencil technique[10]. The 3-D points were calculated as above to provide the 3-D vessel tree. The centroid of the 3-D tree was positioned at (0, 0, 50 cm) in the unprimed frame, and the 3-D centerlines were projected onto the unprimed image plane. Each 3-D point was then transformed according to Eq. 1, and projected onto the primed image plane. A uniformly-distributed random error of up to 2 pixels was added to the endpoint pixel position of each vessel segment.

Our technique was applied in five different trials. For each trial, the errors in the components of $\mathbf{R}$ and $\mathbf{t}$ were selected from a uniform random distribution with maxima given in Table 1. The errors in R_z and t_y were chosen to be smaller than the other components by a factor of 10 to reflect the typical errors in biplane gantry information. Since the magnitude of $\mathbf{t}$ is assumed known, t_z was not varied. Each trial included 100 instances in which the geometry and reconstructed 3-D vessel tree were calculated. The results were evaluated using several methods.

Trial	ΔR_x (deg.)	ΔR_y (deg.)	ΔR_z (deg.)	Δt_x (cm)	Δt_y (cm)
1	1	1	0.1	1	0.1
2	2	2	0.2	2	0.2
3	3	3	0.3	3	0.3
4	4	4	0.4	4	0.4
5	5	5	0.5	5	0.5

Table 1: Maximum errors in the components of $\mathbf{R}$ and $\mathbf{t}$, for the five trials conducted.

In order to reconstruct a 3-D point using a specified geometry, the epipolar line corresponding to an image point in one image must intersect the corresponding vessel in the other image (see Methods). In each case, we determined the fraction of the total number of 3-D points which resulted in such intersections. This fraction was compared to the fraction of intersections obtained when only the initial gantry information was used to provide the geometry.

The calculated 3-D data were compared to the true data using a Procrustes algorithm[14,15], which determines the rotation, $\mathbf{P}_R$, translation, $\mathbf{P}_t$, and scaling (relative magnification), P_M, required to map one 3-D data set to another in a least-squares sense. The magnitude of $\mathbf{P}_R$ gives an indication of the size of the angular errors in the calculated $\mathbf{R}$. $\mathbf{P}_t$ indicates the translation of the centers-of-mass of the reconstructed and true data. The amount by which P_s differs from unity indicates the magnification error in the reconstructed data. For comparison, the vessel tree was also reconstructed based on the initial gantry information only, and these 3-D data were also compared to the true data.

The curvature at each point in the true 3-D vessel tree was calculated. A similar calculation was employed for one of the above instances using only gantry information with random errors in $\mathbf{R}$ and $\mathbf{t}$ of 4° and 4% maximum, respectively. This calculation was performed before and after application of our technique. For each reconstruction, the absolute difference and relative errors between the calculated and true curvature values were determined for each 3-D point and averaged over the entire tree.

3. RESULTS

3.1 Comparison of fractions of intersections found

An intersection of the epipolar line and the vessel centerline is necessary in order to reconstruct a 3-D point, and thus missed intersections will result in an incompletely reconstructed vessel tree. The total number of points in the 3-D vessel tree was 124. Figure 4 presents the fraction of the points for which intersections between epipolar lines and corresponding vessels were found. Two cases are shown: the results of employing only the initial gantry information ("uncorrected" data), and the results of employing our technique to solve for **R** and **t** ("corrected" data). The fraction of intersections found for the uncorrected data decreases from about 94% to about 78%, but remains relatively constant at about 97% for the corrected data.

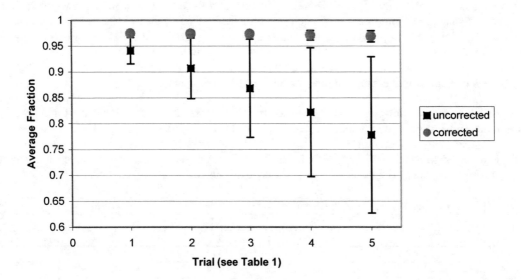

Figure 4: Fraction of intersections found, before and after correction. The fraction for the uncorrected 3-D tree decreases from 0.94 to 0.78, while remaining relatively constant at 0.97 for the corrected tree.

3.2 Comparison of 3-D data sets

Figures 5-8 show the comparisons of the reconstructed 3-D vessel tree to the original tree. The error bars represent the standard deviation of the results for the 100 instances. The rotational error in the uncorrected data increases from ~1° to more than 4°, indicating that the rotational error is correlated with the initial gantry angle error. In the corrected data, this error only increases from ~1° to ~1.5°. Similarly, the translation error increases in the uncorrected data from ~1cm to ~5cm, whereas in the corrected data, the increase is only from ~1 cm to ~1.5cm. The magnification error in the uncorrected data increases from 1% to about 5%. In the corrected data, the magnification error remains relatively constant at about 1%. This small magnification error indicates that our technique can determine 3-D points with an error in magnification of only 1%, even when the initial error in the gantry angle is as large as 5°.

Figure 7 shows the average configuration error for the corrected and uncorrected reconstructed 3-D data sets. The average configuration error is the absolute average 3-D Euclidean distance between the reconstructed 3-D points, after application of the Procrustes technique, and the true 3-D points. The configuration error is related to how well the shape of the 3-D vessel tree is preserved. The average configuration error for the uncorrected data increases from about 0.4 mm to 1.4 mm. In the corrected data, the average configuration error remains relatively constant at about 0.2mm. These results indicate that our technique preserves the shape of the 3-D vessel tree to a much higher degree than does reconstruction from the gantry information alone.

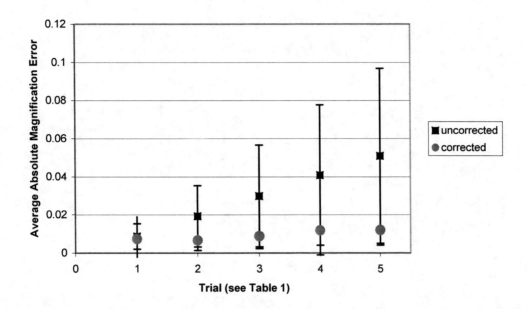

Figure 5: Absolute magnification error of the reconstructed 3-D data set, before and after correction. The magnification error increases from 1% to 5% for the uncorrected 3-D tree, while remaining relatively constant at 1% for the corrected tree.

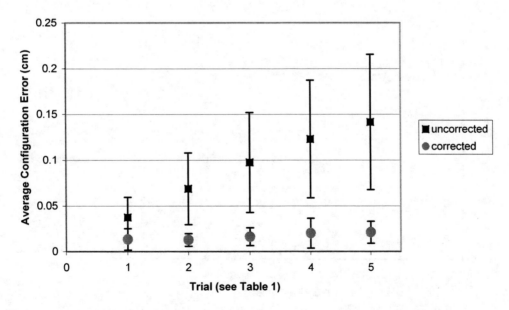

Figure 6: Configuration error, before and after correction, between true 3-D data and reconstructed data after application of the Procrustes algorithm. The configuration increases from 0.4 mm to 1.4 mm error for the uncorrected 3-D tree, while remaining relatively constant at 0.2 mm for the corrected tree.

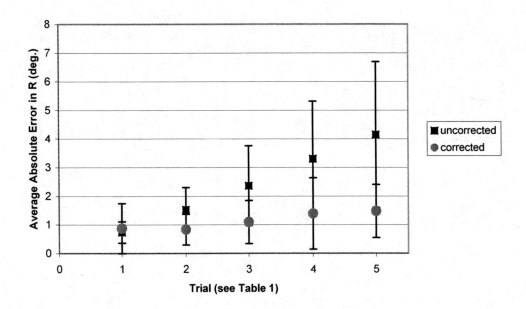

Figure 7: Rotation relating the reconstructed 3-D data set and the true 3-D data set, before and after correction. The rotational error increases from 1° to 4° for the uncorrected 3-D tree, while only increasing from 1° to 1.5° for the corrected tree.

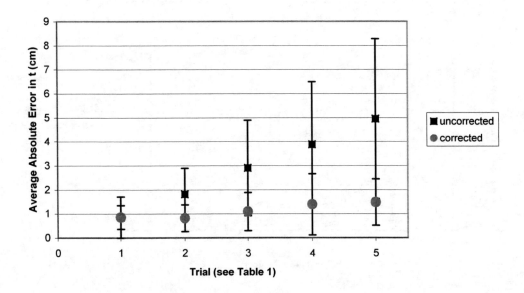

Figure 8: Translation relating the reconstructed 3-D data set and the true 3-D data set, before and after correction. The translation increases from 1 cm to 5 cm error for the uncorrected 3-D tree, while only increasing from 1 cm to 1.5 cm for the corrected tree.

3.3 Comparison of curvature calculations

The average curvature of the true 3-D vessel tree was 2.02 cm^{-1} ± 1.4 cm^{-1}. The average absolute difference between the true curvature and that determined from the uncorrected 3-D data was 0.836 cm^{-1} ± 0.8 cm^{-1}. This error was reduced to 0.230 cm^{-1} ± 0.5 cm^{-1} when the corrected 3-D data were used. The relative error in curvature was reduced from 0.990 ± 3.1 to 0.136 ± 0.3.

4. CONCLUSIONS

We have developed a technique for determining the biplane geometry from biplane images of a 3-D network of curves. Unlike existing techniques, our method does not require indicated correspondences between vessel bifurcation points. Instead, the user is required to identify corresponding vessel regions. The gantry angles, object magnifications and SID's are also required.

Simulation studies were conducted using random errors in gantry information and user indication. The results indicate that our technique provides a significant improvement over use of gantry information alone. By comparing the reconstructed 3-D vessel tree to the true 3-D vessel tree, we have shown that our technique is accurate to within 1° in rotational accuracy, 1 cm in center-of-mass accuracy, 1% in magnification accuracy and 0.2 mm in average configuration error, for indication errors of 0.2 mm. In addition, our technique provides intersections between epipolar lines and corresponding vessels for about 97% of the points. This large fraction allows the reconstruction of almost every 3-D point in the true vessel tree.

Our technique also facilitates calculation of the curvature at any point along the 3-D vessel tree, with a relative accuracy of about 14%. This may be useful in assessing catheter accessibility during interventional procedures.

ACKNOWLEDGMENTS

This work was supported by NIH Grants HL52567 and NS38746, an equipment grant from the Toshiba Corporation and an operating grant from the John R. Oishei Foundation.

REFERENCES

1. G. P. M. Prause, S. C. DeJong, C. R. McKay, and M. Sonka: Semi-automated segmentation and 3-D reconstruction of coronary trees: Biplane angiography and intravascular ultrasound data fusion. Proc. SPIE 2709: 82-92, 1996.
2. A. Wahle, E. Wellnhofer, I. Mugaragu, H. U. Sauer, H. Oswald, and E. Fleck: Assessment of diffuse coronary artery disease by quantitative analysis of coronary morphology based upon 3-D reconstruction from biplane angiograms. IEEE Transactions on Medical Imaging 14: 230-241, 1995.
3. D. Parker, D. Pope, R. Van Bree, and H. Marshall: Three-dimensional reconstruction of moving arterial beds from digital subtraction angiography. Comp. and Biomed. Res. 20: 166-185, 1987.
4. M. J. Potel, J. M. Rubin, S. A. MacKay, A. M. Aisen, J. Al-Sadir, and R. E. Sayre: Methods for evaluating cardiac wall motion in three dimensions using bifurcation points of the coronary arterial tree. Invest Radiol 8: 47-57, 1983.
5. K. Kitamura, J. M. Tobis and J. Sklansky: Estimating the 3D skeletons and transverse areas of coronary arteries from biplane angiograms. IEEE Trans. Med. Imaging 7: 173-187, 1988.
6. Y. Bresler and A. Macovsky: Estimation of the 3D shape of blood vessels from X-Ray Images. Proc. IEEE Comput. Soc. Int. Symp. Med. Images Icons, Arlington, Texas: 251-258, 1984.
7. S. Y. J. Chen, C. E. Metz: Improved determination of biplane imaging geometry from two projection images and its application to three-dimensional reconstruction of coronary arterial trees. Med. Phys. 24: 633-654, 1997.
8. K. R. Hoffmann, A. Sen, C. E. Metz, K. G. Chua, B. B. Williams, J. Esthappan, M. Fiebich, M. Mazzucco, K. Doi: Determination of 3D vessel trees from biplane coronary images. Proc. Computer Assisted Radiology '97, H. U. Lemke, M. W. Vannier, K. Inamura, eds. (Elsevier, New York, 1997), pp. 162-165.
9. C. E. Metz and L. E. Fencil: Determination of three-dimensional structure in biplane radiography without prior knowledge of the relationship between the two views. Med Phys 16: 45-51, 1989.

10. K. R. Hoffmann, C. E. Metz, Y. Chen: Determination of 3D imaging geometry and object configurations from two biplane views: an enhancement of the Metz-Fencil technique. Med Phys 22: 1219-1227, 1995.

11. G. Xu and Z. Zhang, *Epipolar geometry in stereo, motion and object recognition: A unified approach.* Kluwer Academic Publishers, Dordrecht, The Netherlands, 1996.

12. Sen A, Li L, Doi K, Hoffmann KR: Quantitative evaluation of a coronary vessel tracking technique on clinical angiographic projections. Med Phys 26:698-706, 1999.

13. W.H. Press, B. P. Flannery, S.A. Teukolsky, and W. T. Vetterling, *Numerical recipes in C: The art of scientific computing.* Cambridge University Press, Cambridge, England, 1992.

14. P. H. Schoeneman: A generalized solution to the orthogonal Procrustes problem. Psychometrika **31**, 1-10 (1966).

15. P. H. Schoeneman and R. M. Carroll: Fitting one matrix to another under choice of a central dilation and a rigid motion. Psychometrika **35**, 245-254 (1970).

A thinning algorithm on 2D gray-level images

Cherng-Min Ma[1], Shu-Yen Wan

Dept. of Information Management, Chang Gung University, Taiwan

ABSTRACT

Thinning on binary images is widely discussed in the past three decades. A binary image can be obtained by thresholding a gray-level image. For preventing possible information losses in the thresholding process, it may be natural to design thinning algorithms directly on the original gray-level images. This paper proposes a two-step template-based thinning algorithm on gray-level images. The first step of the algorithm is to extract 4-connected gray-level skeletons from gray-level objects. The second step is to extract 8-connected gray-level skeletons from the consequent result of the first step.

Keywords: thinning, gray-level image, parallel processing, reduction operator, topology preserving operator

1. PRELIMINARY

An *image* can be represented as a 2D array in which each cell represents a pixel of the image. A *gray-level image* can be represented in such a way that each cell of the array is assigned an integer from 0 to m where $m > 0$. A typical representation of a gray-level image is to use a byte to denote 256 (from 0 to $m = 255$) different gray-levels for each pixel of the image. A pixel assigned the greatest possible value m is colored white and is called an *object pixel*; a pixel assigned value 0 is colored black and is called a *background pixel*.

Binary images is a special case of gray-level images where a *binary image* can be represented in such a way that each cell of the array is assigned a value of either 0 or 1 ($= m$). For easier explanation, 3D graphs for the example images in this paper are provided as well where the height of each bar represents the gray-level of the pixel at the corresponding coordinate. Traditionally, thinning, as a preprocessing operation of image processing, is applied to binary images [4]. A thinning algorithm is to iteratively *reduce* object pixels to background pixels. For a parallel thinning algorithm, a number of object pixels are reduced in each iteration. A thinning algorithm terminates when no object pixels can be reduced. Noticed that a parallel thinning algorithm may reduce all pixels in the outmost layer of an object to background pixels at the same time.

The set of object pixels in the resulting image after the thinning process is called the *skeletons* of the original objects. Thinned results are easier to trace and hence are easier to recognize. Generally, thinning on binary images should satisfy three criteria: (i) a skeleton is approximately in the middle of the original object; (ii) a skeleton should "look like" the original object, and (iii) a skeleton maintains the same connectivity structure of the original object. The second criterion concerns the geometry property of the images, and the third criterion concerns the topology property of the images. Generally, a binary thinning algorithm satisfies the first and the second criteria if the algorithm is applied to reduce an object layer by layer. The satisfaction of a thinning algorithm on binary images to the third criterion can be justified mathematically.

Consider a gray-level image. It is not surprised if one defines that a pixel with gray-level 0 is absolutely not an object pixel,

---

[1] address: 259 Wen-Hua 1st Rd., Guei-Shan, Tao-Yuan 333, Taiwan; e-mail: minma@mail.cgu.edu.tw

and is absolutely a background pixel. The strength (or degree) for a pixel being an object pixel or a background pixel is function of it gray-level (from 0 to the highest possible value of all gray-levels). The gray-level of a pixel determines the relations between the pixel itself and its neighboring pixels. For example, let p_1 and p_2 be two gray-level pixels next to each other and let q_1 and q_2 be two gray-level pixels next to each other. If the gray-levels of p_1, p_2, q_1, and q_2 are 255, 255, 0, and 255, respectively, then p_1 and p_2 have a stronger relation than q_1 and q_2 does. Furthermore, the boundary of an object in a gray-level image can be rather vague. It is not straightforward to see whether a pixel belongs to an object or to the background in a gray-level image (see Figure 4.1).

The traditional thinning theories on binary images are not enough to handle thinning on gray-level images. Rosenfeld introduced the concept of *digital topology* in [9] that discussed the operations on binary images. Many papers contain topology-preserving operations on binary images based on Rosenfeld's work. He also introduced the concept of fuzzy digital topology in [7-8] for the operations on gray-level images based on the fuzzy theory introduced by Zadeh in 1965 [10]. More consequent results were proposed in [3, 6]. A number of gray-level thinning algorithms were proposed (see [1-2, 5]).

2.   2D GRAY-LEVEL IMAGES

An image is defined on a 2D array in which each cell represents a pixel. Each cell of the array is assigned a value indicating the "color" of the corresponding pixel. In this paper, when we compare a pixel with a value t or assign a value t to a pixel, we actually mean to compare the value in the cell corresponding to the pixel with a value t and assign a value t to the cell corresponding to the pixel, respectively. A gray-level image is an image in which each pixel is assigned a non-negative value indicating its gray-level. For example, in an 8-bit gray-level image, a pixel with gray-level 0 is a black pixel, and a pixel with gray-level 255 is a white pixel. A black pixel is absolutely a background pixel, and a white pixel is absolutely an object pixel. A pixel with greater gray-level has a stronger possibility to be an object pixel than a pixel with smaller gray-level does. Let p and q be two pixels of a gray-level image. We define the neighborhood of p as follows:

p_{nw}	p_n	p_{ne}
p_w	p	p_e
p_{sw}	p_s	p_{se}

Then p is 8-*adjacent* to every pixel in $\{p_n, p_{ne}, p_e, p_{se}, p_s, p_{sw}, p_w, p_{nw}\}$, and p is 4-*adjacent* to every pixel in $\{p_n, p_e, p_s, p_w\}$. Two pixels are 8- or 4-*neighbors* to each other if they are so adjacent. The immediate neighborhood of a pixel p, denoted $N(p)$, is the union of p and all p's 8-neighbors. Let $N^*(p)$ be $N(p) - \{p\}$. We use $g(p)$ to denote the gray-level of p. If p has exactly one 8-neighbor whose gray-level is greater than $g(p)$, then p is called an *8-end* pixel; if p has exactly one 4-neighbor whose gray-level is greater than $g(p)$, then p is called a *4-end* pixel. If p has at least one 4-neighbor whose gray-level is smaller than $g(p)$, then p is called a *border* pixel. If every 8-neighbor of p has smaller gray-level than $g(p)$, then p is called an *8-peak* pixel; if every 4-neighbor of p has smaller gray-level than $g(p)$, then p is called a *4-peak* pixel.

An 8- or 4-*path* from p to q, denoted $\pi(p, q)$, is a sequence of pixels, $p = p_0 - p_1 - p_2 - ... - p_n = q$, from p to q where all two consecutive pixels in the sequence are 8- or 4-adjacent, respectively. Let $\min(\pi(p, q))$ be the minimum in the set of $g(p_i)$, for every p_i in $\pi(p, q)$. Then the *degree of connectedness* of p and q, denoted $C(p, q)$, is defined to be maximum in the set of $\min(\pi_j(p, q))$ for every 8- or 4-path $\pi_j(p, q)$ from p to q [7-8]. Two pixels p and q are *connected* if $C(p, q)$ is greater than or equal to $\min(g(p), g(q))$. A gray-level pixel p is called *simple* if its reduction (i.e., reducing its gray-level) does not reduce the degree of connectedness of pixels in $N^*(p)$ (with paths lie in $N^*(p)$) [8].

Consider Figure 2.1. Let p be neither a peak pixel nor an end pixel. Then

- p is called a *diagonal ridge* pixel if for each of the configurations Figure 2.1.(a-d), $g(p)$ is greater than both $g(u_1)$ and $g(u_2)$, and $g(s)$ is greater than both $g(u_1)$ and $g(u_2)$, and
- p is called a *straight ridge* pixel if for either of the configurations Figure 2.1.(e-f), $g(p)$ is greater than both $g(u_1)$ and $g(u_2)$, $g(s_1)$ is greater than both $g(u_1)$ and $g(u_2)$, and $g(s_2)$ is greater than both $g(u_1)$ and $g(u_2)$.

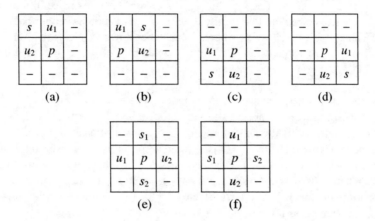

Figure 2.1. Simple and non-simple reductions of gray-level pixels.

Consider Figure 2.2 (shown below). Each cell denotes a gray-level pixel, and the value in each cell represents the gray-level of the corresponding pixel. In Figure 2.2.(a), the gray-level of the central pixel is reduced from 20 to 0, and the template of Figure 2.2.(b) shows the result of such a reduction. It is not difficult to see that the degrees of connectedness between any two pixels that surround the central reducing pixel of Figure 2.2.(a) remain unchanged after the reduction (by the connectedness in the 3 by 3 neighborhood). Thus, the reduction of the gray-level of the central pixel from 20 to 0 in Figure 2.2.(a) is simple. The template in Figure 2.2.(d) is obtained from the template in Figure 2.2.(c) by reducing the gray-level of the central pixel from 20 to 0. Clearly, the degree of connectedness of the north and south neighbors of the central pixel of the template in Figure 2.2.(c) are weaken from 20 to 15 as shown in the template of Figure 2.2.(d). Such reduction is then non-simple.

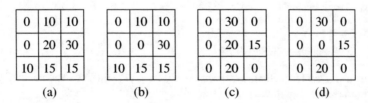

Figure 2.2. Simple and non-simple reductions of gray-level pixels.

A possible approach for thinning on gray-level images is to extract gray-level skeletons from gray-level objects, that is, the skeleton of a set of brighter pixels should be brighter than the skeleton of a set of darker pixels. A general problem of gray-level thinning algorithm is to reduce a set of pixels of the same gray-level where the set of pixels is surrounded by a set of pixels with much higher gray-level. A gray-level thinning algorithm may be applied to binary images. When that happens, the resulting image after the application of a gray-level thinning algorithm is still a binary image and should preserve the topology of the original binary image. Thinning algorithms on gray-level images has been discussed in [1-3, 5-6].

3. THE ALGORITHM AND ITS APPLICATIONS

A parallel thinning algorithm on binary images can be represented as a set of templates in which each object pixel matches any of these templates is reduced to a background pixel. A parallel thinning algorithm consisting of eight templates on binary images was shown in [4]. Each of the eight templates contains three different symbols: 0 (matches background pixels), 1 (matches object pixels), and "–" (called *don't-care*, and matches either background pixels or object pixels). In this paper, "–" is called don't-care as well where "–" matches any possible gray-level. Thus, when discussing the neighborhood configuration of a particular pixel p, if any 8-neighborh x of p is represented by "–", then one of the following three statement holds: $g(x) > g(p)$, $g(x) = g(p)$, or $g(x) = g(p)$.

Our algorithm contains two sets of templates, denoted Ω_4 (see Figure 3.1) and Ω_8 (see Figure 3.2). Ω_4 is stimulated by the approach proposed in [1] and is to extract 4-connected skeletons from original objects, and Ω_8 is to extract 8-connected skeletons from the results extracted by Ω_4. If the neighborhood configuration of a pixel p of a gray-level image matches any template in Ω_8 or Ω_4 by the following rules, then $g(p)$ is reduced accordingly. Moreover, let X and Y be two non-empty disjoint sets of gray-level pixels. When we say "$X < Y$" we mean that the gray-level of every pixel in X is smaller than the gray-levels of all pixels in Y. When either $X = \{g(x)\}$ or $Y = \{g(y)\}$ is a singleton set, we may write "$X < g(y)$" or "$g(x) < Y$", respectively. Other comparisons between X and Y are defined similarly. We introduce the rules related to Ω_8 in Rule 3.1 and the rules related to Ω_4 in Rule 3.2 as follows.

Rule 3.1. Let p be a pixel in a gray-level image and let Ω_4 be a set of templates shown in Figure 3.1. Then $g(p)$ is *replaceable* if p is in a configuration that matches any of the following templates of Ω_4:
1. in Figure 3.1.(a, c),
    a. $X = \{g(u_1)\}$, and $X < g(p) \leq \{g(r_1), g(r_2), g(r_3), g(r_4), g(s_1)\}$, and
    b. $g(s_1) = g(p)$ implies $g(s_2) \geq g(p)$,
2. in Figure 3.1.(b, d, i, j),
    a. $X = \{g(u_1), g(u_2), g(u_2)\}$, and $X < g(p) \leq \{g(r_1), g(r_2), g(s_1)\}$, and
    b. $g(s_1) = g(p)$ implies $g(s_2) \geq g(p)$,
3. in Figure 3.1.(e, g), $X = \{g(u_1)\}$, and $X < g(p) \leq \{g(r_1), g(r_2), g(r_3), g(r_4), g(r_5)\}$,
4. in Figure 3.1.(f, h, l), $X = \{g(u_1), g(u_2), g(u_2)\}$, and $X < g(p) \leq \{g(r_1), g(r_2), g(r_3)\}$,
5. in Figure 3.1.(k),
    a. $X = \{g(u_1), g(u_2), g(u_2)\}$, and $X < g(p) \leq \{g(r), g(s_1), g(t_1)\}$,
    b. $g(s_1) = g(p)$ implies $g(s_2) \geq g(p)$, and
    c. $g(t_1) = g(p)$ implies $g(t_2) \geq g(p)$,
where the maximum of X is a candidate for replacing $g(p)$.

Rule 3.2. Let p be a pixel in a gray-level image and let Ω_8 be a set of templates shown in Figure 3.2.. Then $g(p)$ is *replaceable* if p is in a configuration that matches any of the following templates of Ω_8:
1. in Figure 3.2.(a),
    a. $X = \{g(u_1), g(u_2), g(u_2)\}$, and $X < g(p) \leq \{g(r_1), g(s_1)\}$,
    b. $g(r_1) = g(p)$ implies $g(r_2) \geq g(p)$, and
    c. $g(s_1) = g(p)$ implies $g(s_2) \geq g(p)$,
2. in Figure 3.2.(b, d),
    a. $X = \{g(u_1), g(u_2), g(u_2)\}$, and $X < g(p) \leq \{g(r_1), g(s_1), g(s_2)\}$,
    b. $g(s_1) = g(p)$ implies $g(s_2) \geq g(p)$,
3. in Figure 3.2.(c), $X = \{g(u_1), g(u_2), g(u_2)\}$, and $X < g(p) \leq \{g(r_1), g(r_2)\}$,
where the maximum of X is a candidate for replacing $g(p)$.

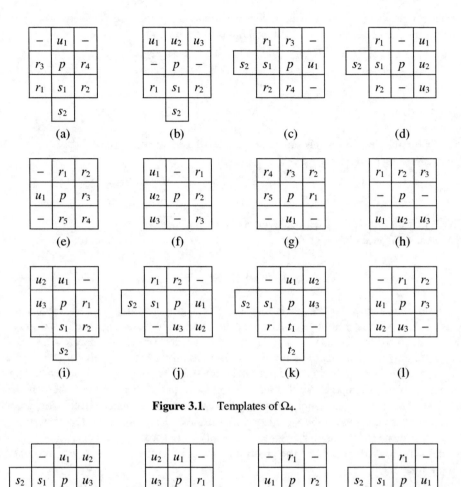

Figure 3.1. Templates of Ω_4.

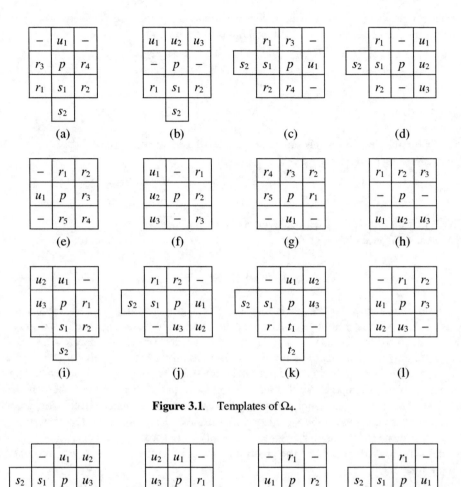

Figure 3.2. Templates of Ω_8.

If p is replaceable by any template in either Ω_4 or Ω_8, respectively, then a candidate generated from that template is stored in a list for replacing $g(p)$. If p is replaceable by more than one template in either Ω_4 or Ω_8, respectively, then the list may contain a number of candidates of different gray-levels that are considered to replace $g(p)$. The following rule is to choose an appropriate value from the set of all candidates to replace $g(p)$.

Rule 3.3. Let p be a pixel in a gray-level image, and let T be the set of all candidates of different gray-levels considered to replace $g(p)$. Then $g(p)$ is replaced by the minimum value in T.

Our algorithm contains two stages where the resulting image of the first stage is the input image to the second stage. Each stage is an iterative process where, in each iteration, a number of pixels are reduced by either Ω_4 or Ω_8, respectively. Each stage terminates when no gray-level pixels can be reduced by either Ω_4 or Ω_8, respectively. The algorithm terminates when both stages are terminate. The structure of our algorithm is as follows.

Algorithm.

> (* stage 1 *)
> input image P
> repeat
> > modify P with all gray-level pixels satisfying Ω_4 are reduced accordingly;
> until no pixel can be reduced from P by Ω_4;
>
> (* stage 2 *)
> repeat
> > modify P with all gray-level pixels satisfying Ω_8 are reduced accordingly;
> until no pixel can be reduced from P by Ω_8;

4. DISCUSSION

The operation of stage 1 is to reduce border pixels in parallel of a gray-level object where each reduced pixel is in a neighborhood configuration that matches at least one template in Ω_4. The resulting image is a gray-level image with gray-level skeletons (in the 4-connectedness sense). Note that no end pixels (in the 4-connectedness sense) can be reduced by Ω_4. This stage can be thought as analogues to thinning operations on (4, 8) binary images (i.e., apply 4-connectedness on object pixels and 8-connectedness on background pixels). Figure 4.2.(a-c) show images corresponding the three images in Figure 4.1.(a-c), respectively. The operation of stage 2 is to reduce pixels in parallel on the boundary of a gray-level object where each reduced pixel is in a neighborhood configuration that matches Ω_8. The second stage follows immediately after stage 1. No end pixels (in the 8-connectedness sense) can be reduced by Ω_8. This stage can be thought as analogues to thinning operations on (8, 4) binary images (i.e., apply 8-connectedness on object pixels and 4-connectedness on background pixels). The resulting image of the algorithm is a gray-level image with gray-level skeletons extracting from the original input image.

An example image of gray-levels from 0 to 255 is given for verifying the performance of the algorithm (see Figure 4.1). 3D bar graphs corresponding to Figure 4.1 are presented as well (see Figure 4.2) where the height of each 3D bar represents the gray-level of the corresponding pixel at that particular position. Note that the skeleton of an object consisting of pixels of different gray-levels is still a set of pixels of different gray-levels. Figure 4.1.(a) shows an image contains a branching object. Figure 4.1.(b) is the result after the application of the stage 1 of the algorithm. It is not difficult to see that the skeleton is 4-connected. Figure 4.1.(c) is the consequent result after the application of the stage 2 of the algorithm. Figure 4.1.(c) shows an 8-connected skeleton. This example demonstrates the geometrical property of the algorithm, i.e., a skeleton should look like the original object.

A special configuration on gray-level images, called *bottom*, is a set of connected pixels of the same gray-level surrounded by a set of pixels with greater gray-levels. Imaging a set X of pixels of gray-level 50 surrounded by a set Y of pixels of gray-level 100 forming a cycle. An ideal skeleton could be a unit-width skeleton reduced from Y and is composed by a set of ridge pixels of gray-level 100, and the pixels in X are completely lowered to 0. Generally, the reduction of the gray-level of a pixel is a function on the neighboring pixels with lower gray-levels. For a pixel in a bottom, all of its neighboring pixels are with equal to greater gray-levels. If the reduction of any pixel in a bottom is allowable, then a "shallow hole" is created. The algorithm proposed in this paper cannot handle this problem. More properties should be established to handle this problem.

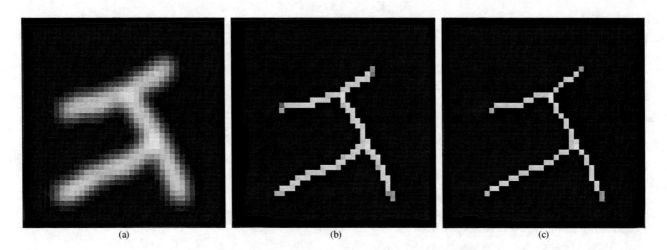

Figure 4.1. A gray-level image containing a branching object.

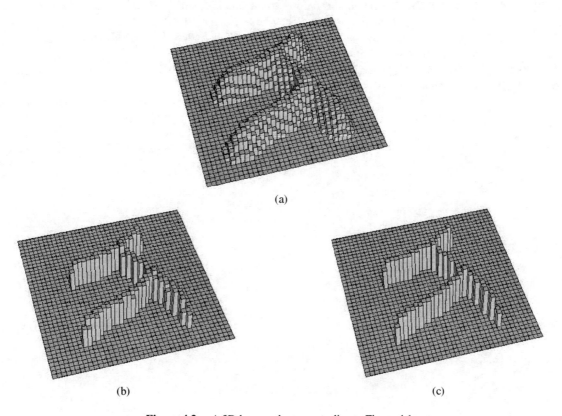

Figure 4.2. A 3D bar graph corresponding to Figure 4.1.

5. CONCLUSION

A gray-level thinning algorithm is applied to gray-level images to reduce the gray-levels of a set of pixels on the image. This paper proposes a thinning algorithm on gray-level images. The algorithm contains two stages where each stage contains reduction templates to reduce pixels on the boundaries of objects. The result of the first stage of the algorithm is an image with 4-connected skeletons. The result of the second stage is a consequent image with 8-connected skeletons. An example is provided for testing the performance of the algorithm. The resulting image that contains skeletons extracted by the algorithm from the original gray-level image is still a gray-level image.

6. REFERENCES

[1] K. Abe, F. Mizutani and C. Wang, *Thinning of gray-level images with combined sequential and parallel conditions for pixel removal*, IEEE Trans. Syst. Man Cybern. **24**, 294-299, 1994.

[2] C. Arcelli and L. Serino, *Parallel reduction operators for gray-level pictures*, Int'l Journal of Pattern Recognition and Artificial Intelligence, **14**-3, 281-295, 2000.

[3] C. Arcelli, *Topological changes in gray-tone digital pictures*, Pattern Recognition, **32**, 1019-1023, 1999.

[4] C. M. Holt, A. Steward, M. Clint, and R. H. Perrott, *An improved parallel thinning algorithm*, Communications of the ACM, **30**, 156-160, 1987.

[5] C. R. Dyer and A. Rosenfeld, *Thinning operations on gray-scale pictures*, IEEE Trans. PAMI,. **1**, 88-89, 1979.

[6] S. K. Pal, *Fuzzy skeletonization of an image*, Pattern Recognition Letters, **10**, 17-23, 1989.

[7] A. Rosenfeld, *The fuzzy geometry of image subsets*, Pattern Recognition Letters, **2**, 311-317, 1984.

[8] A. Rosenfeld, *Fuzzy digital topology*, Information and Control, **40**, 76-87, 1979.

[9] A. Rosenfeld, Digital Topology, *The American Mathematics Monthly*, **86**, 621-630, 1979.

[10] L. Zadeh, *Fuzzy sets*, Information and Control, **8**, 338-353, 1965.

3D-Imaging Using Mobile Low-End C-Arm Systems

Jörn Lütjens[ab], Reiner Koppe[a], Erhard Klotz[a], Michael Grass[a], and Volker Rasche[a]

[a]Philips Research Laboratories, Hamburg, Germany
[b]University of Surrey, Guildford, UK

ABSTRACT

During the last years, three-dimensional X-ray imaging has become a well-established imaging modality, setting the golden standard for spatial resolution in three-dimensional X-ray imaging. Firstly introduced on a motorized C-arm system, it gained benefit from the high spatial resolution of the image intensifier. Using cone-beam reconstruction, it provided fast access to truly three-dimensional imaging with isotropic voxel dimensions.

However, the non-rigid mechanics and the image distortion in the image intensifier required dedicated calibration processes and obligated the developers to use the most stable and reliable system in the C-arm device family. The need for system calibration also required the system to be able to reproducibly adjust the C-arm to the pre-calibrated positions, which seemed only possible with the motorized movement of a high-end system. On mobile, non-motorized C-arm systems, which are often used for guiding surgical procedures, however, 3D application has not been feasible due to the non-reproducibility of the mechanical movement.

In this paper, first results regarding the feasibility of this approach are presented. The data were acquired on a Philips BV 26 surgical C-arm. This device is fully movable. The "C" arc is adjusted manually.

Keywords: Low-end C-Arm Systems, Cone-Beam Reconstruction

1. INTRODUCTION

In 1995, a new modality in medical imaging, three-dimensional X-ray imaging, was introduced by the Philips Research Laboratories.[1] This new development became possible after the first vascular C-arm, the Integris V 3000 gantry (PMS, Best, the Netherlands) had been equipped with an option for a 180° rotational fluoroscopy run. Since it became commercially available in 1999, it has established itself among the classical modalities CT, MR, and PET/SPECT for volume imaging.[2]

Vascular C-arm systems like the Integris had originally been designed for interventional fluoroscopy from arbitrary viewing angles, e.g. in monitoring the progress of a catheter treatment. Their image intensifier-based X-ray projections did not possess the high dynamical resolution of CT but provided a significant improvement in spatial resolution against the semiconductor elements in standard CT gantries. Moreover, the use of a two-dimensional detector enabled reconstruction to isotropic voxels.

Its low dynamical resolution restricted the new modality to the imaging of high X-ray contrast objects, such as bones or contrast agent-filled vessels. On the other side, this restriction enabled the use of the easily applicable Feldkamp algorithm[3] without large trade-offs in the image quality.

Other attention-demanding aspects were the non-rigid mechanics and the image distortion in the image intensifier, which is due to magnetic influences of the Earth's magnetic field. These effects had to be compensated by elaborate calibration processes. An important feature of a suitable gantry was therefore that the positioning had to be reproducible. The Integris gantry, being mounted to the ceiling, provided these features and needed only one calibration run per installation.

In the meantime, however, there have been attempts to make the 3D-functionality available on smaller, non-motorized movable C-arms too. While offering an inferior rigidness and thus a limited reproducibility of the C-arm positioning, these devices would be very flexible tools in the operation room. First research into this area was pursued by Philips on a Philips BV 26 C-arm gantry, which was enhanced to a proto-type C-arm suitable for 3D imaging. In this paper, the first reconstruction results are presented.

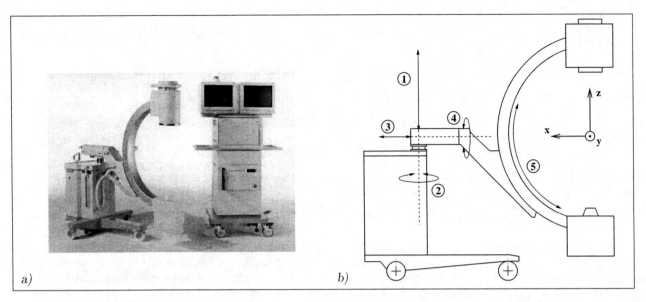

Figure 1. *a)* Picture of the BV 26 surgical C-arm by Philips, taken from the operator's manual. ©Philips Medical Systems Netherlands, 1993. *b)* Sketch of the C-arm BV 26 and its degrees of freedom. Particularly relevant for the application to 3D reconstruction are numbers 4 and 5. They move the X-ray tube and the image intensifier, placed on opposite ends of the "C" on a sphere around a common iso-center.

2. METHODS

The reconstruction of attenuation values in a volume from X-ray projections requires knowledge on the line integrals of the attenuation coefficients and on the exact positions, at which the line integrals were measured. The data acquisition device, in this case the BV 26 C-arm, must therefore provide the projection images as well as the positions and orientations of the X-ray tube and the detector. Furthermore, the image distortion, spoiling our knowledge on the ray locations, must be accounted for in order to avoid severe artefacts in the reconstructed image. Position and distortion correction are subject to a dedicated calibration. This necessitated some changes to the BV 26 C-arm, which are described in the next sections.

The calibrated data are then fed into a reconstruction algorithm. Offering a good compromise between complexity, computing time, image artefact level, and C-arm trajectory requirements, the Feldkamp method[3] has been the method of choice for most products using circular trajectories in the domain of 3D X-ray so far. We used a variant of this algorithm too for the present work.

2.1. The PHILIPS BV 26 C-arm

The experimental set-up comprises the BV 26 C-arm gantry, provided with X-ray tube and image intensifier, adjustable by five degrees of freedom and movably suspended on wheels. The two important degrees of freedom are measured with two angle meters, which are hooked up to the system. Further items are a video interface, needed to obtain the projection images and to store them on a hard disk, as well as a set of X-ray calibration phantoms. Each of the components will be presented shortly in the following section.

The BV 26 (Fig. 1 a) is a standard medical imaging device by PHILIPS Medical System, Best, the Netherlands. It was designed primarily for applications in the field of surgery and interventional procedures, where its advantages are maneuverability, a 15 cm field of view, and imaging quality. However, it is also suitable for use as a mobile diagnostic unit to support other hospital disciplines.

2.1.1. Geometry of the BV 26 C-arm

Figure 1 b presents a rough sketch of the C-arm BV 26. The C-arm gantry provides a suspension for the actual "C". The X-ray source (tube) and the detector (image intensifier) are mounted at opposite ends of the "C", respectively.

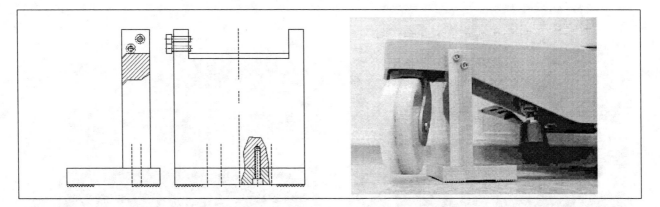

Figure 2. A drawing (left) and a photograph of the jacks that have been constructed in order to keep the BV 26 in a fixed spatial relation to the laboratory.

The C-arm can be rolled to any position in the operating theatre. Additionally, there are five degrees of freedom:

1. vertical displacement;
2. rotation around vertical z-axis;
3. horizontal displacement;
4. rotation around horizontal x-axis (hereinafter called "Angulation");
5. rotation around horizontal y-axis (referred to as "Rotation" below);

The numbering corresponds to the numbers in Fig. 1 b.

While the first one uses an electric motor for displacement, the other four have to be adjusted by hand. The last two move X-ray detector and source on opposite sides of a sphere. For the trajectories used in 3D reconstruction these are the most important degrees of freedom. For the purpose of showing the feasibility of the approach, it is therefore sufficient to set the other degrees of freedom to fixed positions and thus simplify the calibration of the positioning.

2.1.2. Ensuring the reproducibility of the positioning

A pre-condition for a successful calibration of the C-arm positioning is that the positions can be reproducibly adjusted at all. This is not the case for the BV 26 since it is supported by wheels, which allows for easy maneuverability in the operating theatre. As a consequence, it must be ensured that the gantry does not move relative to the ground during the image acquisition. Moreover, the C-arm must possess a defined spatial relation to an exterior magnetic field because the image distortion has not been calibrated for arbitrary magnetic fields. As a first approach the C-arm was mounted on jacks, as shown in Fig. 2. This allowed to show the sufficient accuracy of the repositioning. Of course, the fixation would have to be solved in a more elegant manner for application in an operating room.

2.1.3. Installation of angle meters on the BV 26

The BV-26 in its original state is not provided with measurement devices for the degrees of freedom. Therefore it was necessary to partly rebuild the C-arm in order to attach the angle meters. As pointed out in section 2.1.1, the number of the C-arm's used degrees of freedom can be reduced to two. We call them "Angulation" angle and "Rotation" angle. In Fig. 1 b, they are referred to as number 4 and 5, respectively. Fig. 3 shows photographs of the angle meters and how they are mounted on the C-arm.

In order to judge the reliability of the angle meters, an accuracy study has been carried out. The results are displayed in table 1. We measured the position of a set of LEDs fixed to the surface of the image intensifier of the BV 26 with an independent device based on optical localization, an Optotrak system by Northern Digital

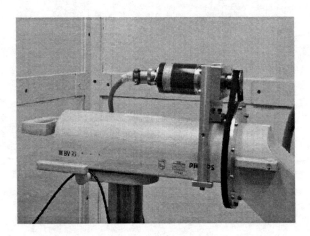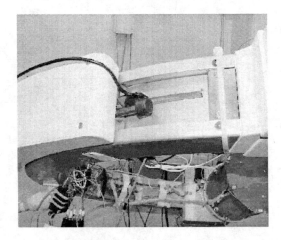

Figure 3. Photographs of the angle meters measuring Angulation (left) and Rotation (right) angles, respectively. The former uses an angle encoder while the latter measures signatures on a magnetic strip.

Type of measurement	RMS
Optotrak (fixed C-arm)	0.0093 mm
Readjustment of Angulation angle	0.22 mm
Readjustment of Rotation angle	0.20 mm
Readjustment of both angles	0.42 mm

Table 1: RMS of the accuracy tests for the repositioning of the BV 26 C-arm

Inc. By measuring the position of the LED object at rest, the intrinsic accuracy of the position measurement with the Optotrak system was determined in a preliminary run to be better than $10 \mu m$ (from a distance of 2.5 m), which is by far enough to judge the accuracy of the angle meters.

Subsequently, the C-arm, having already been heaved onto the jacks, was readjusted to a certain position a number of times. This was done three times, once for testing each angle, Rotation and Angulation, separately while the other was held fixed, and once for testing the readjustment according to both angle meters. The result was encouraging in that the repositioning accuracy was always better than ± 0.4 mm, or ± 0.2 mm for each angle alone. We consider this sufficient for the targeted application.

2.2. System calibration

With the Angulation and Rotation angles measured, it would in principle be possible to compute the locations of both detector and X-ray source according to a geometrical model. The geometry of an individual ray from the source to a detector element could then be calculated. However, in reality this geometry will deviate from the model prediction because of two effects.

1. **Static bending of the gantry under the influence of gravity**

   Due to its asymmetric suspension, C-arms are inflected in a complex manner. It would be far too complicated to model this behaviour, because it itself depends on a large number of parameters (such as the elasticity tensors and masses in various parts of the gantry), which are mostly unknown.

   We have seen that the gravitation-induced inflection of the gantry can be considered reproducible. Hence, a calibration is feasible. The measured angles then serve as a parameterization of the spherical space of the C-arm orientation. The actual measurement of the gantry parts must be stored in a look-up table together with the corresponding angles.

2. Image distortion due to external magnetic fields

External magnetic fields, such as that of the Earth, induce a distortion to the projection image of the image intensifier. It is rather difficult and supposedly not as accurate to determine the distortion online, e. g. from a set of markers at the edge of the images. An alternative is to calibrate the specific image distortions of a number of C-arm orientations in advance. This imposes not much extra effort, since a calibration step is necessary for the position measurement anyway.

In the following sections, the procedures and objects needed for a full system calibration are described.

2.2.1. Image distortion correction

Empirical studies[1][4][5] have shown that there are basically two types of distortions produced by magnetic influences: S-shaped distortions caused by a magnetic field vector parallel to the image intensifier normal and translations in one direction if the magnetic field vector is perpendicular to the image intensifier normal. These distortions are of order 3 or 2, respectively.

Additionally, a constant distortion is caused by the curved entrance window of the II. This effect is termed pincushion distortion. It depends on the II geometry only and does not change with the magnetic field. It can be described with a second order polynomial.

The two effects, magnetic distortion and pincushion distortion, impose each other. They can be accounted for in one calibration step. In order to correct the distortion, a transformation $D : \mathbb{R}^2 \mapsto \mathbb{R}^2$ is needed which defines the relation between any point in the original image to its distorted position. Since the combined distortions are at most of order three, a third order polynomial is used to model D.

Grid phantom Similar to the Integris distortion correction, we used a marker phantom consisting of X-ray opaque spheres, arranged on a rectangular grid on a plate directly in front of the detector. Fig. 4a shows a drawing of the phantom, which is combined with the ring phantom for focus calibration.

The rectangular distribution guarantees a uniform spacing of the distortion measurement. The spherical geometry of the markers is convenient for the segmentation routine that must locate them in the image.

Another positive aspect of this calibration method is that no camera model is needed to relate the pixels in the projection images to the measurement locations on the detector. The images are transformed into a form where the grey values measured at the locations of the grid points correspond directly to the measurement of a virtual detector element located in the physical marker in the phantom. Thus, the detector plane can be identified for calibration purposes with the grid phantom plane.

A superposition of X-ray projection of the grid phantom from many orientations of the C-arm has showed that the magnitude of the image distortion is in the order of 2 . . . 5 mm if not corrected for.

Determination of the image distortion coefficients The evaluation of the X-ray projections of the grid phantom is done semi-automatically. Using a sensible set of start parameters, the positions of the grid bullets in the image are determined by a segmentation routine.

Each pair of co-ordinates yields a piece of information on the image distortion in one specific location of the image. The entire distortion, being of order three, can be modeled by a polynomial of the same degree. For each calibrated position l with original co-ordinates (x_u^l, y_u^l) the distorted co-ordinates (x_d^l, y_d^l) are calculated as

$$x_d^l = f(x_u^l, y_u^l) = \sum_{i=0}^{9} a_i \, p(x_u^l, y_u^l, i) \tag{1}$$

$$y_d^l = g(x_u^l, y_u^l) = \sum_{i=0}^{9} b_i \, p(x_u^l, y_u^l, i).$$

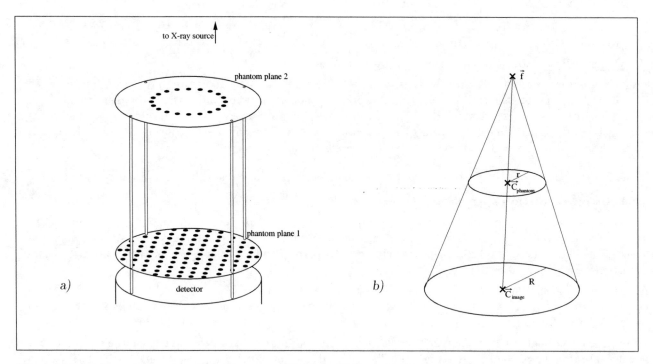

Figure 4. *a)* Schematic drawing of the phantom used for focal spot calibration and distortion correction. It consists of two X-ray-transparent planes containing metal spheres. Plane 1 in front of the detector contains spheres on a grid. A second plate (plane 2) containing spheres arranged on a circle is mounted at a certain distance to the detector. It is used for the focal spot measurement as shown in *b)*.

Here, the x_u and y_u denote the undistorted co-ordinates, the x_d and y_d their distorted counterparts, and $p(x, y, i)$ is a function defining the different powers of x and y in the polynomial, as shown in table 2.

i	0	1	2	3	4	5	6	7	8	9
p(x, y, i)	1	x	y	xy	x^2	y^2	x^2y	xy^2	x^3	y^3

Table 2: Definition of the function $p(x, y, i)$

The set of distorted and undistorted co-ordinates can now be fed into a maximum likelihood calculation to obtain a least-square-fit of the a_i and b_i.[6]

2.2.2. Geometry calibration

The geometry calibration has been achieved by evaluating X-ray projections of two further phantoms. The first is used to measure the focal spot positions with respect to the detector. This is necessary since the position of the anode within the tube case cannot be measured from the outside. The second phantom provides the measurement of the relative position and orientation of the detector to a reference point on the patient table.

Focal spot calibration The detector-mounted phantom used for focal spot calibration is depicted in Fig. 4 a. The focal spot can be measured by using the ring of spheres in the upper part of the phantom. Therefore, the center and radius of the circle of spheres in the projection image are determined. The geometrical consideration for the focus calculation is shown in Fig. 4 b. It is worth noting that the projection images must be corrected for the inherent distortion before evaluating the focal spot phantom.

Geometry measurement using a dodecahedron phantom The absolute shift and rotation of both detector and tube with respect to the iso-center of the gantry is finally measured with a third phantom, which consists of X-ray opaque markers at the vertices of a dodecahedron, plus some additional markers breaking its symmetry.

For each position to be calibrated, one projection must be taken. It must be corrected for image distortion, and the focal spot position relative to the detector must be determined. Then – using some a priori knowledge on the first positions of the gantry – the supposed positions of the markers are calculated according to a geometrical model, thus defining search windows. Final segmentation of the spheres in the image is applied to find the centers of the markers.

The measured positions of the markers in the image are used to numerically calculate the shift and rotation of the dodecahedron phantom relative to the detector in a least-squares sense.

2.3. Volume reconstruction using the Feldkamp method

Most 3D X-ray application currently available use the Feldkamp algorithm[3] for reconstructing the volume attenuation values. This algorithm is a cone-beam version of the commonly known filtered back-projection used in CT systems to generate slice images. Although complete information for volume reconstruction requires more sophisticated trajectories[7][8][9], it runs on projections from a circular trajectory only, compromising little of the image quality. This brings about a great simplification in the data acquisition. We will not describe the Feldkamp method in more detail, since it is a standard method.

2.4. Description of the data acquisition process

Now that all parts of the imaging chain have been mentioned, the procedure for generating a calibrated reconstructed volume data set of attenuation values will be described.

1. The first step is to mount the C-arm onto the jacks (see section 2.1.2). Since the BV 26 gantry weighs about 245 kg, this is only possible using a heavy crowbar. From now on, the C-arm must be kept on the jacks until the end of the data acquisition.

2. Then the ring/grid phantom is screwed on the entrance window of the image intensifier. Since we are aiming for a circular trajectory, the Rotation angle is set to about $90°$. The Angulation angle is subsequently adjusted by hand to a number of values with a constant increment. In our case we used 100 projections and an angular increment of $2°$. Image distortion is determined for each position. The undistorted images of the ring phantom provide the focus positions.

3. For the next step, the ring/grid phantom must be removed. The dodecahedron phantom must be placed in the iso-center of the gantry on the patient table. The correct position can be recursively approximated using projections from perpendicular directions. Projections are taken from the same set of positions as in the previous step, corrected for distortion and evaluated as described in section 2.2.2. The correct positions are found by comparing the Angulation values.

4. Now the dodecahedron phantom can be removed and the patient or other object of interest be placed in the iso-center. Projections are taken from the same positions as before and distortion correction is applied.

5. The calibrated images and position vectors are finally passed to the reconstruction algorithm, which returns a volume data set after successful completion.

As a 6th step, the volume data must be visualized, e. g. by looking at slices through the volume or by volume-rendering the data.

The calibration procedure (steps 1–3) needs to be performed only once if the gantry remains on the jacks, or if it can be placed to the same position after removal. If the position is changed, the image distortion will possibly yield incorrect results. The amount of the degradation depends on the variability of the magnetic field within the room and on the rotation angle between the old and the new orientation of the gantry.

The manual adjustment of the C-arm is very cumbersome, especially since the final image quality crucially depends on the exactness of the repositioning, which has to be performed twice during the calibration and another time for each clinical acquisition run. In the present experimental set-up, the Angulation is measured with an accuracy of $1/100°$. The positioning on such a fine scale takes about 10 s alone per projection for an experienced operator. Under these circumstances, the recording of 100 projections takes hat least 15–20 minutes, more likely even longer. This is certainly unacceptable for a clinical application.

The solution would be to motorize the movement of the Angulation. A simplification of the acquisition can also be achieved by interpolation, eliminating the need to exactly readjust the each angle during the clinical acquisition run.

2.5. Interpolative calibration

If the domain of calibration can be extended from the separately recorded positions to the one-dimensional range spanning these positions, or even to the region in-between the positions, then the positioning need not be very accurate. In fact, any position in the calibrated range would then be valid, and it would suffice to guarantee a certain uniformity of the distribution of the projection locations, provided that the interpolation does not observably spoil the final image quality.

We considered two variants, one-dimensional and two-dimensional interpolation. While 1D-interpolation certainly suffices for a circular trajectory, the 2D-interpolation can be used to ensure that projections from *any* direction are calibrated. This would in principle enable arbitrary trajectories as is required by potentially exact reconstruction algorithms (such as e.g. by Defrise and Clack[10]) that might be implemented in the future.

2.5.1. 1D-interpolation

1D-interpolation makes use of the recorded Angulation values. If the angle of the current position is φ, it must be determined which are the two nearest calibrated positions. Let them be recorded at φ_1 and φ_2, respectively. The interpolation coefficients c_1 and c_2 can be calculated straightforward as $c_1 = (\varphi_2 - \varphi)/(\varphi_2 - \varphi_1)$ and $c_2 = (\varphi_1 - \varphi)/(\varphi_1 - \varphi_2)$. They can be used to calculate the distortion coefficients as e.g. $a_i^{int} = c_1 a_i^1 + c_2 a_i^2$.

However, a simple linear interpolation does not yield a good approximation of the geometry data. Since we are dealing with vectors pointing to positions on the surface of a sphere, the interpolated vectors may more or less point to the correct directions but will be shorter than the measured vectors at φ_1 and φ_2. This can be solved by a higher order interpolation kernel, such as the cubic spline or the cubic convolution kernel[11] [12] [13]. However, we chose to use a different method making use of the a priori information that the position vectors are found on a spherical surface. This can be exploited by stretching the interpolated vector to the weighted sum of the original vectors. Thus, if v_1 and v_2 are the vector used for interpolation, then $\tilde{v}$ is the linearly interpolated vector, which is stretched to $|v| = c_1|v_1| + c_2|v_2|$.

2.5.2. 2D-interpolation

The 2D-interpolation is more complicated. While the circular path in 1D-interpolation can be mapped onto a line, the spherical surface encountered in the variation of both angles, Angulation and Rotation, cannot be mapped conservatively onto a plane. Additionally, the surrounding calibrated positions must be found among a larger, possibly unordered set of positions.

While the latter task is commonly addressed by triangulating the point set, and interpolating by calculation of the *barycentric co-ordinates*[14] of the position to be calibrated, we adapted this scheme to something we call *spherical Delaunay triangulation* and *spherical barycentric co-ordinates*. This method is based on replacing the cardinal lengths in the planar case with the corresponding spherical quantities, such as arc lengths etc.

Again, the interpolation of vectors was performed with the length correction as pointed out in the previous section.

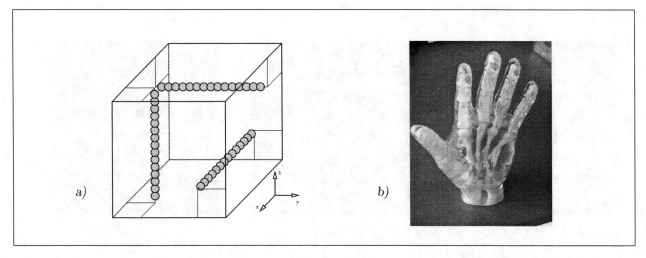

Figure 5. The investigated X-ray phantoms. *a)* Drawing of the triple-rod-phantom. *b)* Photograph of a hand phantom by 3M.

3. RECONSTRUCTION RESULTS

For the first reconstructions, three objects have been used. The first object is something we call the triple-rod-phantom, of which a drawing is presented in Fig. 5 a. It consists of three "rods", each rod being constituted by 15 metal balls of ≈ 3 mm diameter. The three rods are arranged in a cube made of X-ray transparent material with a side length of $a = 48$ mm. With a Cartesian co-ordinate system placed in the center of the cube, each rod is parallel to one axis. The rod $i = 1, 2, 3$ is placed on the line $x_{i+1} = -x_{i+2} = d/4$, understood as $i \mod 3$. The triple-rod-phantom was chosen because of its simple geometry and because it facilitates the judgment of the final spatial resolution.

The second object was a hand phantom made by 3M. It is a casting of a hand with a material of medium X-ray opacity and the bones of the hand ingrained in it.

Finally, the projections of the dodecahedron phantom, which are taken during the calibration phase, can be used to judge the quality of the calibration in terms of spatial resolution. For this, the dodecahedron projections are passed to the reconstruction algorithm. Since the geometrical model parameters were fitted to the markers of the phantom, the reconstructed markers are good indicators for the consistency of the parameters.

3.1. Reconstructions of the triple-rod-phantom

Figs. 6 a–c shows maximum-intensity-projections (MIP) of the reconstructed triple-rod-phantom in the direction of the cardinal axes. It was generated from 100 projection on an angular range of 200°. The plane of the trajectory, i.e. the plane, in which both detector and tube were rotating during the acquisition is identical to the x-z-plane in the reconstructed volume. That is why we can see a clearer separation of the spaces between the spheres in the rod that is parallel to the x-axis (see Fig. 6 a and c).

3.2. Reconstructions of the dodecahedron phantom

Passing the projections of the dodecahedron phantom, which were originally used to measure the positions of the detector and the source, back to the reconstruction algorithm, a volume data set containing the marker balls is obtained. The degree of distortion of the individual markers is an indicator for the quality of the calibration. In Fig. 7 a, a slice through the reconstructed volume is shown. The grey values have been inverted in this case. Fig. 7 b shows a close-up of the right-most marker in Fig. 7 a. One can see that the shape of the markers is to a good degree circular.

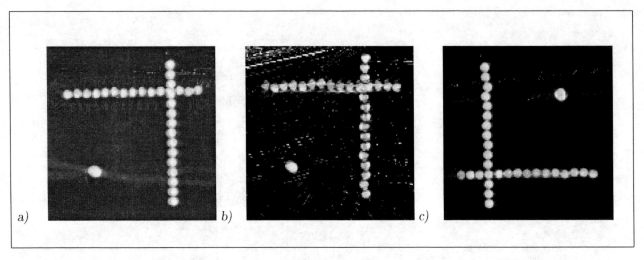

Figure 6. Maximum-intensity-projections of the reconstructed triple-rod-phantom. The reconstruction was made from 100 projections on a circular trajectory. *a)* view from x-direction; *b)* view from y-direction; *c)* view from z-direction;

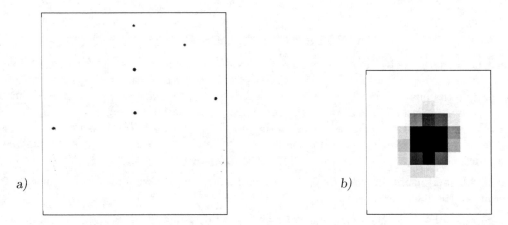

Figure 7. *a)* Slice through the reconstructed dodecahedron phantom. The reconstruction was made from 100 projections on a circular trajectory. One can see the distribution of the metal spheres (dark disks) within the phantom. *b)* Zoom of the right-most marker. The small deviation from the circular shape is an indicator for a good calibration quality.

3.3. Reconstructions of a hand phantom

The volume data set of the hand phantom was obtained from 100 projections over an angular range of 200°. Figs. 8 and 9 show volume-rendered views of the data set. The grey value window has been adjusted in order to separate the bones from the surrounding voxels. One can clearly see the distinct bones of the wrist, separated by small spaces. While the images reveal a high spatial resolution, the grey values differ comparably much due to the poor photon statistics of the image intensifier.

In Fig. 9, a cut through the rendered volume is presented. Here we can see that even the inner fine structure of the bones could be partly reproduced.

4. CONCLUSION

The feasibility of the use of a surgical image intensifier based C-arm system for 3D X-ray reconstruction has been proven. It has been shown that the BV 26 C-arm can be reproducibly adjusted to pre-calibrated positions. The quality of the calibration, including image distortion correction, geometry measurement and gantry fixation, is high enough to preserve a high spatial resolution in the reconstructed volume data set. The application of the technology to a medical test phantom with bones of a human hand has produced promising results.

While some aspects of the current data acquisition, such as the fixation using jacks or the manual readjustment, are not yet suited for the use in an operating room, there are no principal obstacles for a development into an easily applicable imaging modality. Especially the interpolated calibration brings about a great simplification, thereby reducing the requirements of the reproducibility of the readjustment by a motorized system. The new system could establish itself in interventional imaging. Additionally, the volume data sets might be used in the future for improved planning and verification of the exact 3D placement of prosthesis and screws in bones.

ACKNOWLEDGMENTS

The author wishes to thank the Philips Research Laboratories Hamburg, Germany and Dr. Walter Gilboy as well as Dr. Ed Morton from the University of Surrey, Guildford, UK, for making this work possible.

REFERENCES

1. R. Koppe, E. Klotz, J. Op de Beck, and H. Aerts, "3D vessel reconstruction based on rotational angiography," 1995. Proceedings of the CAR'95.

2. M. Grass, R. Koppe, E. Klotz, R. Proksa, M. Kuhn, H. Aerts, J. O. de Beek, and R. Kemkers, "3D-reconstruction of high contrast objects using c-arm image intensifer projection data," *Computerized Medical Imaging and Graphics* (23), pp. 311–321, 1999.

3. L. A. Feldkamp, L. C. Davis, and J. W. Kress, "Practial cone-beam algorithms," *J. Opt. Soc. Am. A* **6**, pp. 612 – 619, June 1984.

4. R. Koppe and E. Klotz, "Automatic measurement of real geometry parameters of rotational scans of INTEGRIS V3000 for performing 3D angiography," Tech. Rep. 817/94, Philips GmbH Forschungslaboratorien, Hamburg, 1994.

5. F. Gläser, "Entwicklung und Implementierung eines Verfahrens zur Kalibration eines C-Arm Röntgengerätes," Master's thesis, Medizinische Universität Lübeck, Jan. 1999.

6. H. R. Schwarz, ed., *Numerische Mathematik*, B. G. Teubner Verlagsgesellschaft, Stuttgart, 1986.

7. H. K. Tuy, "An inversion formula for cone-beam reconstructions," *SIAM J. Appl. Math.* **43**, pp. 546 – 552, Jan. 1983.

8. B. Smith, "Image reconstruction from cone-beam projections: Necessary and sufficient conditions and reconstruction methods," *IEEE Trans. Med. Imag.* **MI-4**, pp. 14 – 25, 1985.

9. P. Grangeat, *Analyse d'un système d'imagerie 3D par reconstruction à partir de radiographies X en géométrie conique*. PhD thesis, Ecole Nationale Supérieure des Télécommunications, Paris, 1987.

10. M. Defrise and R. Clack, "A cone-beam reconstruction algorithm using shift-variant filtering and cone-beam backprojection," *IEEE Trans. Med. Imag.* **13**, pp. 186 – 195, Mar. 1994.

11. R. G. Keys, "Cubic convolution interpolation for digital image processing," *IEEE Transactions on Acoustics, Speech, and Signal Processing* **ASSP-29**, pp. 1153 – 1160, Dec. 1981.

12. J. A. Parker, R. V. Kenyon, and D. E. Troxel, "Comparison of interpolation methods for image resampling," *IEEE Trans. Med. Imag.* **MI-2**, pp. 31 – 39, Mar. 1983.

13. E. Maeland, "On the comparison of interpolation methods," *IEEE Trans. Med. Imag.* **7**, pp. 213 – 217, Sept. 1988.

14. I. N. Bronstein and Semendjajew, *Taschenbuch der Mathematik*, B. G. Teubner Verlagsgesellschaft, Leipzig, 1989.

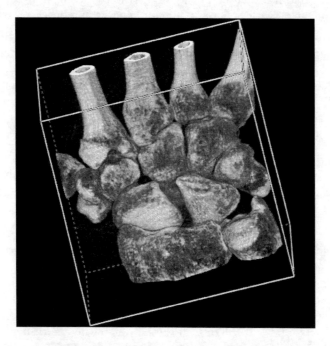

Figure 8: Volume-rendered view of the reconstructed hand phantom.

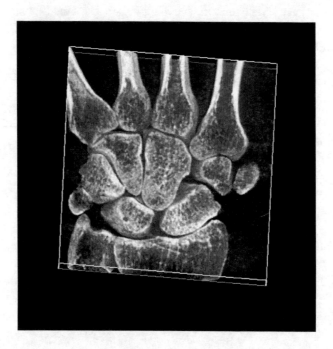

Figure 9: Cut through the volume-rendered view of the reconstructed hand phantom.

Feasibility of an automated technique for detection of large misregistrations

Claudia E. Rodríguez-Carranza[a,c] and Murray H. Loew[b,c]

[a]Department of Computer Science
[b]Department of Electrical and Computer Engineering,
[c]Institute for Medical Imaging and Image Analysis
The George Washington University,
Washington DC 20052, USA

ABSTRACT

Before a retrospective registration algorithm can be used routinely in the clinic, methods must be provided for distinguishing between registration solutions that are clinically satisfactory and those that are not .[1] One approach is to rely on a human observer. Here, we present an *algorithmic* procedure for assessing quality that discriminates between badly misregistered pairs and those that are clinically useful.

Keywords: misregistration, detection

1. INTRODUCTION

The lack of ground truth in the clinical setting makes it essential to find methodologies to assess automated retrospective registration techniques, which sometimes converge at clinically unsatisfactory values.[1]

It has been postulated that visual analysis of registered images may be a useful and practical means to evaluate image misregistration[2]; that is, to rely on a human observer to assess the registration results visually and to reject images that have been registered with insufficient accuracy. Little has been done, however, to study the upper limits of human visual detection.

Holton et al.[3] were the first to attempt measuring quantitatively the ability of observers to determine 3D registration accuracy from a colorwash superposition of images. They used receiver operating characteristic (ROC) analysis to evaluate the ability of observers to discriminate between correctly and incorrectly registered images.

For a first set of experiments, their study used five patient MRI studies from which simulated match images were created. The following three types of misregistrations were used: pure translation (multiaxes), simple rotation and translation, and multiple-axis rotation. The degree of misregistration was estimated by the position of eight markers in each base image; the mean Euclidean distance between coordinates of the markers, prior to and after misregistration, was used as a measure of the state-of-registration. Each of ten observers viewed a total of 150 images, of which half were registered, half were misregistered; half were high resolution, and half were low resolution. They were asked to classify each pair as: (1) probably misregistered, (2) possibly misregistered, (3) equivocal, (4) possibly registered, (5) probably registered. The second set of experiments used MRI-SPECT image pairs from the same patients. There was a single session of 50 images, and the observers were asked to identify the more misregistered image (i.e., the reference image perturbed by a known amount).

Prior to the experiments, there was a training session during which both registered and misregistered images were shown to the observer. A training image was shown after five test images, for recalibration.

Each image volume was classified by its mean marker distance value, and classes defined by the magnitude of this value. ROC curves were generated from observer responses for each class. The results showed that a

---

Further author information:
C.E.R.C. : E-mail: claudia@seas.gwu.edu
M.H.L. : E-mail: loew@seas.gwu.edu

threshold exists somewhere between 4 mm and 6 mm above which it becomes easier for the observer to detect misregistration. There was no indication of which of the three types of misregistrations were more difficult to identify by the observers.

Wong et al.[2] were the first to investigate the amount of error an observer could distinguish by visual assessment. The study used a single MR and PET image pair that had been misregistered by translational $(1, 2, 3, 4 \text{ mm})$ and rotational $(1, 2, 3, 4°)$ displacements, a single axis at a time, and either in negative or positive direction (i.e., the study did not include misregistrations having a combination of translational and rotational displacements). A total of fifty-four pairs were presented to five observers: forty eight misregistered pairs mixed with six copies of the correctly registered pair. They were asked to classify each pair into one of four categories: (1) no detectable misregistration, (2) possible misregistration, (3) definite small misregistration, or (4) definite large misregistration. The gold standard consisted of the pair registered with a mutual information-based algorithm.

All five observers classified the six copies of the correctly registered pair either as "no detectable misregistration" or "possible misregistration". All observers identified translations larger than 2 mm in the x and y axes, and larger than 3 mm for the z axis as "definite misregistrations" (either small or large). With rotational misregistrations, rotation around the z-axis was detectable by all at 2° or greater; rotation around the y-axis was detected by all at $+3°/-4°$ or greater, and rotation around the x-axis at $+2°/-4°$ or greater. Observers were able to detect all rotations of 4° of rotational displacement or greater, and 80% of rotations of 3° of rotational displacement or greater.

The observers consistently used contours to identify misregistrations; the absence of good edge distinction made some misregistrations more difficult to identify. That was the case for the z-axis translations and rotations around the $x-$ and $y-$axes.

As for information given to the observers prior to the study, they were first familiarized to the display format and the effect of various misregistrations; this also helped to set a uniform categorization of different magnitudes of image registration detected among observers. They were told that there were best registered as well as misregistered images, and that any misregistrations were purely translational or rotational.

The study by Fitzpatrick et al.[1] was more elaborate, as they intended to provide a preliminary methodology for the evaluation of the effectiveness of visual assessment of registration accuracy as a clinical tool. The image volumes were from CT and MR, and the observers were evaluated against a gold standard obtained using external fiducial markers. Fourteen misregistrations, with errors distributed uniformly between 0 and 10 mm, were assessed by two observers for five image pairs at five anatomical locations; therefore, the total was 700 *direct assessments* (see below), and fifty *point localizations* (five anatomical locations per image per observer). In this study, error referred to target registration error (TRE).[4]

The tools for measuring quality of visual assessment were: (1) *agreement rate*, which is the ratio of observers' true positives and true negatives to total cases; (2) the *Kappa statistic*, which measures the degree to which agreement between raters exceeds chance*; and (3) receiver operating characteristic (ROC) area.

The study evaluated the ability of two observers to classify misregistration errors using three methods of assessment. The observers were asked to identify (1) registration error in the vicinity of a set of points marked in an overlay of the boundary of one image to the other (direct assessment), or (2) corresponding MR points on the CT image (single- and multiple-point assessment). The estimated errors were compared with errors as measured by the gold standard to determine agreement relative to each of six thresholds ("is the error above k mm?", where $k \in \{1, \ldots, 6\}$). Agreement means that errors are on the same side of the threshold.

Using the three assessment methods, the observers were compared to the gold standard; some of the findings were: (1) no assessment performed well at 1 mm; (2) all methods showed fair agreement $(0.4 < \kappa < 0.75)$ for all thresholds of 2mm and higher (except single-point at 2 mm, which showed poor agreement); (3) for 2 mm and higher, agreement rates for the three methods lay between 76% and 90%; (4) for 2 mm and higher, the mean ROC areas for the three methods lay between 0.82 and 0.95; (5) the multiple-point method either matched or

---

*Values below 0.40 are considered to represent poor agreement; values between 0.40 and 0.75 to represent fair to good agreement, and values greater than 0.75 to represent excellent agreement.

out-performed the direct method for all thresholds at 3 mm and higher; (6) the results are strongly influenced by the distribution of misregistration errors.

The information provided to the observer prior to the test included imaging protocols and the knowledge that registration errors ranged "approximately uniformly" from zero to an upper limit of "around 10 mm" (according to a gold standard). They were blinded to the actual misregistrations, which were presented in random order.

An early reference to the limits of visual assessment of misregistration appeared in Pietrzyk et al..[5] In their study about interactive alignment of MR and PET images, they tilted the image plane and resliced the MR tomograms and observed that translations of 4 mm (2 pixels) in either direction resulted in clearly visible mismatch, and that rotations of 3° were detectable.

The time required to identify anatomical landmarks and register the images depends on a variety of factors, such as modalities involved, resolution of both modalities, proficiency of the operator, software tools used, distribution of misregistration error generated, target points used, etc. In the MR to CT study by Fitzpatrick et al.,[1] the average time to localize a point was 30 sec/point for one observer and 60 sec/point for the other. Therefore, for a five-point visual assessment (for two images, the total number of points to be found is then 10) it would take those observers an average of 5 and 10 minutes, respectively, to localize the points.

In summary, one study indicated that errors (with respect to marker positions) above the range of $4-6$ mm are more easily detected by observers; another study found that displacements of 4 mm and rotations of 3° are detected. Another indicated that the minimum *individual* translation displacements an observer can detect are 3 mm and rotations of 4°. The fourth study found that two visual assessment methods had agreement rates of at least 80%, mean ROC areas between 0.84 and 0.95, and fair agreement with the gold standard (kappa statistics) for errors of 2 mm and higher.

The above studies were concerned with determining the minimum error an observer can detect. On average then, it would take about 5 minutes for the visual assessment of registration accuracy, by a trained observer. It would be desirable that an alternative assessment method existed that would do an automatic or semi-automatic evaluation that would reduce the amount of work the observer needs to do by either improving the quality or reducing the number of badly misregistered pairs he will be asked to assess. A first step in that direction is to devise an algorithm that would classify registration results into two categories: "greatly misregistered" and "possibly correctly registered". Therefore, we propose and demonstrate an algorithmic assessment technique for 3D CT-MR brain registration based on contours.

2. METHODOLOGY

The purpose of these experiments was to determine the feasibility of three registration quality measures for assessing accuracy on retrospective 3D CT-MR brain registration. The quality measures were based on both brain and scalp contours, and the assumption was that the closer those contours are the more accurate the alignment is. The assessment algorithm consisted of two steps: (1) the extraction of the brain and scalp contours in the pair of registered images and (2) the computation of the registration quality measures.

We used CT-T1 and CT-T2 images of three patients, with ground truth available for each pair (section 2.4). The six image pairs were registered using the ground truth information, and misregistration transformations were applied to each of them to construct a set of misregistered cases. Each misregistered case belonged to one of two classes: "acceptable accuracy" and "unacceptable accuracy" (section 2.6). Each case is then segmented (section 2.1) and evaluated by the new registration quality measures (section 2.2).

The purpose of the measures of registration quality is to permit the labeling of a misregistered pair as being either "possibly correctly registered" or "greatly misregistered". A perfect measure would assign a "possibly correctly registered" label to each of the misregistered pairs belonging to the class "acceptable accuracy", and a "greatly misregistered" label to each pair of the class "unacceptable accuracy". We used ROC analysis (section 2.7) to compare the performance of the three new measures of registration quality .

2.1. Brain and head extraction

Here we describe the strategies used for segmenting the brain and head of the CT and MR images. The output of the segmentation was a binary image, and we assumed that the brain (or head) region corresponded to the largest connected region. That region was isolated using a connected-component algorithm. The final stage was to extract a one-pixel thick contour from the identified connected-component.

Brain extraction. For the CT brain, the mean gray level and the standard deviation within a $11 \times 11 \times 11$ cube at the center of the image were calculated; that cube was assumed to lie within the brain region. Any gray value in the range $[\mu - 5\sigma, \mu + 20\sigma]$ was considered to belong to the brain.

For the MR brain we used BET (Brain Extraction Tool) developed at the Oxford Centre for Functional Magnetic Resonance Imaging of the Brain (FMRIB).[6] Its basis is a deformable model which evolves to fit the brain's surface by the application of a set of locally adaptive model forces. The method is very fast and requires no pre-registration or other pre-processing before being applied.

Head extraction. The thresholding strategy for the CT image simply consisted of defining the background as the lowest ten percent of the gray level range.

For the MR image, we used an in-house segmentation method that consisted of Gaussian smoothing followed by a thresholding process, which used some definitions from BET.[6] We computed the threshold for the image background from the robust intensity extremes of the image[†]. The robust intensity minimum, t_2, was calculated as the intensity below which 2% of the cumulative histogram lies; the maximum, t_{98}, is computed similarly, but at a 98% cutoff. The threshold to identify the background in the smoothed image was set to lie 8% of the way between t_2 and t_{98}.

2.2. Measures of registration quality

The following measures were applied to the superimposed contour images.

Average 0-1 Fraction (A01F). This measure of registration quality was applied to the brain contours and consisted of the average proportion of CT contour voxels, over a set of n slices, that had an MR contour voxel within a distance of zero or one voxels *in the x-y plane*. Note that this procedure requires that only a 3×3 neighborhood centered at each CT contour voxel be examined to find the closest MR contour voxel. A01F ranges between 0 and 1, and small values correspond to large misregistrations. The set of n slices constituted the central 25% of the total image volume.

Sum of Large Distances (SOLD). This measure consisted of the sum of distances larger than a threshold (set to three for this work), weighted by the fraction of voxels that had a distance larger than the threshold (over n slices). It was applied to the scalp contours. The assumption was that for large misregistrations, many voxels in the CT contour would be far from the nearest MR voxel; this is in comparison to small misregistrations, which might have few such voxels. Therefore, SOLD is expected to be larger for large misregistrations than for small misregistrations. This measure was applied only to 15% of the slices at, and superior to, the nose level.

In SOLD, the search for the closest voxel was restricted to a small set of directions and within a range of twenty voxels. First, from each CT voxel, the search direction is along a perpendicular line from the CT contour, to within a radius of 20 voxels in each direction away from it. If an MR voxel was found, the Euclidean distance was annotated; if not, then an MR voxel was searched for along a vertical, horizontal, and a diagonal (45°) line. The minimum of these three distances was annotated as the distance between the current CT contour voxel and the MR contour. If there was no MR contour voxel found in any of those directions, an arbitrary distance of 20 was assigned, and the next CT voxel examined (this means that any MR voxel outside the searched neighborhood was given the same distance value). The MR voxels that were identified as being closest to a CT voxel were deleted, so that they would not be identified more than once.

From the above, the values of SOLD ranged between 0 and $20 \times n\times$ maximum length of contour.

Ratio SOLD/A10F. We also tested the potential of a measure that consisted of the ratio of the two described above. In section 2.7 we provide the details for such choice.

[†]The word robust here means that small numbers of voxels with extreme values will be ignored.

2.3. Data

The registration quality measures were tested on CT, T1, and T2 images of three patients (practice set, patient 1, and patient 5) from the Vanderbilt study.[4] The dimensions of the CT were $512 \times 512 \times \{28, 29, 33\}$ slices (voxel size of $0.65 \times 0.65 \times 4$ mm), and all six MR images were $256 \times 256 \times 26$ (voxel size of $1.25 \times 1.25 \times 4$ mm).

2.4. Validation

The gold standard from the image pairs in the Vanderbilt study is a system based on the implantation of fiducial markers into the skull of the patient. Since the dataset was developed for a blind study, ground truth is available for only one Vanderbilt image pair (the practice set). This ground truth consists of a *transformation table* with the coordinates of the eight corner voxels in the "From" volume (e.g. CT in the case of CT to MR), and the transformed positions of these eight points relative to the origin of the "To" modality.[4]

For the image volumes of the other two patients (patients one and five) the gold standard was an edge-based registration algorithm developed by Hsu et al.[7] That registration algorithm had been tested previously on the Vanderbilt images, and the errors reported by them (computed over a set of ten anatomic landmarks) were less than 2 mm. Again, a transformation table was given to us as ground truth. This work aims at detection of large misregistrations. Therefore a reference registration method that yields small uncertainties (approximately 2 mm) will have minimal effect on the results. This fact guided our validation process.

In this paper, *registration error* was defined as the RMS distance between the two sets of eight corner points of CT produced by its registration to MR using (1) the gold standard and (2) a given registration transformation. Note that the definition of registration error used here is different from the one used in the earlier visual accuracy validation papers.[1,2]

2.5. Misregistration

For this study, various magnitudes of misregistering transformation vectors were used. The magnitudes of the resultant translational and rotational vectors were confined to $0-8$ mm and $0-8°$. Misregistering transformation vectors in those ranges generated registration errors of $0 - 35$ mm.

Rotational and translational magnitudes were randomly selected from the ranges $[0, 1], [1, 2], [2, 3], \ldots, [7, 8]$ mm or degrees. Misregistrations with all combinations of translational and rotational magnitudes were created, for a total of $8 \times 8 = 64$ combinations. In addition, misregistrations with only translations or rotations were created, which added $8 + 8 = 16$ more cases; hence the total number of misregistration options was $64 + 16 = 80$. Ten random misregistrations were constructed for each range, so there were 800 misregistrations per image pair per patient, to which a perfectly registered pair was added. A01F and SOLD were computed for each of the total 801 cases.

2.6. Defining what is acceptable accuracy

Based on two previous studies[2,8] we defined the following two classes of registrations:

- *Acceptable accuracy*: Registrations with translation vector of less than or equal to 3 mm and rotation vector of less than or equal to 4° from ground truth.

- *Unacceptable accuracy*: Registrations with translation vector of more than 3 mm and/or rotation vector of more than 4° from ground truth.

Each of the generated misregistered pairs were assigned the appropriate class. In our study, we pooled the CT-T1 cases of the three patients in one set, and the CT-T2 cases in another. Each set consisted of 2403 misregistered pairs (801×3), from which 76% of the cases were of class "unacceptable accuracy" and 24% were of class "acceptable accuracy".

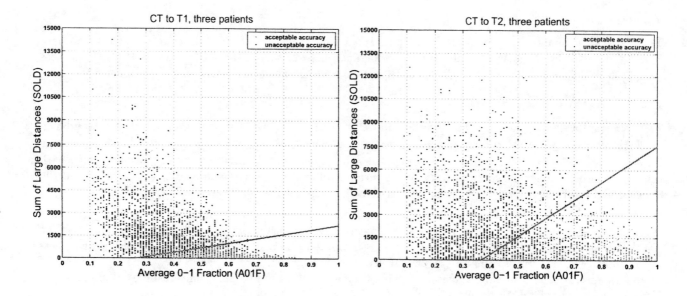

Figure 1. Feature space for the 2403 misregistered CT-T1 and CT-T2 pairs, showing the two classes of registration : "acceptable accuracy" and "unacceptable accuracy".

2.7. Comparison with Receiver Operating Characteristic Analysis

Comparison with ROC Analysis. Receiver operating characteristic (ROC) analysis and its associated indices are valuable tools for the assessment of the accuracy of diagnostic tests.[9] They are being used to judge the discrimination ability of various statistical methods for predictive purposes. A ROC curve is a plot of a test's true positive rate (or sensitivity) against its false positive rate (or 1-specificity). It is constructed by varying the test threshold defining "positive" and estimating the sensitivity and specificity imposed by that threshold. The ROC curve provides a concise description of the trade-offs available between sensitivity and specificity.

In this work, we chose to compare the performance of the registration quality measures with an ROC analysis. An ROC was constructed by varying the threshold at which a given misregistered pair would be labeled "possibly correctly registered" or "greatly misregistered" by a given measure. Although not shown, those thresholds correspond to a vertical partition (for A01F) or a horizontal partition (for SOLD) in the plots of Figure 1. The plots show the distribution of "acceptable accuracy" and "unacceptable accuracy" cases in the two-dimensional feature space created by A01F and SOLD. In addition, we also explored diagonal partitions as the one shown in the same figure; the measure is then of the form SOLD = $m \times$A01F + b. In this case, the ROC was constructed by fixing the slope and changing the intercept.

Given any linear partition of the feature-space, the number of misregistered pairs belonging to class "acceptable accuracy" that were labeled as "possibly correctly registered" corresponded to the true positives; similarly, the true negatives corresponded to the number of pairs of class "unacceptable accuracy" that were labeled as "greatly misregistered". The true positive rate is computed as true positives divided by true positives plus false negatives. The false positive rate is computed as false positives divided by false positives plus true negatives.

The area under the curve is one of the measures of accuracy associated with the ROC curve.[10] Statistical comparisons between two areas can be made by testing their difference using the formula[11]

$$ z = \frac{\hat{A}_1 - \hat{A}_2}{SE(\hat{A}_1 - \hat{A}_2)} \qquad (1) $$

where $\hat{A}_1$ and $\hat{A}_2$ are the two estimated ROC areas [‡], and SE the standard error. The quantity z is then

---

[‡]We use the general symbol $\hat{A}$ instead of A_z, since A_z is used only when the ROC curve is fitted with the conventional

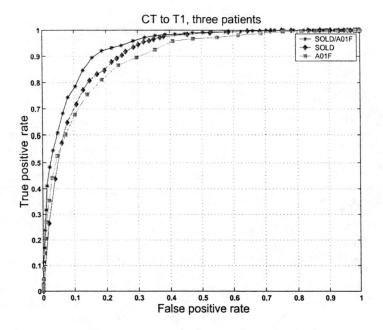

Figure 2: ROC curves of the classification performance of A01F, SOLD, and SOLD/A01F for CT-T1 pairs

referred to the tables of the normal distribution and values of z above some cutoff are taken as evidence that the "true" ROC areas are different.

The standard error of the difference between two ROC areas is calculated as[10, 13]:

$$SE(\hat{A}_1 - \hat{A}_2) = \sqrt{SE^2(\hat{A}_1) + SE^2(\hat{A}_2) - 2rSE(\hat{A}_1)SE(\hat{A}_2)} \tag{2}$$

where r represents the estimated correlation between $\hat{A}_1$ and $\hat{A}_2$ (for non-correlated cases, $r = 0$).

A conservative estimate[10] of the standard error of a ROC area value is:

$$SE(\hat{A}) = \sqrt{\frac{\theta(1 - \theta) + (n_A - 1)(Q_1 - \theta^2) + (n_N - 1)(Q_2 - \theta^2)}{n_A n_N}} \tag{3}$$

where Q_1 and Q_2 are two distribution-specific quantities, θ is the "true" area under the ROC curve, and n_A and n_N are the number of "abnormal" and normal (in this paper, "unacceptable accuracy" and "acceptable accuracy", respectively) samples, respectively. The estimate $\hat{A}_i$ is used as an estimate of θ. The quantities Q_1 and Q_2 are expressed as functions of θ:

$$Q_1 = \theta/(2 - \theta) \qquad Q_2 = 2\theta^2/(1 + \theta) \tag{4}$$

3. RESULTS

Figures 2 and 3 show the ROC curves for the three measures: A01F, SOLD, and SOLD/A01F. The ROC curve for the SOLD/A01F measure that is shown in the figure corresponds to the best curve that was obtained (in terms of area under the curve).

---

binormal model,[12] which is not the case in this paper.

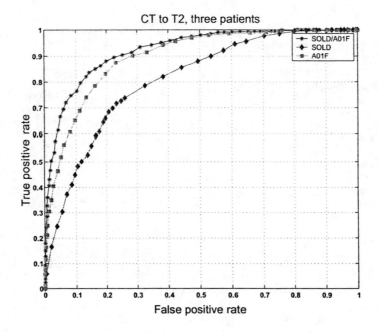

Figure 3: ROC curves of the classification performance of A01F, SOLD, and SOLD/A01F for CT-T2 pairs

The area under the curve was computed using the trapezoid rule. Table 1 shows the estimated areas for the three measures for both the CT-T1 and CT-T2 cases. Table 2 shows the results for the z-statistic test when comparing SOLD/A01F against the other two measures. We used a two-tailed test for statistical significance. The null hypothesis was that the two observed ROC areas are the same. A critical range of $z > 2.58$ or $z < -2.58$ (a level of significance p=0.01) indicated that the null hypothesis could be rejected.

Method of Classification	$\hat{A}$	
	CT to T1	CT to T2
A01F	0.8949	0.8965
SOLD	0.9093	0.8072
SOLD/A01F	0.9352	0.9262

Table 1: Areas under the curves for the ROC plots in Figures 2 and 3.

Method 1 vs Method 2	z statistic	
	CT to T1	CT to T2
A01F vs SOLD/A01F	5.11	3.54
SOLD vs SOLD/A01F	3.47	11.23

Table 2: Statistical test for differences in areas under the ROC curves.

4. DISCUSSION

As a measure of the quality in performance of the three proposed measures of registration quality we used the area under the ROC curve. The results from Table 2 indicate that the differences in area under the curve for SOLD/A01F against A01F or SOLD are statistically significant (p < 0.01). Even though we are comparing the same images across measures, the standard errors were calculated assuming no correlation (i.e., $r = 0$ in equation 2); but that was sufficient since the null hypothesis was rejected at $p < 0.01$. The ROC area for SOLD for both image sets was above 0.92.

Looking at the cases that corresponded to false positives, we observed that a large portion of those misregistrations had large translations in the z axis, or large rotations around the x and y axes.

The measure SOLD had a poorer performance for the CT-T2 images than for the CT-T1 images. Looking at the ROC curves of the CT-T2 images of each patient separately, we noted that it was patient 5 for which SOLD attained the smaller true positive rates and influenced the pooled ROC curve. The performance on patient 5 can be explained by the fact that there were discrepancies in the segmentation of CT and T2 in the region of the eyes and nose. Even small transformations that pulled contours in that region further apart led to at least twice as many voxels having large distances (i.e. large values of SOLD) than similar transformations for other patients. Hence some CT-T2 misregistered cases belonging to class "acceptable accuracy" had a large value for SOLD and were labeled incorrectly as "greatly misregistered" instead of "possibly correctly registered". This was reflected in the reduced true positive rate.

This raises the question of how important is the accuracy of segmentation to the measures' usefulness. Large segmentation errors such as having one whole region appearing in one image but not in the other will result in a measure value equivalent to a bad registration. On the other hand, for small registration errors the dependence is small because for registrations far from correct alignment the actual distance between contours will be much larger than the error induced by segmentation. Work is underway on a general proof of this observation.

The work done by Wong et al.[2] studied single-axis perturbations only. Our work included perturbations in all axes, such as in Fitzpatrick et al.[1] Comparing the results for that study to ours is not straightforward since the misregistration error ranges differ. Nevertheless it is interesting to note that our statistical measures of quality lay in the same ranges. In our study, the ROC areas for SOLD/A01F were 0.92 and 0.93, which are in the range of ROC areas in their study (0.73-0.95). We computed agreement rates at three points (FP=0.1, 0.15, 0.2) in the best SOLD/A01F curve, and the results were: 0.873. 0.856, 0.829 for CT to T1 and 0.866, 0.849, 0.820, for CT to T2. . This numbers lay in the agreement rate range ($[0.80, 0.90]$) obtained in that study.

The $\hat{A}$ index may not be the best measure of the performance of measures of registration quality. In practice, we would want to maximize the number of registrations with acceptable accuracy reaching the physician, and at the same time filter as many registrations with unacceptable accuracy as possible. That means that we are seeking measures of high sensitivity and high specificity. Therefore, a registration quality measure would not be particularly useful for false-positive rates larger than, say, 0.2. Using the work of McClish,[14] our next step is then to compare our ROC curves only in the range between FP=0 and FP=0.2. In looking for improvements on the measure, that is also the range that we will focus on.

5. CONCLUSIONS

We proposed an automated measure of registration quality based on brain contours as an aid to labeling registrations as either "possibly correctly registered" or "greatly misregistered". The results of the present study indicate that the use of the SOLD/A01F may be a good first step to reduce the number of badly registered images reaching the clinician.

REFERENCES

1. J. M. Fitzpatrick, "Visual assessment of the accuracy of retrospective registration of MR and CT images of the brain," *IEEE Transactions on Medical Imaging* **17**(4), pp. 571–585, 1998.
2. J. C. H. Wong, C. Studholme, D. J. Hawkes, and M. N. Maisey, "Evaluation of the limits of visual detection of image misregistration in a brain F-18 FDG PET-MRI study," *European Journal of Nuclear Medicine* **24**(6), 1997.
3. K. S. Holton, R. A. Robb, U. Taneja, and J. E. Gray, "The evaluation of 3D multimodality image registration using ROC analysis," in *SPIE Proceedings in Medical Imaging, Image Perception*, H. Kundel, ed., **2436**, pp. 90–104, 1995.

4. J. West, M. Fitzpatrick, M. Wang, and et al., "Comparison and evaluation of retrospective intermodality brain image registration techniques," *Journal of Computer Assissted Tomography* **21**(4), pp. 554–566, 1997.

5. U. Pietrzyk, K. Herholz, and W. D. Heiss, "Three-dimensional alignment of functional and morphological tomograms," *Journal of Computer Assissted Tomography* **14**(1), pp. 51–59, 1990.

6. S. M. Smith, "BET : Brain extraction tool," in *FMRIB Technical Report,* **TR00SMS2a**, Oxford Centre for Functional Magnetic Resonance Imaging of the Brain (FMRIB).

7. L. Hsu and M. H. Loew, "Automated registration of brain images using edge and surface features," *IEEE Engineering in Medicine and Biology* **18**(6), pp. 40–47, 1999.

8. C. Studholme, D. L. G. Hill, and D. Hawkes, "Automated three-dimensional registration of magnetic resonance and positron emission tomography brain images by multiresolution optimization of voxel similarity measures," *Medical Physics* **24**(1), pp. 25–35, 1997.

9. C. E. Metz, "Basic principles of ROC analysis," *Semin. Nucl. Med* **8**, pp. 283–298, 1978.

10. J. A. Hanley and B. J. McNeil, "The meaning and use of the area under a receiving operating characteristic (ROC) curve," *Radiology* **143**(April), pp. 29–36, 1982.

11. B. J. McNeil and J. A. Hanley, "Statistical approaches to the analysis of receiver operating characteristic (ROC) curves," *Medical Decision Making* **4**(2), pp. 137–150, 1984.

12. Y. Jiang, C. E. Metz, and R. M. Nishikawa, "A receiver operating characteristic partial area index for highly sensitive diagnostic tests," *Radiology* **201**(3), pp. 745–750, 1996.

13. J. A. Hanley and B. J. McNeil, "A method of comparing the areas under receiving operating characteristic curvecs derived from the same cases," *Radiology* **148**(September), pp. 839–843, 1983.

14. D. K. McClish, "Analyzing a portion of the ROC curve," *Medical Decision Making* **9**, pp. 190–195, 1989.

Mixture of principal axes registration: a neural computation approach

Rujirutana Srikanchana[a], Jianhua Xuan[a], Kun Huang[a], Matthew Freedman[b], and Yue Wang[a]

[a]Department of Electrical Engineering and Computer Science,
The Catholic University of America, Washington, DC 20064, USA
[b]Department of Radiology,
Georgetown University Medical Center, Washington, DC 20007, USA

ABSTRACT

Non-rigid image registration is a prerequisite for many medical imaging applications such as change analysis in image-based diagnosis and therapy assessment. Nonlinear interpolation methods may be used to recover the deformation if the correspondence of the extracted feature points is available. However, it may be very difficult to establish such correspondence at an initial stage when confronted with large and complex deformation. In this paper, a mixture of principal axes registration (mPAR) is proposed to tackle the correspondence problem using a neural computation method. The feature is to align two point sets without needing to establish the explicit point correspondence. The mPAR aligns two point sets by minimizing the relative entropy between their probability distributions resulting in a maximum likelihood estimate of the transformation mixture. The neural computation for the mPAR is developed using a committee machine to obtain a mixture of piece-wise rigid registrations. The complete registration process consists of two steps: (1) using the mPAR to establish an improved point correspondence and (2) using a multilayer perceptron (MLP) neural network to recover the nonlinear deformation. The mPAR method has been applied to register a contrast-enhanced magnetic resonance (MR) image sequece. The experimental results show that our method not only improves the point correspondence but also results in a desirable error-resilience property for control point selection errors.

Keywords: M ixture of Principal Axes Registration, Non-Rigid Image Registration, Change Analysis, Neural Computation, Multilayer Perceptron, Control Points Selection.

1. INTRODUCTION

Image registration is an essential step for many medical image analysis applications such as image fusion, quantitative change analysis in image-based diagnosis and therapy assessment.[1,2] For example, medical diagnosis often benefits from the complementary information in images of different modalities. Multimodality imaging of breast is regarded as a powerful diagnostic tool. In breast imaging, different modalities offer different diagnostic information. In order to fuse the complementary information, the alignment of the images is the first step to be performed to overcome the complication of misregistrations caused by patient motion and physical change. Image registration consists of aligning the images by scaling, rotating, and translating, one or both images so that they are of the same size and have the same orientation and location. Mathematically, image registration can be formulated as to estimate the transformational geometry from two feature point sets, i.e., to recover a matrix representation requiring a set of correspondence matches between features in the two coordinate system. Arun *et. al.*[3] present an algorithm for finding the least-squares solution of the transformation matrix, which is based on the decoupling of translation and rotation and the singular value decomposition (SVD) of a cross-covariance matrix.

Further author information: (Send correspondence to Rujirutana Srikanchana)
E-mail: 55srikanchan@cua.edu, Telephone: 1 202 319 5243
Address: EE/CS Department, The Catholic University of America, Washington, D.C., U.S.A.

The major limitation of the above method is twofold: (1) while feature matching methods can give quite accurate solutions, obtaining correct correspondences of features is a hard problem, especially in the case of images acquired using different modalities or from inter-subjects; and (2) a rigidity assumption is heuristically imposed that is usually not valid in medical images with non-rigid human organs such as breast.[2,4] One popular method that does not require feature correspondence is the principal axes registration (PAR) method.[1] The PAR method is based on the relatively stable geometric properties of image features, i.e., the geometric information contained in these stable image features is often sufficient to determine the transformation between images.[2] However, the PAR method results in a rigid body transform with scaling coefficients. The transform works effectively if the objects to be registered have orientation differences within a certain limit, dependent on the objects' shape and if their shapes are well matched. If their orientations are too different, the transform may arrive at the wrong rotation angle due to problems with object symmetry. Once again, the method cannot handle the cases with non-rigid objects.

In this paper, we present a neural computation based non-rigid image registration method using piece-wise rigid transformation. In other words, rather than using a single transformation matrix that gives rise to a large registration error, we attempt to interpolatively apply a mixture of transformations to minimize the registration error. By generalizing PAR to a mixture of principal axes registration (mPAR) scheme, the mixture is fit using the expectation-maximization (EM) algorithm by performing a soft partitioning of the data set. The registration process consists of two steps: (1) using the mPAR to establish an improved point correspondence and (2) using a multilayer perceptron (MLP) neural network to recover nonlinear deformation based on the established point correspondence. A finite mixture of transformations is obtained through aligning the two point sets by minimizing the relative entropy between their probability distributions resulting in a maximum likelihood estimate of the transformation matrix. Specifically, a probabilistic adaptive principal components extraction (PAPEX) algorithm[10] is developed to estimate the transformation matrix using the orthogonal set of eigenvalues and eigenvectors of the auto covariance matrix. A committee machine is then used to combine multiple transformations for the recovery of the total transformational geometry of the non-rigid object. An accurate point correspondence can be established by applying the finite mixture of transformations to the two point sets. Finally, an MLP neural network is adopted to recover the nonlinear deformation by the polynomial mapping function based on the point correspondence.

The mPAR method has been applied to register a contrast-enhanced breast magnetic resonance image (MRI) sequence. With MRI, the breast is usually imaged functionally using a contrast agent. The rate of uptake of the contrast agent is used to characterize a given breast tissue. This rate is studied by observing the change in gray level of the tissue at several instants of time after injection of the agent. However, the non-rigid nature of breast tissue almost guarantees that these different images would be misregistered. To study the uptake process effectively and to also make a quantitative estimate of change in uptake, it would be necessary to align or register these different images. Image registration is thus an important problem. To align these different images, we first extract the control objects of the image using a stochastic segmentation method. With the extracted control objects, we then apply our mPAR method to recover the total transformational geometry of the contrast-enhanced MRI. An accurate point correspondence can be established by applying the mixture of transformations to the two point sets. As a final step, we apply an MLP neural network to recover the nonlinear deformation in the form of the polynomial transformation using the established point correspondence. The experimental results shows that the image differencing after registering two images by applying our mPAR method can greatly improve the accuracy in extraction of the enhanced area compared to that of without any registration.

2. THEORY AND METHOD

Assume two 3-D data point sets $\{\mathbf{p}_{iA}\}$ and $\{\mathbf{p}_{iB}\}$, $i = 1, 2, ..., N$, are related by

$$\mathbf{p}_{iB} = \mathbf{R}\mathbf{p}_{iA} + \mathbf{T} + \mathbf{N}_i \tag{1}$$

where $\mathbf{R}$ is a rotation matrix, $\mathbf{T}$ a translation vector, and $\mathbf{N}_i$ a noise vector. Given $\{\mathbf{p}_{iA}\}$ and $\{\mathbf{p}_{iB}\}$, Arun et. al. present an algorithm for finding the least-squares solution of $\mathbf{R}$ and $\mathbf{T}$ by decoupling translation and rotation and using the singular value decomposition (SVD) of a 3×3 cross-covariance matrix.[3]

Suggested by information theory,[5] we can consider the feature point sets in two images as two separate realizations of the same random source. Hence, to align two sets of feature points, we do not need to establish point correspondences to extract the transformation matrix. Instead, we can aligning the two point sets by minimizing the relative entropy between their probability distributions. In other words, if $P_{\{\mathbf{p}_i\}}$ denotes the distribution of the feature point set in an image, we have the simple probabilistic relationship to describe the transformation between two point sets:

$$P_{\{\mathbf{p}_{jB}\}} = P_{\{\mathbf{R}\mathbf{p}_{iA}+\mathbf{T}\}} + \epsilon \tag{2}$$

where ϵ is the noise component. Since the probability distributions can be computed independently on each image without the need to establish feature correspondences, and given the two distributions of the control point sets in the two images, we can recover the transformation matrix in a simple fashion,[2] as we now sketch.

2.1. Registration

For observation of the distributions, we can estimate $\mathbf{R}$ and $\mathbf{T}$ by minimizing the relative entropy (Kullback-Leibler distance) between $P_{\{\mathbf{p}_{jB}\}}$ and $P_{\{\mathbf{R}\mathbf{p}_{iA}+\mathbf{T}\}}$. The least relative entropy estimator is defined as

$$\arg\min_{\mathbf{R},\mathbf{T}} D(P_{\{\mathbf{p}_{jB}\}} || P_{\{\mathbf{R}\mathbf{p}_{iA}+\mathbf{T}\}}) \tag{3}$$

where D denotes the relative entropy measure. Following the same strategy to decouple translation and rotation as in,[3] we can define a new data point by $\mathbf{q}_{iA} = \mathbf{p}_{iA} - \mathbf{p}_A^0$ and $\mathbf{q}_{jB} = \mathbf{p}_{jB} - \mathbf{p}_B^0$, where $\mathbf{p}_A^0$ and $\mathbf{p}_B^0$ are the centroids of $\{\mathbf{p}_{iA}\}$ and $\{\mathbf{p}_{jB}\}$, respectively. Then the optimal geometric transformations, $\mathbf{R}$ and $\mathbf{T}$, can be computed as

$$\mathbf{R} = \mathbf{U}_B \mathbf{H} \mathbf{U}_A^t \tag{4}$$

$$\mathbf{T} = \mathbf{p}_B^0 - \mathbf{R}\mathbf{p}_A^0 \tag{5}$$

where the superscript t denotes matrix transposition, $\mathbf{U}_A$ and $\mathbf{U}_B$ are 3×3 orthonormal matrices, and $\mathbf{H}$ is a 3×3 diagonal matrix with element $h_m = \sqrt{\lambda_{mB}/\lambda_{mA}}$. Note that the transformation $\mathbf{U}$ consists of the orthonormal set of eigenvectors and h_m is the squared root of the eigenvalues λ_m of the auto-covariance matrix $\mathbf{C}$ for $m = 1, 2, 3$ and for $\{\mathbf{p}_{iA}\}$ and $\{\mathbf{p}_{jB}\}$, respectively.

However, because of its global linearity, the application of PAR is somewhat limited to deal with rigid objects only.[6] An alternative paradigm is to model a multimodal control point set with a collection of local linear models. The method is a two-stage procedure: a soft partitioning of the data set followed by estimation of the principal axes within each partition.[7] Recently there has been considerable success in using standard finite normal mixture (SFNM) to model the distribution of a multimodal data set. The association of a SFNM distribution with PAR offers the possibility of being able to register two images through a mixture of probabilistic principal axes transformations.[7] Assume that there are K_0 control point clusters, where each control point cluster defines a transformation $\{\mathbf{R}_k, \mathbf{T}_k\}$. For a point $\mathbf{p}_{nA}$, its new locations corresponding to each of the transformations are $\mathbf{p}_{nk} = \mathbf{R}_k \mathbf{p}_{nA} + \mathbf{T}_k$ for $k = 1, ..., K_0$. Further assume that the control point set defines a SFNM distribution

$$f(\mathbf{p}_i) = \sum_{k=1}^{K_0} \pi_k g(\mathbf{p}_i | \boldsymbol{\mu}_k, \mathbf{C}_k) \tag{6}$$

where g is the Gaussian kernel with mean vector $\boldsymbol{\mu}_k$ and auto-covariance matrix $\mathbf{C}_k$, and π_k is the mixing factor proportional to the number of control points in cluster k. For each of the control point sets $\{\mathbf{p}_{iA}\}$ and $\{\mathbf{p}_{iB}\}$, the mixture distribution is fit using the expectation-maximization (EM) algorithm. In principle, the E step involves assigning to the linear models responsibilities, i.e., the posterior Bayesian probability, from the control points; the M step involves re-estimating the parameters of the linear models from the above assignment.[7]

Thus the statistical membership of point $\mathbf{p}_{nA}$ belonging to each of the control point clusters can be derived by

$$z_{nk} = P(\mathbf{R}_k, \mathbf{T}_k | \mathbf{p}_{nA}) = \frac{\pi_{kA} g(\mathbf{p}_{nA} | \boldsymbol{\mu}_{kA}, \mathbf{C}_{kA})}{f(\mathbf{p}_{nA})} \tag{7}$$

i.e., the posterior probability of $\{\mathbf{R}_k, \mathbf{T}_k\}$ given $\mathbf{p}_{nA}$. We can define the mPAR transformation as

$$\mathbf{p}_n = \sum_{k=1}^{K_0} z_{nk} \mathbf{p}_{nk} \tag{8}$$

$$= \sum_{k=1}^{K_0} \frac{\pi_{kA} g(\mathbf{p}_{nA}|\boldsymbol{\mu}_{kA}, \mathbf{C}_{kA})}{f(\mathbf{p}_{nA})}(\mathbf{R}_k \mathbf{p}_{nA} + \mathbf{T}_k) \tag{9}$$

where $\{\mathbf{R}_k, \mathbf{T}_k\}$ is determined based on $\{\mu_{kA}, \mathbf{C}_{kA}\}$ and $\{\mu_{kB}, \mathbf{C}_{kB}\}$, which we have estimated in the previous step using the EM algorithm. This philosophy for recovering transformational geometry of the non-rigid objects is similar in spirit to the *divide-and-conquer* principle,[6] under which the relative entropy between the two point sets reaches its minimum

$$\arg \min_{\mathbf{R}_k, \mathbf{T}_k} D(P_{\{\mathbf{p}_{jB}\}} || P_{\{\sum_{k=1}^{K_0} z_{ik}(\mathbf{R}_k \mathbf{p}_{iA} + \mathbf{T}_k)\}}) \tag{10}$$

both globally and locally.

Based on a mixture of probabilistic principal axes transformations, the next section describes a neural computation using a committee machine to obtain a mixture of piece-wise rigid registrations, which gives a reliable point correspondence using multiple extracted object control points.

2.2. Neural Computation

There are many numerical techniques to perform the maximum likelihood estimation. The most popular method is the EM algorithm. The EM algorithm first calculates the posterior Bayesian probabilities of the data through the data observations and the current parameter estimates (E-Step) and then updates parameter estimates (M-Step). The procedure cycles back and forth between these two steps. A neural network interpretation of the EM algorithm is given in.[8] Because of its reputation of being slow in which new information acquired in the expectation step is not used immediately, on-line versions of the EM algorithm are proposed for large-scale sequential learning. We adopt a fully unsupervised and incremental stochastic learning algorithm to implement the EM algorithm. The scheme provides winner-takes-in probability (Bayesian "soft") splits of the control points, hence allowing the data to contribute simultaneously to multiple clusters. The incremental stochastic learning EM algorithm can be described as follows:

$E - Step$

$$z_{(i+1)k} = \frac{\pi_k^{(i)} g(\mathbf{p}_{i+1}|\boldsymbol{\mu}_k^{(i)}, \mathbf{C}_k^{(i)})}{f(\mathbf{p}_{i+1}|\pi_k^{(i)}, \boldsymbol{\mu}_k^{(i)}, \mathbf{C}_k^{(i)})} \tag{11}$$

$M - Step$

$$\boldsymbol{\mu}_k^{(i+1)} = \boldsymbol{\mu}_k^{(i)} + a(i)(\mathbf{p}_{i+1} - \boldsymbol{\mu}_k^{(i)})z_{(i+1)k}, \tag{12}$$

$$\mathbf{C}_k^{(i+1)} = \mathbf{C}_k^{(i)} + b(i)[(\mathbf{p}_{i+1} - \boldsymbol{\mu}_k^{(i)})(\mathbf{p}_{i+1} - \boldsymbol{\mu}_k^{(i)})^T - \mathbf{C}_k^{(i)}]z_{(i+1)k}, \tag{13}$$

$$\pi_k^{(i+1)} = \frac{i}{i+1}\pi_k^{(i)} + \frac{1}{i+1}z_{(i+1)k} \tag{14}$$

for $k = 1, ..., K_0$ and for $\{\mathbf{p}_{iA}\}$ and $\{\mathbf{p}_{iB}\}$, respectively. In the above equations, $a(i)$ and $b(i)$ are introduced as the learning rates that converge to zero, ensuring unbiased estimates after convergence. This procedure is termed as neural computation of the EM algorithm. At each complete cycle of the algorithm, we first use "*old*" set of parameter values to determine the posterior probabilities $z_{(i+1)k}$. These posterior probabilities are then used to obtain "*new*" values $\pi_k^{(i+1)}, \boldsymbol{\mu}_k^{(i+1)}, \mathbf{C}_k^{(i+1)}$. The algorithm cycles back and forth until the value of relative entropy between the data histogram and mixture model reaches its minimum

$$\arg \min_{\pi_k, \boldsymbol{\mu}_k, \mathbf{C}_k} D(P_{\{\mathbf{p}_i\}} || f(\mathbf{p}_i)) \tag{15}$$

for $\{\mathbf{p}_{iA}\}$ and $\{\mathbf{p}_{iB}\}$, respectively.

With a soft partitioning of the data set using Eqs. (11-14), control points will now effectively belong to more than one cluster spatially. Thus, the effective input values are $\mathbf{p}_{ik} = z_{ik}(\mathbf{p}_i - \boldsymbol{\mu}_k)$ for an independent registration transformation k in the committee machine.[9] We then extend an adaptive principal components extraction (APEX) algorithm to a probabilistic version, i.e., PAPEX,[10] to determine $\mathbf{U}_k$ for $\{\mathbf{p}_{iA}\}$ and $\{\mathbf{p}_{iB}\}$, respectively, summarized as follows.

1. Initialize the feedforward weight vector $\mathbf{u}_{mk}$ for $m = 1, 2, 3$, and the feedback weight vector $\mathbf{a}_{mk}$ to small random values for $m = 2, 3$, at time $i = 1$. Assign a small positive value to the learning rate parameter η.

2. Set $m = 1$, and for $i = 1, 2, ...$, compute

$$y_{1k}(i) = \mathbf{u}_{1k}^T(i)z_{ik}(\mathbf{p}_i - \boldsymbol{\mu}_k) \tag{16}$$

$$\mathbf{u}_{1k}(i+1) = \mathbf{u}_{1k}(i) + \eta[y_{1k}(i)z_{1k}(\mathbf{p}_i - \boldsymbol{\mu}_k) - y_{1k}^2(i)\mathbf{u}_{1k}(i)] \tag{17}$$

For large i we have $\mathbf{u}_{1k}(i) \longrightarrow \mathbf{u}_{1k}$, where $\mathbf{u}_{1k}$ is the eigenvector associated with the largest eigenvalue of the cluster k, and $\lambda_{1k} = \frac{1}{N}\sum_{i=1}^{N} y_{1k}^2(i)$.

3. Set $m = 2$, and for $i = 1, 2, ...$, compute

$$\mathbf{y}_{(m-1)k}(i) = [y_{1k}(i), y_{2k}(i), ..., y_{(m-1)k}(i)]^T \tag{18}$$

$$y_{mk}(i) = \mathbf{u}_{mk}^T(i)z_{ik}(\mathbf{p}_i - \boldsymbol{\mu}_k) + \mathbf{a}_{mk}^T(i)\mathbf{y}_{(m-1)k}(i) \tag{19}$$

$$\mathbf{u}_{mk}(i+1) = \mathbf{u}_{mk}(i) + \eta[y_{mk}(i)z_{ik}(\mathbf{p}_i - \boldsymbol{\mu}_k) - y_{mk}^2(i)\mathbf{u}_{mk}(i)] \tag{20}$$

$$\mathbf{a}_{mk}(i+1) = \mathbf{a}_{mk}(i) - \eta[y_{mk}(i)\mathbf{y}_{(m-1)k}(i) + y_{mk}^2(i)\mathbf{a}_{mk}(i)] \tag{21}$$

For large i we have $\mathbf{u}_{2k}(i) \longrightarrow \mathbf{u}_{2k}$, where $\mathbf{u}_{2k}$ is the eigenvector associated with the second largest eigenvalue of the cluster k, and $\lambda_{2k} = \frac{1}{N}\sum_{i=1}^{N} y_{2k}^2(i)$.

4. Set $m = 3$, go to step 3. For large i we have $\mathbf{u}_{3k}(i) \longrightarrow \mathbf{u}_{3k}$, where $\mathbf{u}_{3k}$ is the eigenvector associated with the third largest eigenvalue of the cluster k, and $\lambda_{3k} = \frac{1}{N}\sum_{i=1}^{N} y_{3k}^2(i)$. The next step is to introduce a committee machine for combining multiple transformations in a mixture fashion.

Consider the modular network nature of Eq. (8), we can easily realize that it is a mixture of local expert model. Each local expert performs supervised learning through our PAPEX algorithm, and the individual responses of the experts are nonlinearly combined by means of a single gating network. This is our committee machine to combine multiple transformations to form the total transformational geometry of the non-rigid object. The neural computation of a committee machine can be achieved by distributing the learning tasks among a number of experts, which in turn partitioning the input space into a set of subspaces. The experts are in theory performing supervised learning in that the individual outputs are combined to model the desired response. There is, however, a sense in which the experts are also performing self-organized learning; that is, they self organize to find a good partitioning of the input space so that each expert does well at modeling its own subspace, and as a whole group they model the input space jointly. It is assume here that the different experts work best in different regions of the input space in accordance with the probabilistic generative model. In our case, the effective input values are $\mathbf{p}_{ik} = z_{ik}(\mathbf{p}_i - \boldsymbol{\mu}_k)$ for an independent registration transformation k in the networks. A committee machine consists of k supervised modules, with a soft partitioning of the data set using EM algorithm and the function PAPEX to determine the transformation of the orthogonal set of eigenvalues and eigenvectors of the auto-covariance matrix among the networks. The output of an integrating unit in our committee machine is a transformational matrix of the image pair.

Based on those correspondences established by applying the transformational matrix between the two images, the control points of two images are obtained. The final step is to recover the deformation of the object by calculating the polynomial transformation using piece-wise interpolation. The goal is to fine tune the alignment achieved in the initial registration by considering the object as a non-rigid body. This allows for the consideration of the non-rigid deformation between the images. The polynomial based transform such as thin-plate spline (TPS) has been shown to be able to handle non-rigid deformations of the object. In our case, we develop a three-layer MLP neural network to acquire the polynomial transform, where the input nodes are fed with the coordinates of the corresponding control points of the image. The MLP is trained by the corresponding control point pairs as its inputs and outputs using the backpropagation algorithm. The three-layer MLP converges to a polynomial transform that captures the relationship between corresponding control point pairs. The MLP neural network further recovers the underlying non-linear deformation between two images by interpolating the learned relationship between corresponding control point pairs. Finally, by applying the MLP polynomial transform to all the pixels in an image followed by a bilinear grey level interpolation method, we can obtain all the pixel intensity values in the image that is our final registered image.

In order to apply our registration method, we need to establish the corresponding objects between two images. We have developed a stochastic segmentation method to extract the corresponding objects in both images. The mPAR uses these corresponding objects to combine multiple transforms recovered by PAR in a mixture form. After the mPAR step, we can easily establish control point correspondence where control points are selected corner points on the boundaries of extracted corresponding objects. Next, we will describe our segmentation method for control point extraction.

2.3. Segmentation

Assume that each pixel in the image can be decomposed into pixel images x and context image l. By ignoring information regarding the spatial ordering of pixels, we can treat context images as random variables and describe them using a multinomial distribution with unknown parameters π_k, $k = 1, ..., K$, which can be interpreted as a prior probability of pixel labels determined by the global context information. In particular, based on the statistical properties of pixel images, where pixel image is defined as the observed gray level associated with the pixel, a SFNM distribution is justified to model the image histogram by determining the optimal parameters with respect to a distance measure of a sum of the following general form $f_r(x) = \sum_{k=1}^{K} \pi_k g(x|\mu_k, \sigma_k^2)$ with $\sum_{k=1}^{K} \pi_k = 1$, $\pi_k \geq 0$, and $g(x|\mu_k, \sigma_k^2) = \frac{1}{\sqrt{2\pi}\sigma_k} \exp(-\frac{(x-\mu_k)^2}{2\sigma_k^2})$ where μ_k and σ_k are the mean and variance of the kth Gaussian kernel, and π_k is the global regularization parameter. We use K to denote the number of Gaussian components and r to denote the parameter vector. This tissue quantification is achieved through three completely unsupervised steps: (1) parameter initialization by optimal histogram quantization, (2) model estimation by histogram based fast EM algorithm, and (3) model selection by minimum description length (MDL) criterion. It is shown that the SFNM model converges to the true distribution when the pixel image are asymptotically independent.[17]

After we obtain the optimal parameters for all components, we use a multiple thresholding procedure for initializing image segmentation based on maximum likelihood (ML) principle, which is followed by contextual Bayes relaxation labeling (CBRL) algorithm to obtain a consistent labeling solution based on localized SFNM formulation for improving initial segmentation by using neighborhood text regularities. We define the component in localized SFNM by the support function:

$$S_i(k) = \pi_k^{(i)} \frac{1}{\sqrt{2\pi}\sigma_k} \exp(-\frac{(x-\mu_k)^2}{2\sigma_k^2}) \tag{22}$$

where $\pi_k^{(i)}$ is the local conditional prior of regions, the support function $S_i(k)$ is a function of the component (tissue type) k. Then tissue segmentation is interpreted as the satisfaction of a system of inequalities as follows $S_i(l_i) \geq S_i(k)$ for all k and for $i = 1, ..., N$, where $l_i, i = 1, ..., N$ is the context images, and a consistent labeling is defined as the one having maximum support at each pixel simultaneously. We further define the average local consistency measure $A(l) = \sum_{i=1}^{N} \sum_k I(l_i, k)S_i(k)$ to link consistent labeling to global optimization.[18]

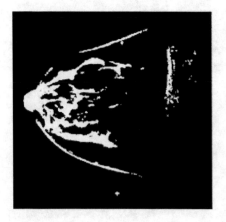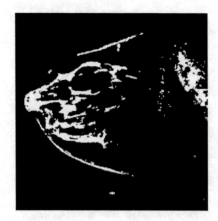

Figure 1: Segmentation result of fibroglandular tissue (left: pre-contrast image; right: post contrast image).

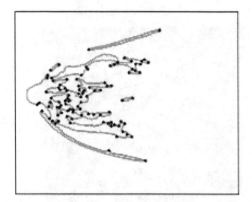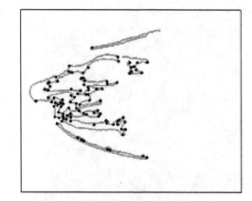

Figure 2: Extracted control points in a pre-contrast image (left) and a post-contrast image (right).

3. RESULT AND DISCUSSION

We applied our mPAR method to register pre- and post-contrast MR breast images. A 3-D breast MRI scan is acquired prior to the injection of contrast agent, followed by a sequence of 3-D breast MRI scan after the agent has been applied. The goal of image registration for this study is to relate any point in the post-contrast sequence to the pre-contrast reference image. The first step of our method is try to correct the global misalignment by performed a pre-registration step using the PAR method. The PAR method uses the extracted skinline as the control objects to globally align images. Since we do not want to change any contents in the post-contrast image, we decide to apply our registration method to the pre-contrast image. After we performed the pre-registration step, we applied our segmentation method to extract the control objects (fibroglandular tissue) in both pre- and post-contrast images. Figure 1 shows the segmented regions of fibroglandular tissue that will be used in our mPAR method as the corresponding control objects for non-rigid registration.

Our mPAR method treats the regions of fibroglandular tissue as multiple objects that can be obtained using the EM soft-partitioning algorithm. We then apply the PAPEX algorithm to determine transformation matrices between all the corresponding objects. A committee machine is then used to combine individual transforms to form a total transformational geometry of the non-rigid object, i.e., resulting in a mixture of individual transforms. After we apply the mixture transformation matrix to pre-contrast image, all the objects (i.e., the regions of fibroglandular tissue) are well aligned. We then apply a corner detection algorithm to extract those high-curvature points on the boundaries of fibroglandular tissue to serve as control points for the

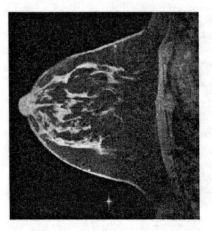 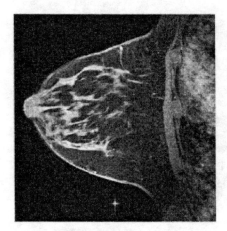

Figure 3. A pair of a contrast-enhanced breast MR images (left: pre-contrast image with global alignment based on PAR method; right: post contrast image).

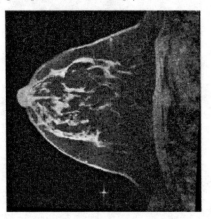 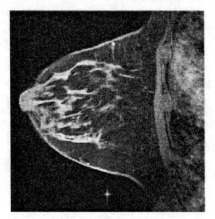

Figure 4. A pre-contrast image (left) and a registered post-contrast (right) image using the mPAR registration method.

MLP. Figure 2 shown the extracted control points in both pre- and post-contrast images. The control point correspondence between pre- and post-contrast images can be conveniently established using a simple correlation method. Finally, an MLP neural network is trained using the corresponding control point pairs to recover the nonlinear deformation between two images. The non-linear deformation is represented by a polynomial mapping function that is interpolated by the neural network based on the control point correspondence. Figure 4 shows a registered pre- and post-contrast image pair using our non-rigid registration method - the mPAR method.

To relate a post-contrast image to a pre-contrast image, we simple do the image difference between the post-contrast image and the pre-contrast image. The difference results are the enhanced area of fibroglandular tissue, i.e., the area that has been highlighted by the contrast agent. Figure 5 (left) shows the difference images between the post-contrast image and registered pre-contrast image. As a comparison, we also show the difference image of the post-contrast image and unregistered (original) pre-contrast image in Figure 5 (right), where false regions of the enhanced area of fibroglandular tissue can be observed due to the misalignment between pre- and post contrast images. The results demonstrate that the mPAR can successfully recover the deformation between pre- and post-contrast images so the enhanced area can be accurately extracted by image differencing between the post-contrast image and registered pre-contrast image.

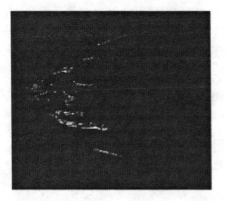 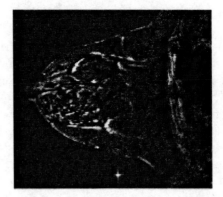

Figure 5. Difference images of the enhanced area (left: difference image with our mPAR registration; right: difference image without registration).

4. CONCLUSION

In this paper, we have presented the theoretical concepts and methods of a neural computation based non-rigid image registration method - the mPAR method. The approach uses a committee machine to recover the total transformational geometry of the non-rigid object. The committee machine combines multiple rigid transforms in a finite mixture registration scheme. Finite mixture transform combination is a novel technique to combine multiple transforms contained in a single image, which yields a lower mean square error (MSE) than that of using any local transform alone. In other word, the mPAR method results in a smooth image while local transforms yield an image containing discontinuities on transform boundaries. In addition, the registration obtained by the committee machine is fine tuned using the nonlinear transform recovered by a MLP network. The MLP neural network is trained by the extracted control point pairs and converges to a polynomial transform that captures the nonlinear deformation between two images.

We have applied our mPAR algorithm to MR breast registration problem. The experimental results have demonstrated that our mPAR method can successfully recover the nonlinear deformation between images. More importantly, our mPAR method aligns two point sets without the need of establishing explicit point correspondence. Instead, it aligns the two point sets by minimizing the relative entropy between their probability distributions. Furthermore, through aligning the two point sets initially by our mPAR method, we can improve the accuracy of establishing the feature point correspondence. The MLP neural network has been introduced to recover the deformation based on established feature point correspondence. The MLP has also resulted in a desirable error-resilience property for control point selection errors. However, some distortion can be observed in the final warped images. We believe that the distortion is largely caused by the errors in control point selection and correspondence. Improvement in this portion should reduce the distortion and yield better registration results. Finally, it is worthy noting that using neural networks in this problem has increased the generality of this approach to allow us to improve the algorithm and adjust performance as imaging conditions change.

ACKNOWLEDGMENTS

This work was supported by the US Army Medical Research and Materiel Command under Grants DAMD17-00-0195 and DAMD17-98-8045.

REFERENCES

1. M. Moshfeghi and H. Rusinek, "Three-dimensional registration of multimodality medical images using the principal axes techniques," *Philips J. Res.*, vol. 47, no.2, pp. 81-97, 1992.

2. V. Govindu and C. Shekhar, "Alignment using distributions of local geometric properties," *IEEE Trans. Pattern Anal. Machine Intell.*, vol. 21, no.10, pp. 1031-1043, October 1999.

3. K. S. Arun, T. S. Huang, and S. D. Blostein, "Least-squares fitting of two 3-D point sets," *IEEE Trans. Pattern Anal. Machine Intell.*, vol. 9, no.5, pp. 698-700, September 1987.

4. A. D.J. Cross and E. R. Hancock, "Graph matching with a dual-step EM algorithm," *IEEE Trans. Pattern Anal. Machine Intell.*, vol. 20, no.11, pp. 1236-1253, November 1998.

5. T. M. Cover and J. A. Thomas, *Elements of Information Theory*, New York: Wiley, 1991.

6. G. E. Hinton, P. Dayan, and M. Revow, "Modeling the manifolds of images of handwritten digits," *IEEE Trans. Neural Nets.*, vol. 8, no.1, pp. 65-74, January 1997.

7. Y. Wang, L. Luo, M. T. Freedman, and S. Y. Kung, "Probabilistic principal component subspaces: A hierarchical finite mixture model for data visualization," *IEEE Trans. Neural Nets.*, vol. 11, no. 3, pp. 625-636, May 2000.

8. L. Perlovsky and M. McManus, "Maximum likelihood neural networks for sensor fusion and adaptive classification," *Neural Networks*, vol. 4, pp. 89-102, 1991.

9. S. Haykin, Neural Networks: A Comprehensive Foundation, 2nd ed., Prentice-Hall, Inc., Upper Saddle River, Ney Jersey, 1999.

10. S. Y. Kung, *Principal Component Neural Networks*, New York: Wiley, 1996.

11. M. I. Jordan and R. A. Jacobs, "Hierarchical mixture of experts and the EM algorithm," *Neural Computation*, vol. 6, pp. 181-214, 1994.

12. D. M. Titterington, A. F. M. Smith, and U. E. Markov, *Statistical analysis of finite mixture distributions*, New York: John Wiley, 1985.

13. K. Woods, et. al., "Patient site model supported change detection," *Proceedings of SPIE Medical Imaging: 2000*, vol.1, no. 24 , pp. 1095-1106, 2000.

14. J. Lu, R. Srikanchana, M. McClain, Y. Wang, J. Xuan, I. A. Sesterhenn, M. T. Freedman, and S. K. Mun, "A statistical volumetric model for characterization and visualization of prostate cancer," *Proc. SPIE Medical Imaging*, vol. 3976, pp. 142-153, 2000.

15. K. Woods, *Image Guided Diagnosis through Change Detection in Image Sequences*, Doctoral Dissertation, The Catholic University of America, 2000.

16. P. Santago and H.D. Gage, "Quantification of MR Brain images by mixture density and partial volume modeling," *IEEE Trans. Med. Imag.*, vol. 12, no. 3, pp. 566-574, Sept. 1993.

17. Y.Wang and T. Adali, "Efficient learning of finite normal mixtures for image quantification," *Proc. IEEE Int. Conf. Acoustic, Speech, and Signal Processing*, Atlanta, GA, 1996, pp. 3422-3425.

18. R. A. Hummel and S. W. Zucker, "On the foundations of relaxation labeling processes," *IEEE Trans. Pattern Anal. Machine Intell.*, vol. 5, May 1983.

The Adaptive Bases Algorithm for Nonrigid Image Registration

Gustavo K. Rohde[1,3], Akram Aldroubi[2], Benoit M. Dawant[1]

[1]Department of Electrical Engineering and Computer Science, Vanderbilt University
[2]Department of Mathematics, Vanderbilt University
[3]Currently with the Section of Tissue Biophysics and Biomimetics, Laboratory of Medical and Integrative Biophysics, NICHD, National Institutes of Health
rohdeg@helix.nih.gov, aldroubi@math.vanderbilt.edu, benoit.dawant@vanderbilt.edu,

ABSTRACT

Nonrigid registration of medical images is an important procedure in many aspects of current biomedical and bioengineering research. For example, it is a necessary step for studying the variation of biological tissue properties, such as shape or diffusion properties across population, compute population averages, or atlas-based segmentation. Recently we have introduced the Adaptive Bases registration algorithm as a general method for performing nonrigid registration of medical images and we have shown it to be faster and more accurate than existing algorithms of the same class [1-3]. The overall properties of the Adaptive Bases algorithm are reviewed here and the method is validated on applications that include the computation of average images, atlas based segmentation, and motion correction of video images. Results show the Adaptive Bases algorithm to be capable of producing high quality nonrigid matches for the applications above mentioned.

Keywords: Adaptive Bases, nonrigid registration, mutual information, atlas-based segmentation, motion correction.

1. INTRODUCTION

The goal in digital image registration is to generate a mapping f relating any point in the domain of a source image $B(\mathbf{x})$ to a point in the domain of a target image $A(\mathbf{x})$ such that a cost function $C(A(\mathbf{x}), B(f(\mathbf{x})), f)$ is optimized. The cost function C contains terms that measure how well images A and B are aligned and may also have additional terms that impose restrictions on f. In nonrigid registration, the mapping f is usually interpreted as the

$$f(\mathbf{x}) = \mathbf{x} + \mathbf{v}(\mathbf{x}), \tag{1}$$

where $\mathbf{v}(\mathbf{x})$ is known as the deformation field.

To this date, one of the most successful concepts in determining how well two images align has been to measure statistical dependence between the source and target images through the Mutual Information measure, a special case of the Kullback-Leibler measure [4,5]. Other measures of statistical dependence include the coefficient of linear correlation and the closely related L^2 norm. Such measures, however, assume that the relationship between the pixel intensities of the source and target images is constant or linear. This assumption cannot always be verified, especially in the case of multimodal image matching. The Mutual Information measure makes no such assumptions about the nature of the relationship between the pixel values of the images. It can be viewed as the evidence for discrimination in favor of the hypothesis that the intensity values in the images are statistically dependent against the hypothesis that they are independent [14]:

$$I(A,B) = H(A) + H(B) - H(A,B) = \sum_{a,b} p_{AB}(a,b) \log \frac{p_{AB}(a,b)}{p_A(a) p_B(b)} \tag{2}$$

where A and B are again the target and source images with marginal probability distributions $p_A(a)$, $p_B(b)$, and joint distribution $p_{AB}(a,b)$. The difficulty in using (2), and other closely related measures [6], is that its estimation can be computationally expensive. Moreover, no analytic maximizer of f for (2) exists. Therefore, when performing nonrigid registration, many researchers have opted to model f using a linear combination of B-splines placed on a regular grid over the domain of the images, tranforming the solution of (1) into an iterative maximization process [7-13]. Such methods are known to be computationally demanding. For example, solving for f using a grid of about 3mm spacing between control points (64 x 64 x 32 points in 3D space for typical MR volumes) generates a 393,216 dimensional parameter search space. Such large optimization problems are not only computationally expensive but are prone to converging to local optima. Recently, we have introduced the Adaptive Bases registration algorithm as a general method for performing nonrigid registration of medical images. We have shown the Adaptive Bases method to be faster and more accurate than existing algorithms of the same class [1-3]. The remaining of this paper presents a brief overview of the Adaptive Bases method and demonstrates it's use in computing average images, atlas based segmentation, as well as motion correction of epicardial fluorescence videos.

2. THE ADAPTIVE BASES IMAGE REGISTRATION ALGORITHM

2.1 Introduction

The major drawback in most B-spline based image registration algorithms [7-13] is that much computation time is wasted in regions where image mismatch may not be present. The approach we have developed addresses this problem by first identifying regions over which the images are not registered correctly. When these regions have been identified the deformation field is adapted locally. This is done by placing basis functions over misregistered regions only and optimizing their coefficients to improve local registration. Because we place our basis functions irregularly over the image we do not use B-splines which are sub-optimal for this purpose but rather compactly supported radial functions. A method for identifying which regions are miss-registered at a particular scale, independently of the cost function being used, is also derived. Finally, a computationally efficient and exact scheme for maintaining the topological consistency of the image being deformed is derived.

2.2 Local Deformation Field Models and Radial Basis Functions

As previously stated, rather than modeling the deformation field with a linear combination of cubic B-splines placed on a regular grid as is usually done [7 -13] we build our deformation field incrementally, region by region, focusing on regions that are misregistered. The method by which we identify the relevant regions is detailed below but the total deformation field $\mathbf{v}(\mathbf{x})$ is modeled as a linear combination of a set of basis functions irregularly spaced over the image domain, i.e.,

$$\mathbf{v}(\mathbf{x}) = \sum_{i=1}^{N} \mathbf{c}_i \Phi(\mathbf{x} - \mathbf{x}_i), \qquad (3)$$

with coefficients $\mathbf{c}_1,...,\mathbf{c}_N \in \Re^d$, where d is the dimensionality of the images, and a function $\Phi: \Re^d \to \Re$ that is *positive definite* on $\Re^d$ in the following sense: for all sets $X = \{\mathbf{x}_1,...,\mathbf{x}_N\}$ of finitely many distinct points $\mathbf{x}_1,...,\mathbf{x}_N$ in $\Re^d$, the matrix $M = \left(\Phi(\mathbf{x}_k - \mathbf{x}_j)\right)_{1 \le j,k \le N}$ is *positive definite* which guarantees the solvability of the system

$$\mathbf{y}_k = \sum_{i=1}^{N} \mathbf{c}_i \Phi(\mathbf{x}_k - \mathbf{x}_i), \quad 1 \le k \le N. \quad (4)$$

This property is important for registration problems for it guarantees that the model allows for the construction of any given deformation field solution prescribed by $\mathbf{y}_k$ at arbitrary locations $\mathbf{x}_k$. For a detailed discussion of radial basis functions and their applications consult Shaback [10].

Since B-splines basis functions do not guarantee the solvability of (4), we cannot use them in an Adaptive Bases algorithm. Thus, in our implementation we have chosen to use one of Wu's compactly supported positive definite radial basis functions:

$$\Phi(\mathbf{x}) = \phi\left(\frac{\|\mathbf{x}\|_2}{s}\right), \quad \mathbf{x} \in \Re^d \quad (5)$$

$$\phi(r) = (1-r)_+^4 (3r^3 + 12r^2 + 16r + 4) \text{ for } r \ge 0, \quad (6)$$

where $(1-r)_+ = \max(1-r, 0)$, s is a predetermined scale for the basis function, and $\|\|_2$ is the usual Euclidean norm on $\Re^d$.

There are several advantages in using a compactly supported basis function such as (6) in registration problems. First, compact support means that for each value of $\mathbf{x}$, the sum in (3) can be reduced to relatively few terms. This also means that under many circumstances optimization can be confined to a finite part of the domain D, improving the computational efficiency of the overall method. Moreover, (6) and therefore (5) have been shown to possess C^2 continuity. Smoothness properties are important in registration problems since the first and second derivatives of the deformation field are often used for the computation of the gradient, and sometimes Hessian, of the cost function with respect to the optimization parameters. These quantities are used in several optimization algorithms applicable to this type of registration problem, e.g., conjugate gradient descent, or Newton methods.

2.3 Multiscale and Multiresolution Approach

The Adaptive Bases method approaches the final deformation field iteratively across scales and resolutions. Here resolution means the spatial resolution of the image while the scale is related to the transformation itself. A standard image pyramid is created to apply the algorithm at different resolutions. At each resolution, the scale of the transformation is adapted by modifying the region of support and the number of basis functions. The scale of the transformation is proportional to the bases' region of support (i.e., a large region of support leads to a transformation at a large scale). Typically the algorithm is initialized on a low-resolution image with few basis functions having large support. As the algorithm progresses to finer resolutions and smaller scales, the region of support of the basis functions is reduced. Following this approach, the final deformation field is computed as

$$\mathbf{v}(\mathbf{x}) = \mathbf{v}_1(\mathbf{x}) + \dots + \mathbf{v}_M(\mathbf{x}). \quad (7)$$

with M the total number of levels (in the remainder of this paper, a level refers to a particular combination of scale and resolution).

2.4 Regions of Miss-registration Identification

One of the key features of the Adaptive Bases algorithm is that it adjusts the transformation only where it needs to be adjusted. This requires identifying regions where the two images are not well registered at the current level and adjusting the deformation field over these regions. To achieve this, the Adaptive Bases algorithm uses a local measure of miss-registration that can be used in conjunction with any measure of similarity. The basic idea is as follows. At each level m a regular grid of basis functions is placed over the domain of the images. The gradient $\mathbf{G}$ of the cost function with respect to the coefficient of the basis function on this grid is evaluated. The value of $\mathbf{G}$ is then used to determine which regions in the images are most likely to be miss-registered at the current level. The idea behind using $\mathbf{G}$ to decide on regions of mismatch is as follows: if the magnitude of the gradient of the cost function with respect to the coefficient c_i is large, then the cost function is not at a minimum with respect to c_i. If the cost function is not at a minimum at the location corresponding to c_i then it is likely that the region where the corresponding basis function is located is miss-registered. Therefore registration in this particular area could be improved at the current level. If, on the other hand, the magnitude of the gradient with respect to coefficient c_j is small, two situations are possible. Either the images are reasonably well registered over that region at the current level or the images could be significantly misregistered at that location but the cost function is at a local extremum. In either case, further gradient-based optimization in this region is unfruitful and should therefore be neglected.

Note that this algorithm is independent of the cost function and therefore represents a general approach for region of mismatch identification. Furthermore, since evaluating **G** is a required part of the gradient ascent optimization method, we can use **G** not only to identify regions of mismatch but also to correct for image mismatch at a global level at little additional cost.

2.5 Local Optimization

Once regions of interest have been identified, the local deformation fields need to be computed. Given a location representing the center of a region of interest $\mathbf{x}^j$ and the current resolution and scale s, the Adaptive Bases approach chooses eight locations $\mathbf{x}^j_{[1,...,8]}$ arranged in the form of a cube around $\mathbf{x}^j$ as centers for the basis functions that will be used for computing the deformation field associated with a particular region of the image. For two-dimensional registrations a square around the center location $\mathbf{x}^j$ is used, in 3D we use a cube. This gives us the ability to build local deformations with 8 degrees of freedom in 2D and 24 degrees of freedom in 3D around location $\mathbf{x}^j$. The support of the basis functions placed around location $\mathbf{x}^j$ is also s. Note that the value for s is obtained from the support of the basis functions used in the automatic region of interest identification algorithm presented earlier. The local deformation field is thus adjusted at the current scale and resolution. A steepest gradient descent algorithm combined with the quadratic interpolation four-point bracketing update method of line minimization is then applied to the coefficients of the cube of basis functions to optimize the cost function chosen.

2.6 Optimization Constraint Scheme

In image registration problems, particularly nonrigid ones, it is often necessary to prevent the optimization from producing deformations that violate the topology constraint of the source image. Previous attempts at constraining spline based deformation field models to produce consistent topological deformations can be found in Rueckert *et. al.* [5] or Studholme *et al.* [3] where the basic idea is to optimize the similarity measure while regularizing the deformation field by minimizing its second derivative. While this technique can reduce folding artifacts, it does not guarantee the positive definiteness of the Jacobian of the transformation. The Adaptive Bases algorithm introduces a novel scheme that explicitly enforces the topological constraint in a computationally efficient manner. The novel approach not only makes explicit the relationship between a smoothness constraint and the Jacobian of the deformation field, but derives precise bounds for the basis functions coefficients c_i in equation (3) that guarantee this positiveness. With knowledge of such precise bounds such constraint scheme can be efficiently implemented by keeping track of only the coefficients being optimized. Consider the following deformation field:

$$T(\mathbf{x}) = \mathbf{x} + \mathbf{v}_1(\mathbf{x}) + \mathbf{v}_2(\mathbf{x}) + ... + \mathbf{v}_N(\mathbf{x}), \qquad (8)$$

from $\Re^3 \to \Re^3$, where N is the number of levels utilized during registration. Let $J(T) = \mathbf{I} + \alpha_1(\mathbf{x}) + \alpha_2(\mathbf{x}) + ... + \alpha_N(\mathbf{x})$ be the Jacobian matrix of the transformation $T(\mathbf{x})$, where $\mathbf{I}$ is the identity matrix and $\alpha_i(\mathbf{x})$ is the Jacobian matrix of the displacement field $\mathbf{v}_i(\mathbf{x})$. In [1, 2] we prove that if the constraint

$$\left\| \alpha_{n+1} \right\|_\infty < \frac{1}{3}\left(1 - 3\left\| \sum_{i=1}^n \alpha_i \right\|_\infty \right) \qquad (9)$$

is satisfied, then the Jacobian matrix remains positive definite. In other words, for any given deformation field (8), a displacement field $\mathbf{v}_{N+1}(\mathbf{x})$ can be added without violating the topology constraint as long as relationship (9) is satisfied for n=1, ..., N. Relationship (9) can be used to design a number of possible constraint schemes for registration procedures that use splines, radial basis functions, or other types of bases. One possible scheme is to compute $\left\| \sum_{i=1}^n \alpha_i \right\|_\infty$ after each level. Then (9) can be used to compute bounds on the basis function coefficients c_i composing the $(n+1)^{th}$ displacement field. This, however, would be computationally expensive since in our registration algorithm the evaluation of $\left\|\sum_{i=1}^{n}\alpha_i(\mathbf{x})\right\|_\infty$ for all coordinates $\mathbf{x}$ would have to be done explicitly through finite differences. Another possible constraint scheme is to use (9) to compute bounds for the basis function coefficients by assuming worst-case estimates for $\left\|\sum_{i=1}^{n}\alpha_i(\mathbf{x})\right\|_\infty$. For example, if the number N of levels is fixed a priori, then (9) will be satisfied if $1-3\left\|\sum_{i=1}^{n}\alpha_i\right\|_\infty$ is positive for any value of n=1, …,N. Using the triangle inequality $\left\|\sum_{i=1}^{n}\alpha_i\right\|_\infty \leq \sum_{i=1}^{n}\|\alpha_i\|_\infty$, we derive the bound

$$\max_{i=1,…,N}\|\alpha_i\|_\infty \leq \lambda < \frac{1}{3N} \qquad (10)$$

In practice, we use (10) to obtain the bounds for the basis function's coefficients at each level of the algorithm. Such bounds are derived in such a way as to guarantee that the Jacobian matrix of the deformation field remains positive definite at all points $\mathbf{x}$, guaranteeing thus that no folding artifacts will be produced throughout the domain of the images. Please refer to [1] for more information about the constraint scheme used in the Adaptive Bases approach.

2.7 Summary of the Adaptive Bases method

Figure 1 summarizes the Adaptive Bases algorithm presented here. At first, input images A($\mathbf{x}$) and B($\mathbf{x}$) are downsampled to the lowest user-specified resolution and a bounding box is computed from the union of the foreground of both images. Initially, $\mathbf{v}$ is set to zero. The parameters needed by the algorithm are the number of resolutions and the scales at which the transformation needs to be computed at each resolution (the scales are specified by the number of basis functions to be used when creating the regular grid Θ; the lower the number of basis functions, the larger the scale). At each resolution and scale, the region of support for the basis functions is calculated as a constant times the distance between two adjacent grid points in Θ (in practice the constant is between 1.5 and 2).

Initialize $A(\mathbf{x})$, $B(f(\mathbf{x}))$, $f(\mathbf{x})$, and Θ at the lowest resolution and scale
For I=1… Number of resolutions
    For J=1…. Number of scales at current resolution
        Create regular grid Θ at current resolution and scale and compute
            Region of support for basis functions
        Identify regions of misregistration
        Optimize each region independently from one another
    End for
    Upsample $A(\mathbf{x})$, $B(f(\mathbf{x}))$, $f(\mathbf{x})$,
End for
Ouput $B(f(\mathbf{x}))$, $f(\mathbf{x})$.

Figure 1: The Adaptive Bases Registration Algorithm

3. APPLICATIONS

Here the Adaptive Bases registration method is validated on three separate applications: creation of average images, atlas based segmentation, and motion correction of epicardial fluorescence video recordings. For all the applications mentioned, rigid body or affine registration is performed prior to nonrigid registration. Mutual Information based cost functions are also used for rigid and affine registration. It has been determined in practice that this pre-processing step approach speeds up convergence of most nonrigid registration algorithms, as well as improving the quality of the results [1,2].

3.1 Creation of image averages

The MR images used here were obtained with high-resolution 3D SPGR pulse sequences (FOV 24 x 24 cm, 256 x 256, 1.3 mm thickness, 0 mm gap, TE = 1.9 ms, flip angle = 20 deg, TI = 450 ms, TR = 11.9 ms, 124 slices). Each contained a 3D image of the head. We have used the Adaptive Bases algorithm to align a set of 10 MR images to a single reference one as accurately as possible. The MRI scans were then averaged onto this common reference system so as to provide insight on the quality of the registrations.

Seven levels were used in the nonrigid registration step, starting from a 2X2X2 set of basis functions, optimized at one fourth of the original resolution, to a 60X60X44 grid of basis functions optimized at full image resolution. The cost function used here was the Normalized Mutual Information described in [9]. 24 bins were used in estimating the joint histograms of the images. During optimization of any particular set of basis functions, an optimum was declared when two successive iterations failed to produce an improvement greater than 0.0005 in the cost function value. The registration of a single volume to the reference image lasted between 6 and 7 hours on a Sun Ultra 10 workstation. Figure 2 shows an example registration obtained with the Adaptive Bases method.

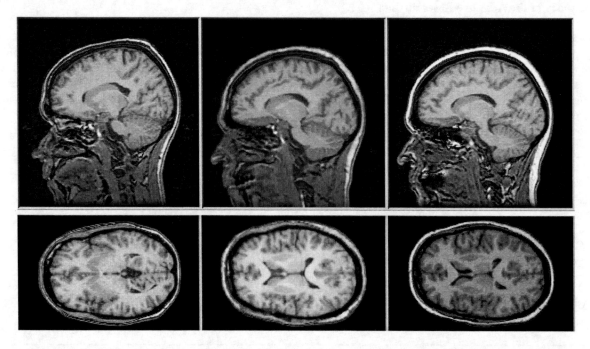

Figure 2: Each row from left to right, the source image, the resulting nonrigid registration between the source and target images, the target image.

It was noticed that two out of the ten registrations attempted failed. Convergence to local minima led the algorithm to produce incorrect transformations around the cerebellum area in these two images. This may have been due to the fact that the 9-degree of freedom registration step did not align the images well enough, or the images were significantly different to begin with. They were therefore excluded from the computation of the average volume. The average volume computed from the eight remaining images is shown in figure 3. For comparison purposes, figure 3 also shows the averages computed from the original images prior to registration, the average computed after the 9-degree of freedom registration, the average computed after nonrigid registration with grids going up to 32X32X28 basis functions, the average computed after nonrigid registration with basis function grids of up to 60X60X44. As can be seen from this figure, the sharpness of the average image increases as the compliance of the transformation used increases. A sharp average volume suggests good quality in all of the registrations.

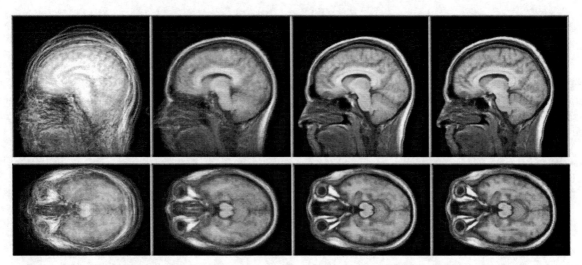

Figure 3: Each row from left to right: average prior to registration, average after affine registration, average after nonrigid registration with 32X32X28 basis function compliance, average after nonrigid registration with 60X60X44 compliance.

3.2 Atlas based segmentation

In this section we evaluate the ability of the Adaptive Bases algorithm to perform automatic atlas based segmentation. The idea in atlas based segmentation is to use the nonrigid registration procedure to obtain an accurate mapping between the coordinate space of the atlas, here defined as a chosen reference image, and an image of a particular subject. Once this transformation is known, any structure that has already been segmented in the atlas can be directly transformed so as to match the same structure in the subject. Segmentation can then be performed by assigning the value of zero to all pixels in the subject image that do not fall within the spatial coordinates of the deformed structure. We tested the ability of our algorithm to perform automatic segmentation of the brain, spine, and eyes on ten test images. Visual results showing the quality of the registration based segmentation procedure are presented. To better assess the error in the segmentation procedure we also computed a similarity index between results obtained through the automatic segmentation procedure and results obtained through manual segmentation.

The images used in the following experiments are the same as the ones used the previous section. Before nonrigid registration was applied all ten images were registered to the chosen reference volume through a Mutual Information based 9-degree of freedom registration. Because we are concerned mainly with assessing the ability of the newly proposed nonrigid registration algorithm to perform atlas based segmentation, the evaluation of the segmentation results was performed on the ten images after 9 degree of freedom registration. From here on we refer to the subject images as being those that were registered to the reference volume through 9 degree of freedom transformations. The nonrigid registration relating all points in the domain of the atlas image to all points in the domain of each subject image was computed using the Adaptive Bases registration algorithm presented earlier. The algorithm settings were the same as those mentioned above.

Figure 4 shows representative segmentations of each organ mentioned. Note that instead of showing only the segmented brain, spine or eyes, figure 4 shows the contour of the organ derived by deforming the manually segmented atlas so as to match each of the 10 subjects. Shown this way, segmentation errors can be identified more clearly.

Further analysis of the segmentation results shown in figure 4 was performed by comparing them to results obtained through manual segmentation. The brain, spine or optic fiber of each patient was manually segmented in four transverse slices chosen at random. Thus four binary 2D images of each organ were obtained for each patient. These were compared with the corresponding binary images generated by warping the atlas brain onto the same patient. The comparison was done by examining the amount of overlap in the two binary images through a similarity index. For two binary images Q and W the similarity index is given by:

$$S(Q,W) = 2\frac{\int_\Omega (Q \cap W)}{\int_\Omega Q + \int_\Omega W} \tag{11}$$

Here Ω refers to domain of the images. Note that the similarity index s falls in the interval [0,1]. It is zero when the intersection of binary images Q and W is zero. It is one when the images are identical. Tables 1-3 give the similarity index statistics computed from four random slices across all ten patients. Table 1 gives the average, minimum and maximum similarity indexes for the four slices, chosen at random, computed in each subject. Tables 2 and 3 report the similarity index for the randomly chosen slice of each subject. The average S computed for each patient shows very good correspondence between the automatically segmented images and the manually segmented ones. This indicates that the automatic segmentation procedure presented here is approximately equivalent to manual segmentation.

Table 1: Average, minimum, and maximum similarity index of the brain computed for the four slices chosen in each subject.

Patient	1	2	3	4	5	6	7	8	9	10
Average S	0.967	0.962	0.960	0.962	0.970	0.970	0.965	0.973	0.962	0.963
Maximum	0.977	0.975	0.967	0.970	0.974	0.974	0.977	0.981	0.978	0.969
Minimum	0.944	0.939	0.942	0.956	0.959	0.965	0.936	0.955	0.952	0.956

Table 2: Similarity index of the spine for each of the 10 subjects.

Patient	1	2	3	4	5	6	7	8	9	10
S	0.931	0.924	0.934	0.915	0.928	0.920	0.912	0.946	0.922	0.923

Table 3: Similarity index for each eye in each subject

Patient	1	2	3	4	5	6	7	8	9	10
Left eye	0.907	0.900	0.900	0.876	0.900	0.860	0.856	0.915	0.912	0.823
Right eye	0.888	0.863	0.805	0.877	0.898	0.823	0.864	0.892	0.918	0.816

3.3 Motion correction in epicardial fluorescence video recordings

Optical recording techniques have been widely applied in cardiac electrophysiology for studies of electrodynamics. By staining the tissue with vital dyes and recording the induced fluorescence from the tissue, it is possible to record with high spatial resolution electrical propagation from a large area on the tissue. The non-invasive, non-contact nature of the optical approach provides many advantages over the traditional recording method using electrodes. On the other hand, the optical method also has limitations. The most significant constraint of using optical recording in cardiac tissue is muscle contraction, which deforms the shape of the recorded signal.

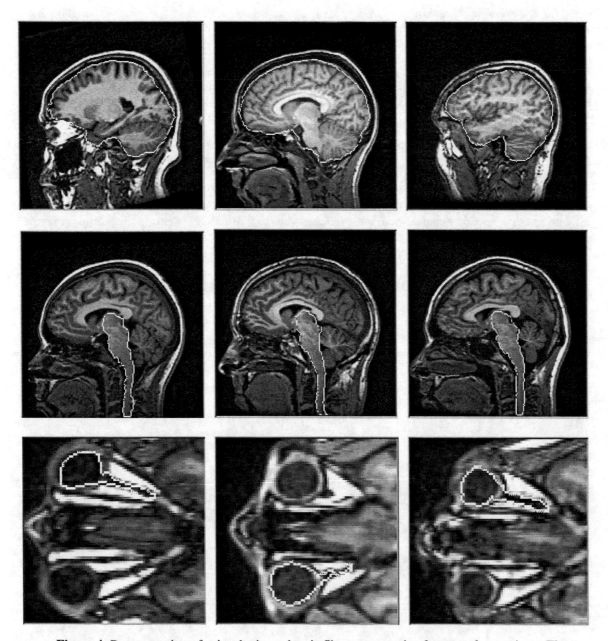

Figure 4: Demonstration of spine, brain, and optic fiber segmentation for a set of ten patients. The contours drawn here were obtained by deforming the atlas mask to each subject.

The basic principle of optical mapping is based on the proportional change of fluorescence intensity resulting from the change in the underlying phenomena, such as transmembrane potential or calcium ion concentration. Ideally, in order to perform such a comparison of fluorescence intensity, each sensing element should record from the same location on the tissue over the entire recording episode. In addition, because the induced fluorescence is roughly proportional to the intensity of the induction light, tissue illumination condition should also remain stable during data acquisition. When the tissue moves during the recording, its relative position with respect to the sensor and the light source changes, resulting in an artificial variation of fluorescence intensity intermingled with the desired signal. Furthermore, quantification of intensity variation is not meaningful if the fluorescence comes from different locations on the tissue.

The data used for this experiment was collected in the following manner. New Zealand white rabbits weighing 4.4-5.5 kg were injected with 1000 units of heparin and 70 mg/kg sodium pentobarbital to induce deep general anesthesia. The heart was excised and the ascending aorta cannulated and secured for retrograde perfusion of the coronaries with a modified HEPES perfusate (108 mM NaCl, 5 mM KCl, 5 mM HEPES, 10 mM glucose, 20 mM NaC2H3O2, 1 mM MgCl2, 2.5 mM CaCl2). The perfusate was filtered through a micropore filter, adjusted to pH 7.35-7.45 with 1 N NaOH, oxygenated with 100% O2, and warmed to 37± 0.5 °C. Coronary perfusion pressure was regulated to 80-95 mmHg. During the experiment, the hearts were exposed to the air. The potential-sensitive dye di-4-ANEPPS (Molecular Probes, OR) at a concentration of 0.5 mM was added to the perfusate for approximately 15 minutes to stain the heart.

Fluorescence from the heart surface was elicited by a solid-state, frequency-doubled laser (Verdi V5, Coherent, Santa Clara, CA) at a wavelength of 532 nm. Laser light was delivered to the heart using multiple 1-mm optical fibers (SP-SF-960, FIS Inc., Oriskany, NY). The root-mean-square variation of laser intensity was 0.02%. The emitting fluorescence was imaged with a high-speed CCD camera (Model CA-D1-0128T, Dalsa Inc., Waterloo, ON, Canada) through a color glass filter with a cut-off wavelength of 590 nm (Schott Glass Technologies, Duryea, PA). The faceplate of the camera was cooled with an ethylene-glycol coolant from a refrigerated waterbath to 15°C. Digitized images from the camera was transferred to a PCI bus-master frame grabber board (IC-PCI, Imaging Technology Inc., Bedford, MA) that was mounted in an IBM-compatible personal computer.

Because of the relative motion between the beating heart and the stationary camera, the movies collected from this setup can contain a significant amount of heart motion artifact. We have used Mutual Information based registration techniques to correct for heart motion in such movie data. For each movie a frame that did not show activation potential was chosen as the reference frame. Prior to registration, the data of each movie was first resampled to one byte intensity resolution. The spatial resolution of each frame was 128X128 pixels and each movie contained 500 frames. Full affine registration (12 degrees of freedom) was computed between each frame and the reference frame using Powel's direction set method. The results obtained from the affine registration step were then used to initialize the nonrigid registration step. The cost function used was the negative of the Mutual Information. Joint histograms with 64X64 bin resolution were used in the computation of the cost function.

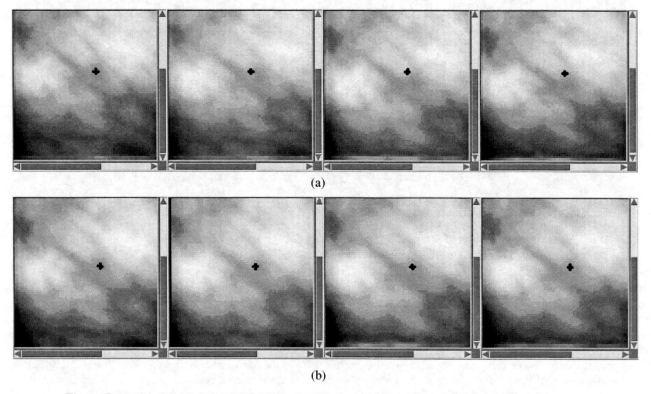

(a)

(b)

Figure 5: (a-top): frames from raw data movie. (b-bottom): frames from movie after nonrigid correction.

Figure 5 (a) shows a sequence of frames from a raw data movie. A dot was drawn above a salient anatomical feature on the tissue of the heart on the first image (top left corner). The dot was copied onto the same image coordinates for each of the three other frames shown in figure 5 (a). Figure 5 (b) displays the corresponding frames of the movie corrected for heart motion through Mutual Information based nonrigid registration. As the images clearly show, the relative motion between the dot and the heart is significantly diminished.

Further analysis of the cardiac data was conducted by plotting the L^2-error between each frame of the movie and the chosen reference frame for that particular movie. These are shown in figure 6. Because the movies contain activation potential information, image noise, and motion artifact, the L^2-error plot should measure biological signal, noise due to nonuniform illumination, as well as motion. Therefore, it is unreasonable to expect that the error between each movie frame and the reference frame will be even close to zero after heart motion correction. If the error due to heart motion is eliminated, however, one would expect the L^2-norm between each frame and the reference frame to decrease. As seen from figure 6, the L^2-error between each frame and the chosen reference frame is significantly decreased after nonrigid registration.

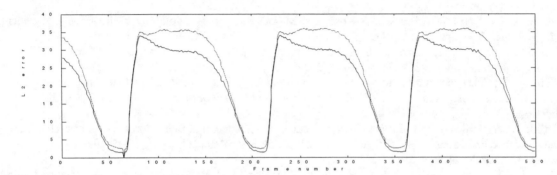

Figure 6: Plot of L^2-error between each frame and the chosen reference frame. The upper curve corresponds to the error present in the uncorrected data, while the lower represents the error of the movie after nonrigid motion correction.

4. DISCUSSION

Previously [1,2], we have shown the Adaptive Bases method to outperform traditional spatially invariant approaches for optimizing a deformation field. Here we have shown that the Adaptive Bases method coupled with an information theoretic similarity measure is a powerful approach applicable to a variety of spatial normalization problems. It should also be noted that since we have introduced the idea of local adaptation of the transformation's compliance, others have proposed techniques by which regular grid B-splines approach can be sped up [15,16]. The approach these authors use is to fix the coefficients of the B-splines whose region of support have been labeled as passive. Criteria used to identify passive regions include local statistical measures such as the joint entropy or the gradient measure we introduced in [2]. Comparative evaluations of this method with ours remains to be done.

5. ACKNOWLEDGMENT

Research of the second author was supported in part by NSF grant DMS-0103104.

6. REFERENCES

1. G. K. Rohde, "The Adaptive Grid Registration Algorithm: A New Spline Modeling Approach for Automatic Intensity Based Nonrigid Registration." Masters Thesis. Vanderbilt University, August 2001.
2. Rohde G. K., Aldroubi A. and Dawant B.M. "Adaptive free-form deformation for inter-patient medical image registration", Proc. SPIE Vol. 4322, p. 1578-1587, Medical Imaging 2001: Image Processing, Milan Sonka; Kenneth M. Hanson; Eds.
3. T. Disenbacher, G. Rohde, D. Harding, A. Aldroubi, and B. Dawant, "Multiscale Nonrigid Data Registration Using Adaptive Basis Functions." SPIE-Wavelet Applications In Signal and Image Processing VIII, A. Aldroubi, A. F. Laine, and M. A. Unser (Eds.), Vol. 4119, pp. 1076-1083, SPIE Press, Bellingham WA, 2000.
4. Maes F., Collignon A., Vanderneulen D., Marchal G., Suetens P. "Multimodality image registration by maximization of mutual information", IEEE Transactions on Medical Imaging, 16(2), pp. 187-198, 1997.
5. Viola, P., W. M., Wells III, "Multi-modal volume registration by maximization of mutual information," Medical Image Analysis, 1(1), pp 35-51, 1996.
6. C. Studholme, D. L. G. Hill, D. J. Hawkes, "An overlap invariant entropy measure of 3D medical image alignment," Pattern Recognition, 32(1), pp. 71-86, 1999.
7. J. Kybic, P. Thévenaz, A. Nirkko, and M. Unser, "Unwarping of Unidirectionally Distorted EPI Images." IEEE Transactions on Medical Imaging, 19 (2), pp 80-93, 2000.
8. C. Studholme, R.T. Constable, and J. Duncan. "Accurate Alignment of Functional EPI Data to Anatomical MRI Using a Physics-Based Distortion Model." IEEE Transactions on Medical Imaging, 19 (11), pp. 1115-1127, November 2000.
9. C. Studholme, V. A. Cardenas, and M. W. Weiner, "Multiscale image and multiscale deformation of brain anatomy for building average brain atlases," Proc. SPIE Vol. 4322, p. 557-568, Medical Imaging 2001: Image Processing, Milan Sonka; Kenneth M. Hanson; Eds.
10. D. Rueckert, L. I. Sonoda, C. Hayes, D. L. G. Hill, M. O. Leach, and D. J. Hawkes, "Nonrigid Registration Using Free-Form Deformations: Application to Breast MR Images." IEEE Transactions on Medical Imaging, 18(8), pp 712-721, 1999.
11. D. Mattes, D. R. Haynor, H. Vesselle, T. K. Lewellen, and W. Eubank, "Nonrigid mutlimodality image registration," Proc. SPIE Vol. 4322, p. 1609-1620, Medical Imaging 2001: Image Processing, Milan Sonka; Kenneth M. Hanson; Eds.
12. T. Rohlfing, C. R. Maurer, Jr., W. G. O'Dell, M. C. Schell, and J. Zhong, "Modeling liver motion and deformation during the respiratory cycle using intensity-based free-form registration of gated MR images," Proc. SPIE Vol. 4319, p. 337-348, Medical Imaging 2001: Visualization, Display, and Image-Guided Procedures, Seong K. Mun; Ed.
13. O. Musse, F. Heitz, J-P. Armspach, "3D deformable image matching: a hierarchical approach over nested subspaces," Proc. SPIE Vol. 3979, p. 458-469, Medical Imaging 2000: Image Processing, Kenneth M. Hanson; Ed.
14. Solomon Kullback, Information Theory and Statistics, Dover Publications, Inc., New York, 1968.
15. T. Rohfing, C.R. Maurer, "Intensity-Based Non-rigid Registration Using Adaptive Multilevel Free-Form Deformation with an Incompressibility Constraint," MICCAI'2001 proceedings, pp 111-119, 2001.
16. J. A. Shnabel, D. Rueckert, M. Quist, J. M. Blackall, A. D. Castellano-Smith, T. Harkens, G. P. Penney, W. A. Hall, H. Liu, C. L. Truwit, F. A. Gerristen, D. L. Hill, D. J. Hawkes, "A Generic Framework for Non-rigid Registration Based on Non-uniform Multi-level Free-Form Deformations," MICCAI'2001, pp.573-581, 2001.

Analysis of a New Method for Consistent Large-Deformation Elastic Image Registration

Jianchun He, Gary E. Christensen, Jay T. Rubinstein and Ge Wang

University of Iowa, Iowa City, IA 52242

ABSTRACT

This paper provides initial analysis of a new consistent, large-deformation elastic image registration (CLEIR) algorithm that jointly estimates a consistent set of forward and reverse transformations between two images. The estimated transformations are able to accommodate large deformations while constraining the forward and reverse transformations to be inverses of one another. The algorithm assumes that the two N-dimensional images to be registered contain topologically similar objects and were collected using the same imaging modality. The image registration problem is formulated in a (N+1)-dimensional space where the additional dimension is referred to as the temporal or time dimension. A periodic-in-time, nonlinear, (N+1)-dimensional transformation is estimated that deforms one image into the shape of the other and back again. Large deformations from one image to the other are accommodated by concatenating the small-deformation incremental transformations from one time instant to the next. An inverse consistency constraint is placed on the incremental transformations to enforce within a specified tolerance that the forward and reverse transformations between the two images are inverses of each other. The feasibility of the algorithm for accommodating nonlinear deformations was demonstrated using 2D synthesized phantom images and CT inner ear images. The effect of varying the number of intermediate templates was studied for these data sets.

Keywords: Elastic image registration, inverse consistency, nonlinear, large deformation

1. INTRODUCTION

This paper presents a preliminary analysis of a new consistent large-deformation elastic image registration (CLEIR) algorithm that was first described in.[1] The CLEIR algorithm registers two images by deforming each image into the shape of the other using a fixed number of incremental small-deformation transformations. The composition of the small deformation incremental transformations produces a large deformation transformation from one image to the other.

An example of a pair of images that require a large-deformation, nonlinear transformation model to be registered is shown in Figure 1. In this case, the "patch" and "C" images can not be registered using a small deformation model since a small deformation model is unable to curve the patch into the shape of the "C" and vice versa. However, it is possible to deform the patch part of the way into the shape of the "C" using a small deformation model. This new shape can then be deformed further into the shape of the "C" using another small deformation model. Continuing this process will finally result in a deformation of the patch into the "C". Likewise, the "C" can incrementally be transformed into the shape of the patch.

The number of incremental transformations used to deform the original images into the shape of each other is referred to as the temporal sampling number. The optimal temporal sampling number required to match two images is a function of the shape differences between the objects contained in the images. As a rule of thumb, the larger the shape differences between the objects, the more incremental transformations that are required to give a good registration. On the other hand, minimizing the temporal sampling number has the advantage of reducing computer computation and storage requirements. This paper investigates the effect of varying the number of incremental transformations that are required to transform one image into the shape of the other.

Send correspondence to Gary E. Christensen

Gary E. Christensen: E-mail: gary-christensen@uiowa.edu, Telephone: (319)-335-6055, Fax: (319)-335-6028

Medical Imaging 2002: Image Processing, Milan Sonka, J. Michael Fitzpatrick, Editors, Proceedings of SPIE Vol. 4684 (2002) © 2002 SPIE · 1605-7422/02/$15.00

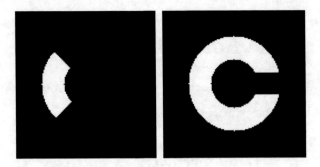

Figure 1: Simple objects used to test the image registration algorithm.

This paper is organized as follows. Section 2 summarizes the CLEIR algorithm that was originally presented in.[1] Mathematical details are presented that describe how two images are registered using the incremental transformations, how the transformations are composed together to create a large deformation transformation, and how the inverse consistency error between the forward and reverse transformations is minimized. Section 3 describes the performance of the CLEIR algorithm for the "patch" to "C" images and for CT images of the inner ear.

2. CONSISTENT LARGE-DEFORMATION ELASTIC IMAGE REGISTRATION (CLEIR) ALGORITHM

Figure 2 illustrates how two images $I_0(x)$ and $I_1(x)$ are registered using the CLEIR algorithm. The two N-dimensional images I_0 and I_1 are registered by constructing a N+1-dimensional image T that is periodic in both the spatial and temporal dimensions. The image T is defined as a sequence of N-dimensional images indexed by time i that smoothly changes shape from image I_0 at time $i = 0$ to the image I_1 at time $i = 4$ and back again at time $i = 8$. Each N-dimensional image T is assumed to be periodic in space to accommodate the Fourier series parameterization of the transformations (see below).

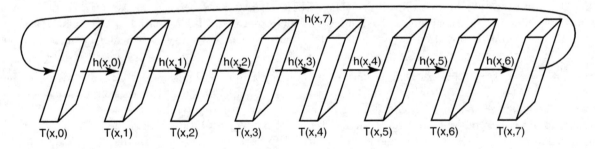

Figure 2: (N+1)D image and associated incremental transformations.

The transformation $h(x, i)$ defines the mapping from incremental image i to image $(i + 1)$, that is, $h(x, i)$ defines the correspondence between the coordinate system of image i and that of image $(i + 1)$. Let $u(x, i) = h(x, i) - x$ denote the displacement field associated with the forward transformation h and let $\tilde{u}(x, i) = h^{-1}(x, i) - x$ denote the displacement field associated with the inverse transformation h^{-1}.

Mathematically, T and h denote the periodic extension of images $I_0(x)$ and $I_1(x)$ such that

$$T(x,0) = I_0(x), \quad T(x,1) = T(h(x,0),0), \quad T(x,2) = T(h(x,1),1), \quad T(x,3) = T(h(x,2),2),$$
$$T(x,4) = I_1(x), \quad T(x,5) = I_1(h(x,4)), \quad T(x,6) = T(h(x,5),5), \quad T(x,7) = T(h(x,6),6)$$

for the case $i = 8$. The spatial transformations $h(x, \cdot)$ can be composed together to produce the intermediate time samples of T from the original images, i.e.,

$$T(h(x,3),3) = I_0(h(h(h(h(x,3),2),1),0)) \quad \text{and} \quad T(h(x,7),7) = I_1(h(h(h(h(x,7),6),5),4)). \tag{1}$$

2.1. Inverse Consistency Constraint

A necessary condition to insure a biologically realistic transformation* between two images is that the forward and reverse transformations are inverses of one another. This is accomplished by placing an inverse-consistency constraint[2] on the transformation h that defines the correspondence between the temporal subimages of T. Eq. 1 implies that the forward and reverse transformations that map I_0 to I_1 and back are given by

$$h_{\text{for}}(x) = h(h(h(h(x,3),2),1),0) \quad \text{and} \quad h_{\text{rev}}(x) = h(h(h(h(x,7),6),5),4), \tag{2}$$

respectively. The inverse-consistency constraint implies that the composition of the forward and reverse transformations produce the identity mapping, i.e., $h_{\text{for}}(h_{\text{rev}}(x)) = h_{\text{rev}}(h_{\text{for}}(x)) = x$.

The inverse consistency constraint for the N+1-dimensional transformation is imposed by enforcing the constraints

$$h(x,i) = h^{-1}(x, N_t - 1 - i) \tag{3}$$

for $0 \leq i < N_t$. These constraints imply that each intermediate image $T(x,i)$ has the approximate appearance of the image $T(x, N_t - i)$ for $0 \leq i < N_t$, i.e., $T(x,i) \sim T(x, N_t - i)$ for $x \in \Omega_x$.

2.2. Parameter Estimation

The N+1 dimensional image registration problem is formulated as the minimization with respect to h of the cost function

$$C(h) = \sigma_e \sum_{i=0}^{N_t-1} \int_{\Omega_x} (T(h(x,i),i) - S(x,i))^2 dx + \sigma_s \sum_{i=0}^{N_t-1} \int_{\Omega_x} (T(h(x,i),i) - T(x, N_t - 1 - i))^2 dx$$

$$+ \sigma_i \sum_{i=0}^{N_t-1} \int_{\Omega_x} ||h(x,i) - h^{-1}(x, N_t - 1 - i)||^2 dx + \sigma_r \sum_{i=0}^{N_t-1} \int_{\Omega_x} ||Lu(x,i)||^2 dx \tag{4}$$

where L can be any symmetric differential operator and is used to help smooth and prevent folding of the transformation. Image S is defined as $S(x,i) = T(x,i+1)$, $0 \leq i < N_t$ and is assumed to be constant during each iteration of the transformation parameter estimation and is updated after each estimation iteration. In this paper, the Laplacian operator was used for regularization and is given by $Lu(x,t) = \alpha_1 \frac{\partial^2 u}{\partial x_1^2} + \alpha_2 \frac{\partial^2 u}{\partial x_2^2} + \alpha_3 \frac{\partial^2 u}{\partial x_3^2} + \alpha_4 \frac{\partial^2 u}{\partial t^2}$.

The displacement field at each temporal sample i is parameterized in terms of a N-dimensional Fourier series. The Fourier series coefficients are estimated that minimize the cost function in Eq. 4. The discrete-time Fourier series representation of the displacement field is given by $u(x,i) = \sum_k \mu_{i,k} e^{j<x,\omega_k>}$ where the coefficients $\mu_{i,k}$ are (3×1), complex-valued vectors with complex conjugate symmetry for a fixed i and $\omega_k = \left[\frac{2\pi k_1}{N_1}, \frac{2\pi k_2}{N_2}, \frac{2\pi k_3}{N_3}, \frac{2\pi k_4}{N_t}\right]$.

3. RESULTS

The proposed algorithm was tested on the synthetic 2D images shown in Fig. 1 and the CT inner ear images shown in Fig. 3. To study the impact of N_t on the registration effect, the time axis of the images was discretized into 2, 4, 8, and 16 equally spaced samples, and the same parameters were applied to experiments with different N_t.

---

*True biological correspondence only makes sense when comparing images from the same individual. A biologically realistic correspondence is a biologically meaningful pointwise correspondence between images of different people and is task dependent.

Inner ear 1(L) Inner ear 1(R) Inner ear 2(L) Inner ear 2(R) Inner ear 3(L) Inner ear 3(R)

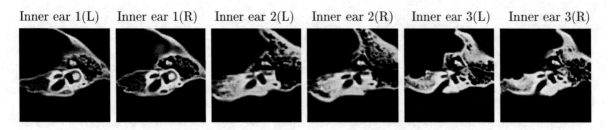

Figure 3: CT slices from left and right ears used for registration.

In the first experiment, the image containing a patch shown in Fig. 1 was deformed into the shape of the "C" and vice versa. The transformation of the patch to the "C" requires a large-deformation, nonlinear transformation. The dimensions of the images were 128×128 pixels. The radii of the outer and inner contour of the "C" object were 41 and 21 pixels, respectively. The two ends of the "C" were separated by 19 background pixels. The patch was a portion of the "C", starting at 135° and ending at 225°. The algorithm was tested for $N_t = 2$, 4, 8 and 16 with the maximum number of iterations set to 8000. But in cases $N_t = 2$ and 4, the minimum Jacobian of the transformation became negative and the program exited before the maximum number of iterations was reached. The results $N_t = 2$, 4, and 8 are shown in Figure 4. Each row of Figure 4 corresponds to a time index starting at time $t = 0$ for the top row and progressing to time $t = N_t - 1$ for the bottom row. The first column shows how the template image T was initialized for the gradient descent procedure; the first half samples $T(x, 0) - T(x, N_t/2 - 1)$ were set equal to image I_0 and the second half samples $T(x, N_t/2) - T(x, N_t - 1)$ were set equal to image I_1. The second column shows the intermediate deformed images $T(h(x, 0), 0)$ to $T(h(x, N_t - 1), N_t - 1)$ (from top to bottom) after the program stopped. The top half of the images in the third column show the absolute difference between the images $T(h(x, 0), 0)$ through $T(h(x, N_t/2 - 1), N_t/2 - 1)$ and the target image I_1. The bottom half images show the absolute difference between the images $T(h(x, N_t/2), N_t/2)$ through $T(h(x, N_t - 1), N_t - 1)$ and the target image I_0. The images of the fourth and fifth columns show the accumulated displacement fields in the x and y dimensions, respectively, where black denotes a negative displacement and white denotes a positive displacement. Columns six and seven show the Jacobian of the accumulated transformations and the result of applying the accumulated transformations to a rectangular grid. See Appendix for details of how the accumulated transformation function and its Jacobian are calculated.

For case $N_t = 2$, which is equivalent to consistent linear elastic registration,[2, 3] we see that the patch was not fully deformed into the shape of the "C" and the "C" was not fully deformed into the shape of the patch. The deformation went a little further for case $N_t = 4$ where one intermediate image for each direction was inserted into the temporal axis. For case $N_t = 8$, the nearly black difference image in the fourth and eighth images of column three show that the patch was transformed into the shape of the "C" and the "C" was transformed into the shape of the patch, respectively. The images in columns 2 demonstrate the periodic nature of the template T in time and show that the shape of the intermediate images are equally spaced in time. The images in columns 3 to 7 also demonstrate that the total deformation was equally distributed in time.

The parameter sets used for this experiment and the other experiments described below are shown in Table 1, where Δt was the gradient descent step size. The parameter sets for each experiment were chosen by experimentation.

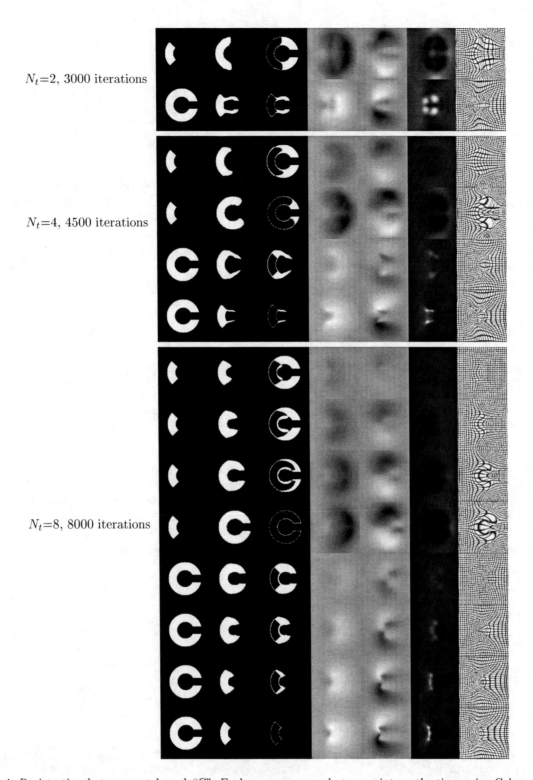

Figure 4. Registration between patch and "C". Each row corresponds to a point on the time axis. Column 1 shows the initialization of the template before gradient descent. Column 2 shows the incrementally deformed template images after registration. Column 3 shows absolute difference images between the incrementally deformed template images and their corresponding target images. Column 4 and 5 shows the accumulated x- and y-displacement fields, respectively. Column 6 shows the accumulated Jacobian images. Column 7 shows the accumulated deformed grid image.

Table 1. Parameter set for experiments. The inner ear 1, 2, and 3 experiments register a patient's left inner ear image with the same patient's right inner ear image.

Experiment	Δt	α_{1-3}	α_4	σ_e	σ_s	σ_i	σ_r
patch to C	0.00002	1.0	1.0	1.0	1.0	1000.0	0.0001
Inner ear 1	0.00005	1.0	5.0	1.0	1.0	1000.0	0.00001
Inner ear 2	0.00001	1.0	1.0	1.0	1.0	1000.0	0.00001
Inner ear 3	0.00001	1.0	1.0	1.0	1.0	1000.0	0.00002

The average value of the absolute intensity difference between the deformed template and target images are given in the first row of table 2, where forward means matching patch to "C" and backward means matching "C" to the patch. A significant decrease in the average value of the absolute difference is observed when N_t was changed from 2 to 4 and from 4 to 8. This is consistent with Figure 4. But the change in difference is not significant when N_t was changed from 8 to 16. This is because $N_t = 8$ is enough to deform the templates to targets and there was little room left for improvement.

Table 2. Average absolute intensity difference between the deformed image and the target image (intensity scale 0 – 100)

Experiment	$ave(|I_0(h_{forward}(x)) - I_1(x)|)$				$ave(|I_1(h_{reverse}(x)) - I_0(x)|)$			
	$N_t=2$	$N_t=4$	$N_t=8$	$N_t=16$	$N_t=2$	$N_t=4$	$N_t=8$	$N_t=16$
patch and C	10.4	4.29	0.900	0.862	3.21	0.846	0.269	0.270
Inner ear 1	2.21	2.16	2.10	2.04	2.07	2.02	1.97	1.91
Inner ear 2	3.20	2.97	2.72	2.48	3.15	2.91	2.63	2.47
Inner ear 3	3.20	2.98	2.81	2.67	3.50	3.25	3.06	2.88

The maximum and average inverse consistency error is reported in the first row of table 3. See appendix for details of how they were calculated. A pattern does not show up in table 3, possibly because the inverse consistency cost is not a dominating factor in the objective function. When inverse consistency contradicts with the interest of the intensity difference, the gradient descent favors reducing the image difference rather than getting the inverse consistency. Another possible reason is that when the transformation function is approximated by only a few number of Fourier coefficients, it might be impossible to drive the transformation functions to a position that minimize the inverse consistency.

Table 3: Comparison of maximum and average inverse consistency error (ICE).

Experiment	Maximum ICE				Average ICE			
	$N_t=2$	$N_t=4$	$N_t=8$	$N_t=16$	$N_t=2$	$N_t=4$	$N_t=8$	$N_t=16$
patch to c	4.13	8.08	3.50	2.71	0.380	0.307	0.196	0.266
Inner ear 1	1.54	1.23	1.40	1.76	0.080	0.068	0.061	0.073
Inner ear 2	2.78	2.19	1.87	3.04	0.197	0.167	0.149	0.154
Inner ear 3	3.09	2.54	5.22	4.96	0.199	0.170	0.163	0.149

The minimum and reciprocal of maximum values of the Jacobian[†] of all intermediate transformation are given in the first row of table 4, and the Jacobians of final accumulated transformations are given in the fifth row of table 4. The entries correspond to patch to "C" experiment with $N_t = 2$ or 4 were the result before the minimum Jacobian went negative. They do not mean much to us because the registration did not converge yet.

[†]The Jacobian values were calculated with respect to a Eulerian coordinate system. In a Eulerian coordinate system, an expansion corresponds to a Jacobian value less than 1 and a shrinking corresponds to a Jacobian value greater than 1.

Table 4: Minimum and reciprocal of the maximum Jacobian of the intermediate and accumulated transformations

Experiment	Minimum Jacobian				1/Maximum Jacobian			
	$N_t=2$	$N_t=4$	$N_t=8$	$N_t=16$	$N_t=2$	$N_t=4$	$N_t=8$	$N_t=16$
Intermediate Transformations								
patch to c	0.067	0.021	0.393	0.506	0.172	0.199	0.415	0.514
Inner ear 1	0.309	0.449	0.561	0.683	0.466	0.577	0.660	0.725
Inner ear 2	0.198	0.333	0.411	0.428	0.365	0.482	0.512	0.549
Inner ear 3	0.219	0.330	0.289	0.494	0.317	0.451	0.453	0.595
Accumulated Transformations								
patch to c	0.067	0.003	0.028	0.030	0.172	0.056	0.043	0.036
Inner ear 1	0.309	0.289	0.236	0.173	0.466	0.384	0.297	0.201
Inner ear 2	0.198	0.167	0.149	0.106	0.365	0.276	0.188	0.136
Inner ear 3	0.219	0.154	0.051	0.045	0.317	0.229	0.105	0.074

In each of the CT image experiment, a slice of a patient's left inner ear CT image was registered with a corresponding slice from the same patient's right inner ear. These experiments are motivated by a potential clinical application in the diagnosis of inner ear disorders due to the fact that many anatomic defects are unilateral and current diagnosis is somewhat subjective. Quantitative measurements provided by the transformation might be used in the future to answer whether the left and right inner ear structures are differ and how they are different.

The dimensions of the CT inner ear images were 256×256 pixels. The slices are selected to cut through ossicles. The intensity windowing for the slices were from 100 to 2200 and the resulting intensity was converted to 256 gray scales. The result of running the algorithm on data of patient 3 for 5000 iterations of gradient descent with $N_t = 4$ is shown in Figure 5. The descriptions of the panels in this figure are similar to those in Figure 4, only without the displacement field columns. The average value of absolute difference image, the inverse consistency errors, and the Jacobians are also given in Tables 2 through 4. Table 4 shows that with more intermediate images, the minimum Jacobians of the intermediate transformations increases, which means each individual image was deformed less in order to register the left and right ear images. Theoretically, if the accumulated transformation matches the images exactly, the minimum of accumulated Jacobian would not change when more intermediate images are used. This is not the case in Table 4, where the minimum of accumulated Jacobian actually decrease when more intermediate images were used. The reason for the minimum accumulated Jacobian to decrease is that with more intermediate images, the algorithm was able to deform each image more to its corresponding image. This is also consistent with the decreasing intensity difference shown in Table 2.

4. SUMMARY

This paper showed that it was possible to use the CLEIR algorithm to accommodate large deformation shape differences between the patch and the "C" images. The patch to "C" experiment clearly showed that a minimum number of intermediate transformations were required for successful mapping. The registration of the left and right inner ear images only required a small deformation for registration. In this case, there were no experimental results that clearly shows that adding any incremental transformations improved the registration.

APPENDIX A. ACCUMULATED TRANSFORMATIONS, DISPLACEMENT FIELDS, AND JACOBIANS

Columns 2, 4, 5, 6 and 7 in Figs. 4 and 5 are related to the accumulated transformations of the final registration. Let $h_a(x, i)$ denote the accumulated transformation of time point i, and $J_a(x, i)$ the Jacobian of $h_a(x, i)$. Let $u_a(x, i) = h_a(x, i) - x$ be the accumulated displacement field.

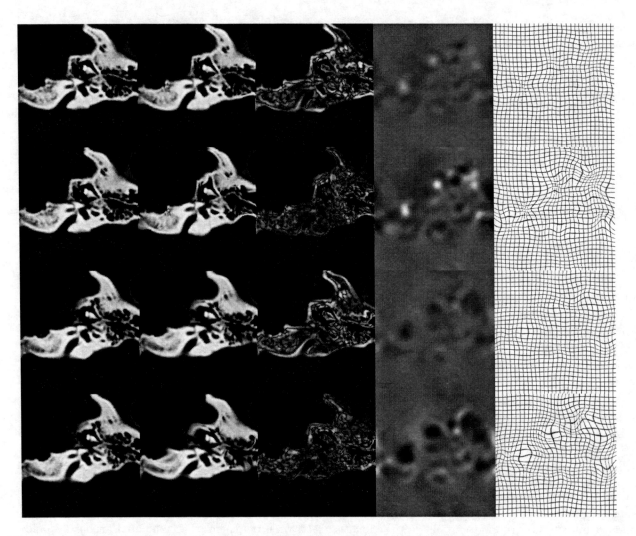

Figure 5. Registration between left and right inner ear CT image of patient 2 with N_t=4. Each row corresponds to a point on the time axis. Column 1 shows the initialization of the template before gradient descent. Column 2 shows the incrementally deformed template images after gradient descent. Column 3 shows absolute difference images between the incrementally deformed template images and their corresponding target images. Column 4 shows the accumulated Jacobian images. Column 5 shows the accumulated deformed grid image.

A.1. Accumulated Transformation

The accumulated transformation of time point i is defined as:

$$h_a(x,i) = \begin{cases} h(...(h(h(x,i),i-1),...),0), & \text{for } 0 \le i < N_t/2 \\ h(...(h(h(x,i),i-1),...),N_t/2), & \text{for } N_t/2 \le i < N_t \end{cases}. \tag{5}$$

In Figs. 4 and 5, the ith row of column 2 corresponds to $T(h_a(x,i),i)$; the ith row of column 3 corresponds to $|I_1(x) - T(h_a(x,i),i)|$ for $0 \le i < N_t/2$ and $|I_0(x) - T(h_a(x,i),i)|$ for $N_t/2 \le i < N_t$; and the ith row of the last column corresponds to a rectangular grid deformed by $h_a(x,i)$.

A.2. Accumulated Displacement Field and Inverse Consistency

Since our parameterization is applied to the displacement field instead of the transformation function itself, all of the calculations are performed on the displacement field. To explain how two displacement fields are concatenated, let $u_{AB}(x)$, $u_{BC}(x)$, and $u_{AC}(x)$ denote the displacement fields that deform image A to B, B to C, and A to C, respectively. Then

$$
\begin{aligned}
u_{AC}(x) &= h_{AC}(x) - x \\
&= h_{AB}(h_{BC}(x)) - x \\
&= u_{AB}(h_{BC}(x)) + h_{BC}(x) - x \\
&= u_{AB}(h_{BC}(x)) + u_{BC}(x)
\end{aligned}
\tag{6}
$$

i.e. the composition of two consecutive displacement fields equals the first displacement field deformed by the second plus the second displacement field. The ith accumulated displacement field is calculated by composing the displacement fields one bye one from $t = 0$ to $t = i$ for $0 \leq i < N_t/2$, or by composing one by one from $t = N_t/2$ to $t = i$ for $N_t/2 \leq i < N_t$.

The inverse consistency error is computed using all the incremental transformations (see table 3). The inverse consistency error starting and ending at time $t = 0$ is computed by concatenating all the incremental displacement fields one-by-one starting from $t = 0$ and ending at $t = N_t - 1$. The inverse consistency error starting and ending at time $t = N_t/2$ is computed by concatenating all the incremental displacement fields one-by-one starting from $t = N_t/2$, wrapping around at $t = N_t - 1$, and ending at $t = N_t/2 - 1$. The Euclidean distance of the resulting displacement fields are calculated and their maximum and mean values are recorded in Table 3.

A.3. Accumulated Jacobian

The Jacobian of the accumulated transformation $h_a(x, i)$ can not be calculated directly from $h_a(x, i)$ for large deformations since it is computed on a discrete lattice. This is because $h_a(x, i)$ is a sampling of an implied continuous large-deformation transformation and the values of the transformation between the samples cannot be recovered from the samples. The loss of information due to sampling causes the Jacobian of $h_a(x, i)$ to be negative in areas of large deformations when computed on a finite grid. This problem is avoided by computing the Jacobian of each incremental transformation and using the result of Theorem A.1 to compute the accumulated Jacobian.

The Jacobian of the accumulated transformation $h_a(x, i)$ as shown in column 6 of Figure 4 and column 4 of Figure 5 are calculated from the Jacobians of the incremental transformations by concatenating them one-by-one.

The following theorem states that when we compose two transformations $g(y)$ and $h(z)$ for $g : R^N \to R^N$ and $h : R^N \to R^N$, the Jacobian of the composite transformation $g(h(z))$ is the multiplication of the Jacobian of the first transformation deformed by the second transformation $J_g(h(z))$ with the Jacobian of the second transformation $J_h(z)$.

THEOREM A.1. *For $g : R^N \to R^N$ and $h : R^N \to R^N$, the Jacobian of $f(z)$, which is the composition of transformations $g(y)$ and $h(z)$ given by $f(z) = g(h(z))$, is equal to*

$$
J_f(z) = J_g(h(z)) \times J_h(z), \qquad \text{For all } z.
\tag{7}
$$

Proof:

Without loss of generality, assume that the images are two dimensional. By definition of the Jacobian,

$$
J_g(y) = \begin{vmatrix} \frac{\partial g_1(y_1, y_2)}{\partial y_1} & \frac{\partial g_1(y_1, y_2)}{\partial y_2} \\ \frac{\partial g_2(y_1, y_2)}{\partial y_1} & \frac{\partial g_2(y_1, y_2)}{\partial y_2} \end{vmatrix} \qquad J_h(z) = \begin{vmatrix} \frac{\partial h_1(z_1, z_2)}{\partial z_1} & \frac{\partial h_1(z_1, z_2)}{\partial z_2} \\ \frac{\partial h_2(z_1, z_2)}{\partial z_1} & \frac{\partial h_2(z_1, z_2)}{\partial z_2} \end{vmatrix}
$$

where $g(y) = \begin{bmatrix} g_1(y_1, y_2) \\ g_2(y_1, y_2) \end{bmatrix}$ and $h(z) = \begin{bmatrix} h_1(z_1, z_2) \\ h_2(z_1, z_2) \end{bmatrix}$.

The Jacobian of $f(z)$ is computed using the chain rule for differentiation as

$$
\begin{aligned}
J_f(z) &= \left| \begin{array}{cc} \frac{\partial f_1(z_1,z_2)}{\partial z_1} & \frac{\partial f_1(z_1,z_2)}{\partial z_2} \\ \frac{\partial f_2(z_1,z_2)}{\partial z_1} & \frac{\partial f_2(z_1,z_2)}{\partial z_2} \end{array} \right| \\
&= \left| \begin{array}{cc} \frac{\partial g_1(y)}{\partial y_1}\big|_{h(z)} \frac{\partial h_1(z)}{\partial z_1} + \frac{\partial g_1(y)}{\partial y_2}\big|_{h(z)} \frac{\partial h_2(z)}{\partial z_1} & \frac{\partial g_1(y)}{\partial y_1}\big|_{h(z)} \frac{\partial h_1(z)}{\partial z_2} + \frac{\partial g_1(y)}{\partial y_2}\big|_{h(z)} \frac{\partial h_2(z)}{\partial z_2} \\ \frac{\partial g_2(y)}{\partial y_1}\big|_{h(z)} \frac{\partial h_1(z)}{\partial z_1} + \frac{\partial g_2(y)}{\partial y_2}\big|_{h(z)} \frac{\partial h_2(z)}{\partial z_1} & \frac{\partial g_2(y)}{\partial y_1}\big|_{h(z)} \frac{\partial h_1(z)}{\partial z_2} + \frac{\partial g_2(y)}{\partial y_2}\big|_{h(z)} \frac{\partial h_2(z)}{\partial z_2} \end{array} \right| \\
&= \left| \begin{array}{cc} \frac{\partial g_1(y_1,y_2)}{\partial y_1} & \frac{\partial g_1(y_1,y_2)}{\partial y_2} \\ \frac{\partial g_2(y_1,y_2)}{\partial y_1} & \frac{\partial g_2(y_1,y_2)}{\partial y_2} \end{array} \right|_{h(z)} \times \left| \begin{array}{cc} \frac{\partial h_1(z_1,z_2)}{\partial z_1} & \frac{\partial h_1(z_1,z_2)}{\partial z_2} \\ \frac{\partial h_2(z_1,z_2)}{\partial z_1} & \frac{\partial h_2(z_1,z_2)}{\partial z_2} \end{array} \right| \\
&= J_g(h(z)) \times J_h(z). \qquad\qquad \text{Q.E.D.}
\end{aligned}
$$

ACKNOWLEDGMENTS

This work was supported in part by the NIH under grants NS35368, CA75371, and DC03590, and a grant from the Whitaker Foundation.

REFERENCES

1. G. Christensen and J. He, "Consistent nonolinear elastic image registration," *IEEE Proceedings of Mathematical Methods in Biomedical Image Analysis* , Dec. 2001.

2. G. Christensen and H. Johnson, "Consistent image registration," *IEEE Transactions on Medical Imaging* **20**, pp. 568–582, July 2001.

3. G. Christensen, "Consistent linear-elastic transformations for image matching," in *Information Processing in Medical Imaging*, A. Kuba and M. Samal, eds., *LCNS 1613*, pp. 224–237, Springer-Verlag, June 1999.

Pose estimation of teeth through crown-shape matching

Vevin W.Y. Mok[†], S.H. Ong[†], Kelvin W.C. Foong[‡], Toshiaki Kondo[†]
[†]Department of Electrical and Computer Engineering, National University of Singapore
[‡]Department of Preventive Dentistry, National University of Singapore

ABSTRACT

This paper presents a technique for determining a tooth's pose given a dental plaster cast and a set of generic tooth models. The ultimate goal of pose estimation is to obtain information about the sizes and positions of the roots, which lie hidden within the gums, without the use of X-rays, CT or MRI. In our approach, the tooth of interest is first extracted from the 3D dental cast image through segmentation. 2D views are then generated from the extracted tooth and are matched against a target view generated from the generic model with known pose. Additional views are generated in the vicinity of the best view and the entire process is repeated until convergence. Upon convergence, the generic tooth is superimposed onto the dental cast to show the position of the root. The results of applying the technique to canines demonstrate the excellent potential of the algorithm for generic tooth fitting.

Keywords: Tooth matching, shape matching, Fourier descriptors, pose estimation

1. INTRODUCTION

Dental casts are often used by orthodontists for clinical analysis during the course of treatment. However, these casts (Figure 1) provide only information about the crowns of the teeth. Information about the positions and sizes of the roots, which lie hidden within the gums, can only be obtained through conventional methods such as X-rays, CT or MRI. X-rays are cheap but they provide only 2D data. While CT and MRI are able to provide 3D volumetric data, both are expensive and CT imaging is radiologically invasive. We thus set out to develop a system that allows orthodontists to visualize the position of a tooth's root without the use of X-rays, CT or MRI. To achieve this goal, we attempted fitting generic tooth models onto real-life dental cast models. We performed shape matching on the crown of a tooth in order to estimate the pose of the tooth and thereby find the position of its root. Although shape matching has been widely researched, its application to tooth matching is relatively new.

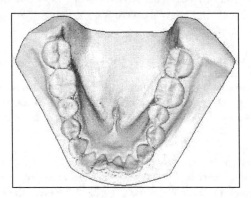

Figure 1: Dental cast model.

The registration of 3D surfaces has been extensively researched in machine vision and its applications range from constructing terrain maps[1] and maps of the sea floor[2] to recognizing objects in a CAD database[3]. Surface registration has also been applied in the medical field[4] to reconcile useful anatomical information in the form of collected surface points, which originate from various complementary biomedical imaging modalities.

Audette et al.[4] classified surface registration techniques into 4 main classes.

(1) Feature-based methods, e.g. Besl and Jain[5], which attempt to represent a surface shape using a compact set of features.

(2) Point-based methods that make use all the surface points in the data set. An example is Besl and Mc Kay's iterative closest point[6] (ICP) method, where two surfaces assumed to be in close proximity to full alignment are registered by iteratively minimizing the sum of squared distances between mutually closest points on both surfaces.

(3) Model-based methods, e.g. Kimmel et al.[7], which model the surface based on its likely shape and dynamic behaviour.

(4) Global shape techniques that register surfaces based on global surface geometry. For example, Johnson and Herbert[8] proposed using spin images to represent the local and some global object information at all vertex points. Point matches are found from highly correlated spin images of model and scene. The best model-scene surface match is then computed using a set of point matches.

Although the above mentioned 3D surface registration techniques have shown excellent results, they are not suitable in our application for the following reasons.

(1) Most surface registration techniques are used to reconcile surface information of the same object acquired by different imaging modalities. However, in our application we are trying to fit a generic tooth model onto real-life samples, i.e. model fitting.

(2) Although each tooth type has a generic shape and size, each tooth has variances in its shape and size that can drastically affect the performance of surface registration.

(3) The ICP method requires users to provide good initial estimates.

(4) Some surface registration techniques require large training data sets, which is difficult to obtain.

A technique that is able to match using the generic shape of each tooth type with less reliance on user input is required. In our approach, we avoided the inconsistencies of 3D tooth shape by attempting to match the 2D crown shape. The 3D space is hierarchically searched for possible poses that will generate 2D crown shapes similar to the target crown shape. Based on the estimated pose, the generic tooth model is scaled and aligned followed by superimposing it onto the dental cast model to show the position of the root. We also envisage the use of a tooth fitting system in the following clinical applications.

(1) Identification of tooth root positioning for orthognathic surgery simulation.

(2) Prediction of tooth shape and size for (a) forensic reconstruction of a missing tooth given the same tooth type or construction of a virtual tooth given a tooth from a different but sequential series, and (b) building up a tooth that is badly broken down or missing using the opposite tooth or a tooth from a different but sequential series as a cross reference.

The following sections are organized as follows. Section 2 describes the method used to perform generic tooth fitting. Section 2.1 presents the iterative process of generating 2D views to converge to an estimated pose. Section 2.2 describes the shape representation and the similarity measure used to select the best matching views. Section 2.2 also details the calculation of rotation, scaling and translation factors for transformation computation in order to perform model fitting. Section 3 shows the results when the technique is applied to canines. The paper is concluded in Section 4.

2. METHODOLOGY

Michel et al.[9] proposed a technique to align projective 2D images, such as X-rays, to 3D volumetric data, such as CT or MRI, by hierarchically searching the 3D space for possible poses based on the notion of shape similarity between the projected 2D view and the target view. The 3D object is placed within a viewing sphere where sample 2D views are obtained and matched against the given 2D image. Shape similarity is measured using the shock graph strategy known as the "graduated assignment algorithm"[10], which represents the shape by its medial axis with associated velocities. One of the limitations of this algorithm is the dependence on the accuracy of the shape matching process. Since the matching scheme relies on the object's topological structure about the medial axis, the algorithm is able to correlate weakly similar shapes but is unable to discern small differences in highly similar shapes.

We propose an extension of the above technique to fit a generic tooth model onto real-life dental cast models. The tooth of interest is extracted from the 3D dental model image through segmentation and is placed at the centre of a viewing sphere, as shown in Figure 2. The viewing sphere is initially coarsely sampled and projected views produced at each of the sample points are matched against the target view. The target view is obtained by projecting the generic tooth with known pose onto a target plane. More projected views are obtained in the vicinity of the best view and the procedure is repeated till convergence to an estimated pose. Matching is based on the similarity between the projected crown shapes and the targeted crown shape. In our approach, we represented the crown shapes using Fourier descriptors as the crown shapes are simple and lack prominent features. Unlike the "graduated assignment algorithm", Fourier descriptors eliminate the needs for users to label feature points and are able to discern small differences in highly similar shapes. Rotation, scaling and translation parameters required in order to align the projected view with the target view can also be found directly from the descriptors.

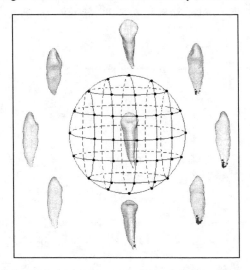

Figure 2: Viewing sphere and different views obtained when a canine is placed at its centre.

2.1 Generation of 2D views

The method proposed here determines a tooth's pose using a dental plaster cast and a set of generic tooth samples. The tooth samples are selected because they are representative of the average shape and size of each tooth type. The dental plaster cast and tooth samples are first scanned using a laser scanner to produce three-dimensional high-resolution images. The tooth of interest is next extracted from the 3D dental cast image through segmentation and is placed at the centre of a viewing sphere. This viewing sphere is centered at the origin of the coordinate system (Figure 3).

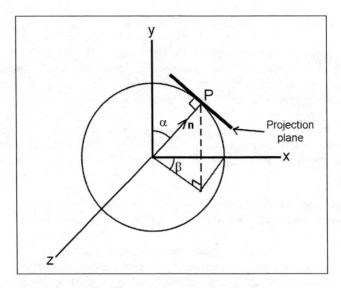

Figure 3: 3D object coordinate system.

At the initialization stage, the sphere is coarsely and uniformly sampled at N points. Each of these N points on the sphere is specified by two angles α and β. As shown in Figure 3, $\tilde{n}$ is the vector joining the sampling point P on the sphere to the origin, α is the angle between the vector $\tilde{n}$ and the y-axis, while β is the angle between the projection of $\tilde{n}$ on the x-z plane and the x-axis. $\tilde{n}$ is also the normal to the projection plane at point P with a 2D image coordinate system (Figure 4).

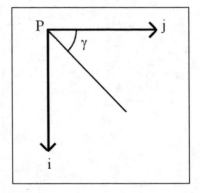

Figure 4: 2D image coordinates of the projection plane at P.

In order to relate the projection plane to the 3D object coordinate system, a third parameter, γ, has to be specified. γ is the rotation of the projection plane about the vector $\tilde{n}$. Therefore, each 2D view that is obtained by projecting the 3D tooth onto the tangential plane at each of the N sample points is described by a set of unique pose parameters (α, β, γ). These pose parameters relate the 3D tooth's pose and the estimated pose that gives the best matching view and will be used for transformation computation when superimposing the generic tooth model on the dental cast. In this technique, we determine α and β through the iterative process of sampling and shape matching, while γ is determined from the angle that brings the most similar projected shape into the best alignment with the target shape.

The projected 2D views are matched against a target view and are ranked according to their extent of crown shape similarity. The target view is obtained by projecting the generic tooth model onto a target plane with known pose parameters. In our application, we assume that the chosen target shape can only be generated with one unique set of pose parameters. As such, only views whose pose parameters are closer to the true pose will generate more similar views.

Next, we chose the grid square whose four corner points generated the best matching 2D views. This square is sub-divided equally and new points are chosen where new 2D views are generated for matching. Figure 5 illustrates the iterative process of sampling and selection. This procedure is repeated until convergence to an estimated pose of desired accuracy.

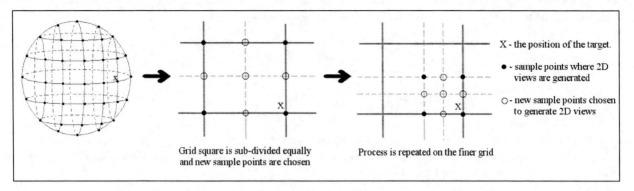

Figure 5: Process of iterative sampling and selection.

2.2 Crown shape matching

Matching is based on the similarity between the projected crown shapes and the targeted crown shape. In our approach we represent the crown shapes using Fourier descriptors. The boundary of the crown is first extracted from each 2D view (Figure 6). In order to form a complete boundary so as to compact the shape information into the lower frequency components of the Fourier descriptors, the incomplete boundary is reflected to form a complete boundary.

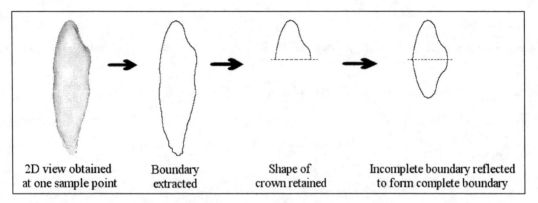

Figure 6: Figure showing the generation of complete boundary.

Each crown shape has an N-point complete boundary in the 2D image plane (Figure 4) and can be written as

$$s(k) = a(k) + jb(k) , \qquad (1)$$

for $k = 0, 1, 2, \ldots\ldots, N - 1$. The discrete Fourier transform (DFT) of $s(k)$ is

$$F(u) = \frac{1}{N} \sum_{k=0}^{N-1} s(k) \exp[- j2\pi uk / N], \qquad (2)$$

for $u = 0, 1, 2,\ldots\ldots, N - 1$, where the complex coefficients $F(u)$ are the Fourier descriptors of the boundary. In our application, we kept N equal to an integer power of 2 and applied the Fast Fourier transform (FFT) on the complete boundary to obtain the shape descriptors.

Shape similarity is then measured using the correlation between the Fourier descriptors of each of the projected crown shapes and the target shape. This is calculated based on the function

$$\zeta = \frac{\sum_u \left[F_{proj}(u) - \overline{F}_{proj}\right]\left[F_{tgt}(u) - \overline{F}_{tgt}\right]}{\left\{\sum_u \left[F_{proj}(u) - \overline{F}_{proj}\right]^2 \sum_u \left[F_{tgt}(u) - \overline{F}_{tgt}\right]^2\right\}^{1/2}}, \tag{3}$$

for $u = 0, 1, 2,\ldots\ldots, N - 1$, where $F_{proj}(u)$ and $F_{tgt}(u)$ are the Fourier descriptors of the projected crown shape and the target crown shape, respectively. Additional views are generated in the vicinity of the view with the highest correlation and the process is repeated until convergence.

Our objective is to fit a generic tooth model onto real-life dental cast models. Rotation, scaling and translation parameters are required in order to align the projected view with the target view. We state below the effects of rotation, scaling and translation on Fourier descriptors.

A boundary that has been rotated by an angle of γ about point P in (Figure 4) is represented by

$$s_r(k) = s(k)e^{j\gamma} \tag{4}$$

and its Fourier descriptors are

$$F_r(u) = F(u)e^{j\gamma}, \tag{5}$$

where γ is one of the pose parameters (α, β, γ) mentioned in Section 2.1 that relates the 2D image coordinates to the 3D object coordinates.

For a boundary that has been scaled such that the new boundary is represented by

$$s_s(k) = \sigma\, s(k), \tag{6}$$

its Fourier descriptors are given as

$$F_s(u) = \sigma\, F(u). \tag{7}$$

When a boundary has been translated such that the new boundary is represented by

$$s_t(k) = s(k) + \left(t_x + jt_y\right), \tag{8}$$

the Fourier descriptors of the new boundary are

$$F_t(u) = F(u) + \left(t_x + jt_y\right)\delta(u). \tag{9}$$

A boundary that has been rotated, scaled and translated will have its coordinates represented by

$$s_{rst}(k) = \sigma\, e^{j\theta}\left[s(k) + \left(t_x + jt_y\right)\right], \tag{10}$$

while its Fourier descriptors are

$$F_{rst}(u) = \sigma\, e^{j\theta} \left[F(u) + \left(t_x + j t_y \right) \delta(u) \right]. \tag{11}$$

Upon convergence of the selection strategy described in Section 2, the projected view can be brought into alignment with the target view by doing the following computations.

The scale of the projected view relative to the target view can be calculated as

$$\sigma = \left| \frac{F_{proj}(u)}{F_{tgt}(u)} \right|, \tag{12}$$

and the angle of rotation as

$$\gamma = \angle \left(\frac{F_{proj}(u)}{F_{tgt}(u)} \right), \tag{13}$$

where $u = 1, 2, \ldots, N-1$. The term $F(0)$ cannot be used for computing σ and γ as the phase and magnitude of $F(0)$ are affected by translation as shown in Equations 10 and 11. Translation of the projected view relative to the target view can be determined by

$$t_x = \mathrm{Re}\left[\frac{1}{\sigma} F_{proj}(0) e^{-j\gamma} - F_{tgt}(0) \right], \tag{14}$$

$$t_y = \mathrm{Im}\left[\frac{1}{\sigma} F_{proj}(0) e^{-j\gamma} - F_{tgt}(0) \right]. \tag{15}$$

Based on the pose parameters (α, β, γ), the scaling factor σ and the translation ($t_x + j t_y$), the generic tooth model is scaled and aligned to superimpose onto the dental cast model to show the position of the root.

3. RESULTS & DISCUSSION

We conducted preliminary tests on a pair of upper-right canines, with one canine serving as the generic tooth model and the other canine sample simulating a tooth extracted from a dental cast. As shown in Figure 7, the target view is first obtained from the generic tooth. 2D views were then generated from the other canine sample and matched against the target view. In the same figure, we show the four best matching 2D views that were selected in the first iteration of the selection process and the final best matching 2D view selected upon convergence of the selection. It can be observed that the best matching 2D view selected in the final iteration of the algorithm is highly similar to the target view. The rotation, scaling and translation parameters required to fit the generic tooth onto the canine sample are calculated and Figure 8 shows the result of superimposing the generic tooth onto the canine sample.

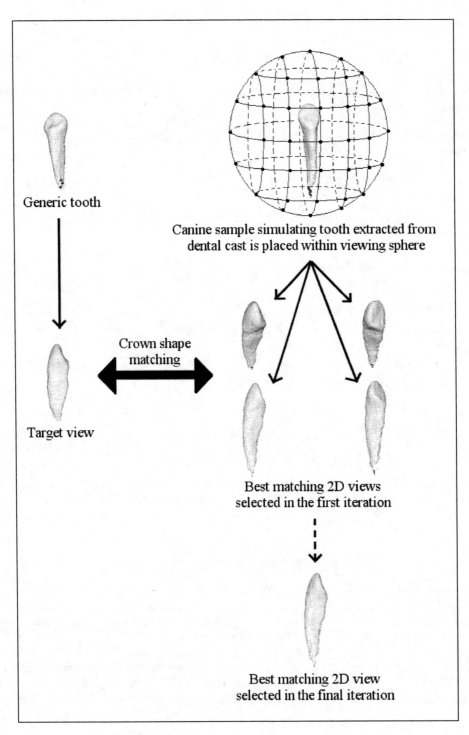

Generic tooth

Canine sample simulating tooth extracted from dental cast is placed within viewing sphere

Crown shape matching

Target view

Best matching 2D views selected in the first iteration

Best matching 2D view selected in the final iteration

Figure 7: Results of crown shape matching.

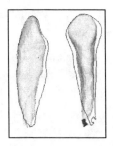

Figure 8: Figure shows the boundary of the generic tooth superimposed onto the canine sample, which simulates a tooth extracted from the dental cast.

From Figure 8, it can be observed that the boundary of the generic tooth closely outlines the boundary of the canine sample. The estimated length of the root is also close to that of the canine sample's root length. Such results show the algorithm is able to accurately estimate the positions and sizes of the root and thus show its potential to reach the ultimate goal of generic tooth model fitting onto real life dental cast models. However, because of the variances inherent in the size of the tooth, there is a larger estimation error in the width of the tooth.

4. CONCLUSION

We have presented a technique for finding the root positions of teeth using dental cast and generic tooth samples, instead of conventional methods such as X-rays, CT or MRI. The method relies on matching the tooth crown in order to estimate the pose of a tooth, and thereby find the position of its root. Multiple projections are generated at different viewing points and matched against a target view. Additional views are generated in the vicinity of the best view and the entire process is repeated until convergence. Experiments on canines have shown that the algorithm is able to closely estimate the position and the length of root and that the algorithm has the potential to perform generic tooth model fitting onto real-life dental cast models. This will be the focus of future work and more experiments on other tooth types are being conducted to confirm the feasibility of the proposed approach.

REFERENCES

1. D.F. Huber and M. Hebert, "A New Approach to 3-D Terrain Mapping", *Proceedings of the 1999 IEEE/RSJ International Conference on Intelligent Robotics and Systems*, pp. 1121-1127, October 1999.
2. B, Kamgar-Parsi, J.L. Jones and A. Rosefield, "Registration of multiple overlapping range images: scenes without distinctive features", *IEEE Transactions on Pattern Analysis and Machine Intelligence*, **13(9)**, pp. 857-871, 1991.
3. T.J. Fan, G. Medioni and R. Nevatia, "Recognizing 3-D objects using surface descriptions", *IEEE Transactions on Pattern Analysis and Machine Intelligence*, **11(11)**, pp. 1140-1157, 1989.
4. Michel A. Audette, Frank P. Ferrie and Terry M. Peters, "An algorithmic overview of surface registration techniques for medical imaging", *Medical Image Analysis*, **4(3)**, pp. 201-217, September 2000.
5. P.J. Besl and R.C. Jain, "Invariant surface characteristics for 3D object recognition in range images", *CVGIP*, **33**, pp. 33-80, 1986.
6. P.J. Besl, and N.D. Mc Kay, "A method for registration of 3D shapes", *IEEE Transactions on Pattern Analysis and Machine Intelligence*, **14(2)**, pp. 239-256, February 1992.
7. R. Kimmel, N. Kiryati and A.M. Bruckstein, "Analyzing and synthesizing images by revolving curves with the Osher-Sethian method", *Computer Vision*, **24(1)**, pages 37-56, 1997.
8. A. E. Johnson and M. Hebert, "Using spin images for efficient object recognition in cluttered 3D scenes", *IEEE Transactions on Pattern Analysis and Machine Intelligence*, **21(5)**, pp. 433-449, 1999.

9. Christopher M. Cyr, Ahmed F. Kamal, Thomas B. Sebastian and Benjamin B. Kimia, "2D-3D registration based on shape matching", *Proceedings of IEEE Workshop on Mathematical Methods in Biomedical Image Analysis*, pp. 198-203, 2000.

10. S. Gold and A. Rangarajan, "A graduated assignment algorithm for graph matching", *IEEE Transactions on Pattern Analysis and Machine Intelligence*, **18(4)**, pp. 377-388, 1996.

Automatic quantification of liver-heart cross talk for quality assessment in SPECT myocardial perfusion imaging

Guo-Qing Wei[a] , Anant Madabushi[b] , JianZhong Qian[a] , and John Engdahl [c]

[a] Imaging Department, Siemens Corporate Research, Inc.
755 College Road East, Princeton NJ 08536
[b] Department of Bioengineering,
University of Pennsylvania, Philadelphia, PA 19104
[c] Siemens Medical Solutions, Inc.
2501 North Barrington Road, Hoffman Estates, IL 60195

ABSTRACT

In the single-photon emission computed tomography (SPECT), it is highly desirable to provide physicians with a measure of the strength of the liver-heart cross talk as a means of assessing the quality of the images, so that appropriate actions can be taken to avoid false diagnosis. Liver-heart cross talk is an phenomenon in which the liver count interferes with the heart count in 3D reconstruction, which generates artifacts in the reconstructed images. In this paper, we propose an automatic method for quantification of such liver-heart cross talk. The system performs heart detection followed by non-heart organ segmentation and quantification of their activities. An appearance-based approach is applied to find the heart center in each image, with invariance to image intensity and contrast. Then heart and non-heart activities are quantified in each image. A measurement formula is proposed to compute the amount of liver-heart cross talk as a function of the size of the non-heart activity regions, of the strengths of the heart and non-heart activities, and of the distance of the non-heart regions to the heart. The method has been tested on 150 patient studies of different isotopes and acquisition types, with very promising results.

Keywords: SPECT, liver-heart cross talk, quality number, heart detection, robust fitting, non-heart activity segmentation, non-heart activity quantification, fusion.

1. INTRODUCTION

In the single-photon emission computed tomography (SPECT) of nuclear medicine, there are many factors that may cause artifacts in the reconstruction of the heart. Among them are attenuation [1], position dependent resolution [2], Compton scatter [2], motion [13,4], and liver uptake [6]. Although correction algorithms exist for most of the artifacts mentioned above, these algorithms themselves may cause additional artifacts or side effects when applied inappropriately. Therefore it is highly necessary to provide an automatic measurement system to quantify the severity of each artifact, so that a corresponding correction algorithm is applied only when the degree of severity is above a certain threshold. In this paper, we attempt to quantify one of the least studied artifacts in SPECT, namely the artifact caused by liver uptakes.

Germanto *et al.* [6] first pointed out that the filtered back-projection algorithm (FBP) [5], which is the most widely used method for heart reconstruction, produces artifactual defects in the inferior/inferoseptal myocardial wall when there are the high uptakes of either liver activities or of other organs. This is reflected in the reduced count in the myocardial wall near the liver. This phenomenon is often called the *liver-heart cross talk*. A direct consequence of that is that this liver-heart artifact may be confused with artifacts of coronary artery diseases, causing false diagnosis by physicians. To remedy this problem, it was suggested in [6] that FBP be performed using a ramp filter and without pre-smoothing of the projection data. Nuyts *et al.* [7] found that the Maximum-Likelihood Expectation-Maximization (ML-EM) algorithm [8] is capable of suppressing the artifacts. If an accurate attenuation map is available, the ML-EM algorithm can nearly eliminate the artifact [7]. The ML-EM algorithm, however, is much slower than the FBP algorithm and some times has problems in convergence. Therefore, it should be applied only when it is needed.

Based on the above analysis, it is highly desirable to devise a method to monitor the liver-heart artifact automatically. The method should give a quantitative measurement about the extent to which the cross talk may be occurring. Therefore based on this quality number, physicians can take appropriate actions, e.g., to switch to the ML-EM algorithm.

2. METHODOLOGY

The first step in quantifying the liver-heart cross-talk is to localize the heart position in each image. Based on the heart position and count, liver activities are then segmented and quantified. A flowchart of the system diagram is shown in Fig.1.

2.1. Heart detection

2.1.1. Region of interest determination

To find the heart position in each image, it is imperative to restrict the search region to some region of interest (ROI), so that not only search time can be substantially reduced, but also a more robust detection can be achieved. In [10], a technique is described to find an upper limit and a lower limit of the heart in the vertical direction of the images. This is based on the 1-D pseudo motion analysis of the image sequence. Since the heart pixels are usually the brightest points in the corresponding scan line, and since the heart follow a fixed pattern of motion, such information can be encoded in a 1D curve called the pseudo motion map. First, the pseudo motion map of an identified heart is extracted as a template. Then this template is matched against the pseudo motion maps of the scan lines. A correlation profile is thus obtained. The scan lines containing the heart produce higher correlation scores than the others.

Since SPECT images are very noisy, the correlation profile obtained may contain high correlation scores that are non-heart. Also, some scan lines containing the heart may produce low correlations. To remove the false peaks and to fill the gaps in the correlation profile, morphological closing operation is performed. The obtained profile is then thresholded to find connected components (segments). Since the approximate heart size is known *a priori*, the segments whose sizes are above a pre-selected threshold or below another pre-selected threshold are discarded. The remaining segments represent possible heart positions in the image sequence.

We also extended the method of [10] by refining the region of interest for each frame independently. In the 1D pseudo motion map, the value at an image frame represents the x-coordinate of the brightest point in the scan line. This information can be used to define the heart range along the x-axis for each frame. Since the maximum intensity on a scan line containing the heart may be not from the heart, errors may occur in determining the x-range of the heart. There are two sources of errors. First, noises may alter the heart count. We use smoothing operations to reduce errors of this kind. Secondly, high liver activity may occur on the same scan line of the heart. In this case, the maximum intensity may be from the liver, instead of the heart. We do not try to avoid errors of this kind at the ROI localization. Instead, we expect the trajectory fitting in the heart detection phase to discard false localization of heart.

2.1.2. Heart detection by a training-based method

The heart detection is based on two steps: off-line training and on-line detection. In the off-line stage, typical heart images are extracted manually. Eigen-heart images are then found by principal component analysis (PCA). In contrast to conventional methods of PCA-based training, there is no brightness and contrast normalization since such normalization is usually based on maximum and minimum intensity values and is very sensitive to noises (SPECT images are very noisy). In the detection stage, an integrated approach is proposed to shift and scale the image under consideration to fit the intensity range of the eigen-images. This is achieved by projecting the intensity-transformed image (with unknown scale and shift parameters) onto the eigen-images and minimizing the error of fit. This leads to a set of equations on both the intensity transformation parameters and the projection coefficients. Based on the orthonormality properties of the eigen-images, these equations can be reduced to a set of linear equations on scale and shift parameters only. By using the least-squares method, these equations can be easily solved for the scale and shift parameters. In this way, the normalization is made robust against noises. Details of the method are presented in [11].

2.1.3. Heart position fitting and refining

The heart positions are detected in each frame independently as described in section 2.1.2. It is known from SPECT imaging, however, that the heart trajectory should follow a sine curve due to the pattern of camera motions. This prior knowledge can be used to correct detection errors in individual frames. Suppose $\{(x_i, y_i), i = 1, 2, \ldots N\}$ are the coordinates of the detected heart positions. Then the x-coordinates should satisfy a sine curve

$$x_i = A \sin(ki + \theta) \tag{1}$$

where $A, k,$ and θ are the parameters of the sine curve. We fit the x-coordinates of the detected heart positions by minimizing the following error function

$$E = \sum_{i=1}^{N} \rho_i(d_i) d_i^2 \tag{2}$$

$$d_i = x_i - A\sin(kx_i + \theta) \tag{3}$$

with respect to the parameters $A, k,$ and θ, where $\rho(d)$ is a weighting function used to exclude outliers, outliers being detected positions whose errors are too large to satisfy a sine curve; d_i is the error of fit for the i-th image. The function $\rho(d)$ is chosen such that when the error d becomes larger, the weight becomes less:

$$\rho(d) = e^{-d^2/\sigma^2} \tag{4}$$

In this way, frames in which the errors of heart positions are too large will have negligible effect on the final fitting result; that is, the fitting is mainly based on the heart positions which satisfy a sine trajectory. The minimization of (2) over $A, k,$ and θ is achieved iteratively as follows. First, an initial estimate of the variables $A, k,$ and θ are obtained based on the detected positions. Then the residual error (3) is calculated for each frame. Based on that, the weight (4) for each frame is determined. The obtained weights are substituted into (2), and the resulting error function E is minimized over $A, k,$ and θ to get a new estimate of the parameters. This procedure repeats until convergence is reached.

After the heart trajectory is fitted, those image frames in which the distances of the detected heart positions to the trajectory are greater than a threshold are identified. The heart positions in these frames need to be refined. Since the trajectory provides an approximate heart position for these frames, the procedure in section 2.1.2 above is applied again to a small neighborhood of these predicted heart positions. An improved heart position is then returned for each of these frames.

2.1.4. Determining heart's bounding circle

After the heart's center is localized, the next step is to determine the bounding circle of the heart. The bounding circle is the minimum circle circumscribing the heart. Starting from the heart center, we grow a circle and computing the average intensity within the circle for each image frame. Since the heart count is usually higher than the surrounding structure, and since the heart shape is nearly circular, the mean intensity will start to increase initially. However, as the circle passes through the middle of the left ventricle ring, the average intensity within the circle will start to decrease, This is true, even in the presence of non-heart structures of high intensity. This is because these high intensity structures do not have a circular shape and are not centered at the heart center. Based on this property, we can determine the heart's outer bounding circle as the one where the average intensity falls below some pre-defined percentage of the maximum average intensity. A more accurate method for determining the heart size would be to find the reflection point in the intensity profile. This is the point where the second derivative shows maximum. Since the heart is usually not clearly visible at the beginning and the end of the image sequence, and since the heart shape at those places are non-circular, we pick only middle 1/3 of the frames for this analysis. The final heart size is computed as the average of the heart sizes in those middle frames.

2.2. Quantifying the liver-heart effect

2.2.1. Non-Heart activity segmentation

From the bounding circles, the average level of the heart activity (intensity) across all the frames can be computed. Non-heart activities, such as liver, whose intensity level are near or above the average heart activity and whose location are within certain range of distance from the heart, will have interference with the heart in 3D reconstruction. These non-heart activities should be segmented. Since the average heart activity has been computed, the segmentation can be done by setting a threshold near the average heart activity. Pixels whose intensities are above the threshold and are lying outside of the bounding circles are segmented as non-heart activities.

2.2.2. Quantification of the liver-heart effect per frame

The strength of liver-heart artifact depends on several factors. First, the higher the level of non-heart activities, the stronger the liver-heart artifact. Secondly, non-heart activities that are closer to the heart will have greater negative effects. Thirdly, the artifact is proportional to the size of the non-heart activities. Based on these relationships we propose to quantify the degree of liver-heart artifact at the i-th frame by the following formula:

$$Q_i = \frac{weighted\_liver\_intensity}{average\_heart\_intensity} \cdot \frac{number\_liver\_pixels}{heart\_area}$$
$$\cdot \frac{\sum distance(liver\_pixels, heart)}{normalization\_factor} \tag{5}$$

where

$$weighted\_liver\_intensity = \frac{\sum_n I_n w_n}{\sum_n w_n}$$

The variable I_n is the intensity level of the n-th non-heart pixel, w_n is the weight assigned to this pixel, which is computed as being inversely proportional to the distance of the pixel to the heart. The value of the variable Q_i is normalized to lie between 0 and 1. A low values means less liver-heart cross-talk, while a value near 1 indicates a strong liver-heart interference.

2.2.3. Fusion of the measurements

Based on (5), the liver-heart cross-talk of the i-th frame can be quantified. The quantifications for all the frames need to be integrated to give a single number indicating the overall quality of the image sequence. Since liver-heart cross-talk usually occurs for consecutive frames, we make local average of the measurements $\{Q_i\}$ to remove any spurious measurement errors. The size of the average window is chosen to be 5. The final quality number is chosen to be the maximum of the smoothed measurements. The above procedure of fusing individual measurements to get the final quality number can be expressed by the following form:

$$Q = \max\{\sum_{k=-2}^{2} Q_i\}$$

In fact, many other forms of integration can be equally applicable. For example, instead of local averaging, the median of the liver activities on a segment of frames can be used.

The quality number obtained can be used by physicians as a guidance as to whether to take appropriate actions. For example, if the quality number is low, other 3D reconstruction methods, instead of the filtered backprojection method, can be used to reduce the artifacts, at the expense of increased computational complexity.

3.EXPERIMENTS

Figure 3 shows an example of quality measure by the proposed technique. Figure 3 (a) is the original image sequence. Fig3 (b) shows the pseudo-motion map of the image sequence. Fig.3(c) is the extracted pseudo-motion map corresponding to the heart. The upper and lower boundaries of the band in Fig.3(c) are the heart position's upper and lower limits used in the heart detection. Fig.3(d) shows the trajectory fitting procedure on the heart positions in the primary detection. Here the x-axis represents the frame number, the y-axis represents the x-coordinates of the detected positions. It can be seen that even large detection errors can still be corrected based on the fitting. Fig.3 (e) illustrates the detected heart positions shown as bounding boxes overlaid on the heart images. The size of the bounding box reflects the estimated heart size. Fig.3 (f) shows the non-heart activity measurement for all the frames. Fig.3 (g) is the quality number extracted from the curve in (f), shown as a bar. The height of the bar is equal to the value of the quality number.

The method of automatic quantification of liver-heart cross talk has been tested on a database of 156 patients. The correct heart detection rate is 96.6% for all the frames. Most detection errors occur at the end of the image sequence where the heart count has become very low. For the purpose of liver-heart artifact quantification, the end of the image sequence almost plays no role, since the liver activities in those frames are low too. From the 156 image sequences, our algorithm is able to give a very reasonable, intuitively good indication of the actual liver activities in the images.

4.CONCLUSIONS

In this paper, we have presented a first automatic method for quantifying the amount of liver activities in SPECT myocardial perfusion imaging. This is an important step toward image quality control. The method provides physicians a single number indicating the degree of liver-heart cross talk that may occur in the image acquisition. With this quality number, the physicians can take appropriate actives to avoid liver-heart artifacts in the 3D reconstruction. Initial experimental results have been very encouraging. Further clinical test and validation are needed to make it practically useful.

REFERENCES:

1. W. Chang, R.E. Henkin, E. Buddemeyer, "The sources of overestimation in the quantification by SPECT of uptakes in a myocardial phantom: concise communication," *Journal of Nuclear Medicine,* Vol.25, 1984, pp.788-791.
2. R.L. Eisner, D.J. Nowsk, W. Fajman, "Fundamentals of 180° acqusition and reconstruction in SPECT imaging," *Journal of Nuclear Medicine,* Vol.27, 1986, pp.1727-1728.
3. R.L. Eisner, ``Use of Cross-correlation function to detect patient motion during SPECT imaging", *Journal of Nuclear Medicine*, Vol.28, No.1, 1987, pp.97-101.
4. G.Q. Wei, J. Qian, E. Chen, J. Engdahl, "A Three-pass Variable-length Correlation Method for Motion Correction in SPECT Myocardial Perfusion Imaging'' , *Proc. SPIE Medical Imaging,* 2000
5. L. Shepp, B. Logan, "The Fourier reconstruction of a head section," *IEEE Trans. Nuclear Sci,* 21, 1974, pp.21-43
6. G. Germano, T. Chua, H. Kiat, J.S. Areeda, D.S. Berman, "A quantitative phantom analysis of artifacts due to hepatic activity in Technetium-99m myocardial perfusion SPECT studies", *Journal of Nuclear Medicine,* Vol.35, No.2, Feb.1994, pp.356-359.
7. J. Nuyts, P. Dupont, V.van den Maegdenbergh, S. Vleugels, P. Suetens, L. Mortelmans, "A Study of the liver-heart artifact in emission tomography," *Journal of Nuclear Medicine,* Vol.36, No.1, Jan.1995, pp.133-139.
8. L. Shepp, Y. Vardi, J.B. Ra, S. K. Hilal, Z.H. Cho, "Maximum likelihood reconstruction for emission tomography," *IEEE Trans. Medical Imaging,* 1, 1981, pp.113-122
9. K. Lange, R. Carson, "EM reconstruction algorithm for emission and transmission tomography," *J. Computer Assist. Tomog.,* 1984, pp.306-316
10. B. Xu, J. Chou, and J. Qian "Determining the position range of the heart from a sequence of projection images using 1-D pseudo motion analysis", US Patent, 5682887, 1997
11. G.Q. Wei, J. Qian, J. Engdahl, "An Integrated Approach to Brightness and Contrast Normalization in Appearance-based Heart Detection in SPECT", *Proc. SPIE Medical Imaging*, 2002

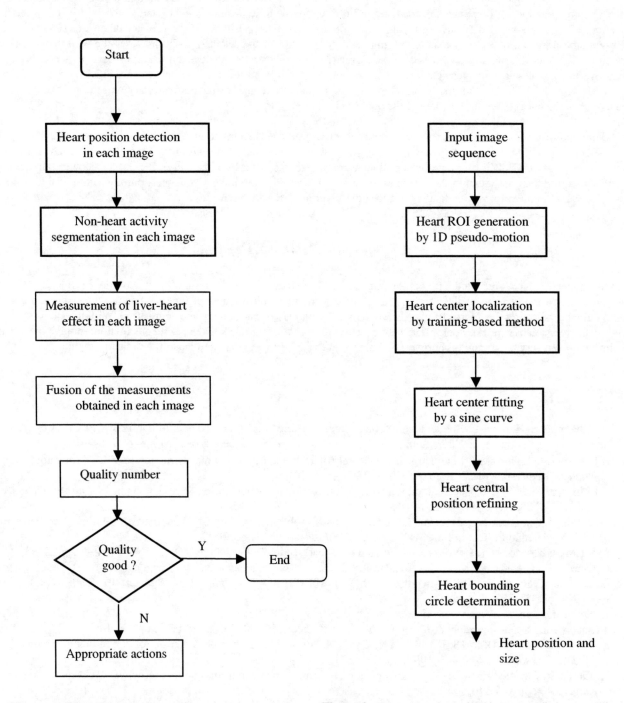

Figure 1: The system diagram of liver-heart artifact quantification.

Figure 2: Heart detection with sine curve fitting, outlier detection, and outlier correction.

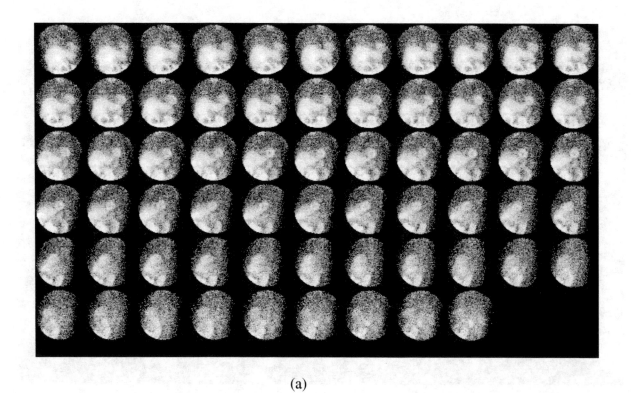

(a)

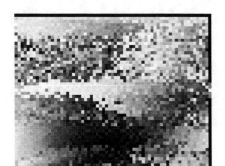

(b)

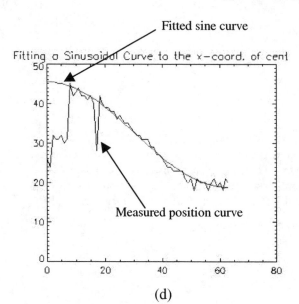

(c)

Fitted sine curve

Fitting a Sinusoidal Curve to the x-coord. of cent

Measured position curve

(d)

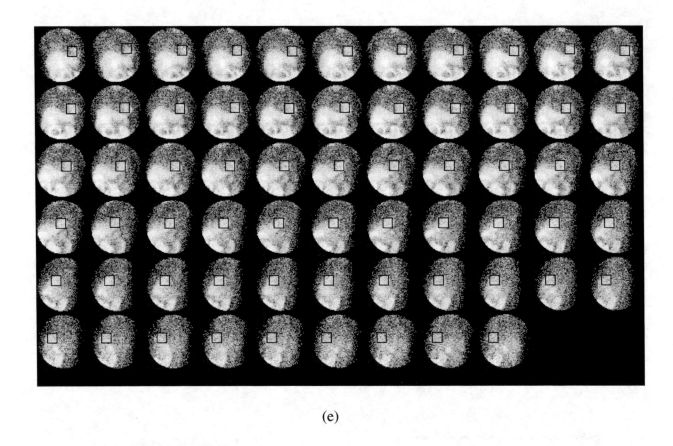

(e)

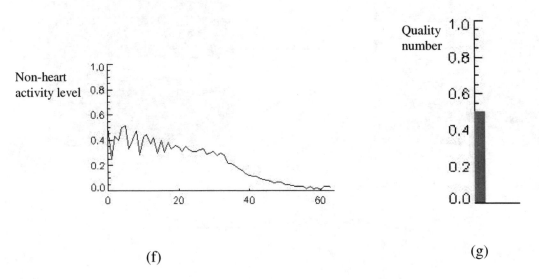

(f)

(g)

Figure 3: An example of SPECT image quality measure. (a) original image sequence; (b) pseudo-motion map; (c) extracted pseudo-motion map corresponding to the heart. The upper and lower boundaries of the band are the heart position's upper and lower limits; (d) detected x-coordinates of the heart and the fitted sine curve; (e) detected heart position shown as bounding boxes overlaid on the heart images; (f) non-heart activity measurement for all the frames; (g) quality number extracted from the curve in (f).

Automatic quality assessment of JPEG and JPEG 2000 compressed images

Walter F. Good[*], Glenn Maitz[†], Xiao Hui Wang[‡]

Department of Radiology, University of Pittsburgh

ABSTRACT

A novel figure-of-merit (FOM) for automatically quantifying the types of artifacts that appear in compressed images was investigated. This FOM is based on task specific linear combinations of magnitude, frequency and "localized" structure information derived from difference images. For each elemental diagnostic task (e.g., detection of microcalcifications) a value is calculated as the weighted linear combination of the output of an array of filters, and the FOM is defined to be the maximum of these values, taken over all relevant diagnostic tasks. This FOM was tested by applying it to a previously assembled set of 60 mammograms that had been digitized and compressed at five different compression levels using our version of the original JPEG algorithm. The FOM results were compared to subjective assessments of image quality provided by nine radiologists. A subset consisting of 25 images was also processed with the JPEG 2000 algorithm and evaluated by the FOM. A significant correlation existed between readers' subjective ratings and FOMs for JPEG compressed images. A comparison between the results of the two compression algorithms reveals that, to achieve a comparable FOM level, the JPEG 2000 images were compressed at a bitrate that was typically 15% lower than that of images compressed with the original JPEG algorithm.

Keywords: mammography, image compression, image quality

1. INTRODUCTION

There are numerous advantages to handling medical images in a digital format, but the large volume of digital data needed to represent many kinds of radiographic images has created difficult challenges for the implementers of image archives, networks and workstations. Image compression is widely advocated as one means of alleviating the problems associated with the large data volume of radiographic images. While the use of lossless compression does not introduce concerns about changes in image quality, the compression ratios that can be achieved with these methods are not sufficient for many applications. To attain practical levels of image compression it is necessary to accept some loss of image fidelity.

Currently there are two international standards for image compression that seem to be capable of providing acceptable image quality while achieving a significant level of lossy compression. The Joint Photographic Experts Group (JPEG) was formed by the International Organization for Standardization to address image compression issues. In 1992 they adopted the original JPEG image compression standard[1-5], and more recently, they defined a wavelet-based standard, JPEG 2000, which is expected to exhibit improved performance[6,7]. Although these standards do not specifically address radiological images, they were designed to be universally applicable to continuous tone images, and there are many practical advantages if they can be adapted for use in radiology.

[*]goodwf@msx.upmc.edu; Phone 412-641-2560; University of Pittsburgh, Department of Radiology, Imaging Research, 300 Halket St., Pittsburgh, PA 15213-3180.

[†]maitzgs@msx.upmc.edu; Phone 412-641-2562; University of Pittsburgh, Department of Radiology, Imaging Research, 300 Halket St., Pittsburgh, PA 15213-3180.

[‡]wangxh@msx.upmc.edu; Phone 412-641-2561; University of Pittsburgh, Department of Radiology, Imaging Research, 300 Halket St., Pittsburgh, PA 15213-3180.

Each of these compression methods introduces a characteristic kind of artifact or loss of image information. A significant difference in these algorithms, as they are applied in this study, is that the original JPEG algorithm requires that images be divided into 8-pixel × 8-pixel blocks, which are compressed independently, creating the potential for artifact at the boundaries between the blocks. The JPEG 2000 algorithm, while permitting the image to be decomposed into tiles, does not require it. When images are represented by a single tile, there is no concern about blocking artifact.

While it is possible to statistically characterize the artifacts produced in ensembles of images compressed at fixed bitrates, this does not insure that individual compressed images are of acceptable quality. When images are being archived in a compressed format, it is necessary to guarantee that the diagnostic quality of each compressed image is acceptable before the system disposes of the original image data. If it is determined that a compressed image has an unacceptable level of artifact, then the original can be compressed at a higher bitrate to preserve more of its diagnostic content. Because performing such a review of each compressed image manually is not generally practical, it is desirable implement automatic methods for assessing changes in the diagnostic quality of an image at the time it is compressed.

It is widely reported in the literature that traditional physical measures such as RMSE are not highly correlated to subjective assessment of image quality[8,9]. Other measures such as the square root integral[10,11], power spectra measures[12], and measures based on characteristics of the human visual system[12-14] have been more successful in some respects, but none have been shown to be adequate for automatically guaranteeing that compressed images are of an acceptable quality.

One inherent problem in most existing measures of quality is that they cannot be related directly to specific kinds of diagnostic information. Different diagnostic tasks are concerned with different aspects of image quality so the figure-of-merit (FOM) needs to be somewhat task dependent. Image quality is multidimensional and it is unlikely that any single simple measure can achieve a high degree of correlation to changes in observer performance over a variety of tasks[15]. Nevertheless, it should be possible to provide a task-dependent mechanism to insure that the loss of diagnostic quality is below some acceptable threshold, particularly when the degradation is held to an almost visually lossless level.

To overcome the limitations of the previous measures, we developed and studied the FOM described below, which can be applied to the original image and the difference between the original image and a degraded version of the original. This measure is based on not only the magnitude of the difference image, but also on the structure in this image as measured, for example, by morphological techniques or by concepts derived from "localized" fractal dimension.

The FOM incorporates task dependent weighting factors that relate to the relative importance of various kinds of artifact for different diagnostic tasks. For this project, it was calibrated for mammography, where the relevant tasks were assumed to be the detection and classification of masses and microcalcifications. The FOM was tested by applying it to a set of digitized mammograms that had been compressed with one or both of the JPEG algorithms.

2. METHODOLOGY

2.1 Development of FOM
We implemented the FOM as a task specific linear combination of the outputs of an array of filters that are applied to an original image and the difference between the original image and a degraded version of the original. For each elementary detection or classification task (e.g., detection of microcalcifications in a mammogram) an array of weighting factors was used to form a linear combination of the outputs of the filters. Different tasks use different weighting factors. These calculated values for elementary tasks are then combined by taking the maximum over all relevant elementary tasks. For the case of mammography presented here, there could potentially be separate weighting factors for detection of microcalcifications, detection of masses, classification of microcalcifications and classification of masses.

To determine weighting factors for mammography, for the results described below, we reanalyzed a previous study of the compression of mammograms in which mammographers had rank-ordered images compressed at 6 different compression ratios, based on image quality for the detection of masses and microcalcifications[16]. Because this data did not allow us to obtain separate weighting factors for the classification tasks, and in many cases the quality factors for classification will likely be similar to those for detection, we based the FOM for mammography on only the image characteristics required for the detection of abnormalities. Basically for mammography, the FOM for masses emphasizes both the low frequency bandpass filters and large-size blob filters while the FOM for microcalcifications emphasizes the high frequency filters, small blob detectors and the texture filter. Thus, only one set of weighting factors was generated for detection and classification of masses and a second set was similarly generated for calcifications. After compression of a mammogram, the filters are applied to the difference image and a value is calculated for each task by using the corresponding weighting factors to form linear combinations of the outputs of the filters. The FOM was taken to be the maximum of these two values.

Provisions have been made in our software for applying a utility function, reflecting the relative clinical importance of the various diagnostic tasks, to the task specific values before the values are combined. Such utility functions do not generally exist and their determination, which has proven to be a very challenging task in itself, is beyond the scope of this project. For the results presented below, all diagnostic tasks have been weighted equally.

We implemented three types of filters: 1) Spatial frequency filters; 2) Size dependent "blob" detectors; and, 3) Texture filters. The filters are applied to difference images. In the case of our optimized version of the original JPEG algorithm, where we set background pixels to a constant value to improve the compressibility of images, we set the corresponding pixels in the difference image to a value of zero. This effectively eliminates the background as a factor in calculating the FOM.

Bandpass filters are calculated by decomposing the power spectra of the difference image into 6 bands whose relative lengths were set at: 32/63 (highest frequency band), 16/63, 8/63, 4/63, 2/63, and 1/63 (lowest frequency band). For each band, the total energy in the band was calculated.

The blob filters operate by adaptively thresholding the squared-difference image and then applying a dilation operator multiple times followed by the application of an erosion operator an equal number of times. This process connects blobs that are physically close but disconnected, and eliminates small holes in blobs. Each of the remaining connected regions is labeled and a histogram of the number of objects as a function of size is calculated. We then decompose this histogram into five equally spaced size ranges, and the integral over each range is used as the value for the corresponding filter.

The primary texture filter we rely on in this study provides a measure of local variance, after correction for any local linear trends. A Gaussian-weighted least-squares fit of a linear function is performed at each pixel in the difference image. The residual weighted-sum-of-squares at the pixel is used as a measure of complexity at that point. Both the maximum and mean, taken over the relevant image area, are retained as measures of complexity.

2.2 Application of FOM to compressed mammograms
To test the FOM, we applied it to a set of mammograms that had been digitized and compressed at various compression ratios. All digitized images had been compressed with the original JPEG algorithm, and a subset was compressed with the JPEG 2000 algorithm.

2.2.1 Mammography case set – As part of a previous observer performance study of the compression of mammograms, sixty cases had been selected and verified by pathology for positive cases, and by follow-up for negative cases. The case set included 23 cases with masses and 27 with clusters of microcalcifications. Fourteen of the cases were malignant.

2.2.2 Image digitization and printing – Original mammograms were digitized using a Lumisys-150 (Lumisys, Sunnyvale, CA) high-resolution, high-contrast sensitivity laser film digitizer that produces a scan matrix of 4,096 x 5,120 pixels for an 8 x 10-inch film, by digitizing at a 50-μm sampling interval. This pixel resolution results in a Nyquist spatial frequency of 10 cycles/mm, which preserved most of the content of the analog film.

Both the compressed versions as well as the original (non-compressed) digitized data, for images evaluated by radiologists in this study, were laser printed onto film with a specially modified Kodak EKTASCAN 2180 laser film printer (Eastman-Kodak, Rochester, NY). This laser printer had been modified to print a 43μm pixel size.

2.2.3 Image compression – All images were compressed using the original JPEG algorithm and a subset was additionally compressed with the JPEG 2000 algorithm. Compression with the original JPEG algorithm was performed using software optimized specifically for the compression of digitized mammograms, that has previously been developed and tested in our laboratory[17-21]. Our software is a 12-bit version of the extended JPEG standard. For this study, Huffman encoding was used to encode the quantized coefficients and all compression ratios were based on this. The Huffman table was derived from the statistics of each individual quantized image rather than from ensemble statistics. Each digitized image was initially compressed at five different compression levels. Quantization matrices required by the JPEG algorithm were derived by scaling a base matrix designed to preserve slightly more accuracy for the lowest frequency components, which produced mean compression ratios of 24:1, 34:1, 51:1, 70:1, 101:1, respectively. The highest level of quantization resulted in a mean compression ratio of 101:1, which is significantly higher than what is required to permit the efficient handling of mammographic images with current digital technology, and it is in the range where studies of other algorithms applied to different image types have shown significant deterioration in image quality[22-26].

Prior to compression all digitized mammograms were preprocessed to improve their compressibility. Our preprocessing operation is divided into two steps – first we segment and crop the image and modify the background pixel values to minimize the storage requirements for the background and then we optionally apply a noise removal filter to the tissue pixels. The actual procedures employed in this process have been described elsewhere[18].

The JPEG 2000 algorithm employed in this study was a version of JJ2000 provided by EPFL, ERICSSON and Canon Research Center France. As utilized here, compression was non-progressive, each image consisted of a single component, and we did not tile images (i.e., each image was considered to be a single tile). The Daubechies 9-tap/7-tap discrete wavelet transform, a non-reversible filter, was used. Because software implementing the JPEG 2000 algorithm has only recently become available, we have not performed the kinds of optimization of this algorithm that we previously did for the original JPEG algorithm.

2.2.4 Radiologists' evaluations – Nine readers, all Board certified radiologists, participated in this project. Each reading session involved having one radiologist review 30 cases, all in the same compression mode. While the primary task in the previous study was the detection of abnormalities, readers were also asked to give a subjective assessment of image quality relative to the detection of masses or microcalcification clusters, for each image.

2.2.5 Comparison between original JPEG and JPEG 2000 – We processed an additional subset of images with the JPEG 2000 algorithm. A subset consisting of 25 JPEG compressed images was randomly identified, with the constraint that their subjective ratings be evenly distributed over the range of reported subjective ratings. The original (non-compressed) image corresponding to each of these images was compressed with the JPEG 2000 algorithm at a bitrate that was selected to produce the same FOM value as the original JPEG compressed image (i.e., the independent variable was FOM and the dependent variable was bitrate).

3. RESULTS

As can be seen in Table 1, average subjective image quality ratings for both mass detection and microcalcification detection decreased monotonically with increasing compression ratio. We calculated the FOM for each image in the previous study and the FOM components corresponding to masses and microcalcifications are also presented in Table 1. The correlation between the FOM values and the averaged subjective ratings was calculated for masses as r=-0.84 (p=0.02) and for microcalcifications as r=-.87 (p=0.01). The FOM appears to be a more sensitive function of compression ratio and image quality than subjective assessment.

At each bitrate the FOM for microcalcifications was higher than that for masses. Thus the FOM for the image as a whole was determined by the impact of compression on the detection or classification of microcalcifications. This is consistent with our previous experiences suggesting that the detectability of masses is considerably less sensitive to the types of artifacts produced by the image compression algorithms studied here.

Figure 1 compares the bitrate for JPEG 2000 to the bitrate for our optimized version of the original JPEG algorithm, for corresponding FOM values. Note that the bitrate for the original JPEG algorithm is the bitrate for the tissue pixels only. The comparison indicates that JPEG 2000 is approximately 20% more efficient at the low bitrate (high compression) end of the plot, but only 10% more efficient at the higher bitrates.

Mode			Mass		Microcalcification		FOM
Compr. Ratio	Bits/Pixel (img avg)	Bits/Pixel (tissue avg)	Subjective Quality	FOM	Subjective Quality	FOM	
Original	12	12	55	0	49	0	0
24:1	0.500	0.823	53	0.9	47	1.3	1.3
34:1	0.353	0.578	53	3.4	47	4.5	4.5
52:1	0.231	0.374	53	4.7	44	5.7	5.7
70:1	0.171	0.275	50	5.1	38	6.5	6.5
101:1	0.119	0.188	50	5.9	33	8.2	8.2

Table 1: Average subjective ratings and FOMs, from mammography compression study, for compression with the optimized JPEG algorithm.

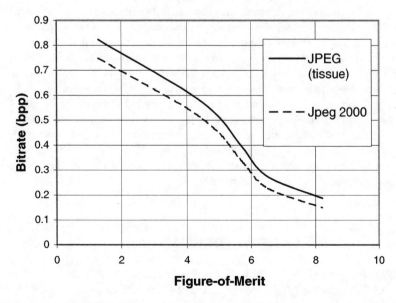

Figure 1: Comparison between JPEG 2000 and the original JPEG algorithm optimized for mammography.

4. DISCUSSION

4.1 Combining task specific outputs

The limitation on compression will generally be determined by either subjective assessment or by the abnormality most sensitive to image degradation induced by compression. In this case, microcalcifications appear to be significantly more sensitive than masses, in terms of subjective assessment, and our previous study indicated this is also true for measures of observer performance. While we have investigated combining task specific values by both summing the values and finding the maximum value, in the absence of a utility function, we adopted the maximum on the assumption that it is the most highly impaired task that is the limiting factor for determining whether an image is acceptable. If the task specific values are calibrated to reflect absolute changes in diagnostic performance, and if a utility function is applied, then summing the task specific values would provide a more reasonable estimate of the change in diagnostic utility.

4.2 Need for additional filters

These filters implemented in this project have been shown to be adequate for the kinds of tasks described below but they are not necessarily optimal. Because this project provides a general mechanism for systematically constructing appropriate FOMs, by incorporating other filters or sets of weighting factors, new filters can easily be added to our software to accommodate the specific features that must be preserved in particular types of images.

4.3 Restriction of original JPEG to tissue pixels

For our optimized version of the original JPEG algorithm, most of the bits in the compressed data stream represent tissue pixels. This is because the background has been set to a constant value and compressed at a very high compression ratio. Since we have not performed such an optimization for the JPEG 2000 algorithm, for the purpose of comparing the two algorithms, we assume that the bitrate for the JPEG 2000 compressed image represents the bitrate for tissues pixels for that image. This may not be entirely accurate because the background in these images, being very dense, results in a higher level of digitizer noise than is present in the less dense tissue areas.

5. CONCLUSIONS

Prior to archiving individual compressed images, it will be necessary to guarantee that diagnostic quality has not been lost in the compression process. This project has demonstrated the feasibility of creating task-specific FOMs that can be used to automatically assess degradation resulting from image compression. The FOM employed here is sufficiently correlated to subjective assessment that it should be possible to establish a threshold for FOM values, below which images will subjectively be considered acceptable. Because our previous study indicated that, for the compression of digitized mammograms, the subjective assessment is reduced before there is a significant decline in observer performance, this should also guarantee that there is no significant loss of observer performance. It is our expectation that a threshold can be identified such that, for compressed images having FOM values below this threshold, it would not be possible to demonstrate a loss of observer performance, due to image compression, in any reasonable kind of observer performance study. If this turns out to be the case, then calculating the FOM and testing it against such a threshold, prior to archiving a compressed image, would allow us to automatically insure that an image is of acceptable quality, or to reprocess it at a lower compression ratio if it is not. This should be sufficient for guaranteeing that a particular image had been unduly degraded by image compression.

ACKNOWLEDGEMENTS

The authors thank Howard Rockette for assisting in the design and performance of this study. This work is sponsored in part by grants CA60259, CA62800 and CA80836 from the National Cancer Institute and LM06236 from the National Library of Medicine, National Institutes of Health, and grant DAMD 17-00-1-0410 from the Department of Defense.

The content of the contained information does not necessarily reflect the position or the policy of the government, and no official endorsement should be inferred.

REFERENCES

1   Joint Photographic Experts Group (JPEG). JPEG Technical Specification, Revision 5 (Document No. JPEG8R5 or JTC1/SC2/WG8 N933). ISO Central Secretariat, 1990.

2   Hudson GP, Yasuda H, Sebestyen I. The international standardization of a still picture compression technique. Proc IEEE Global Telecommunications Conference & Exhibition, November 28-December 1, 1988, Vol. 2, 1016-1021.

3   Wallace G, Vivian R, Poulsen H. Subjective testing results for still picture compression algorithms for international standardization. Proc IEEE Global Telecommunications Conference & Exhibition, November 28-December 1, 1988, Vol. 2, 1022-1027.

4   Leger A, Mitchell JL, Yamazaki Y. Still picture compression algorithms evaluated for international standardization. Proc IEEE Global Telecommunications Conference & Exhibition, November 28-December 1, 1988, Vol. 2, 1028-1032.

5   Pennebaker WB, Mitchell JL. *JPEG: Still Image Data Compression Standard*. Van Nostrand Reinhold, 1993.

6   Christopoulos C, Skodras A, Ebrahimi T. The JPEG2000 still image coding system: an overview. IEEE Trans on Consumer Electronics, 2000, 46(4):1103-1127.

7   Santa-Cruz D, Ebrahimi T, Askelof J, Larsson M, Christopoulos CA. JPEG2000 still image coding versus other standards. Proc SPIE 2000; 4115:446-454.

8   Stein CS, Watson AB, Hitchner LE. Psychophysical rating of image compression techniques. Proc SPIE 1989; 1077:198-208.

9   Girod B. What's wrong with mean-squared error? [Chapter]. Watson AB, Editor. Digital Images and Human Vision. 1st ed. Cambridge, Massachusetts: MIT Press 1993; 207-220.

10   Barten PGJ. The Square root integral (SQRI). Proc SPIE 1989; 1077:73-82.

11   Barten PGJ. Evaluation of the effect of noise on subjective image quality. Proc SPIE 1991; 1453:2-15.

12   Nill NB, Bouzas BH. Objective image quality measure derived from digital image power spectra. Optical Engineering 1992; 31(4):813-825.

13   Daly S. The visible difference predictor. Proc SPIE 1992; 1666:2-15.

14   Lu HQ. Quantitative evaluation of image enhancement algorithms. Proc SPIE 1991; 1453:223-234.

15   Ahumada AJ, Null CH. Image quality: a multidimensional problem [Chapter]. Watson AB, Editor. Digital Images and Human Vision. 1st ed. Cambridge, Massachusetts: MIT Press 1993; 141-148.

16   Good WF, Sumkin JH, Dash N, Johns CM, Zuley ML, Rockette HE, Gur D. Observer Sensitivity to Small Differences: A Multipoint Rank-Order Experiment. AJR 173 Aug 1999; 275-278.

17   Good WF, Gur D. Quantization techniques for the compression of chest images by JPEG type algorithms. Proc SPIE 1992; 1652:114-121.

18   Good WF, Maitz G, Gur D. JPEG compatible data compression of mammograms. Digital Imaging 1994. 7(3):123-132.

19   JM Holbert, M Staiger, TS Chang, JD Towers, CA Britton: Selection of processing algorithms for digital image compression -- a rank order study. Academic Radiology 1995; 2:273-6.

20   Good W, Lattner S, Maitz G. Evaluation of image compression using plausible "non visually weighted" image fidelity measures. Proceedings of SPIE 1996; 2701:301-309.

21   Lattner S, Good W, Maitz G. Visually weighted assessment of image degradation resulting from image compression. Proceedings of SPIE 1996; 2701:507-518.

22   T Ishigaki, S Sakuma, M Ikeda, Y Itoh, M Suzuki, S Iwai: Clinical evaluation of irreversible image compression: Analysis of chest imaging with computed radiography. Radiology 1990; 175:739-743.

23   H MacMahon, K Doi, S Sanada, SM Montner, ML Giger, CE Metz, N Nakamori, FF Yin, XW Xu, H Yonekawa, H Takeuchi: Data compression: Effect on diagnostic accuracy in digital chest radiography. Radiology 1991; 178:175-179.

24   DR Aberle, F Gleeson, JW Sayre, K Brown, et al: The effect of irreversible compression on diagnostic accuracy in thoracic imaging. Invest Radiol 1993; 28(5)398-403.

25   GG Cox, LT Cook, MF Insana, MA McFadden, TJ Hall, LA Harrison, DA Eckard, NL Martin: The effects of lossy compression on the detection of subtle pulmonary nodules. Med Phys 1996; 23:127-132.

26   Good WF, Maitz G, King J, Gennari R, Gur D. Observer performance assessment of JPEG-compressed high-resolution chest images. Proceedings of SPIE (1999) 3663:8-13.

JPEG domain watermarking

Wenbin Luo[a†], Gregory L. Heileman[a,b‡], Carlos E. Pizano[b⋆]

[a]Department of Electrical & Computer Engineering, University of New Mexico
[b]Elisar Software Corporation

ABSTRACT

In this paper, a JPEG domain image watermarking method that utilizes spatial masking is presented. The watermarking algorithm works in the compressed domain, and can be implemented efficiently in real-time (only 50ms is required for a 512×512 24-bit color image on a 700MHz computer). In many applications, particularly those associated with delivering images over the Internet, the ability to watermark images in real-time is required. In order to achieve a real-time watermarking capability, the proposed technique avoids many of the computation steps associated with JPEG compression. Specifically, the forward and inverse DCT do not need to be calculated, nor do any of the computations associated with quantization. Robustness to JPEG compression and additive noise attacks is achieved with the proposed system, and the relationship between watermark robustness and watermark position is described. A further advantage of the proposed method is that it allows a watermark to be detected in an image without referencing to the original unwatermarked image, or to any other information used in the watermark embedding process.

Keywords: JPEG compression, image watermarking, spatial masking, compressed domain, DCT, quantization

1. INTRODUCTION

The need for developing watermarking techniques that protect electronic information has become increasingly important due to the widespread availability of methods for disseminating exact copies of this information (e.g., via the Internet), and the ease with which this information can be reproduced.[1] Digital watermarking is increasingly being used for the purposes of protecting digital content against unauthorized usage or theft, and for documenting or ensuring (i.e., verifying, guaranteeing, or proving) the integrity of multimedia content. Digital image watermarking involves the embedding of additional information into an image in a manner that is imperceptible to the human observer, but which can be discovered by watermark detection algorithms. Digital image watermarking is typically performed in either the frequency or spatial domain. Early digital image watermarking methods used the spatial domain to perform watermark embedding by simply changing the least significant bit of each pixel in order to encode a message. It has been found that transform domain watermarking schemes are typically much more robust to image manipulation as compared to spatial domain schemes. The method proposed here belongs to frequency domain watermarking category, and in particular involves modifications to the discrete cosine transform (DCT) domain coefficients.

In the DCT domain, watermarks should be embedded in those coefficients that meet the following requirements in order for the watermarks to be invisible and also robust against attacks aimed at removing them.[2] First, watermark embedding should target those coefficients having large perceptual capacity, allowing strong watermarks (strong against attacks) to be embedded without perceptual distortion. Second, the embedding should focus on those coefficients that will change little when common image processing and noise corruption attacks are applied. This should include both intentional and unintentional attack possibilities.

[†]wbluo@eece.unm.edu; Dept. of Electrical & Computer Engineering, University of New Mexico Albuquerque, NM 87131. [‡]heileman@eece.unm.edu; Dept. of Electrical & Computer Engineering, University of New Mexico Albuquerque, NM 87131. [⋆]cpizano@elisar.com; Elisar Software Corp., 2500 Louisiana Blvd. NE, Suite 400, Albuquerque, NM 87110

Medical Imaging 2002: Image Processing, Milan Sonka, J. Michael Fitzpatrick, Editors, Proceedings of SPIE Vol. 4684 (2002) © 2002 SPIE · 1605-7422/02/$15.00

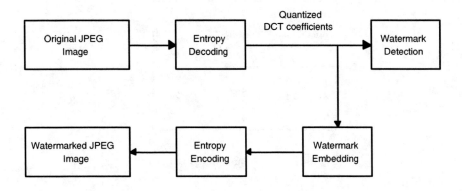

Figure 1: The proposed watermarking system.

In many applications related to Internet-based delivery of images, particularly those associated with large image databases, there are requirements for real-time watermark insertion and extraction. The method described in this paper was developed with these requirements in mind. In particular, this method is capable of embedding a watermark in a 512×512 24-bit color JPEG image in approximately 50ms using a 700MHz computer. Watermark detection and extraction are similarly fast, and do not require access to the original (unwatermarked) image, or to any other information used in the watermark embedding process, in order to detect and extract the watermark. Thus, costly searches through an image database can be avoided during the watermark detection/extraction process.

2. WATERMARKING METHOD

The JPEG compression method starts by dividing an image into disjoint 8×8 blocks of pixels. Next, for each block, the forward DCT is calculated, producing 64 DCT coefficients. Let us denote the (x,y)-th DCT coefficient of the k-th block as $d_k(x, y)$, $0 \leq x, y \leq 7$, $k = 1, \ldots, B$, where B is the total number of blocks in the image. In each block, all 64 coefficients are further quantized to integers $D_k(x, y)$ using a JPEG quantization matrix Q:

$$D_k(x, y) = R\left(\frac{d_k(x, y)}{Q(x, y)}\right),\tag{1}$$

where R denotes the integer round operation. The quantized coefficients are then arranged in a zig-zag manner denoted by $Z_k(i)$, $0 \leq i \leq 63$, $k = 1, \ldots, B$, and compressed using a Huffman coder. The resulting compressed stream, together with a header, forms the JPEG compressed image file. For robustness and simplicity reasons, the method described here embeds watermarks in the luminance (Y) component of an image, leaving the chromatic components $(C_b$ and $C_r)$ intact. The general model for the watermarking system is shown in Figure 1. Note that for the watermark detection/extraction process, we assume that the input to the system (i.e., the "original JPEG image") is the watermarked, and possibly attacked, image.

The specific computations performed at each step in the watermarking embedding process are as follows:

1. Read the original JPEG image, and for each block k, perform entropy decoding in order to obtain the quantized DCT coefficients $Z_k(i)$, $0 \leq i \leq 63$, $k = 1, \ldots, B$.

2. Let i_0 denote the initial coefficient within the coefficient block (in zig-zag order) where watermark insertion begins. Then, in four adjacent DCT coefficient blocks, as shown in Figure 2, a single bit w is embedded as follows:

   if $w = 1$ **then**
       if $Z_1(i_0) < \overline{M} + \delta$ **then**

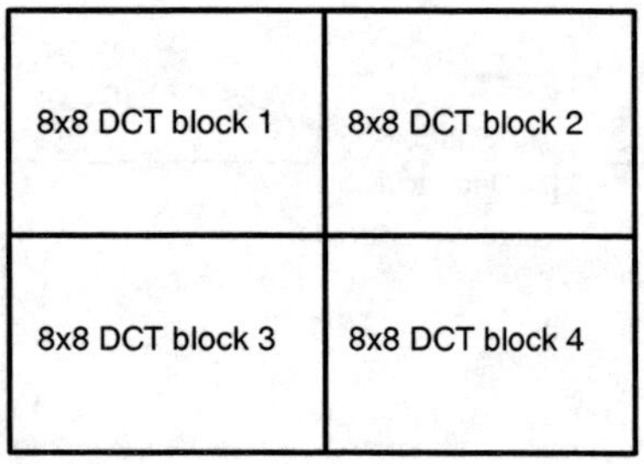

Figure 2: An embedding unit.

$$Z_1^*(i_0) = \overline{M} + \delta$$

else $(w = 0)$

    if $Z_1(i_0) > \overline{M} - \delta$ **then**

        $$Z_1^*(i_0) = \overline{M} - \delta$$

where $\overline{M} = R((Z_2(i_0) + Z_3(i_0) + Z_4(i_0))/3)$, and δ is determined by the local characteristics of the image. Specifically, let $M_{max} = \max\{Z_1(i_0),\ Z_2(i_0),\ Z_3(i_0),\ Z_4(i_0)\}$, $M_{min} = \min\{Z_1(i_0),\ Z_2(i_0),\ Z_3(i_0),\ Z_4(i_0)\}$, and assume T_1 and T_2 are two adjustable threshold values with $T_1 < T_2$. Then, δ is computed as follows:

$$\delta = \begin{cases} 1, & \text{if } (M_{max} - M_{min}) \leq T_1 \\ 2, & \text{if } T_1 < (M_{max} - M_{min}) \leq T_2 \\ 3, & \text{if } T_2 < (M_{max} - M_{min}) \end{cases}$$

The algorithm uses the fact that the relationship between DCT coefficients at the same position in different 8×8 blocks of an image will hold even if these coefficients are quantized by an arbitrary quantization table in the JPEG compression process.[3] The algorithm also exploits the fact that $Z_1(i_0)$ is usually close to $\overline{M}$.

Since the visibility of the superimposed watermark signal is affected by the background texture,[2] the stronger the texture in the background, the lower the visibility of the embedded signal will be (this is texture masking).[4] The method therefore embeds a stronger watermark signal in stronger texture areas.

3. Replace $Z_1(i_0)$ with the new coefficients $Z_1^*(i_0)$. The above procedure is applied to all four DCT coefficient adjacent blocks. The final watermarked image I^* is then obtained by entropy encoding these modified DCT blocks.

Watermark extraction is the inverse of the watermark embedding procedure. Suppose that I^* is the signal-distorted or maliciously-attacked watermarked image. To extract the watermark from I^*, $\overline{M}^*$ is calculated from $Z_1^*(i_0)$ in the same way as in step 2 above. Then, the watermark w is extracted according to following rule:

if $Z_1^*(i_0) > \overline{M}^*$ **then**

    $w = 1$

else $(Z_1^*(i_0) \leq \overline{M}^*)$

    $w = 0$

The experiments detailed in the following section were used to quantify the performance of this watermarking system.

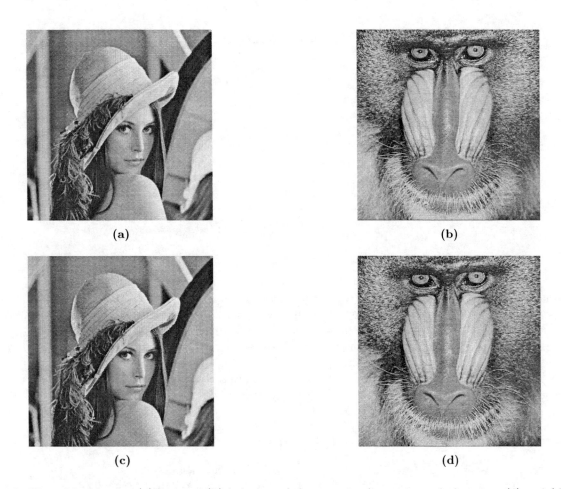

Figure 3: The original images **(a)** lena and **(b)** baboon and the corresponding watermarked versions **(c)** and **(d)**.

3. EXPERIMENTAL RESULTS

The experiments described here compare the performance of different embedding strategies in terms of robustness against JPEG compression and additive noise attacks. The two standard color images shown in Figure 3, *lenna* and *Baboon*, were used in our experiments. All watermarked images derived from these test images were 512×512 pixels and 24-bits in color.

First the two test images were JPEG compressed by quality factor 75. Next, the same watermark was embedded into these two compressed images using parameters $T_1 = 15$, $T_2 = 30$, and at various coefficient locations determined by i_0, $0 \leq i_0 \leq 63$. The average watermarking time of the proposed system was approximately 50ms using a 700MHz computer. A single bit was embedded in a 2x2 block, and in total 1024 bits were embedding in an image. Figure 3 shows the original and the watermarked images, respectively, when $i_0 = 10$. The method does not cause perceptible changes to be introduced into the watermarked images.

The first experiment studies the effects of watermark embedding at various position, ($i_0 = 0, 2, 4, 6, 8, 10$, and 12) on the peak signal-to-noise ratio (PSNR), which is calculated as the difference between the original test image and the watermarked image.

From Figure 4, we see that images containing stronger texture features, e.g., *baboon*, will yield a lower PSNR. This is exactly what we want to achieve with texture-based watermarking. That is, the goal is to always embed stronger watermark signals into rich texture areas.

The next set of experiments details watermark robustness to JPEG compression. The watermarked images, embedded with parameters $i_0 = 0, 2, 6$, and 10, were attacked by JPEG compression at different quality levels.

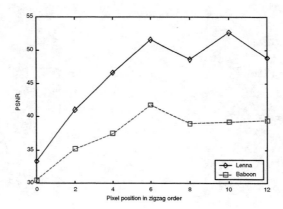

Figure 4: The effects of watermark embedding on PSNR.

The results are shown in Figures 5 (a), (b), and (c). From Figures 5 (a) and (b), it is obvious that watermarks embedded at lower frequencies are more robust than watermarks embedded at higher frequencies. Also, Figure 5 (c), with $i_0 = 10$, shows that the watermark in *baboon* is more robust to JPEG compression attacks than the one in *lena*. This is because the watermark in *baboon*, as described above, is embedded stronger due to the spatial masking used during watermark embedding. The final experiment studies watermark robustness to additive noise attacks. The watermarked images ($i_0 = 10$) are attacked by additive Gaussian noise at different energy levels. The results are presented in Figure 5 (d). It is easy to see from this figure that the watermarked images are very robust to additive noise attacks.

4. CONCLUSIONS

In this paper, we have proposed a fast and robust JPEG domain image watermarking method. The proposed method can be implemented very efficiently, requiring approximately 50ms to embed or extract a watermark using a 700MHz computer. The embedded watermark was experimentally shown to be robust to JPEG compression and additive noise attacks, and can be extracted without reference to the original (unwatermarked) image and embedding parameters. Also, the experiments described here show that embedding watermarks in coefficients, which are "important" for the image, are more likely to retain embedded watermark data, despite attacks that result in visually unimportant distortions. Correct choices for the threshold values T_1 and T_2 are of fundamental importance for watermark invisibility and good detector/extractor performance. It is possible to adjust the threshold values according to different image features, and even add additional threshold level. Methods for automatically selecting threshold values based on image parameters is a direction for future research.

REFERENCES

1. G. L. Heileman, C. E. Pizano, and C. T. Abdallah, "Image watermarking for copyright protection," in *Lecture Notes in Computer Science 1619, Algorithm Engineering and Experimentation: International Workshop ALENEX 99*, M. T. Goodrich and C. C. McGeoch, eds., pp. 226–245, Springer-Verlag, Berlin, 1999.
2. J. Huang, Y. Q. Shi, and Y. Shi, "Embedding image watermarks in DC components," *IEEE Trans. on circuits and systems for video technology* **10**, pp. 974–979, 2000.
3. C. Y. Lin and S. F. Chang, "A robust image authentication method distinguishing JPEG compression from malicious manipulation," *IEEE Trans. on circuits and systems for video technology* **11**, pp. 153–168, 2001.
4. G. C. Langelaar and R. L. Lagendijk, "Optimal differential energy watermarking of DCT encoded images and video," *IEEE Trans. on image processing* **10**, pp. 148–158, 2001.

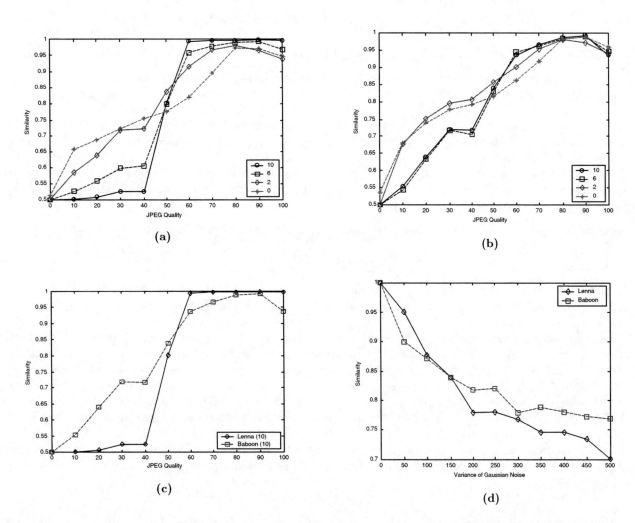

Figure 5. Comparison of watermark robustness to JPEG compression relative to watermark position in (a) lena and (b) baboon. (c) Comparison of watermark robustness to JPEG compression relative to specific images (with different texture components). (d) Comparison of watermark robustness to additive noise attack for the watermarked *lenna* and *baboon* images.

Optimizing feature selection across a multimodality database in computerized classification of breast lesions

Karla Horsch[a], Alfredo Fredy Ceballos[a], Maryellen L. Giger[a], Ioana Bonta[a],
Zhimin Huo[a], Carl J. Vyborny[a], Edward Hendrick[b] and Li Lan[a]

[a]Department of Radiology, University of Chicago, Chicago, IL
[b]Lynn Sage Breast Center, Northwestern University, Chicago, IL

ABSTRACT

Linear step-wise feature selection is performed for computerized analysis methods on a set of mammography features using a database of mammography cases, a set of ultrasound features using a database of ultrasound cases, and a set of mammography and sonography features using a multi-modality database of lesions with both mammograms and sonograms. The large mammography and sonography databases were randomly split 20 times into three subdatabases for feature selection, classifier training and independent validation. The average validation A_z value over the 20 random splits for the mammography database was 0.82 ± 0.04 and for the sonography database was 0.85 ± 0.03. The average consistency feature selection A_z value for the mammography and sonography databases were 0.87 ± 0.02 and 0.88 ± 0.02, respectively. For the mulit-modality database, the consistency feature selection A_z value was 0.93.

Keywords: feature selection, computer-aided diagnosis, mammography, ultrasound

1. INTRODUCTION

Feature selection is an important part of defining successful classifiers. Previously, we developed features for differentiating malignant and benign breast lesions on mammography[1,2] and on sonography.[3,4] In both studies, fifteen features were developed and a subset was selected based on individual A_z values and judgement of the researchers. In this study, we present results of formal feature selection for computerized analysis methods on the fifteen mammography features using the mammography database, the fifteen ultrasound features using the ultrasound database, and a subset of the mammography and sonography features using a combined database of lesions with both mammograms and sonograms. For each of the feature sets and databases, linear step-wise feature selection using the Wilks lambda criterion was performed. The individual databases for mammography and sonography are large and thus each could be randomly split into three subdatabases: one for feature selection, one for training the classifier (linear discriminant) and one for performing independent validation. The combined database is not currently large enough to split into three subdatabases and obtain meaningful results. Therefore, only feature selection was performed with this multi-modality database.

2. DATABASES

The mammography database consists of 369 biopsy proven cases, including 193 benign lesions and 176 malignant lesions. The ultrasound database consists of 458 biopsy proven cases, including 143 complex cysts, 208 benign solid lesions and 107 malignant lesions. The common database having cases with both mammograms and sonograms of the breast consists of 102 cases including 25 complex cysts, 35 benign solid lesions and 42 malignant lesions.

3. FEATURES

The fifteen mammographic features include 8 spiculation features, 5 density features, 1 shape feature and 1 margin sharpness feature.[1] The fifteen sonographic features include 3 shape features, 4 margin features, 4 texture features and 4 posterior acoustic behavior (PAB) features, some of which are described in the references.[3,4] The features are computed for each image. For classification, a particular feature value for a given lesion is the average of that feature over all the views available for the lesion.

Medical Imaging 2002: Image Processing, Milan Sonka, J. Michael Fitzpatrick,
Editors, Proceedings of SPIE Vol. 4684 (2002) © 2002 SPIE · 1605-7422/02/$15.00

Mammographic Database

Lesion Type	Entire Database	Feature Selection Database	Classifier Training Database	Validation Database
Benign Lesions	193	80	57	56
Malignant Lesions	176	70	53	53
Total	369	150	110	109

Sonographic Database

Lesion Type	Entire Database	Feature Selection Database	Classifier Training Database	Validation Database
Cysts	143	48	48	47
Benign Solid Lesions	208	69	69	70
Malignant Lesions	107	36	36	35
Total	458	153	153	152

Table 1. Random selection for splitting the mammographic and sonographic databases in three: the feature selection database, the training database and the validation database.

4. FEATURE SELECTION

Stepwise features selection was employed using the Wilks lambda criterion,[5, 6] with linear discriminant analysis (LDA) being used to determine the classifier in the task of distinguishing malignant and benign lesions. In general, if there are a total of P features, step-wise feature selection involves:

- Step 1

  - Determine the performance of each of the the P features.
  - The feature that has the best performance is selected.

- Step n

  - Assume that m is the number of features that have at one time been added to the feature set. Determine $P - m$ linear discriminants by adding each of the remaining $P - m$ features to the selected feature set.
  - Add a feature: The feature whose addition most improves the performance of the linear classifier is added to the selected feature set if its contribution to the performance is statistically significant.
  - Remove a feature: The feature that contributes least to the performance of the linear classifier is removed from the selected feature set if the contribution of that feature is not statistically significant.

- Repeat the procedure described in step n until no more features are added or removed.

The statistic that we use to measure the performance of the linear classifier is the Wilks lambda statistic[5]:

$$\Lambda = \frac{\sum_{j=1}^{N_t} (t_j - \bar{t})^2 + \sum_{j=1}^{N_f} (f_j - \bar{f})^2}{\sum_{j=1}^{N_t} (t_j - a)^2 + \sum_{j=1}^{N_f} (f_j - a)^2} \tag{1}$$

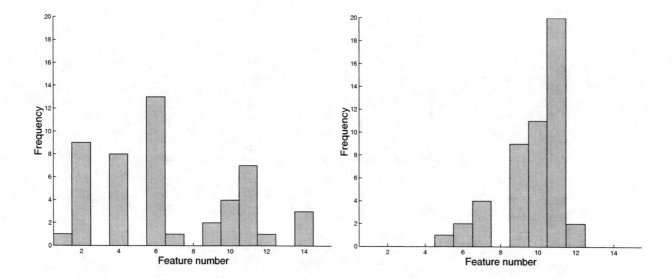

Figure 1. 1. Histogram of the selected mammographic features for the 20 feature selection subdatabases. Features 1-8 are spiculation features, 9-13 are density features, 14 is a margin sharpness feature and 15 is a size feature. 2. Histogram of the selected sonographic features for the 20 feature selection subdatabases. Features 1-4 are margin sharpness features, 5-8 are posterior acoustic behavior features, 9-11 are shape features and 12-15 are texture features.

where t_j and f_j are the discriminant scores for the malignant and benign cases, respectively, and N_t and N_f are the number of malignant and benign cases, respectively. The mean discriminant scores for the malignant, benign and all cases are $\bar{t}$, $\bar{f}$ and a, respectively. The smaller the Wilks lambda value, the greater the separation between the mean discriminant scores of malignant and benign cases. Therefore, in step n, the feature i that may be added to or removed from the feature selection set is the feature whose corresponding Wilks lambda is a minimum. During the "add a feature" phase of step n, Λ is computed from the discriminant scores that merge all the selected features *plus feature i*. During the "remove a feature" phase of step n, Λ is computed from the discriminant scores that merge all the selected features *except feature i*. To determine whether a particular feature i contributes significantly to the performance of the linear classifier in step n, we use the test statistic[5]

$$F_i = (N - 1 - k) \left(\frac{1 - \frac{\Lambda}{\Lambda_i}}{\frac{\Lambda}{\Lambda_i}} \right) \qquad (2)$$

where N is the total number of cases, Λ is determined from the the discriminant function that merges all k features and Λ_i is determined from the discriminant function that merges all but feature i. The value F has an F distribution with 1 and $N - 1 - k$ degrees of freedom. Large values of F indicate a large gain in separation when feature i is added or large loss in separation when feature i is removed. At a confidence level of 0.95, $F(1, N - 1 - k) \approx 4$ for $k = 1, 2, \cdots, 15$ and $N = 150$ (with the mammography cases) or $N = 153$ (with the sonography cases). Therefore, in step n,

- If $F_i > 4$, feature i is added to the selected feature set.

- If $F_i < 4$, feature i is removed from the selected feature set.

5. RESULTS AND DISCUSSION

The mammography database was randomly split 20 times into 3 subdatabases, one each for feature selection, classifier training and validation. The split roughly preserved the proportions of benign and malignant lesions

Split	Selected Mammographic Feature Set				Λ	A_z	A_z (Training)	A_z (Validation)
1	4 (Spiculation) (7.70)	6 (Spiculation) (6.49)	11 (Density) (5.85)		0.57	0.89	0.89	0.76
2	4 (Spiculation) (7.58)	6 (Spiculation) (4.41)			0.61	0.87	0.87	0.78
3	6 (Spiculation) (7.54)	10 (Density) (4.35)	4 (Spiculation) (4.12)		0.61	0.87	0.85	0.84
4	4 (Spiculation) (9.12)	10 (Density) (5.89)	6 (Spiculation) (4.39)		0.60	0.88	0.87	0.82
5	4 (Spiculation) (95.35)				0.61	0.87	0.83	0.79
6	2 (Spiculation) (29.74)	1 (Spiculation) (6.79)			0.62	0.87	0.82	0.81
7	2 (Spiculation) (13.89)	6 (Spiculation) (6.06)	9 (Spiculation) (5.07)		0.54	0.91	0.86	0.78
8	6 (Spiculation) (13.21)	14 (Margin) (12.42)	4 (Spiculation) (6.31)	7 (Spiculation) (4.95)	0.54	0.84	0.82	0.83
9	11 (Density) (15.20)	6 (Spiculation) (7.84)	2 (Spiculation) (3.91)		0.67	0.84	0.86	0.90
10	6 (Spiculation) (97.38)	10 (Density) (8.45)			0.58	0.89	0.79	0.87
11	2 (Spiculation) (77.65)				0.61	0.84	0.83	0.83
12	6 (Spiculation) (8.15)	2 (Spiculation) (6.81)	11 (Density) (5.42)		0.85	0.87	0.89	0.79
13	4 (Spiculation) (66.82)	10 (Density) (11.75)	9 (Spiculation) (5.89)		0.71	0.86	0.87	0.81
14	2 (Spiculation) (79.92)	11 (Density) (4.6)			0.71	0.85	0.82	0.86
15	2 (Spiculation) (118.89)				0.55	0.90	0.76	0.81
16	6 (Spiculation) (92.16)	14 (Margin) (9.24)	11 (Density) (7.16)		0.57	0.90	0.79	0.86
17	11 (Density) (15.79)	6 (Spiculation) (7.57)	12 (Density) (5.86)	2 (Spiculation) (5.21)	0.60	0.87	0.90	0.84
18	4 (Spiculation) (8.69)	11 (Density) (7.36)	6 (Spiculation) (5.48)		0.56	0.89	0.86	0.78
19	2 (Spiculation) (87.81)	14 (Margin) (10.33)			0.60	0.88	0.81	0.83
20	6 (Spiculation) (64.00)				0.70	0.83	0.89	0.81
Mean						0.87 ± 0.02	0.84 ± 0.04	0.82 ± 0.04

Table 2. Results of feature selection from the 15 mammographic features for each of the 20 randomized splits of the mammographic database. The A_z value of the linear classifier that merges the selected features is given for the feature selection, classifier training and validation databases. The numbers in parentheses are the F values associated with deleting that particular feature from the linear classifier.

Split	Feature Selection				Training	Validation
	Selected Sonographic Feature Set		Λ	A_z	A_z	A_z
1	10 (Shape) (29.78) 11 (Shape) (29.14)			0.75	0.83	0.87	0.89
2	9 (Shape) (53.78) 11 (Shape) (21.73)			0.66	0.89	0.88	0.83
3	10 (Shape) (42.44) 11 (Shape) (32.59)			0.69	0.88	0.87	0.83
4	9 (Shape) (17.53) 11 (Shape) (17.46) 7 (PAB) (13.58) 5 (PAB) (6.37) 12 (Texture) (4.23)			0.62	0.90	0.89	0.84
5	10 (Shape) (25.09) 11 (Shape) (21.75) 6 (PAB) (4.01)			0.63	0.91	0.83	0.86
6	9 (Shape) (13.13) 11 (Shape) (12.79) 7 (PAB) (7.45) 6 (PAB) (4.46)			0.71	0.86	0.88	0.90
7	9 (Shape) (41.47) 11 (Shape) (16.27)			0.71	0.86	0.83	0.90
8	9 (Shape) (18.85) 11 (Shape) (6.59) 7 (PAB) (4.47)			0.73	0.85	0.90	0.87
9	10 (Shape) (50.45) 11 (Shape) (37.64)			0.67	0.88	0.85	0.86
10	10 (Shape) (42.20) 11 (Shape) (36.64)			0.66	0.89	0.84	0.84
11	10 (Shape) (36.28) 11 (Shape) (20.42)			0.74	0.86	0.89	0.85
12	10 (Shape) (50.87) 11 (Shape) (43.10) 12 (Texture) (5.26)			0.65	0.90	0.82	0.87
13	9 (Shape) (41.37) 11 (Shape) (15.72)			0.71	0.86	0.88	0.86
14	11 (Shape) (23.82) 10 (Shape) (17.56) 7 (PAB) (4.92)			0.71	0.89	0.85	0.87
15	9 (Shape) (35.80) 11 (Shape) (18.60)			0.72	0.85	0.88	0.84
16	9 (Shape) (35.16) 11 (Shape) (18.34)			0.72	0.85	0.86	0.88
17	11 (Shape) (45.97) 10 (Shape) (33.03)			0.69	0.88	0.80	0.90
18	10 (Shape) (45.95) 11 (Shape) (21.37)			0.71	0.86	0.91	0.82
19	9 (Shape) (61.63) 11 (Shape) (32.87)			0.62	0.89	0.85	0.82
20	10 (Shape) (92.72) 11 (Shape) (38.18)			0.56	0.93	0.87	0.78
Mean					0.88 ± 0.02	0.86 ± 0.03	0.85 ± 0.03

Table 3. Results of feature selection from the 15 sonographic features for each of the 20 randomized splits of the sonographic database. The A_z value of the linear classifier that merges the selected features is given for the feature selection, classifier training and validation databases. The numbers in parentheses are the F values associated with deleting that particular feature from the linear classifier.

Initial feature set	Selected feature set			Wilks	Consistency A_z
15 Mammographic features	Mammo 4 (Spiculation) (42.97)			0.70	0.82
15 Sonographic features	US 10 (Shape) (51.74)	US 11 (Shape) (37.27)		0.55	0.90
All 30 features	US 9 (Shape) (33.89)	Mammo 4 (Spiculation) (21.47)	US 11 (Shape) (15.15)	0.47	0.93
Mammo 4, 9, 10 US 9, 10, 11	US 9 (Shape) (33.89)	Mammo 4 (Spiculation) (21.47)	US 11 (Shape) (15.15)	0.47	0.93

Table 4. Results of feature selection on different inital feature sets using the multi-modality database of 102 cases. The Wilks lambda and consistency A_z values of the linear classifier that merges the selected features are given. The numbers in parentheses are the F values associated with deleting that particular feature from the linear classifier.

as shown in Table 1. The sonography database was also randomly split 20 times into 3 subdatabases roughly preserving the proportions of cysts, benign solid lesions and malignant lesions as shown in Table 1.

For each of the 20 random splits, for both the mammographic and sonographic databases, feature selection, classifier training and validation was performed. The Wilks lambda value was computed for the selected features for each of the 20 random splits. In addition, the F values associated with deleting a feature from the linear classifier were computed. Receiver operating characteristic (ROC) analysis[7] was used to evaluate the performance the linear classifier in the task of distinguishing benign from malignant lesions. The area under the ROC curve (A_z) was used as an indicator of merit. Consistency A_z values were computed for the linear classifier trained on the "feature selection" database and for the linear classifier trained on the "classifier training" database. Finally, the A_z value for the linear classifier trained on the training database and tested on the validation database was determined. These results are given for the mammography database in Table 2 and for the sonography database in Table 3.

Shown in Figure 1 are histograms giving the selection frequency of each of the mammographic features and each of the sonographic features. The top three most selected mammographic features were, from most often selected to least often selected, two spiculation features and a texture feature. The top three most selected sonographic features were a shape feature quantifying the average orientation of gray level gradients along the margin, and two lesion depth-to-width ratio shape features.

We then performed feature selection on the initial feature set of 30 multi-modality features using the combined, multi-modality database of 102 cases. The selected features were a mamographic spiculation feature, a sonographic lesion depth-to-width ratio shape feature and a sonographic shape feature quantifying the average orientation of gray level gradients along the margin. The Wilks lambda statistic for these selected features was 0.47 and the consistency A_z value was 0.93. As the probability of selecting an optimal set of features from such a large inital feature set is small,[8] we also performed feature selection on an initial feature set of six consisting of the top three most selected mammographic and sonographic features. The same features were chosen as when the inital feature set consisted of all 30 multi-modality features. As a basis for comparison, using the mulit-modality database, feature selection was performed on the fifteen mammographic features and on the fifteen sonographic features to yield consistency A_z values of 0.82 and 0.90, respectively. These results are shown in Table 4.

6. SUMMARY

We have investigated linear step-wise feature selection on a set of mammography features, a set of ultrasound features and a subset of mammography and sonography features. Feature selection, linear classifier training and validation performed on the mammographic features using the mammographic database produced average A_z values of 0.87, 0.84 and 0.82, respectively. The two mammographic features most often selected were measures of spiculation. Feature selection, linear classifier training and validation performed on the sonographic features using the sonographic database produced average A_z values of 0.88, 0.86 and 0.85, respectively. The two sonographic features most often selected were two shape features: one quantifying the lesion depth-to-width ratio and the other quantifying the average orientation of gray level gradients along the margin. Feature selection performed on the multi-modality features produced a consistency A_z value 0.93. For the feature sets considered in this study, the multi-modality features selected using the multi-modality database were a subset of the mammographic and sonographic features most often selected using the mammographic and sonographic databases. The results of this study suggest that using both mammographic and sonographic features improves the performance of linear classifiers in the task of distinguishing malignant from benign lesions.

Acknowledgement Some of the results in this paper were generated using a linear stepwise feature selection code written in Matlab by M. A. Kupinski. This work was supported in parts by USPHS grants CA 89452 and T32 CA09649 and by US Army Medical Research and Material Command grant 97-2445.

M. L. Giger Z. Huo and C. J. Vyborny are shareholders in R2 Technology, Inc. (Los Altos, CA). It is the University of Chicago Conflict of Interest Policy that investigators disclose publicly actual or potential significant financial interest which would reasonably appear to be directly and significantly affected by the research activities.

REFERENCES

1. Z. Huo, *Computerized methods for classification of masses and analysis of parenchymal patterns on digitized mamograms.* PhD thesis, University of Chicago, 1988.

2. Z. Huo, M. L. Giger, C. J. Vyborny, and et el, "Analysis of spiculation in the computerized classification of mammographic masses," *Med Phys* **22**, pp. 1569–1579, 1995.

3. M. L. Giger, H. Al-Hallaq, Z. Huo, C. Moran, D. E. Wolverton, C. W. Chan, and W. Zhong, "Computerized analysis of lesions in us images of the breast," *Acad Radiol* **6**, pp. 665–674, 1999.

4. K. Horsch, M. L. Giger, L. A. Venta, and C. J. Vyborny, "Computerized diagnosis of breast lesions on ultrasound," *Medical Physics* , in press.

5. C. J. Huberty, *Applied Discriminant Analysis*, John Wiley and Sons, Inc., 1994.

6. P. L. Lachenbruch, *Discriminant Analysis*, Hafner, London, England, 1975.

7. C. E. Metz, "Some practical issues of experimental design and data analysis in radiological roc studies," *Invest Radiol* **24**, pp. 234–245, 1989.

8. M. A. Kupinski and M. L. Giger, "Feature selection on limited databases," *Med Phys* **26**, pp. 2176–2182, 1999.

Fuzzy clustering of fMRI data: towards a theoretical basis for choosing the fuzziness index

Martin Buerki[a], Helmut Oswald[b], Gerhard Schroth[a]

[a]University Hospital of Berne, Department of Neuroradiology, 3010 Bern, Switzerland
[b]T-Systems Health Care Systems AG, 3007 Bern, Switzerland

ABSTRACT

The fuzzy clustering algorithm (FCA) is a promising approach for the unsupervised analysis of complex fMRI studies with unknown input functions. Among the few parameters required by the FCA, the fuzziness index m plays an important role and the outcome of the clustering depends strongly on it. Unfortunately, there is no theoretical basis currently known for choosing the value of m and so far, empirical approaches have been carried out to find a reasonable value. The theoretical approach presented here calculates the probability distribution of the membership values u_{ij} during one iteration of the FCA and judges the regularity of this distribution, therefore indicating the degree of fuzziness of the resulting partition. This allows us to estimate the compactness of the clusters. It turns out that this probability does not only depend on the fuzziness index m, but also on the length of the time courses, a fact that was until now not noticed. Consequently, a reasonable choice of the fuzziness index depends on the signal to noise ratio and the temporal dimension of the data.

Keywords: functional MRI, fuzzy clustering, fuzziness index

1. INTRODUCTION

In functional MRI, activation patterns are usually retrieved by voxel-wise testing for correlation of the measurements with a paradigm-defined input function (e.g. SPM[1]). In contrast to these standard analysis tools, the fuzzy clustering algorithm[2] (FCA) is a way of investigating complex data without imposing prior assumptions on the results that are searched for. It has been shown that the FCA can reliably detect activation patterns[3,4], even under hard conditions and in complex studies where several different functional components are involved[5]. Furthermore, the FCA has been extended to a multiresolution algorithm in the context of medical imaging to improve stability and performance[6,7].

The FCA based analysis of fMRI time series considers each of the N voxel time-course as a P-dimensional vector $x = (x_1, ..., x_P)$, where N is the number of voxels making up the volume of one MR acquisition and P is the number of acquisitions. The algorithm aims to find C vectors $v_1, ..., v_C$ – the prototypes or centroids for C different clusters – such that the objective function

$$J_m(U,V) = \sum_{i=1}^{N} \sum_{j=1}^{C} (u_{ij})^m d^2(\mathbf{x}_i, \mathbf{v}_j)$$

(1)

is minimized. The scalars $u_{ij} \in [0, 1]$ describe the degree of membership of the time-course x_i to the j-th cluster , where $u_{ij} = 1$ means exclusive membership and $u_{ij} = 0$ is no membership.

d^2 is any inner product metric on $\mathbf{R}^P$ and V represents the set of centroids $v_1, ..., v_C$. The real number $m>1$ is called the fuzziness index. This parameter regulates the fuzziness of the clustering and will be discussed in detail in the main sections of this paper.

Necessary conditions for minimizing J_m are:

$$u_{ij} = \frac{1}{\sum_{k=1}^{C} \left(\frac{d_{ij}}{d_{ik}} \right)^{2/(m-1)}} , \quad 1 \le i \le N, \ 1 \le j \le C, \qquad \text{where } d_{ij} = d(\mathbf{x}_i, \mathbf{v}_j),$$

(2)

and

Corresponding author: M. Buerki. E-mail: martin.buerki@insel.ch

$$\mathbf{v}_j = \frac{\sum_{i=1}^{N}\left(u_{ij}\right)^m \mathbf{x}_k}{\sum_{i=1}^{N}\left(u_{ij}\right)^m} \ , \qquad 1 \le j \le C \ . \tag{3}$$

A local minimum is found by iteratively computing the centroids $\mathbf{v}_1, \ldots, \mathbf{v}_C$ and the membership matrix $U = [\ u_{ij}\ ]$ by equations (2) and (3) until the distance between two consecutively calculated membership matrices $U^{(k)}$ and $U^{(k+1)}$ is less than a defined threshold, i.e.

$$\Delta U = \left\| U^{(k+1)} - U^{(k)} \right\| \le \varepsilon \ , \tag{4}$$

where the threshold is a small number, e.g. $\varepsilon = 0.01$.

2. FINDING THE OPTIMAL CHOICE FOR THE FUZZINESS INDEX

Among the few parameters involved with the FCA, the fuzziness index m plays an important role. It is well known and easily verified that small values for m (i.e. m near 1) lead to a hard partitioning of the data while for $m \rightarrow \infty$, all centroids tend towards the center of the whole dataset. To illustrate this point, consider a 2D-dataset $X = X_1 \cup X_2$ of two normally distributed subsets $X_1, X_2 \subset \mathbf{R}^2$, $|X_1| = |X_2| = 200$, with centers (0/0) and (2/0), respectively. Thus, the mean distance between the subsets is $d = 2$.

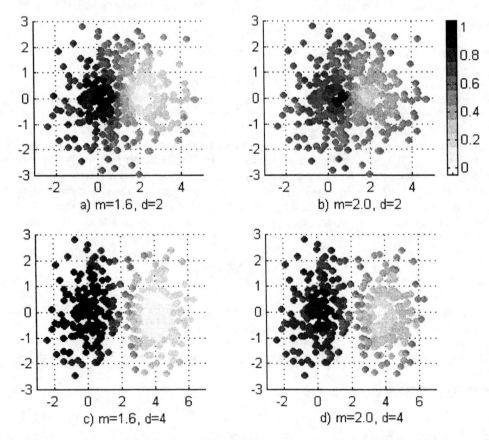

Figure 1. Membership maps of cluster 1 for the dataset X described in the text. Dark colors indicate a high degree of membership. A high contrast in grayscales corresponds to a well separation of the clusters. a) Fuzziness index m=1.6, distance between centers of subsets d=2, b) m=2.0, d=2, c) m=1.6, d=4, d) m=2.0, d=4.

The outcome of the FCA applied to X with different fuzziness indices is shown in Figure 1a) and Figure 1b). When choosing a fuzziness index $m = 1.6$, the FCA yields two well-separated clusters, but setting $m = 2.0$ results in two largely overlapping clusters without significant distinction. As shown in Figure 1c) and Figure 1d), the situation changes when the SNR is altered. Here X_2 has the center (4/0), i.e. the mean distance between the subsets is $d = 4$. The influence of the fuzziness index m to the resulting clustering is again clearly visible. When setting m = 1.6, the boundaries between the clusters are sharp and the classification of the data points between both centroids is too binary. With m = 2.0, the boundaries of the clusters are smoother, but they are still well separated. Note that for both choices of m, the regions with high and low membership values are growing when the SNR increases. This shows that the choice of the fuzziness index depends on the SNR of the dataset under investigation.

Unfortunately, there is no theoretical basis currently known for choosing the value of m and so far, empirical approaches have been carried out to find a reasonable value[8]. The outcome of this was that the widely used value around 2.0 is a good choice. But depending on the metric used in the FCA, others have found lower values to be a good choice[9]. In this work, we propose a theoretical approach for this problem and discuss the parameters that affect an optimal choice for the fuzziness index. We currently restrict ourselves to the case with number of clusters $C = 2$, leaving the general case for future work.

To start, consider a set $X_1 \subset \mathbf{R}^P$ of P-dimensional normally distributed random vectors with mean $\mathbf{m}_1$ and standard deviation s_1, $|X_1| = N_1$. Note that $\mathbf{m}_1$ is again a vector of dimension P. Analogous, consider a set $X_2 \subset \mathbf{R}^P$ of normally distributed random vectors with mean $\mathbf{m}_2$ and standard deviation s_2, $|X_2| = N_2$.

Thus, X_1 and X_2 are two classes of time courses with some gaussian noise added. The assumption of gaussian noise is commonly used, but not mandatory for our approach. As will be clear from what follows, any noise model could be used provided that the probability density function of the noise is known.

Let $X = X_1 \cup X_2$ be the dataset to be clustered by the FCA. Without loss of generality, we can – after a possible translation and rotation of the dataset – assume that $\mathbf{m}_1 = \mathbf{0}$ and $\mathbf{m}_2 = (d, 0, ..., 0)$, where d is the mean distance between the sets X_1 and X_2.

Now we aim to estimate the probability that the membership value u_{ij} will fall within a certain range when calculated by equation (2). In order to have clearly defined conditions, we initialize the algorithm by $v_j = \mathbf{m}_j, j = 1,2$, i.e. we start with the centroids corresponding to the centers of the subsets X_1 and X_2.

For any $\mathbf{x}_i \in X_1$, the membership value $u = u_{i1}$ is

$$u = \cfrac{1}{1 + \left(\cfrac{\displaystyle\sum_{j=1}^{P} x_j^2}{(x_1 - d)^2 + \displaystyle\sum_{j=2}^{P} x_j^2} \right)^{\frac{1}{m-1}}} \tag{5}$$

where each component x_j from $\mathbf{x}_i$ is a normally distributed random variable and thus, u is a function of P independent random variables, $u = f(x_1, ..., x_P)$.

Lemma 1. Let $X = X_1 \cup X_2$ as defined above and let $v_j = \mathbf{m}_j, j = 1,2$. Set $q = \left(\cfrac{1}{U} - 1 \right)^{m-1}$. Then for $u = f(x_1, ..., x_P)$ defined by equation (5), the following holds:

a) if $0 < U < 0.5$:

$$P_{X_1}(u \leq U) = \int\limits_{x_1 \in A_1} \cdots \int\limits_{x_P \in A_P} \frac{1}{(2\pi)^{P/2} s_1^P} e^{-\frac{1}{2s_1^2} \sum_{j=1}^{P} x_j^2} dx_P .. dx_1 . \tag{6}$$

where the domain of integration is given by

$$A_1 = \left[\frac{d(q-\sqrt{q})}{q-1}, \frac{d(q+\sqrt{q})}{q-1} \right],$$

(7)

$$A_i = \left\{ x_i \;\middle|\; |x_i| \leq \sqrt{\frac{q(2dx_1 - d^2) + (1-q)\sum_{j=1}^{i-1} x_j^2}{q-1}} \right\}, \qquad i = 2, \ldots, P,$$

Thus, the domain of integration is a P-dimensional spheroid containing the vector v_2.

b) if $U = 0.5$:

$$P_{X_1}(u \leq 0.5) = \int\limits_{x_1 \geq \frac{d}{2}} \int\limits_{x_2 = -\infty}^{\infty} \cdots \int\limits_{x_P = -\infty}^{\infty} \frac{1}{(2\pi)^{P/2} s_1^P} e^{-\frac{1}{2s_1^2} \sum_{j=1}^{P} x_j^2} \, dx_P \ldots dx_1,$$

(8)

and the domain of integration is the P-dimensional half space $x_1 \geq \dfrac{d}{2}$.

c) if $0.5 < U \leq 1$:

$$P_{X_1}(u \leq U) = 1 - P_{X_1}(u \geq U) = 1 - \int\limits_{x_1 \in A_1} \cdots \int\limits_{x_P \in A_P} \frac{1}{(2\pi)^{P/2} s_1^P} e^{-\frac{1}{2s_1^2} \sum_{j=1}^{P} x_j^2} \, dx_P \ldots dx_1$$

(9)

where the domain of integration is again given by equations (7).

Proof. From the theory of probability, the cumulative probability of a function of P independent gaussian random variables with standard deviation s is

$$P(u \leq U) = \int\limits_{x_1 = -\infty}^{\infty} \cdots \int\limits_{x_{P-1} = -\infty}^{\infty} \int\limits_{x_P \in A_U} \frac{1}{(2\pi)^{P/2} s^P} e^{-\frac{1}{2s^2} \sum_{j=1}^{P} x_j^2} \, dx_P \ldots dx_1,$$

where $A_U = \left\{ x_P \;\middle|\; f(x_1, \ldots, x_P) \leq U \right\}$. Setting $q = \left(\dfrac{1}{U} - 1 \right)^{m-1}$ and solving

$$f(x_1, \ldots, x_P) = \frac{1}{1 + \left(\dfrac{\sum_{j=1}^{P} x_j^2}{(x_1 - d)^2 + \sum_{j=2}^{P} x_j^2} \right)^{\frac{1}{m-1}}} \leq U$$

for x_p yields

$$x_P{}^2(q-1) \leq q(2dx_1 - d^2) + (1-q)\sum_{j=1}^{P-1} x_j{}^2 \qquad (10)$$

Since U<0.5 and positive, $(q-1)$ is strictly positive. Therefore,

$$|x_P| \leq \sqrt{\frac{q(2dx_1 - d^2) + (1-q)\sum_{j=1}^{P-1} x_j{}^2}{q-1}}$$

for the innermost boundaries of integration. The expression above is only defined, if

$$q(2dx_1 - d^2) + (1-q)\sum_{j=1}^{P-1} x_j{}^2 \geq 0.$$

From this, we get the boundaries for each component x_i, $i=2,\ldots,P$, iteratively as

$$|x_i| \leq \sqrt{\frac{q(2dx_1 - d^2) + (1-q)\sum_{j=1}^{i-1} x_j{}^2}{q-1}}, \qquad i = 2, \ldots, P.$$

For the boundaries for x_1, we finally have to solve the quadratic equation

$$q(2dx_1 - d^2) + (1-q)x_1{}^2 \geq 0$$

to find the solution stated in the lemma.

b) For the special case $U = 0.5$, which is equivalent to $(q - 1) = 0$, equation (10) reduces to $0 \leq 2dx_1 - d^2$. Thus, the domain of integration is the P-dimensional half space $x_1 \geq \dfrac{d}{2}$.

c) Due to the topology of the domain of integration, it is more convenient to calculate the probability for $U > 0.5$ indirectly. To determine the domain of integration, we now have to solve $A_U = \{x_P \mid f(x_1,\ldots,x_P) \geq U\}$ for x_P. This yields

$$x_P{}^2(q-1) \geq q(2dx_1 - d^2) + (1-q)\sum_{j=1}^{P-1} x_j{}^2.$$

Note that this time, $(q - 1)$ is strictly negative. Thus we get again

$$|x_P| \leq \sqrt{\frac{q(2dx_1 - d^2) + (1-q)\sum_{j=1}^{P-1} x_j{}^2}{q-1}}.$$

The rest is similar to part a) and this finishes the proof.

On the other hand, for any $x_i \in X_2$, the membership value $u = u_{i1}$ is

$$u = \cfrac{1}{1 + \left(\cfrac{(x_1 + d)^2 + \sum\limits_{j=2}^{P} x_j^2}{\sum\limits_{j=1}^{P} x_j^2} \right)^{\frac{1}{m-1}}} \tag{11}$$

Similar to the case $x_i \in X_1$ discussed above, we can express the probability $P_{X_2}(u < U)$.

Lemma 2. Set $q = \left(\dfrac{1}{U} - 1 \right)^{m-1}$.

a) If $U < 0.5$, then

$$P_{X_2}(u \leq U) = \int\limits_{x_1 \in A_1} \cdots \int\limits_{x_P \in A_P} \frac{1}{(2\pi)^{P/2} s_1^P} e^{-\frac{1}{2s_2^2} \sum\limits_{j=1}^{P} x_j^2} \, dx_P \ldots dx_1 \tag{12}$$

with the domain of integration given by

$$A_1 = \left[\frac{d(1 - \sqrt{q})}{q - 1}, \frac{d(1 + \sqrt{q})}{q - 1} \right],$$

$$A_i = \left\{ x_i \,\middle|\, |x_i| \leq \sqrt{\frac{2dx_1 + d^2 + (1 - q)\sum\limits_{j=1}^{i-1} x_j^2}{q - 1}} \right\}, \quad i = 2, \ldots, P, \tag{13}$$

b) if $U = 0.5$:

$$P_{X_2}(u \leq 0.5) = \int\limits_{x_1 \leq -\frac{d}{2}} \int\limits_{x_2 = -\infty}^{\infty} \cdots \int\limits_{x_P = -\infty}^{\infty} \frac{1}{(2\pi)^{P/2} s_1^P} e^{-\frac{1}{2s_2^2} \sum\limits_{j=1}^{P} x_j^2} \, dx_P \ldots dx_1 . \tag{14}$$

c) if $0.5 < U \leq 1$:

$$P_{X_2}(u \leq U) = 1 - P_{X_2}(u \geq U) = 1 - \int\limits_{x_1 \in A_1} \cdots \int\limits_{x_P \in A_P} \frac{1}{(2\pi)^{P/2} s_1^P} e^{-\frac{1}{2s_2^2} \sum\limits_{j=1}^{P} x_j^2} \, dx_P \ldots dx_1 \tag{15}$$

where the domain of integration is again given by equations (13).

The proof is analogous to the proof of lemma 1.

Combining the results above, we get the probability $P_X(u < U)$ for any $x_i \in X = X_1 \cup X_2$ as

$$P_X(u \leq U) = \frac{N_1 \cdot P_{X_1}(u \leq U) + N_2 \cdot P_{X_2}(u \leq U)}{N_1 + N_2}.$$ (14)

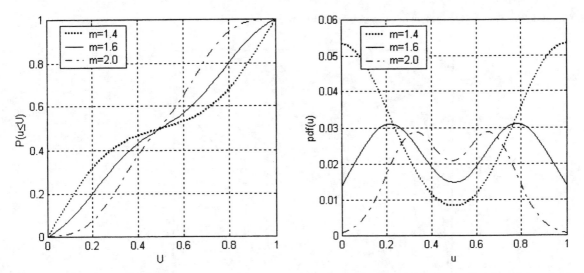

Figure 2. $P_X(u \leq U)$ for a 2-dimensional dataset (left graph) and the corresponding probability density function (right graph). $d = 2$, standard deviation $s_1 = s_2 = 1$, and $N_1 = N_2$.

Figure 2 above illustrates the shape of this function for a 2-dimensional dataset with $d = 2$ and $N_1 = N_2$ together with the derivative, which is the probability density function (pdf). We can see that there are two classes of curves represented by the dotted and the dash-dotted lines. The solid line belongs to a kind of transition zone. Recall that equation (14) yields the distribution of the membership values after the first iteration of the FCA when initialized with the centroids $v_i = m_i$. But interestingly, the shape of the function rests essentially the same during all iterations, in particular, it will always belong to the same class. For the moment, there is no rigorous proof to this conjecture, but we have not yet met any counterexample.

The dotted curve describes a distribution with a lot of very low and very high values for the degrees of membership u_{ij} and only a few intermediate values. Thus, the resulting fuzzy partitions are rather hard. The dash-dotted curve on the other hand corresponds to a distribution with most of the values being in the intermediate range. In this case, the clusters tend to have large overlap and the separation will be insufficient. The closer the curve is to the diagonal, the more evenly distributed are the membership values. Encouraged by many tests, we believe that this is the best solution. Therefore, choosing the optimal value for the fuzziness index m is equivalent to determining m such that the probability function defined in equation (14) is as close to the diagonal as possible.

We now return to the example from the beginning of this chapter. From the graphs in Figure 2, we would suggest a fuzziness index value $m \approx 1.6$ for the dataset with $d = 2$. And indeed, Figure 1 affirms this choice. For $d = 4$, our theory would suggest $m \approx 2$, which is again affirmed by Figure 1.

3. DISCUSSION AND FUTURE WORK

We have presented a theoretical approach to the problem of finding a good choice for the fuzziness index m. It is based on the estimation of the probability distribution of the fuzzy membership values calculated by equation (2) and is an *a priori* choice that depends on the expected (or estimated) SNR of the dataset. But from equations (6) and (12), it is clear that the fuzziness index not only depends on the SNR, but also on the dimension P of the time courses. This is an important fact that was not noticed until now. A noise-only dataset consisting of low-dimensional time courses can easily be separated into different clusters. To see this, consider the squared distance $d^2 = d(x,y)^2$ between two $N(0,\sigma)$-

normally distributed vectors x and y of dimension n. Since the squared norm of a random vector follows a gamma distribution, we have

$$P(d^2 \leq x) = \frac{1}{(2\sigma)^n \Gamma\left(\dfrac{n}{2}\right)} \int_0^x t^{\frac{n}{2}-1} e^{\frac{-t}{4\sigma^2}} \, dt \; .$$

The dependence of $P(d^2 \leq x)$ on the dimension n is shown in Figure 3.

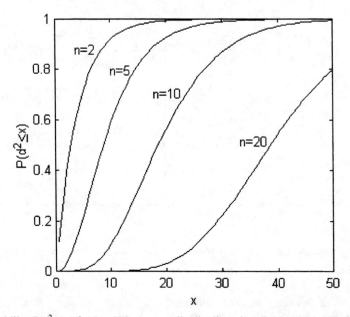

Figure 3. Probability $P(d^2 \leq x)$ for two $N(0,\sigma)$-normally distributed random vectors with dimension n and $\sigma=1$.

Another way to understand this intuitively is to consider the correlation of two vectors. The higher correlated they are, the smaller is the euclidean distance. But the probability for high correlation decreases with increasing dimension of the vectors.

Finally, we point out that this theoretical approach is on principle not limited to the case of gaussian noise. For any noise model other than gaussian noise, equations (6) and (12) simply must be altered to reflect the proper random distribution.

Currently, we are working on the following problems:

For calculating the probabilities in equation (14), we need to implement sufficiently accurate algorithms for numerical integration in high dimensions. Moreover, for practical use of the theory, we think it would be advantageous to tabulate the optimal fuzziness indices for different signal to noise ratios and dimensions. Then the theory should be extended to an arbitrary number of clusters. We should expect that this will also affect the choice of m. Third, the conjecture that the shape of the probability function keeps essentially the same through all iterations should be demonstrated.

4. REFERENCES

1. Friston K., Holmes A.P., Worsley K.J., Pioline J-B., Frith C.D., Frackowiak R.S.J., "Statistical parametric maps in functional imaging: A general linear approach.", *Human Brain Mapping* **2**, pp 189-210, 1995.
2. Bezdek J.C., *Pattern Recognition with Fuzzy Objective Function Algorithms*, Plenum Press, New York, 1981.
3. Scarth G., McIntyre M., Wowk B., Somorjai R., "Detection of novelty in functional images using fuzzy clustering", *Proc. ISMRM*, 3rd Annual Meeting, Nice, p.238, 1995.

4. Somorjai R., Jarmasz M., Baumgartner R. *EVIDENT: A Two-Stage Strategy for the Exploratory Analysis of Functional MRI Data by Fuzzy Clustering*, 2000. http://zeno.ibd.nrc.ca/informatics/pubs/2stagestrategy.pdf

5. Buerki M., Oswald H., Lovblad K. O., Schroth G., Gutbrod K., Schnider A., "Evaluation of complex fMRI designs with fuzzy clustering analysis", *ISNIP*, 6th World Congress, Bern, Switzerland, 2001.

6. Buerki M., Oswald H., Lovblad K. O., Schroth G., "Additional speed up technique to fuzzy clustering using a multi-resolution approach", *Proc. of the SPIE*, pp.1141-1150, 2001.

7. Buerki M., Kiefer C., Oswald H., Lovblad K. O., Schroth G., „Ein Vergleich verschiedener Multiresolution-Pyramiden für die Fuzzy Cluster basierte Auswertung von fMRI Studien", *ISMRM,* 4. Jahrestagung der Deutschen Sektion, Zürich, Switzerland, 2001.

8. M.J. Fadili, S. Ruan, D. Bloyet, B. Mazoyer, "A multistep unsupervised fuzzy clustering analysis of fMRI time series", *Human Brain Mapping* **10**, pp. 160-178, 2000.

9. Golay X., Kollias S., Stoll G., Meier D., Valavanis A., Boesiger P., "A New Correlation-Based Fuzzy Logic Clustering Algorithm for fMRI", *Magn. Reson. Med.* **40**, pp. 249-260, 1998.

Quantitative study of Renormalization Transformation method to correct the inhomogeneity in MR images

Qing Ji, Wilburn E. Reddick, John O. Glass, Evgeny Krynetskiy

Department of Diagnostic Imaging, St. Jude Children's Research Hospital, 332 N. Lauderdale St., Memphis, TN 38105-2794

ABSTRACT

The purpose of this work is to evaluate the effectiveness of using a newly proposed renormalization transformation (RT) technique to correct nonuniformity in MR images. Simulated brain T1, T2 and PD weighted images with two types of bias fields and Gaussian white noise were created using the average signal intensities of white matter, gray matter, and CSF from segmented masks of actual patient examinations. These images were then corrected by the RT method and quantitatively compared with the original non-biased simulated images. This study demonstrated that a single optimal correction exists for the RT method. At the optimal correction, the RT method can remove more than 75 percent of the bias field without significant loss of useful contrast in the images. Unfortunately, this optimal correction can not be directly determined for actual patient images where the truth is not known. However, simulated images showed that the optimal correction could be estimated from changes in the contrast ratio map, where the contrast ratio is the ratio of the local intensity standard deviation and local average intensity. Using the contrast ratio map, the optimal correction can be reliably applied in patient images.

Key Words: MR images, Inhomogeneity, Renormalization Transformation, Image Filter, Image Segmentation

1. INTRODUCTION

Intensity based brain tissue segmentation techniques have been used to study many clinical diseases and abnormalities. However, the performance of those techniques is significantly deteriorated by the intensity inhomogeneity of MR images particularly with newer phased-array coils. The correction techniques for the intensity inhomogeneity in MR images are usually classified into two basic categories: pre-processing and post-processing. In pre-processing techniques, the inhomogeneity, which is caused by the sensitivity profile of the coil is usually calculated based on the knowledge of the coil geometry, shape and relative position to the patient or object measured using a homogenous phantom before or after clinical imaging.[1-3] With post-processing techniques, the bias field is usually obtained from the MR image itself. Low-pass filters were commonly used in post-processing techniques.[4-5] Based on the fact that the sensitivity profile is smoothly varying within the coil, the bias field can be determined by using the low-pass filters to blur the anatomic contrast in the images. However in clinical images, the bias field always partially overlaps with the anatomic information in spatial frequency making it very difficult to separate the overlapped portion of the bias field from that of the anatomic details based on the information of the image alone. The trade-off is either loses the anatomic information or under-estimate the bias field. The ideal filtering scheme for best separating the bias field from the anatomic details in the post-processing methods is to select a proper filtering band to cover the lowest frequency portion of the bias field and exclude the majority of the anatomic details in the spatial frequency domain. The implementation of this optimal filtering scheme is very difficult with most of the previously reported low-pass filters because of the inflexibility of the filtering kernel size.

The renormalization transformation (RT) method is a newly proposed post-processing technique.[6] In contrast to previously reported low-pass filtering schemes in which the kernel size of the filters were pre-selected and fixed, the RT scheme applies a broadband low-pass filter (regional nearest neighboring average filter) multiple times to an image system. The number of the transformations determines the kernel size of the final low-pass filter. By repeatedly applying RT to an image system, the image is gradually transformed into its "equilibrium" state, which is the state that all the pixel values have the same intensity level and are equal to the global mean. In the "equilibrium" state, all the anatomic details and bias field are removed. On the other hand, for each consecutive transformation the change of the filter band is very small. The RT scheme provides a wide range of filtering band searching with a finite step size.

Even though it is possible to implement a filtering band searching scheme in the RT technique, finding the optimal filter is still an unsolved problem. The optimal filter depends on the bias field and anatomic details on each individual image. In clinical images, the bias field and the true anatomic details are unknown. To solve this problem, we propose the concept of a local contrast ratio map. The local contrast ratio is the local intensity standard deviation divided by the local average intensity. Here "local" means a specific pixel and its four nearest neighbor pixels. A 2D local contrast ratio map can be calculated from a 2D image. The local contrast ratio map records the significant contrast information in the original image. The most important characteristic of the local contrast ratio is that it is almost independent of the bias field meaning the difference between the local contrast ratio maps of a biased image and an unbiased image is very small. By monitoring the change of the local contrast ratio map for the corrected image, one may be able to maximize the recovery of useful anatomic contrast information during the correction process.

In this study, an optimal inhomogeneity correction scheme is proposed combining the RT filtering technique with the local contrast map. This scheme was tested by correcting the artificially created bias fields in simulated T1, T2 and PD weighted images. Since the bias fields in the simulated images are known, the effectiveness of this correction scheme can be evaluated quantitatively. The practical realization of this techinique was then demonstrated for an actual clinical MR image.

2. METHOD AND MATERIALS

2.1 Simulated MR Images

Simulated T1, T2 and PD weighted MR images were created from average signal intensity values in clinical images. Masks for white matter, gray matter and CSF were created from segmented images in which the scalp was striped and the partial volumes were redistributed into white matter, gray matter and CSF. The typical intensity values assigned to the white matter, gray matter and CSF tissues in T1, T2 and PD weighted images are listed in Table 1. Two types of

Table 1. The intensity values assigned to each tissue in the simulated images.

	White Matter	Gray Matter	CSF	Others
T1	570	450	310	460
T2	400	550	1100	750
PD	880	1080	1200	1030

bias fields were then created. The first bias field was obtained from an image of a uniform water phantom taken with a phased array head coil. The image was resized to match the dimension of the T1, T2 and PD weighted simulation images. The second bias field is a simple linear bias field that increases from front to back with a total variation of about 60%. Both bias fields were applied as a multiplicitive factor in the simulation images. Zero-mean Gaussian white noise was then added to the final images (Figures 1 and 2).

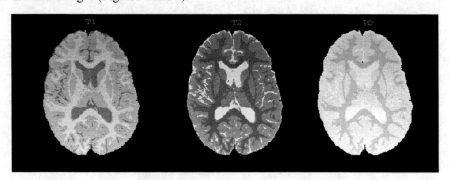

Figure 1. Simulated T1, T2 and PD images with linear bias field.

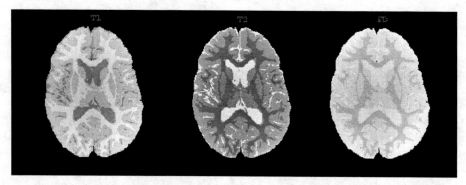

Figure 2. Simulated T1, T2 and PD images with phased array bias field.

2.2 RT Correction Scheme

As described in [6], RT is a linear transformation. If S denotes the region of interest (ROI) in an image and contains N pixels with intensity distribution $I\{I_1, I_2, ...I_N\}$, RT to the system S generates a new intensity distribution $I'\{I'_1, I'_2, ...I'_N\}$ in S.

$$I'_j = \frac{\sum_{i \in s_j} I_i}{n} \tag{1}$$

where s_j is the pixel j and its nearest neighbor pixels, n is the number of pixels in s_j. The ROI in an image can be determined by a binary mask.

The observed image is the product of the bias field $g(x,y)$ and the real tissue image $u(x,y)$ plus the noise. In the case of a noiseless system, the observed image can be expressed:

$$v(x, y) = g(x, y)u(x, y) \tag{2}$$

The bias field can be estimated by applying RT multiple times to the observed image. If T_n denotes the n times transformation, the estimated bias field $\hat{g}_n(x,y)$ can be written:

$$\hat{g}_n(x, y) = T_n(v(x, y)) \tag{3}$$

The corrected image can then be expressed:

$$\hat{u}_n(x, y) = \frac{v(x, y)}{\hat{g}_n(x, y)} v_m \tag{4}$$

where v_m is the global mean of the observed image. If the real tissue image $u(x,y)$ is known, the corrected image can be evaluated by calculating the root mean square (RMS) difference between the true image and the corrected image:

$$RMS = \sqrt{\frac{1}{N} \sum_{(x,y) \in S} (u(x, y) - \hat{u}_n(x, y))^2} \tag{5}$$

2.3 Local Contrast Ratio

For the pixel j in S, the local contrast ratio r_j can be defined:

$$r_j = \frac{\sigma_j}{\bar{I}_j} \tag{6}$$

where $\bar{I}_j$ is the average intensity of s_j and σ_j is the standard deviation. The local contrast ratios of all the pixels in an image form a 2D local contrast ratio map. It is noted that the local contrast ratio is less dependent on the bias field and reflects local intensity variation. The local contrast ratio map records the important anatomic information of the image especially in the tissue transition region. In this study, the local contrast ratio map was used to monitoring the correction process.

2.4 Test Strategy

In this study, a procedure for the evaluation of the quality of the corrected image was designed. In this procedure, the RT was applied to the biased image multiple times; after each transformation, the estimated bias field was used to correct the biased image and the corrected image was compared with the original image by calculating the RMS difference. For each corrected image, the corresponding local contrast ratio map was also generated and the total contrast ratio was immediately calculated. The number of transformations in this procedure was run 1 to 5000 times continuously. The total contrast ratio is calculated by the formula:

$$C = \sum_{(x,y)\in S} r(x, y) \tag{7}$$

3. RESULTS AND DISCUSSIONS

3.1 The Optimal Correction

The root mean square difference between the corrected image and the original image can be used to estimate the quality of the corrected image. The RMS difference is zero for a perfect correction. Figures 3 and 4 illustrate that the quality of

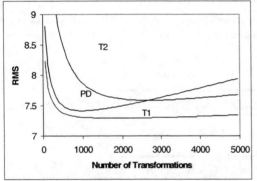

Figure 3. RMS difference versus the number of transformations for linear simulated bias field

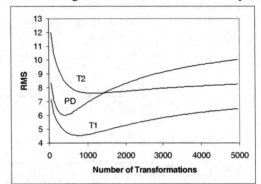

Figure 4. RMS difference versus the number of transformations for simulated phased-array coil bias field

the corrected images depends on the number of transformations used to estimate the bias field. For each image, a single optimal correction exists and is dependent on the image intensity distribution and the bias field type. The optimal numbers of transformations used for the correction are listed in Table 2.

Table 2. Optimal Number of Transformations

Image Type	Linear bias field	Phased-array coil bias field
T1	1900	750
T2	2550	1150
PD	1050	400

There are three cases when using the bias field estimated by multiple RTs. Figure 5 shows the mid-line (x = 130) intensity profiles of three corrected images with three different numbers of transformations. Figure 5 (a) shows that 200 transformations are less than optimal as the corrected image loses some anatomic contrast, and is over-corrected. Figure

5 (b) shows an under-corrected image, as the bias field was not effectively removed. This occurred because the number of transformations was greater than optimal (3000). Figure 5 (c) shows the optimal case and represents the optimal compromise between the removal of the bias field and the preservation of the contrast information of the original image. It is very important to note that even at the optimal case, the bias field is not completely removed. The removal of the bias field can be evaluated by calculating the correction rate in the corrected image. The correction rate is defined as:

$$R = \frac{n_r}{N} \tag{8}$$

Figure 5. Intensity profiles of three corrected PD images with varying number of transformations:

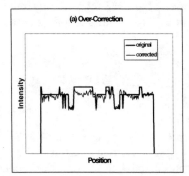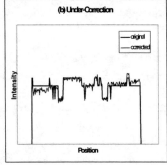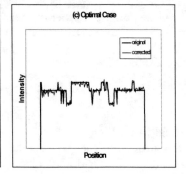

where N is the total number of pixels in the ROI, and n_r is the number of corrected pixels. A corrected pixel is a pixel whose intensity level is within 3% of the pixel value in the original image with no bias field. The correction rates at optimal correction for all corrected images are listed in Table 3.

Table 3. Correction Rate At Optimal Correction (%)

Image Type	Linear bias field	Phased Array Coil bias field
T1	85	92
T2	79	85
PD	95	98

3.2 Optimal Filtering Scheme

Over-correction and under-correction are two cases that we must avoid in using low-pass filtering technique to remove the bias field. In a real clinical image, both the true image and the bias field are unknown; therefore it is very difficult to design an optimal low-pass filter. A local contrast ratio map of the corrected image, although it is generated from the image itself, may provide additional information for the analysis of the quality of image. In Figure 6, the total contrast ratio of the corrected image is plotted as a function of the number of transformations used to correct the image. The

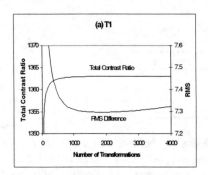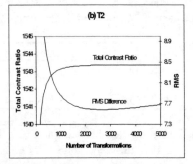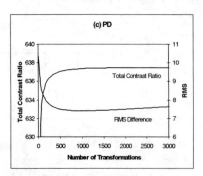

Figure 6. Total contrast ratio versus the number of transformations for (a) T1, (b) T2 and (c) PD simulated images with a linear bias field.

RMS difference dependence on the number of transformations is also plotted in the diagram. Figure 6 shows that the total contrast ratio changes in two stages: at the first stage the total contrast ratio gains rapidly with the increase of the number of transformations. This stage represents the contrast restoration process in the corrected image. In the second stage, the gain of the total contrast ratio is very slow and the total contrast ratio trends to a constant value with the increase of the number of transformations. This stage represents that most of the contrast information in the image has been restored. The transition point between stage 1 and stage 2 is not very easy to distinguish. For the convenience, we arbitrarily defined the transition point as the first arrival of the relative difference of total contrast ratio between two consecutive transformations less than a small number:

$$\frac{C_{n+1} - C_n}{C_n} \leq \varepsilon \qquad (9)$$

Since the value chosen for ε is arbitrary, the value of ε can be select to make the transition point close to the optimal correction. In this study, ε was equal to 1/2000. Table 4 lists the number of transformations for the transition points in

Table 4. Number of transformations for transition points

Image Type	Linear bias field	Phased Array Coil bias field
T1	1822	684
T2	2409	1055
PD	955	394

all the simulated images. A comparison between Table 4 with Table 2 reveals that the turning points are very close to the optimal corrections for all the simulated images. The RMS difference between the turning points and the optimal corrections are less than an intensity level of 0.3. These results support the supposition that the transition point of the total contrast ratio can be used as a criterion for optimal correction in a clinical image as demonstrated in Figures 7 and 8.

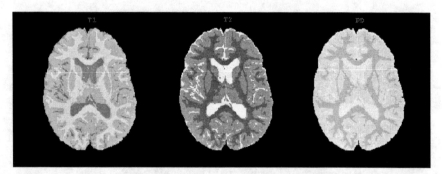

Figure 7. Corrected images for linear bias field

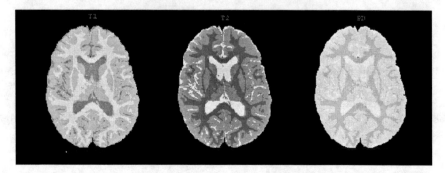

Figure 8. Corrected images for phased-array coil bias field

3.3 Correction of Clinical Data

Using the procedure mentioned above, a clinical MR image (PD-weighted) was corrected. The transition point defined above determined the number of transformations used for the correction. Figures 9 and 10 show the uncorrected and corrected images. Much of the obvious bilateral bias field contamination in the posterior portion fo the images is removed by the developed methodology. It should be noted that, as in the simulated images, not all the bias field is removed. Residual hyperintensity of the posterior gray matter on the patient left can still be observed. Figure 11 shows the curve of the total contrast ratio versus the number of transformations for the clinical image.

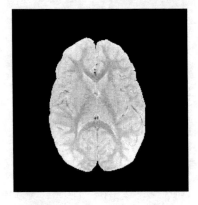 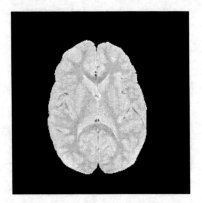

Figure 9. Original clinical PD weighted MR image

Figure 10. Corrected clinical PD weighted MR image

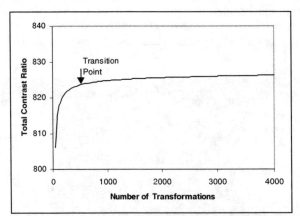

Figure 11. Total contrast ratio versus the number of transformations in clinical PD weighted MR image with a transition point at 565 transformations.

4. CONCLUSIONS

The effectiveness of the renormalization transformation technique for the correction of inhomogeneity in MR images has been quantitatively evaluated in this study. The simulation study shows that there is a single optimal correction in applying the RT technique. At the optimal correction, the bias field can be effectively removed (over 75%). The optimal correction depends on each individual image. To achieve the optimal correction in a clinical image, a transition point of in the curve of the total contrast versus number of transformations was defined. Using the combination of the transition point and the RT technique, the optimal correction for the clinical MR image can be approached.

5. REFERENCES

1. B. R. Condon, J. Patterson, and D. Wyper, "Image nonuniformity in magnetic resonance imaging: Its magnitude and methods for its correction:, *Br. J. Radiol.*, vol. **60**, pp 83-87, (1987)

2. D. A. G. Wicks, G. J. Barker, and P. S. Tofts, "Correction of intensity nonuniformity in MR images of any orientation*", Magn. Reson. Imaging* Vol. **11**, pp. 183-196 (1993)

3. A. Simmons, P. S. Tofts, G. J. Barker, and S. R. Arridge, "Sources of intensity nonuniformity in spin echo images at 1.5 T", *MRM* **32** pp 121-128, (1994)

4. L. Axel, J. Costantini, and J. Listerrud, "Intensity correction in surface-coil MR imaging", *AJR*, **148**, pp 418-420, (1987)

5. B. H. Brinkmann, A. Manduca, and R. A. Robb, "Optimized homomorphis unsharp masking for MR grayscale inhomogeneity correction", *IEEE. Trans. Med. Imag.*, vol. **17**(2), pp 161-171 (1998)

6. D. Chen, L. Li, D. Yoon, J. H. Lee and Z. Liang, "A renormalization method for inhomogeneity correction of MR images", *Proceedings of SPIE* Vol. **4322** pp 939-942 (2001).

Spatiotemporal multiscale vessel enhancement for coronary angiograms

Til Aach[a], Claudia Mayntz[a], Peter Rongen[b], Georg Schmitz[c], and Herman Stegehuis[b]

[a]Institute for Signal Processing, Medical University of Lübeck, D-23538 Lübeck, Germany
[b] Philips Medical Systems, P.O.Box 10000, 5680 DA Best, The Netherlands
[c] Philips Research Laboratories, Weisshausstr. 2, D-52066 Aachen, Germany

ABSTRACT

In coronary angiography, coronaries are imaged filled by a contrast medium which is injected through a catheter. To increase vessel visibility relative to surrounding structures, a background-less, subtraction-like appearance of the angiograms may be desired. This paper describes algorithms to increase vessel contrast and to attenuate background. Due to the strong motion in coronary angiograms, direct subtraction of a mask image acquired initially without contrast agent cannot be applied. We therefore distinguish vessels from background by their contrast, their size and their motion. These criteria are evaluated on a multiscale structure. Enhancement is then applied at locations which are likely to contain vessels. To avoid unacceptable noise boosting, we integrate a multiscale noise reduction filter into this concept. Both performance and computational simplicity make our algorithms attractive.

Keywords: Angiography, cardiology, multiscale processing, vessel visualization, motion, quantum noise

1. INTRODUCTION

In diagnostics and therapy of coronary heart disease, series of projection X-ray images of the moving coronary arteries play a crucial role. These coronary angiograms are acquired in real time with a dose rate about two to three times higher than that of normal fluoroscopy, where image intensifier/camera-chains or large area solid state X-ray detectors are used.[1-5] To make the coronary arteries visible in such coronary angiography, a so-called positive (i.e. radio-opaque) contrast medium is injected by means of a catheter placed for instance in the entrance (ostium) to the left or right coronary artery. The coronary arteries then appear darker than adjacent body tissue. An example angiogram is shown in Fig. 1. Preinterventional coronary angiograms showing the coronary arteries for several heart cycles firstly serve to diagnose e.g. stenoses. Secondly, they are used as roadmaps during therapy like percutaneous transluminal coronary angioplasty (PTCA), where a balloon catheter is pushed towards the stenosis and dilated. Postinterventional coronary angiograms are needed to verify the success of an intervention.

Often in angiography, an increased visibility of vessels is desired for given doses of contrast medium and X-ray exposure. When imaging static vessels, e.g. of the extremities or in the brain, a mask image recorded previously without contrast medium is subtracted in real time from the live angiogram in a modality called digital subtraction angiography (DSA) (see, e.g., Ref. 6). Common background information of mask and live angiogram is then subtracted out, leaving only the vessels filled by contrast medium in the difference images. In addition to showing the vessels free of superpositions by other tissues, DSA also allows to make better use of the available dynamic range of the display. Similarly, the visibility of catheters, guidewires or stents can be improved by the subtraction method.

Further author information: (Send correspondence to T.A.. C.M. is now with Ericsson Eurolab, D-52134 Aachen, Germany. G.S. is now with University of Applied Sciences, Rheinahrcampus, D-53424 Remagen, Germany.)
T.A.: E-mail: aach@isip.mu-luebeck.de, Telephone: +49 451 3909556, Fax: +49 451 3909 555
C.M.: E-mail: claudia.mayntz@eed.ericsson.se
P.R.: E-mail: peter.rongen@philips.com
G.S.: E-mail: schmitz@rheinahrcampus.de
H.S.: E-mail: herman.stegehuis@philips.com

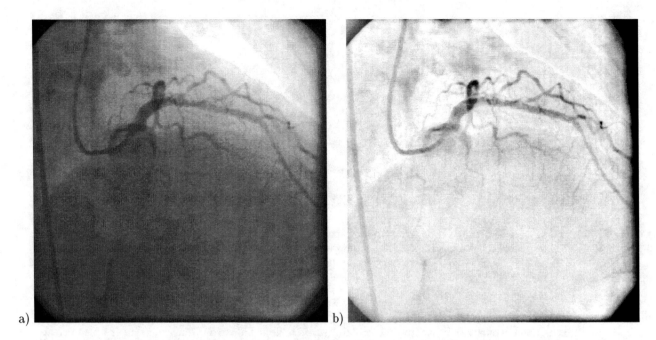

a)   b)

Figure 1: Original frame from a coronary angiogram (a), and its processed version (b).

In coronary angiography, subtraction of a mask image does in general not lead to the desired results. The reason for this is that due to strong motion induced by the beating heart and by respiration, the background information in the mask and the live angiogram is not identical, thus creating artifacts in the difference images. In this paper, we therefore describe an alternative approach to attenuate background and to increase vessel contrast. More specifically, we seek to give coronary angiograms a subtraction-like, background-less appearance with enhanced visibility of vessels and of man-made objects like catheters and guidewires. The basic idea of our algorithm is to identify locations which are likely to contain vessels by evaluating contrast, size and motion using a multiscale decomposition. In addition, we propose a computationally simple filter which prevents unacceptable amplification of quantum noise and which is straightforwardly integrated into our multiscale concept.

2. MULTISCALE VESSEL ENHANCEMENT

2.1. Algorithmic background

When filled by a positive contrast medium, coronary arteries appear darker than their immediate neighbourhood. In a highpass residual image, small vessels therefore tend to appear with negative-valued grey levels. A similar observation holds to a lesser degree for objects like catheters. Also, arteries can roughly be described as elongated objects of small or medium diameter, whose structure is repeated in a "fractal-like" manner across several scales. It is therefore reasonable to decompose coronary angiograms into multiscale residual images using e.g. the Laplacian pyramid.[7] On each scale, we apply a nonlinear gain such that negative valued grey levels are enhanced, while positive ones are attenuated. Unlike our earlier multiscale radiography enhancement algorithm,[8,9] the gain curve is hence nonsymmetric. In addition, arteries move strongly over large distances compared to their diameter due to the heart cycle. In temporal pixelwise difference images between the current and the previous frame, moving vessels therefore generate dark, negative-valued differences at their present positions, and bright, positive-valued ones at their positions in the previous frame. Based on multiscale difference images, we hence increase the gain at pixels with negative-valued temporal differences. Fig. 2 illustrates these vessel clues.

Unlike vessels, background information can be approximately characterized as containing structures of predominantly large size, like diaphragm and lung in Fig. 1. Moreover, background structures may strongly differ

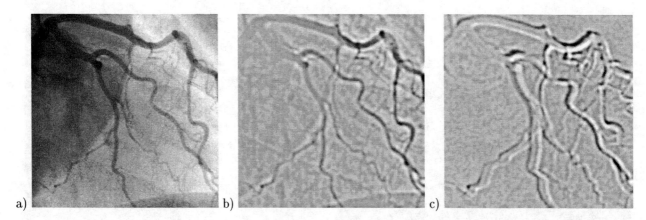

Figure 2. Illustration of spatiotemporal clues to coronary arteries: portion of an original coronary angiogram (a), scale 2 of a multiscale decomposition (b) and scale 2 of the temporal difference image between the depicted and the previous frame. In b) and c), the locations of coronary arteries are clearly discernible as black, tree-like regions. In the temporal difference image c), the coronary arteries also appear in white at their location in the previous frame.

in their absorptions (cf. Refs. 8, 9), and hence require a large dynamic range for display. When examining coronary angiograms or live coronary fluoroscopy in clinical routine, bright background areas of large size may even annoy the observer. Some commercial systems therefore allow manual selection and brightness attenuation of such regions by means of shaping the X-ray beam with shutters or wedges. To reduce background information, we therefore attenuate the lowpass image of the multiscale decomposition. Furthermore, as already mentioned above, bright contrasts are reduced consistently over all scales.

2.2. Spatial algorithm component

Fig. 3 shows the spatial component of our algorithm. Each coronary angiogram frame is decomposed into a number of subband residual images and a lowpass image. We use a Laplacian pyramid[7] of typically about seven levels, using separable binomial lowpass kernels[10] of size 3×3 or 5×5 pixels. Naturally, other hierarchical decompositions like QMF-banks, wavelets[11,12] or morphological pyramids[13] could alternatively be thought of. We favour the Laplacian pyramid because it reconstructs the output image using only lowpass filters. When enhancing strongly, this introduces less visible artifacts compared to a filter bank where also highpass filters are required (cf. Ref. 14).

The Laplacian pyramid decomposes an input image $s(m, n)$ into subbands $d_0(m, n)$, $d_1(m, n)$, ... by recursive lowpass filtering and subtraction. On each level j of the pyramid, the first lowpass is followed by downsampling, i.e. by leaving out every other row and every other column of the image matrix. These operations are summarized as REDUCE in Fig. 3. For subtraction, the reduced image is expanded to the same size as the input image $s_j(m, n)$ to this level, which is achieved by upsampling and interpolation by another lowpass. To reconstruct the input image $s(m, n)$ from this decomposition, the subbands are recursively upsampled, interpolated and added. Clearly, if the subbands are not processed, this pyramid reconstructs $s(m, n)$ perfectly, provided the interpolation lowpass filters used for decomposition and reconstruction are identical.

The bandpass and highpass levels ("detail images") are then subjected to a contrast dependent gain function $h(d_j(m, n))$, which amplifies negative contrasts and attenuates positive contrasts. In the diagram, the gain function is realized by a lookup-table (LUT). The multiscale decomposition ensures that both contrast enhancement and contrast compression are applied uniformly over all scales, i.e. to objects of different sizes. To further attenuate background, the lowpass image in the pyramid is attenuated by a factor a, with $0 \le a \le 1$. The resulting loss of brightness is compensated by adding a certain fraction (by default, $1 - a$) of the global average of the original lowpass image to its attenuated version. The filtered image $g(m, n)$ is then reconstructed from the filtered detail and lowpass images.

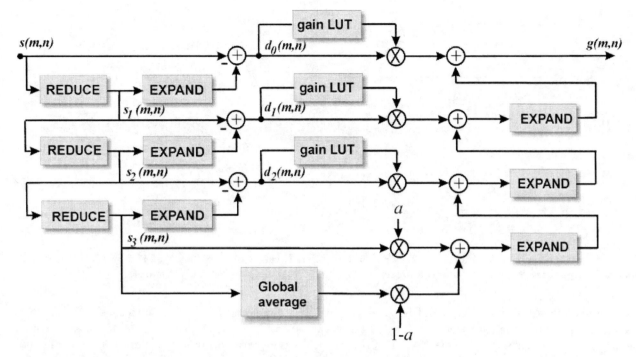

Figure 3. Block diagram of the spatial part of our algorithm. For convenience, only four levels are shown. Also for notational convenience, the pyramid decomposition and reconstruction operations of lowpass filtering and downsampling are summarized as REDUCE, while upsampling and interpolation are depicted as EXPAND.

2.2.1. The gain function

According to the above considerations, the gain function $h(d_j(m,n))$ should be larger than one for negative values of $d_j(m,n)$, and less than one for positive values. There are obviously a lot of choices to design $h(x)$. In this paper, we use the following function:

$$h(x) = \begin{cases} c > 1 & : \quad x < m \\ \frac{1}{x^p} & : \quad x > 1 \quad p \in [0; 0.5] \\ c + \frac{(1-c) \cdot (x-m)}{1-m} & : \quad m \leq x \leq 1 \end{cases}, \tag{1}$$

which is depicted in Fig. 4 a). This gain function enhances grey levels smaller than m by multiplication with $c > 1$. Therefore, m should for each subband be larger than the subband grey levels of vessels. Grey values larger than one are compressed by the factor $1/x^p$. Between $x = m$ and $x = 1$, the gain function decreases linearly. In total, fitting together the enhancement part and attenuation part $1/x^p$ of $h(x)$ at $x = 1$ means that negative contrasts are indeed amplified, while positive ones are reduced depending on the parameter p. At the same time, the singularity of $1/x^p$ at $x = 0$ is avoided.

Instead of looking at the gain function $h(x)$, one could alternatively consider the equivalent point transform $y = f(x)$, with the remapping function $f(x)$ given by $f(x) = h(x) \cdot x$. Fig. 4 b) illustrates this input-output relation for the same parameter values as in Fig. 4 a). Clearly, negative x are converted into output values further away from zero, while positive x are turned into output values closer to zero.

2.2.2. Determining the number of pyramid levels

Fig. 3 shows that each level j of the pyramid carries out a two-channel decomposition of its input $s_j(m,n)$ into a lowpass component $s_{j+1}(m,n)$ and a highpass component $d_j(m,n)$ (where for $j = 0$, we set $s(m,n) = s_0(m,n)$ for consistency of notation.). The entire pyramid can hence be viewed as a recursively continued two-channel composition known as unsharp mask.[8] Compared to the unsharp mask, however, the multiscale pyramid

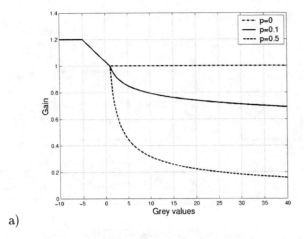
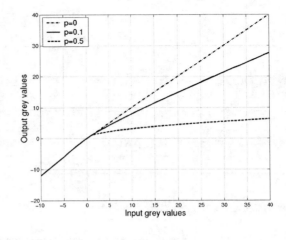

a)   b)

Figure 4. a) Gain function $h(x)$ for $c = 1.2$, $m = -5$, and different values of p. b) Relation $f(x) = h(x) \cdot x$ between input and output grey levels of the subband processing by $h(x)$ in Fig. 4, viewed as a point transform $y = f(x)$.

has two advantages: first, the pyramid is considerably less redundant than the unsharp mask. While the unsharp mask doubles the data volume to be processed, the subbands $d_0(m, n)$, $d_1(m, n)$, ..., together increase the original data volume by no more than a third. Secondly, the pyramid provides a finer decomposition of the input image $s(m, n)$ into subbands representing objects of different sizes (or scales), which are separately accessible for (potentially nonlinear) processing.

As already shown in Refs. 8, 9, the number K of pyramid levels can be related to the size of a moving average filter which is sufficiently large to remove the coronary arteries from the angiograms. The number K of pyramid levels is derived by a comparison of this large area moving average and the pyramid decomposition in the spectral domain. The amplitude spectrum of a discrete moving average of size N is given by

$$H(u) = \left| \frac{1}{N} \cdot \frac{\sin(N \cdot \pi \cdot u)}{\sin(\pi \cdot u)} \right| \ , \tag{2}$$

where u denotes spatial frequency. The lowpass filter LP used in the pyramid (Fig. 3) for both decomposition and reconstruction is a separable binomial filter of size 3×3, formed from the 1D-kernel [0.25 0.5 0.25]. The spectrum $LP(u)$ of this kernel is

$$LP(u) = \{\cos(\pi \cdot u)\}^2 \ . \tag{3}$$

Applying this kernel recursively in a K-level pyramid, and including the effects of subsampling, yields the following transfer function $G(u)$ for the lowpass level (aliasing is neglected in this analysis):

$$G(u) = \prod_{i=0}^{K-2} LP(2^i \cdot u) \ . \tag{4}$$

Experimentally, it turned out that filtering by a moving average with a size of $N = 101$ removes vessels completely. Taking into account that the reconstruction path of the pyramid applies the same sequence of filters again for interpolation, we have evaluated $G^2(u)$, which is the pyramid transfer function for the lowpass level interpolated to its original size. As shown in Fig. 5, the spectrum of the moving average can be approximated with reasonable accuracy by a pyramid utilizing the 3×3 filter kernel and consisting of $K = 7$ levels. $G^2(u)$ then obeys

$$G^2(u) = (LP(u) \cdot LP(2u) \cdot LP(4u) \cdot LP(8u) \cdot LP(16u) \cdot LP(32u))^2 \ . \tag{5}$$

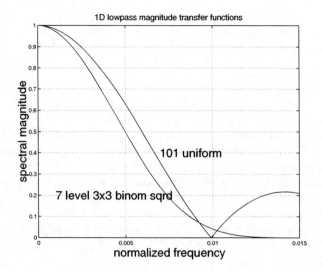

Figure 5. Comparison of the amplitude spectrum of a moving average of size 101 to a pyramid reconstruction from a Laplacian pyramid utilizing only the lowpass level. The pyramid consists of 7 levels, and employs 3×3 binomial filter kernels.

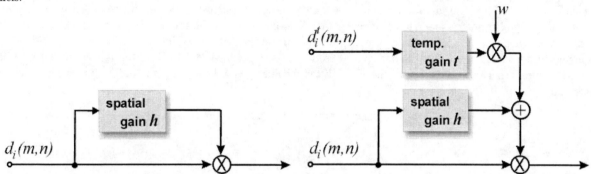

Figure 6. Spatial and spatiotemporal processing of the i-th subbands $d_i(m, n)$ and $d_i^t(m, n)$. In the spatial algorithm, only the spatial gain $h(d_i(m, n))$ is applied. In the spatiotemporal approach, a temporal gain $t(d_i^t(m, n))$ is derived from the i-th subband $d_i^t(m, n)$ of the temporal difference image, weighted by w and added to $h(d_i(m, n))$.

2.3. Temporal algorithm component

As discussed in the introduction, motion prevents us from simply subtracting an empty mask image from the coronary angiograms. In this section we describe how to turn motion into an advantage by extending our algorithm to consider the differences between temporally successive frames as well.

In Fig. 3, the gain function $h(d_j(m, n))$ depends on the contrast values as specified in (1). Additionally, we now make the gain dependent on the *temporal difference image* between current and previous frame. To this end, the temporal difference image is also decomposed in the pyramid, yielding the subbands $d_j^t(m, n)$. As already illustrated in Fig. 2, in these difference images moving vessels show up strongly positive (at their location in the previous image) as well as strongly negative (at their new positions in the currently processed frame). This observation holds for vessels which move between two frames over more than their size, i.e. particularly for small and usually difficult to enhance vessels. We therefore implemented an additional gain function, which is zero for positive temporal differences, while it is equal to one for negative temporal differences smaller than m. Between zero and m, the gain curve is linear. The gain $t(d_j^t(m, n))$ is added to the spatial gain $h(d_j(m, n))$ in (1), yielding for the total gain h_t

$$h_t(d_j(m, n), d_j^t(m, n)) = h(d_j(m, n)) + w \cdot t((d_j^t(m, n))) \ . \tag{6}$$

The parameter w allows to control the influence of the temporal gain. Clearly, $t(x)$ is without effect if no motion occurs, but provides vessel-selective enhancement in the presence of moving vessels. A block diagram of the spatiotemporal subband processing is given in Fig. 6.

2.4. Multiscale noise containment

Since only rather low X-ray dose rates are permitted for acquisition of coronary angiograms and interventional coronary fluoroscopy, the image data discussed here exhibit relatively high levels of quantum noise.[1] Suppression of background information, subband amplification and the use of subsequent frames to calculate the temporal differences tend to further decrease the signal-to-noise ratio. (Note that, similarly, DSA doubles the noise power due to the subtraction of uncorrelated noise realizations.) To compensate for this effect, we have therefore combined the described enhancement algorithm with the multiscale quantum noise reduction filter described in Ref. 15. The central ingredient of this approach is the so-called FIR-median-hybrid (FMH) filter of Ref. 16, which we have applied to the subband images of a Laplacian pyramid. The FMH filter operates with a sliding window of 5×5 pixels. As its name implies, the FMH filter is a hierarchical combination of eight directional two-point linear averaging operations with a cascade of three-point median operations.[16] Equivalently, the filter output can be computed by comparing the grey level of the pixel in the window centre to the eight directional two-point averages (Fig. 7). If the grey level in the window centre exceeds the maximum of the eight directional averages, it is replaced by the maximum. If it is lower than the minimum of the directional averages, it is replaced by the minimum. If it falls between minimum and maximum, it is left unchanged. The FMH filter thus completes interrupted lines and corners, and removes impulse-like noise. Since quantum noise has a lowpass-shaped noise power spectrum,[1] direct FMH filtering is not reasonable. The hierarchically repeated filtering and downsampling operations of the Laplacian pyramid, however, select successively lower frequency components and convert these into higher spatial frequencies, for which the FMH-filter is well suited.[15] An idea close at hand therefore is to apply the FMH-filter within each subband of our algorithm except for the lowpass image, where filtering is not needed.

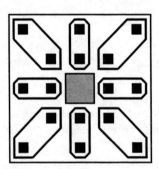

Figure 7. Schematic diagram of FMH filtering. First, the eight directional two-point averages over the pixel pairs to the north, south east, west etc. of the central pixel are taken. The maximum and the minimum of these averages are then compared to the grey level in the window centre.

3. RESULTS

All results in this section were calculated with a pyramid of $K = 7$ levels, and the following settings for p in (1):

level	0	1	2	3	4	5
exponent	0.1	0.1	0.1	0.5	0.5	0.5

These means that compression of positive contrasts is stronger for larger scales (see Fig. 4), i.e. large bright areas in the original image are stronger reduced in brightness. The parameter c in (1) was set to $c = 1.2$, and, for 8-bit images, m was set to $m = -5$. Since the contrast compression and, in particular, the compression of the lowpass image reduces the dynamic range, all images presented here are rescaled such that they again fill the full range available for display. The original images are otherwise raw in the sense that no postprocessing was applied.

Fig. 8 a) shows a 512×512-portion of an original frame of a coronary angiogram. Fig. 8 b) gives the processing result for purely spatial enhancement, i.e. $w = 0$ in (6). The background suppression was set to a value of $a = 0.5$. A comparison with the original frame reveals that background structure is indeed attenuated, while vessel contrast is visibly boosted. Also, background areas which in the original appear brighter than their surroundings are now attenuated, thus allowing a better use of the available dynamic range for vessel display without clipping of image intensities. Fig. 9 a) depicts the same result, but additionally with multiscale noise containment by the 5×5-FMH filter (section 2.4). The processing results with noise containment are visibly less noisy than those without, while at the same time small vessels and other details are well preserved.

Fig. 9 b) shows the frame processed by the spatiotemporal algorithm together with multiscale noise containment. The weights for the influence of the temporal gain were set to $w = 0.3$. The background suppression a was set to its strongest value of $a = 0$. Even under the limited reproduction quality available here, it is evident that particularly small vessels are enhanced compared to the purely spatial algorithm. The noise filter ensures that the vessel contrast boost is not paid for by a comparable boost of noise.

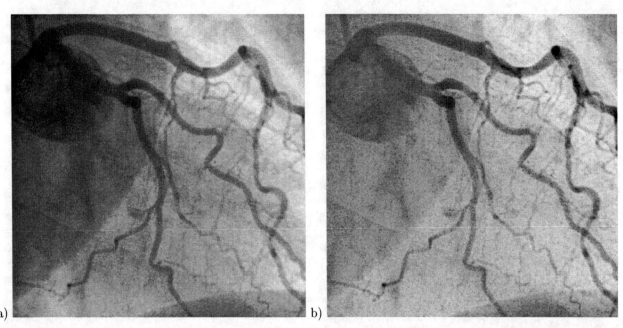

a)   b)

Figure 8. a) Portion of size 512×512 pixels of a frame taken from a coronary angiogram. b) Processing result obtained by purely spatial enhancement without noise containment.

An original frame of another coronary angiogram is shown in Fig. 10 a). Fig. 10 b) gives the processing result as obtained by spatiotemporal filtering with multiscale noise containment. An earlier frame of the same sequence is depicted in Fig. 11 a). The same region for the processed sequence is shown in Fig. 11 b), where the processing was the same as in Fig. 10.

Finally, another frame from a third angiogram was already shown in Fig. 1 a). The processing result as obtained by spatiotemporal noise-contained filtering is given in Fig. 1 b). Fig. 12 a) shows the same angiogram shortly before the contrast medium is injected, where a catheter and a guidewire can be seen. As before, the background and strong positive contrasts are attenuated by our algorithm, while catheter and guidewire are well visible. For comparison, an original *fluoroscopy* frame from the same intervention is shown in Fig. 13 a), and its processing result in Fig. 13 b).

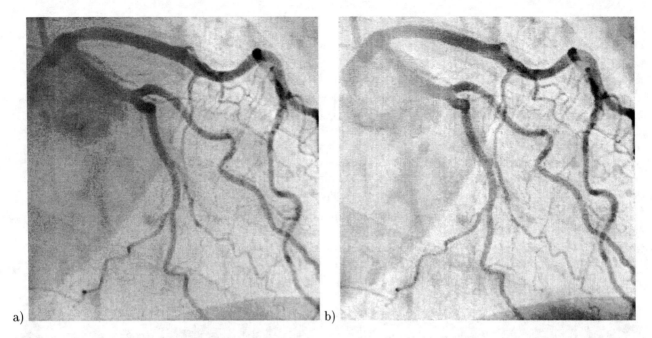

Figure 9. a) Processing result obtained by purely spatial enhancement with noise containment. b) Processing result obtained by spatiotemporal enhancement with noise containment.

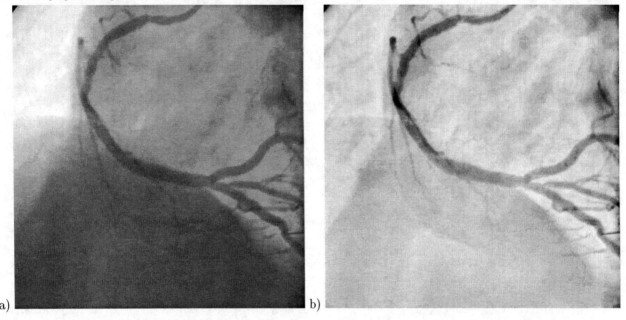

Figure 10: Original frame from another angiogram (a) and its processing result (b).

4. DISCUSSION AND CONCLUSIONS

The results show that our algorithms indeed reach the objective of giving coronary angiograms a DSA-like, vessel-enhanced appearance. Furthermore, processing results on images with interventional instruments, like catheters and guidewires, look promising. Apart from multiscale decomposition and reconstruction, the enhancement requires only point operations, what makes our algorithms also attractive from a computational point of view. The multiscale enhancement can be optionally combined with a spatial multiscale (quantum) noise containment filter, which can be applied within the same multiscale decomposition. Naturally, other noise filters — e.g.

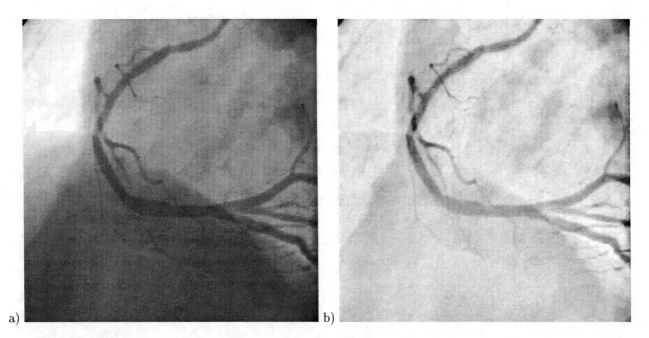

Figure 11. a) Another original frame from the vessel sequence of Fig. 10. b) Processing result as obtained by spatiotemporal enhancement and noise containment.

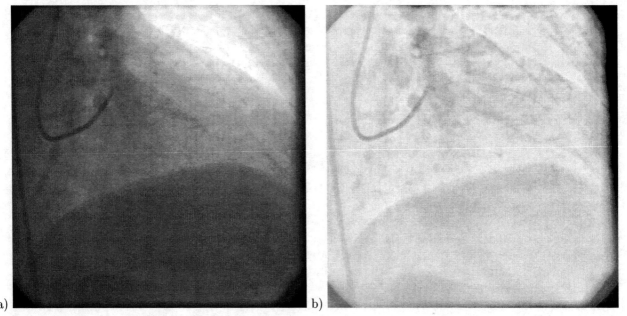

Figure 12. a) An earlier frame from the angiogram of Fig. 1, taken before the contrast medium is injected, and its processed version (b).

temporally recursive filters[17, 18] — may also be used. Algorithm performance with respect to interventional instruments together with the option of noise containment mean that our concept is not only of interest for coronary angiograms, but also for interventional fluoroscopy. Also, increased vessel contrast could help in the analysis of coronary arteries, e.g. for 3D rotational angiographic reconstruction.

The selections of the processing parameters do not appear to be critical. The one parameter which is most dependent on the input images is the parameter m of the gain functions $h(x)$ and $t(x)$, which serves to

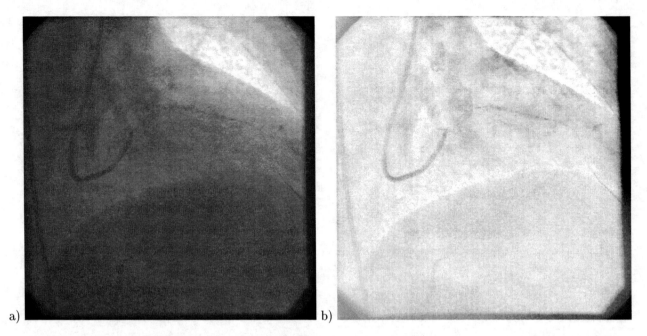

Figure 13. a) A fluoroscopy frame from the same intervention where the coronary angiogram in Figs. 12 and 1 was taken, and its processed version (b).

discriminate between small vessels and noise. We have set this parameter manually here. Automatic adaptation of m could for instance be based on (subband) histogram analysis. Since the value for m is not likely to vary quickly, it could be updated with a rate considerably lower than the frame rate.

4.1. Acknowledgments

We thank the graduate student Tobias Hahn for his help with developing the simulation software and with some of the experiments.

REFERENCES

1. T. Aach, U. Schiebel, and G. Spekowius, "Digital image acquisition and processing in medical x-ray imaging," *Journal of Electronic Imaging* **8**(Special Section on Biomedical Image Representation), pp. 7–22, 1999.

2. J. A. Rowlands and J. Yorkston, "Flat panel detectors for digital radiography," in *Handbook of Medical Imaging*, J. Beutel, H. L. Kundel, and R. L. van Metter, eds., pp. 223–328, Springer Verlag, 2000.

3. U. Schiebel, N. Conrads, N. Jung, M. Weibrecht, H. Wieczorek and T. Zaengel, "Fluoroscopic X-ray imaging with amorphous silicon thin-film arrays", in *Physics of Medical Imaging*, SPIE Vol. 2163, pp. 129-140, 1994.

4. F. Busse, W. Rütten, B. Sandkamp, P. L. Alving, R. Bastiaens, "Design and performance of a high-quality cardiac flat panel detector", in *Physics of Medical Imaging*, SPIE Vol. 4682, to be published, 2002.

5. P. Granfors, D. Albagli, J. Tkaczyk, R. Aufrichtig, H. Netel, G. Brunst, J. Boudry, D. Luo, "Performance of a flat panel cardiac detector", in *Physics of Medical Imaging*, SPIE Vol. 4320, 77-86, 2001.

6. T. M. Buzug, J. Weese, and K. C. Strasters, "Motion detection and motion compensation for digital subtraction angiography image enhancement," *Philips Journal of Research* **51**(2), pp. 203–229, 1998.

7. P. J. Burt and E. H. Adelson, "The Laplacian pyramid as a compact image code," *IEEE Transactions on Communications* **31**(4), pp. 532–540, 1983.

8. M. Stahl, T. Aach, and S. Dippel, "Digital radiography enhancement by nonlinear multiscale processing," *Medical Physics* **27**(1), pp. 56–65, 2000.

9. M. Stahl, T. Aach, S. Dippel, T. Buzug, R. Wiemker, and U. Neitzel, "Noise-resistant weak-structure enhancement for digital radiography," in *SPIE Medical Imaging 99: Image Processing*, K. M. Hanson, ed., pp. 1406–1417, SPIE Vol. 3661, (San Diego, USA), February 20–26 1999.

10. B. Jähne, *Digital Image Processing*, Springer, Berlin, 1997.

11. S. Ranganath, "Image filtering using multiresolution representations," *IEEE Transactions on Pattern Analysis and Machine Intelligence* **13**(5), pp. 426–440, 1991.

12. A. N. Akansu and R. A. Haddad, *Multiresolution Signal Decomposition*, Academic Press, Boston, 1992.

13. J. Goutsias and H. J. A. M. Heijmans, "Multiresolution signal decomposition schemes - part I: Morphological pyramids," *IEEE Transactions on Image Processing* **9**(11), pp. 1862–1867, 2000.

14. S. Dippel, M. Stahl, R. Wiemker, and T. Blaffert, "Multiscale enhancement of digital radiographs: A comparison of Laplacian pyramid and fast wavelet transform," in *Proceedings Computer Assisted Radiology and Surgery CARS'2000*, H. Lemke, M. Vannier, K. Inamura, A. Farman, and K. Doi, eds., pp. 507–512, (San Francisco), 2000.

15. T. Aach and D. Kunz, "Multiscale linear/median hybrid filters for noise reduction in low-dose x-ray images," in *Proceedings ICIP-97*, pp. 358–361, IEEE, (Santa Barbara, CA), October 26–29 1997.

16. A. Nieminen, P. Heinonen, and Y. Neuvo, "A new class of detail-preserving filters for image processing," *IEEE Transactions on Pattern Analysis and Machine Intelligence* **9**(1), pp. 74–90, 1987.

17. E. Dubois and S. Sabri, "Noise reduction in image sequences using motion compensated temporal filtering," *IEEE Transactions on Communications* **32**(7), pp. 826–831, 1984.

18. T. Aach and D. Kunz, "Bayesian motion estimation for temporally recursive noise reduction in x-ray fluoroscopy," *Philips Journal of Research* **51**(2), pp. 231–251, 1998.

EM-IntraSPECT Algorithm With Ordered Subsets (OSEMIS) for Non-Uniform Attenuation Correction in Cardiac Imaging

Andrzej Krol[a][**], Ifeanyi Echeruo[b], Roberto B. Salgado[a,c], Amol S. Hardikar[b], James E. Bowsher[d], David H. Feiglin[a], F. Deaver Thomas[a], Edward Lipson[c], Ioana Coman[b]

[a]SUNY Upstate Medical University, Department of Radiology, Syracuse, NY
[b]Syracuse University, Department of Electrical Engineering and Computer Science, Syracuse NY
[c]Syracuse University, Department of Physics, Syracuse NY
[d]Duke University Medical Center, Department of Radiology, Durham, NC

Keywords: iterative reconstruction, ordered subsets, attenuation compensation, myocardial SPECT

ABSTRACT

Performance of the EM-IntraSPECT (EMIS) algorithm with ordered subsets (OSEMIS) for non-uniform attenuation correction in the chest was assessed. EMIS is a maximum-likelihood expectation maximization (MLEM) algorithm for simultaneously estimating SPECT emission and attenuation parameters from emission data alone. EMIS uses the activity within the patient as transmission tomography sources, with which attenuation coefficients can be estimated. However, the reconstruction time is long. The new algorithm, OSEMIS, is a modified EMIS algorithm based on ordered subsets. Emission Tc-99m SPECT data were acquired over 360° in non-circular orbit from a physical chest phantom using clinical protocol. Both a normal and a defect heart were considered. OSEMIS was evaluated in comparison to EMIS and a conventional MLEM with a fixed uniform attenuation map. Wide ranges of image measures were evaluated, including noise, log-likelihood, and region quantification. Uniformity was assessed from bull's eye plots of the reconstructed images. For the appropriate subset size, OSEMIS yielded essentially the same images as EMIS and better than MLEM, but required only one-tenth as many iterations. Consequently, adequate images were available in about fifteen iterations.

Keywords: Iterative reconstruction, ordered subsets, attenuation compensation, myocardial SPECT

1. INTRODUCTION

Recently we have derived a maximum-likelihood expectation maximization algorithm called EM-IntraSPECT[1] (EMIS) for simultaneously estimating SPECT emission and attenuation parameters from emission data alone. EMIS uses the activity within the patient as transmission tomography sources, with which attenuation coefficients can be estimated. However, the reconstruction time is long as compared to a conventional maximum-likelihood expectation maximization algorithm (MLEM)[2-3]. It is well known that ordered subset approach results in accelerating of image reconstruction with acceptable image quality deterioration[4-6]. The purpose of this study was to evaluate performance of the EM-IntraSPECT (EMIS) algorithm with ordered subsets (OSEMIS) for non-uniform attenuation correction in the chest. The new algorithm, OSEMIS, is a modified EMIS algorithm based on ordered subsets and it has been used in order to accelerate execution of EMIS.

The OSEMIS reconstruction algorithm can be written as:

$$\lambda_k^{n+1} = \lambda_k^n \frac{1}{\sum_{i \in S_0} c_{ik}} \sum_{i \in S_0} \left\{ c_{ik} \cdot \gamma_{ikJ}^n \frac{Y_i}{\sum_{m \in P_i} \lambda_m^n \cdot c_{im} \cdot \gamma_{imJ}^n} + c_{ik}(1 - \gamma_{ikJ}^n) \right\} \quad (1)$$

[*] krola@mail.upstate.edu; phone (315) 464-7054; fax: (315) 464-7068, SUNY Upstate Medical University, Department of Radiology, Syracuse, 750 E. Adams St., NY 13210

$$\mu_{k,lower}^{n+1} = \frac{\sum_{\substack{i \in R \\ k0}} \sum_{\substack{j \in P_i, j \leq k}} \lambda_j^n c_{ij} (\gamma_{ijk}^n - \gamma_{ijk+1}^n)}{\frac{1}{2} \sum_{\substack{i \in R \\ k0}} \sum_{\substack{j \in P_i, j \leq k}} \left\{ 2\lambda_j^n c_{ij} \gamma_{ijj}^n [\frac{Y_i}{\sum_{n \in P_i} \lambda_n^n c_{in} \gamma_{inJ_i}^n} - 1] + \lambda_j^n c_{ij} (\gamma_{ijk}^n + \gamma_{ijk+1}^n) \right\} l_{ijk}} \qquad (2)$$

The meaning of used symbols is as follows:

i — projection subscript,

J_i — number of pixels in the ray I

j — pixel subscript ($j < J_i$),

P_i — set of pixels contributing to projection i,

S_0 — subset of the projection bins corresponding to a particular set of views,

R_{k0} — subset of projections that belongs to S_0 to which pixel k contributes,

Y_i — total (random) number of photons recorded by the detector bin i,

λ_j^n — current estimate of source intensity of pixel j (i.e. the mean number of photons emitted by pixel j),

μ_j^n — current estimate of linear attenuation coefficient of pixel j,

l_{ijm} — the path length in the pixel m, i.e. the length of the line j-i intercepted by pixel m (in ray-tracing we assume that $l_{ijm} \cong l_{im}$ where l_{im} is the fraction of the ray from the center of bin i intercepted by pixel m)

γ_{ijm}^n — probability of surviving attenuation between the source in the center of pixel j and the boundary of pixel m, for the photon heading towards the detector bin i, evaluated using the current vector of parameter estimates μ^n,

c_{ij} — known probability (corrected for the decay rate and the time interval of ith projection) that photon leaving pixel j is directed toward detector bin i.

We want to emphasize that summation in Eqs. 1 and 2 is performed over a subset S_0 of the projection bins corresponding to a particular set of views. The images are updated after user-specified number of projection views (OS size) that form the subset S_0. The OS size may vary from unity (the smallest possible) to the number of acquired views (the largest possible).

2. METHODS

Emission Tc-99m SPECT data were acquired over 360° in a non-circular orbit (pixel size 7.12 mm, 64x32 matrix, 120 views, 10 s/view) from a physical chest phantom. The phantom contained cold "lungs" and "spine" and hot "thorax" cavity, and hot left ventricle "myocardium". Total activity in the "thorax" cavity was 5.1 mCi (0.85 µCi/ml) and 1 mCi in the "myocardium". A normal heart was modeled.

OSEMIS was quantitatively evaluated in comparison to EMIS and a conventional MLEM with a fixed uniform attenuation map. The following measures image measures were evaluated: (i) log-likelihood for a selected slice containing "heart", (ii) three-channel-wide lateral and A-P (anterior-posterior) profiles, (iii) regional quantification for the modeled lungs, spine, soft tissue and bone, (iv) image noise, using a standard deviation in 100 pixels in the center of the "thorax" cavity, (v) uniformity of the activity distribution in the modeled myocardium was evaluated using bull's eye plots of the reconstructed images. The EM-IntraSPECT with OS=120, OSEMIS were used for image reconstruction. A conventional MLEM[2-3] with OS=120 was also used for comparison.

3. RESULTS

A qualitative evaluation of reconstructed images demonstrates that OSEMIS converges much faster than original EMIS code. EMIS required about 100 iterations to produce adequate image (low-resolution), whereas only two iterations of OSEMIS with OS=5 produced quite similar images. The quality of the reconstructed images improved with the OS size, however more iterations were required to obtain adequate

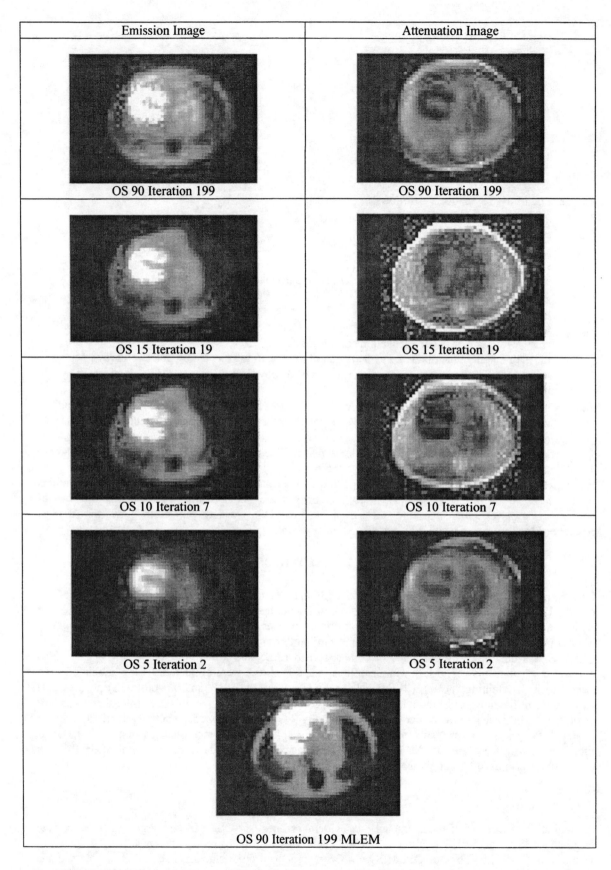

Fig. 1. Reconstructed Transaxial images of slice 9 after iteration 199, 19, 7 and 2 obtained for OS 90, 15, 10, and 5, respectively.

images. He have determined that for the current experimental conditions the reconstruction has to be stopped at iteration 2, 7, 19 and 199 for OS size 5, 10, 15, and 90 (i.e. maximum), respectively. The obtained transaxial images are shown in Fig. 1. For comparison, we reconstructed also the full set of views (OS=90) using MLEM.

The log-likelihood calculated for slice 9 containing the "heart" is shown in Fig. 2. It was calculated at each update denoted here as a subiteration. Generally, increased loglikelihood implies higher resolution, more accurate ROIs, and more image noise. We observe that loglikelihood increases monotonically in EMIS (i.e. OS=90) and MLEM. However, it is much higher for EMIS as compared MLEM. For all smaller subsets the loglikelihood is a non-monotonic function of subiteration. It can be seen that for OS=15 at low iterations it is actually higher than OS=90.

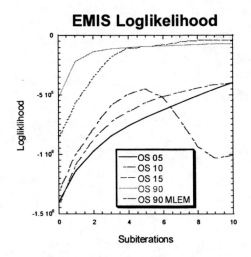 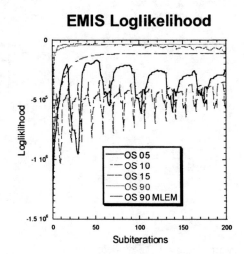

Fig. 2. The log-likelihood calculated for slice 9.

Image noise, obtained using a standard deviation in 100 pixels ROI located in the center of the "thorax" cavity is shown in Fig. 3. For EMIS (OS=90) and OS=5 it increases monotonically with iterations while for OS=10 and OS=15 at low iterations we observe decrease of noise followed by the increase in noise at higher iteration. OS=5 exhibits the highest noise level.

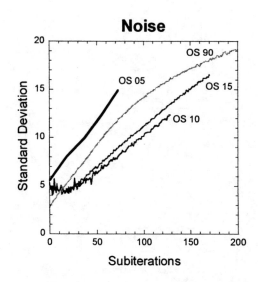

Fig. 3. Image noise, obtained using a standard deviation in 100 pixels ROI.

The three-channel-wide lateral and A-P (anterior-posterior) are shown in Fig. 4. It shows that OS=15 at 20 iterations creates profiles that are quite close to OS=90 at iteration 200.

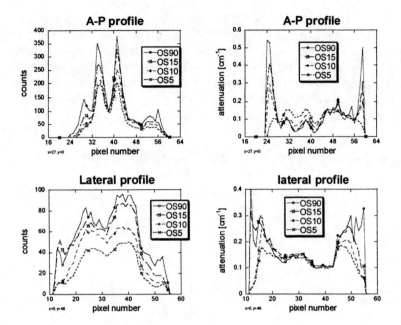

Fig. 4. The three-channel-wide lateral and A-P (anterior-posterior) and lateral profiles.

Regional quantification for the modeled heart and bone is shown in Fig. 5. It demonstrates that only EMIS (OS=90) converges to a mean total activity in the heart and in the spine. The smaller OS size results in monotonically increasing total activity in these ROIs.

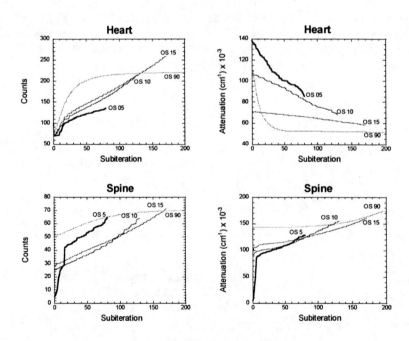

Fig. 5. Regional quantification for the modeled heart and bone.

Uniformity of the activity distribution in the modeled myocardium was evaluated using bull's eye plots of the reconstructed heart images. We observe improved uniformity in EMIS as compared to MLEM. The uniformity deteriorates with decreasing OS size.

CONCLUSIONS

For the appropriate subset size, OSEMIS yields essentially the same images as EMIS and better than MLEM. Consequently, adequate images might be available in about fifteen to twenty iterations.

REFERENCES

1. A. Krol, J.E. Bowsher, S.H. Manglos, M.P., Tornai, D.H. Feiglin and F.D. Thomas. "An EM algorithm for estimating SPECT emission and transmission parameters from emission data only," *IEEE Trans. Med. Imaging*, **20**, pp. 218-232, 2001.
2. L.A. Shepp and Vardi "Maximum likelihood reconstruction for emission tomography," *IEEE Trans. Med. Imag.* **1**, pp. 113-121, 1982.
3. K. Lange and R. Carson "*EM* reconstruction algorithm for emission and transmission tomography," *J. Comp. Assist. Tomog.* **8**, pp. 306-316, 1984.
4. S.H. Manglos, G.M. Gagne, A. Krol , F.D. Thomas and R. Narayanaswamy "Transmission maximum-likelihood reconstruction with ordered subsets for cone-beam CT," *Phys. Med. Biol.* **40**, pp.1225-1241, 1995.
5. D.S. Lalush, B.M. Tsui, "Performance of ordered-subset reconstruction algorithms under conditions of extreme attenuation and truncation in myocardial SPECT," *J. Nucl Med.* **41**, pp 737-44, 2000.
6. A.R. De Pierro, M.E. Beleza Yamagishi "Fast EM-like methods for maximum 'a posteriori' estimates in emission tomography," *IEEE Trans. Med. Imaging.* **20**, pp. 280-8, 2001.

Adaptive robust filters in MRI.

F.A. Barrios[a], L. González-Santos[a], G.R. Favila[a,b] and
R. Rojas[c]

[a]Centro de Neurobiología, UNAM, Campus Juriquilla UNAM,
Querétaro, QRO. 76230, MEXICO.

[b]Departamento de Ingeniería Eléctrica, UAM Iztapalapa,
Mexico D.F. 09340, MEXICO.

[c]División de Imagenología, Hospital ABC, Calle Sur 136 No 116,
Las Américas, México D.F. 01120, MEXICO.

ABSTRACT

An adaptive noise filter that can be used in MRI for noise reduction is presented. The algorithm is mainly based on the robust estimator, *mode*. Using the mode as the gray scale value estimator it is possible to differentiate the structures of interest form the background noise. Noise reduction is one of the most common image correction procedures, used in the enhancement of digital images. Wildly used noise reduction filters for digital imaging are based on median estimation, median filters. Every time noise reduction filters are applied to an image there is a general softening or blurring of it, in particular mean filters are characterized by a strong softening effect for the case of high amplitude noise levels, practically destroying all the fine features in the filtered image. This problem is significantly reduced when median filters are used. The adaptive mode filter proposed in this work have very good noise reduction effect without a strong softening effect and is comparable in CPU time to the median filters. This fine resolution is achieved because the filter changes the mode estimator according to the difference of the deviation of the mode calculated for each the neighborhood of pixels with the global deviation of the mode for each class in the image. We consider it robust, because it uses the mode of gray-scale intensity distribution of the pixels neighborhood and its mode deviation.

Keywords: Image enhancement, adaptive image filters, ROI statistics, robust statistics, mode filters, head MRI

1. INTRODUCTION

An adaptive mode noise filter that can be used in MRI for noise reduction and data softening is presented. Noise reduction is one of the most common image correction procedures used in the enhancement of digital images.[1] MRI is considered as the medical imaging with highest anatomical resolution, and provides with a very high signal to noise ratio information form the tissue been studied. Noise filters and their application range from the most general to specific processes. Wildly used noise reduction filters for digital imaging are based on median estimation, median filters.[2] Every time noise reduction filters are applied to an image there is a general softening or blurring of it, in particular mean filters are characterize by a strong softening effect and also by the extreme changes in grey-scale values for the case of high amplitude noise levels, practically destroying all the fine features in the filtered image. This problem is significantly reduced when median filters are used, as it is well know. For this reason median filters are some times characterized as noise reduction filters. Adaptive filters have been presented in the literature before,[3],[4] with good noise reduction properties for different acquisition techniques. Mode filters can provide with good noise reduction and less softening effect in particular they are effective in image boundary areas. Robust techniques based on mode estimators have been

---

Send correspondence to F.A.B. Email: barrios@mail.cnb.unam.mx; Telephone: (5255)5623-4053; Fax: (5255)5623-4005. R. R. present address: Section of Neuroradiology, Health Sciences Center, School of Medicine in New Orleans, 1542 Tulane Av., Room 211. New Orleans, Louisiana 70112

successfully used in MRI segmentation.[5] Noise reduction is an important field of study for medical imaging, because MRI data some times it is characterized by the nonuniformity of its intensity values , therefore making it difficult to apply automatic processes for feature recognition, like classification of grey-scale values for image segmentation,noise correction, automatic tissue classification, etc..[6] The adaptive mode filters proposed in this work have very good noise reduction effect without a strong softening effect and are comparable in CPU time to the median filters. Robust estimation has been used successfully in applications of image analysis and image segmentation, in particular has been used in MRI for grey-scale value classification as means of image segmentation and in the estimation of intensity distribution in MRI.[7] In this work we propose mode as a region of interest statistical estimator for noise reduction particularly useful in images with nonuniform intensity values.

2. METHODS

2.1. MRI image parameters

All the images used in this work were obtained on a $1.5T$ GE SIGNA LX scanner, (version 8.3, Milwaukee, WI) using different pulse sequences in particular $T1$, $T2$, Fast FALIR and $SPGR$ pulse sequences. All the high resolution images used in this work were obtained from healthy volunteers with a $T1$ weighted $SPGR$ pulse sequence[8] acquisition, using the standard quadrature headcoil, with the following parameters; $TR = 24ms$, $TE = 5ms$ and flip angle of $40°$ with two excitations over a $FOV = 24cm$ and a slice thickness of $1.5mm$ and zero separation. Images were taken using a 256×192 matrix and reconstructed to 256×256, in 124 coronal slices. The head was securely fastened to avoid movement. Images were copied from the patient data base to the operating system as flat files using a G.E. system "insite" propietary tool and then were transferred to an offline analysis workstation. All the proprietary G.E. information, as the image header for example, was striped out and a binary stack of 256×124 images of $16bits$ was build using a simple program developed in our laboratory.

2.2. Filter algorithm

A simple mode filter is calculated from a distribution of grey-level pixel values from the original image $I(x, y)$ and a fixed radius r value for the kernel window $(3x3, 5x5, \ldots)$, the filtering process builds a new image assigning to each new pixel the mode value $M(x, y)$, estimated from the neighborhood of radius r, around the pixel $I(x, y)$ in the original image, we use the mode and variance from the mode defined by Rousseeuw.[9] An identical process using the *median* is done, the resulting images will be used to compare with the adaptive filter. For the adaptive filter the filtering process is slit in to steps; first the estimation of the original image $I(x, y)$, histogram to do a first noise estimate using the mode filter described above and second, a recursive estimation for the recalculation of each pixel marked in the first step utilizing the *local* recalculated mode and deviation form the mode. The filtering procedure can be described in the following steps:

STEP 1 Loading the original image $I(x, y)$, we build a new image IT following

1. $IT = I$.

2. For each pixel $I(x, y)$ the gray-scale mode (m) and deviation (σ) are estimated from the gray-scale values at the eight first neighbors ($3x3$ kernel). And the gray-scale value p at (x, y) is substituted by the mode value m if $|p - m| \geq 2 * \sigma$.

3. The image difference $|IT - I|$ histogram is estimated ($hist$).

4. The image difference histogram derivative is calculated ($D(hist)$).

5. A new estimator is calculated based on the mode (m_D and deviation (σ_D) from all the values that form the pixels in the derivative of the histogram ($D(hist)$). With this new estimator the pixels p reclassified as noise can be estimated from the condition $|D(hist(p) - m_D| > f * \sigma_D$, were f is an external constant adjusting parameter, which in our particular case is $f = 12.0$. At the end of this step we have a pixel set R of the noise pixels.

STEP 2 For each pixel p in the mode filtered image R it is decided if it is noise and if it can be corrected with the best possible gray-scale value. For each $p \in R$ twenty four neighbors are taken (5x5 kernel) and the mode (m^*) and deviation (σ^*) of these gray-scale values from the original images are estimated, the original value at this pixel p is substituted by this robust estimator m^* if the $|p - m^*| \geq 2 * \sigma^*$ condition is satisfied, if not the value at the pixel p in IT is left as the filtered value.

This adaptive robust statistical filter was coded in C and used in an effective way to reduce noise in grey-scale images, in particular in brain $T1$ waited high resolution head MRI

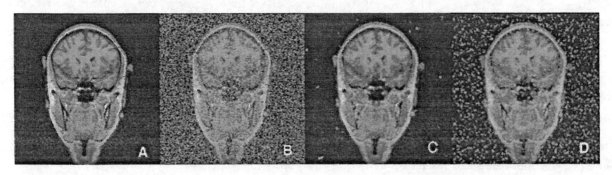

Figure 1. MRI restoration, (A) Original image, (B) Original image contaminated with 20% noise values (C) Filtered image B, using the adaptive mode filter (D) Filtered image B, using a regular median filter.

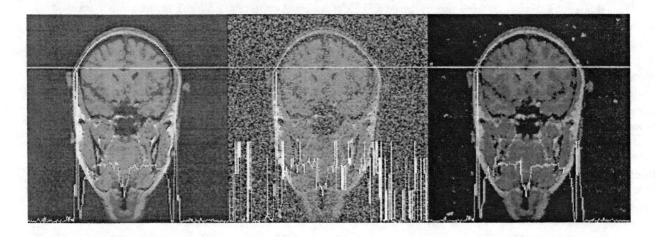

Figure 2. MRI restoration, (A) Original image with histogram superimposed, (B) Original image contaminated with 20% noise values and histogram superimposed (C) Filtered image B, using the adaptive mode filter with the resulting histogram superimposed

3. RESULTS

To evaluate filter execution we contaminated with random noise, with different grey-level intensity in 20% of the pixels distributed all over a series of MR images, median and mode filters of two different radius were used as noise reduction transformations. The processing time of the adaptive mode filter was always approximately a 40% longer than the median filter processing time, but the noise reduction results were superior. As we measure the value dispersion at the background the results show better resolution for the adaptive mode filter since mode filters blurring effect is smaller that the median filers figure 1. The results for the adaptive filer are superior in particular with areas of boundaries and smaller structures, the better behavior of the histogram can be appreciated in the the comparison in figure 2. An important contribution of this work is that, in this communication we present a mode filter with an adaptive process that have proven to be efficient and very effective in noise reduction of gray-scale images, in particular when it is applied to head MRI. Test image analysis shows a stable behavior in the border of regions that change gray level intensity. With a minimal blurring effect of the boundaries and good fine structure resolution.

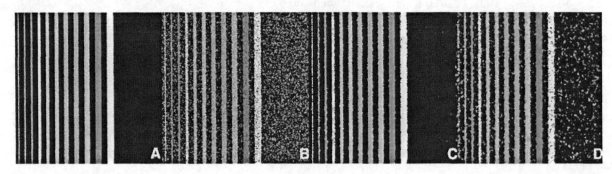

Figure 3. Constructed line test image restoration, (A) Original test image, (B) Original test image contaminated with 20% noise values (C) Filtered test image B, using the adaptive mode filter (D) Filtered test image B, using a regular median filter.

4. CONCLUSIONS

Intensity nonuniformities in MRI are also other limiting source of noise that can be corrected using robust parameters.[7] These nonuniformities sometimes can be treated by applying a mode noise reduction filter. Adaptive median filters have been applied to medical imaging with very good results,[4] .[3] Adaptive mode filters, to our knowledge, have not been wildly used as explicit noise reduction filters and have the same or better response compared to the adaptive median ones. He have found that this kind of filter softens the data and helps in reducing different levels of nonuniformities in the MRI data. Adaptive mode filter shows a better border detection and correction (Figure 3), because in the second step of the process it corrects using a larger radios for the neighborhood (larger kernel). Adaptive mode noise filters are effective for softening the image and compare to the median filters and other adaptive filters and they are not CPU intensive.

ACKNOWLEDGMENTS

We want to thank S. Estrada, RT. and G. Reynoso, RT. for their help during image acquisition. And GE Medical Systems Mexico, Schering Mexicana, S.A. as well as the Imaging Department at the ABC Hospital in Mexico City for their support. This work was partially supported by CONACyT R31162-A.

APPENDIX A. PSEUDOCODE

The adaptive mode filter process can be better understood with the pseudocode for each of the steps described at the methods:

```
STEP 1. Data is a gray scale image I sice NX x NY,
a mode filtered image IT is constructed:

IT = I
FOR i=1, NX-2 DO
   FOR j=1, NY-2 DO BEGIN
   np=0
   FOR k=i-1, i+1 DO
```

```
    FOR n=j-1, j+1 DO BEGIN
        VEC[np] = IR(k, n)
    np = np+1
    ENDFOR
    MODA  = DetecMode(VEC) (The mode is calculated here)
    IF(ABS(IR(i,j) - MODA[0]) GE 2.0*MODA(1))
    THEN IT(i, j) = MODA[0]
    ENDFOR
MODAD =  DetecMode(DERHIST)
(The derivative of the histograme is calculated)
np = 0
(The real noise candidates are estimated here)
FOR i=0, size(DERHIST) DO
IF ABS(DERHIST(i) - MODAD[0]) GT 12.*MODA[1] THEN BEGIN
    R[np] = i
    np = np+1
    ENDIF
```

STEP 2. The real noise pixels are estimated here and the desition to correct them is taken depending on the local value of the mode in a 5 x 5 kernel neighborhood.

```
    FOR k=0, np DO
    FOR i=1, NX-2 DO
        FOR j=1, NY-2 DO IF (IR(i,j) EQ R(k)) THEN BEGIN
    npun = 0
    FOR l=i-2, i+2 DO
    FOR m=j-2, j+2 DO BEGIN
    VEC[npun] = IR(l, m)
    npun = npun
    ENDFOR
MODAN = DetectMode(VEC)
IF (ABS(IR(i, j) - MODAN[0]) GE 2.*MODAN[1])
THEN IT(i,j) = MODAN[0]
ENDIF
```

REFERENCES

1. J. C. Russ, *The Image Processing Handbook*, CRC Press, Boca Raton, FL, 2nd ed., 1994.

2. A. K. Jain, *Fundamentals of Digital Image Processing*, Prentice Hall, Englewood Cliffs, NJ 07632, 1989.

3. C. B. Ahn, Y. C. Song, and P. D. J., "Adaptive template filtering for signal-to-noise ratio enhancement in magnetic resonance imaging," *IEEE Trans. Med. Imag.* **18**(6), pp. 549–556, 1999.

4. A. Sawant, H. Zeman, D. Muratore, S. Samant, and F. DiBianca, "An adaptive median filter algorithm to remove impulse noise in x-ray and ct images and speckle in iltrasound images.," in *Proccedings of SPIE, Medical Imaging 1999, Image Processing*, K. M. Hanson, ed., **3661**, pp. 1263–1274, 1999.

5. L. González-Santos, R. Rojas, J. H. Sossa-Azuela, and F. A. Barrios, "Mri segmentation based on region growing with robust estimation," in *Proccedings of SPIE, Medical Imaging 1999, Image Processing*, K. M. Hanson, ed., **3661**, pp. 880–885, 1999.

6. J. G. Sled, A. P. Zijdenbos, and A. C. Evans, "A nonparametric method for automatic correction of intensity nonuniformity in mri data," *IEEE Trans. Med. Imag.* **17**, pp. 87–97, February 1998.

7. M. Garza-Jinich, V. Medina, P. Meer, and O. Yañez, "Automatic correction of bias field in magnetic resonance images," *Proccedings International Conference on Image Analysis*, pp. 752–756, (Venecia), 1999.

8. R. J. Prorok and A. M. Sawyer, *Fast Imaging Techniques, Signa Advantage Applications Guide*, vol. IV E8804DC, G. E. Medical Systems, Milwaukee, U.S.A., 1992.

9. P. J. Rousseeuw and A. M. Leroy, *Robust Regression and Outlier Detection*, John Wiley and Sons, New York, 1987.

Contrast improvements in digital radiography using a scatter reduction processing algorithm

Kent M. Ogden [a], Charles R. Wilson [b], and Robert Cox [c]

[a] SUNY Upstate Medical University, Syracuse, NY 13210
[b] Medical College of Wisconsin, Milwaukee, WI 53226
[c] NIMH Bethesda, MD 20892

ABSTRACT

An expectation maximization (EM) algorithm has been developed based on a model of radiographic imaging that accounts for scatter radiation and resolution degradation. Digital radiographs of a chest phantom were acquired, and the amount of scatter in several regions was computed using the known radiographic exposure and the known material properties. Contrast and noise were measured in a step wedge in the phantom. The phantom images were processed by the EM algorithm for up to 8 iterations, and the image intensity and noise values were measured at each iteration step. These values were used to compute the scatter reduction properties of the algorithm and its effect on the contrast-to-noise ratio. The algorithm removed over 90% of the scattered radiation in the image. Image noise values were reduced an average of 50% in the first iteration, but then increased to values equal or above unprocessed images. The contrast-to-noise ratio was initially increased substantially, but gradually decreased as further iterations caused the image noise to increase. With proper selection of processing parameters, this algorithm could provide considerable qualitative enhancement of clinical images with a single iteration as well as numerically accurate scatter reduction.

Keywords: Image quality, contrast enhancement, maximum likelihood estimation, expectation maximization, digital radiography.

1. INTRODUCTION

The use of maximum-likelihood estimation (MLE) in medical imaging is best known from its application to image reconstruction in emission computed tomography, as originally described by Shepp and Vardi.[1] In this application of MLE the parameters that define the probability density function describing the observed data are the activities (mean number of decays per unit time) in each of the volume elements that define the image. The reconstructed image is then obtained as the maximum likelihood estimate of these activities. MLE has also been applied to the correction of projection data in CT[2], reconstruction of CT and magnetic resonance images[3,4], restoration of images obtained with optical systems[5,6], and to the restoration of radiographic images. For example, Brailean et al. have applied this technique to recover a de-blurred estimate of the recorded radiographic image.[7] In that application, the point spread function of the imaging system is interpreted as a probability density function that describes the detection of the incident photons. The advantage of using MLE in this way is that most any physical process that degrades the image may be corrected for by incorporating it into the probabilistic model of the image formation process.

In the application of MLE to image reconstruction and restoration problems such as this, the maximum likelihood estimates of the image information usually cannot be calculated analytically, due to the complexity of the likelihood function. In these cases it is necessary to apply a numerical estimation technique to calculate the MLE. The standard approach is to employ an iterative technique such as the expectation maximization (EM) algorithm. The EM algorithm was first described by Dempster, Laird, and Rubin[8] as a general method to compute maximum likelihood estimates from incomplete data. This algorithm has been shown to converge monotonically. It is, however, a computationally intensive technique and the convergence rate can be relatively slow. Work has been done to improve the speed of the algorithm[9,10], and alternative statistical image processing algorithms have been developed that have advantages over the EM algorithm.[11,12,13,14]

Medical Imaging 2002: Image Processing, Milan Sonka, J. Michael Fitzpatrick, Editors, Proceedings of SPIE Vol. 4684 (2002) © 2002 SPIE · 1605-7422/02/$15.00

A technique for scatter reduction using statistical modeling of the imaging process has been developed by Floyd, et al.[15] This is essentially the same technique used by Brailean for de-blurring an image; However, the model is slightly different. This approach models the radiographic image as a scatter image added to a primary image, with the scatter image modeled as a weighted convolution of the primary image with a scatter kernel. A scatter-reduced image is then found by MLE, using the EM algorithm to calculate the maximum likelihood estimate of the primary image given the observed image, and known scatter kernel and (fixed) scatter-to-primary ratio. Floyd reports increases in the signal-to-noise ratio (SNR) in the resulting image, as well as increases in the contrast. The scatter model uses a radially symmetric kernel, however, and it is shown in this work that the detected scatter is not isotropic when a grid is part of the imaging chain. The particular form of the imaging model used also limits the algorithms accuracy, since the scatter to primary ratio is fixed for all locations in the image.

In this work, a new EM algorithm is presented that is derived specifically for radiographic imaging. The derivation follows from a model of the imaging process that incorporates blurring due to a non-ideal imaging system as well as the presence of scatter radiation. This algorithm has an advantage over previously reported applications of EM to radiographic imaging in that the scatter to primary ratio may vary across the image, thus allowing more accurate scatter removal in images where there is a large range of transmissions and therefore scatter to primary ratios, such as in chest imaging.

2. IMAGING MODEL AND EM ALGORITHM

The imaging model used in the development of the EM algorithm is similar to that employed by Floyd, and a schematic illustrating the key features is shown in Fig. 1. The most important assumptions made in the imaging model are described briefly. First, it is assumed that the input x-ray beam is described by a Poisson distributed random variable with mean fluence per unit area that is constant over the patient. The mean number of photons per unit area, No, denotes this incident fluence.

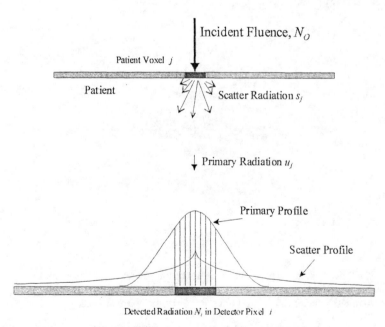

Fig. 1: Schematic illustrating the imaging model. The total detected radiation in each pixel is subdivided into a primary component and a scatter component. The total signal in each pixel is the sum of these components.

The incident fluence then interacts with the patient. The patient is considered subdivided into discrete voxels, and these are indexed with the subscript j, as shown in Fig. 1. There is a one-to-one geometric correspondence between a patient voxel, j, and its corresponding image pixel, which are denoted with the subscript i. The probability of transmission through a given voxel, denoted p_j, is the quantity we are interested in recovering. Given this quantity, we can calculate a scatter- and blur-free image.

Radiation entering a given voxel j is either attenuated (scattered or absorbed) or transmitted. Attenuation is therefore a binomial process, giving rise to primary (unattenuated) radiation exiting the patient that is again described by a Poisson distributed random variable[16] with mean N_op_j. This is shown as u_j in Fig. 1. This primary radiation interacts with the detector, and is 'blurred' due to the non-ideal detector response. This blurring is described by the detectors point spread function (PSF), but in this model the PSF is interpreted as a probability density function describing the probability that primary radiation emanating from voxel j will be detected in pixel i.

Radiation that is attenuated by the patient contributes to the scatter component of the detected x-rays. In this model, it is assumed that the *detected* scatter radiation that is generated in a patient voxel j is again a Poisson distributed random variable with a mean value related to the transmission in that voxel. The mean value of the detected scatter generated in a given voxel is then some function $s(p_j)$. It has been determined experimentally that good scatter reduction can be achieved by using a simple scatter generation function such as $s(p_j) = \alpha\, p_j + \beta$ where α and β are experimentally determined parameters. The mean value of the detected scatter radiation emanating from voxel j is then $N_o(\alpha p_j + \beta)$.

The scatter radiation reaching the detector in a typical imaging system has passed through a scatter rejecting grid, which reduces the intensity and also imposes a unique geometric characteristic on the spatial distribution of the scatter radiation. We expect, in the absence of a grid, that scatter radiation generated by a pencil beam of radiation impinging a uniform slab of material would have a radially symmetric distribution when it reaches a detector such as a film cassette placed behind the material. In the presence of a linear grid, however, the scatter is not radially symmetric, since the probability of scatter penetrating the grid depends on the azimuthal angle between the scatter photon trajectory and the linear grid. An example of this type of distribution is shown in Fig. 2.

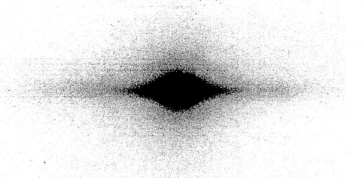

Fig. 2: Scatter radiation produced by a thin beam of x-rays at 80 kVp and incident on 20 cm of acrylic. The grid ratio is 8:1. The image width is approximately 5 cm, and the grid lines are horizontal in this image.

An elliptically weighted exponential was used to model this scatter distribution. This is stated mathematically as

$$K = e^{-\sqrt{a^2x^2 + b^2y^2}}. \tag{1}$$

In this equation, a represents the decay rate of the scatter response function in the x direction, and b represents the decay rate in the y direction. It should be noted that the scatter response function, K, has some dependence on the thickness of the material generating the scatter, and is not spatially invariant when the object generating the scatter is non-uniform, which is certainly the case when imaging a patient. Nevertheless, these assumptions are made to allow the use of Fourier techniques in the calculation of the MLE of the transmission probabilities. Without this assumption, the calculation time required would be prodigious.

With this imaging model, an EM algorithm has been derived that will calculate the MLE of the transmission probabilities given an observed image and measured PSF, scatter response function, and scatter generation function parameters. The mathematical statement of the algorithm is

$$
p = \frac{p^o}{1+\alpha} \left[\frac{I}{I_o(p^o **PSF + (\alpha p^o + \beta)**K)} \right] **PSF
$$
$$
+ \frac{\alpha p^o + \beta}{1+\alpha} \left[\frac{I}{I_o(p^o **PSF + (\alpha p^o + \beta)**K)} \right] **K - \frac{\beta}{1+\alpha}. \tag{2}
$$

All of the variables in this equation except for α, β and I_o, represent two-dimensional distributions. I_o represents the mean value of the intensity of the incident x-ray beam, and p^o represents an initial estimate of the transmission. This is shown without the subscript j for simplicity. I represents the observed image. The double asterisk denotes a two-dimensional convolution. What this equation calculates, then, is a best estimate (in the maximum likelihood sense) of the transmission distribution, p, given the observed image and an *initial* estimate of the transmission distribution. This becomes an EM algorithm when the output of an iteration is used as the input for the next iteration.

Although equation (2) is complex, it can shed some light on the goal of an EM algorithm such as this. Examining the term in the square brackets, we have the observed image divided by an *estimate* of the observed image. The estimate of the observed image is just the current estimate of the transmission distribution (p^o) subjected to the process describing the imaging model. Stated in words, the estimated image is the sum of a primary image convolved with the point spread function with a scatter source image convolved with a scatter response function. It is easy to show that when this estimate of the observed image exactly equals the observed image (I), the output of the algorithm p will be exactly equal to the initial estimate p^o. This is the goal of the EM algorithm, to produce an estimate of an unobservable quantity (the transmission distribution) that will exactly produce the observed image given the imaging model.

3. EXPERIMENTAL METHODS

The data for this project were acquired using a prototype installation of a flat panel digital detector manufactured by General Electric Medical Systems[17] (Milwaukee, WI). This detector is of the indirect detection type, using CsI as the primary converter of x-ray energy to light. The detector has 2k x 2k pixels 200 μm on a side. The total area of the detector is approximately 41cm x 41cm.

Some preliminary image processing is performed on data acquired by this system. First, a map of defective pixels is used to replace 'bad' pixel data with values derived from the nearest neighbors. Then, a flat-field image is used to scale the image to remove the effects of variable amplifier gain and other system generated non-uniformities. There is no other image processing applied to the data at this point, which preserves the highly linear response and wide dynamic range of the system.

In order to implement the EM algorithm and verify its performance, information is needed concerning the scatter response function K, the system point spread function *PSF*, the scatter generation function, and the attenuation of the phantom materials. The latter is required so that the scatter-free values in the phantom images may be calculated for comparison with the phantom images that are processed by the EM algorithm. Although there are good published numbers for the attenuation properties of acrylic, the polychromatic x-ray beam would still require measurements to determine the effective energy, and so it was decided to simply measure the material attenuation properties.

To allow calculation of the expected intensities in the phantom images, attenuation measurements of the acrylic material were made using the same x-ray tube/generator used to acquire the phantom images. The measurements were made using a tightly collimated beam of x-rays projecting through a varying thickness of acrylic. The intensity of the attenuated beam was measured with an MDH model 1015 dosimeter and an MDH 6cc ionization chamber. The acrylic was positioned as close as possible to the x-ray tube, and the ionization chamber positioned 3m from the tube to reduce the detected scatter radiation to negligible levels. Multiple exposures were taken and integrated by the dosimeter, and unattenuated intensity measurements were also made to allow calculation of the linear attenuation coefficients.

3.1 PSF and Scatter Response Determination

To find the *PSF* of the system, measurements are made of the systems line-spread function (LSF) and these measurements are used to generate the two dimensional PSF. This approach assumes that the system PSF is radially symmetric. The LSF of the system is measured using a tungsten strip with a high quality machined edge placed on the image receptor cover. The tungsten is radiographed with a technique that allows reasonably good penetration of the tungsten without saturating the detector with the primary radiation. The images acquired in this way (as well as all the other data acquired with this system) are written to CD-R media and transported to the analysis computer.

Scatter response measurements are made with an acrylic phantom and collimated x-ray beam as shown in Fig. 3.

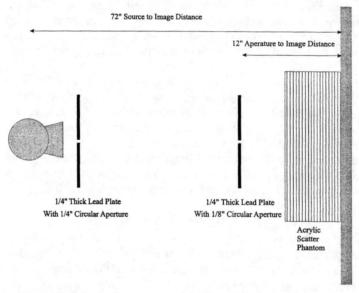

Fig. 3: Experimental arrangement for determining scatter response function.

The two collimators form a thin beam of radiation, and varying amounts of acrylic are inserted into the beam to produce varying amounts of scatter radiation. The acrylic is then removed, and an exposure made at a low technique to produce a primary radiation image. With knowledge of the attenuation properties of the acrylic at the beam energy used, it is then possible to scale the primary image to the appropriate value so that it may be subtracted from the scatter + primary image. The decay rates of the scatter in the directions perpendicular and parallel to the grid lines are then measured using the scatter-only images.

3.2 Phantom Measurements

To test the performance of the algorithm, images were acquired with a chest phantom constructed of acrylic and aluminum. A radiograph of the phantom is shown in Fig. 4. This phantom contains cutout areas for the lung and ¼" aluminum bars to simulate the ribs. The mediastinum also has a ¼" aluminum insert to simulate the bone in the sternum and spine.

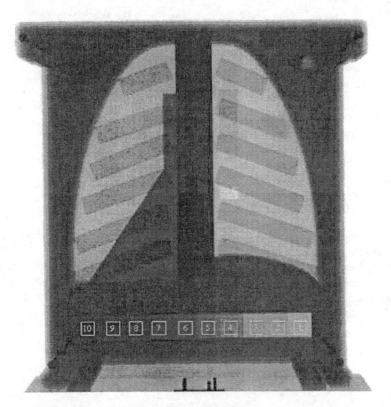

Fig. 4: Radiograph of the chest phantom used to test the performance of the EM algorithm. The numbered regions in the step wedge were used to measure scatter reduction over a range of thickness.

4. RESULTS

4.1 Imaging System Characterization

The edge response data was used to calculate the LSF as shown in Fig. 5. This LSF was then rotated about the central

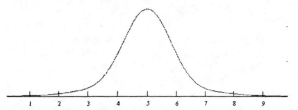

Fig. 5: System line spread function. The x axis units are pixels. This represents the average of ~2800 independent measurements of the LSF.

axis to form the two dimensional PSF. Because of the high quality of the LSF data no further processing was performed, such as fitting with a Gaussian. The full width at half maximum value of 2 pixels agrees well with published values for this detector[17].

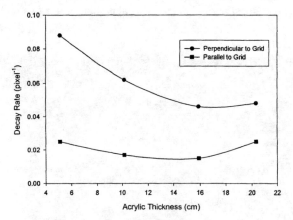

Fig. 6: Scatter decay rates in the horizontal and vertical directions at 80 kVp.

The scatter measurements show that the decay rate of the scatter response is dependent on the thickness of the material generating the scatter. It is also expected that there will be an energy dependence since the effective energy of the scattered radiation will increase as the kVp increases. This allows the scatter radiation to penetrate the grid more readily than scatter generated at lower energies. Fig. 6 shows the measured scatter decay rates for a varying thickness of acrylic at 80 kVp. The decay rates in the direction perpendicular to the grid are greater than those for the parallel direction since the grid is less effective in removing scatter photons whose trajectories are parallel with the grid lines.

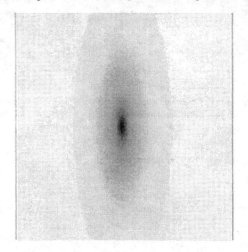

Fig. 7: Scatter kernel constructed using the average decay rates. The extent of the image is 5cm x 5 cm.

In order to produce a single scatter response function for a given x-ray energy (kVp), the averages of the decay rates were used. For the parallel direction, the average is 0.021 pixel^{-1} and for the perpendicular direction the average value is 0.061 pixel^{-1}. Using these decay rates, we construct a scatter response kernel shown graphically in Fig. 7.

The scatter generation function parameters, α and β, were found experimentally by iterating the EM algorithm with a phantom image as the input until the algorithm converged, and comparing the image intensity in the step wedge regions with the expected intensity calculated using the incident image intensity and the measured attenuation properties of the acrylic. In this way, parameters were found that were able to remove over 90% of the scatter radiation from the image. The values of the scatter parameters found were $\alpha = 1.15$ and $\beta = 0.0085$.

4.2 Algorithm Convergence

An important feature of an EM algorithm such as this is that it converges monotonically. The measure of convergence is usually expressed as the calculated values of the log-likelihood function of the system in question. In this case, the log-likelihood function is

$$l = \sum_i \left[-\sum_j \left(I_o[\alpha p_j + \beta]K(i,j) + I_o p_j PSF(i,j) \right) + I_i \ln \sum_j \left(I_o[\alpha p_j + \beta]K(i,j) + I_o p_j PSF(i,j) \right) \right]. \quad (3)$$

In this equation, $K(i,j)$ and $PSF(i,j)$ are the scatter response function and the point spread function, and the (i,j) nomenclature indicates that these are the probabilities that a photon initially emanating from patient voxel j will be detected in pixel i. Because of the nature of Eq. (3), it is not possible to use Fourier techniques in its calculation, and the large size of the data set would result in computation times of several days with the available computing equipment. It is therefore necessary to find another measure of convergence. To provide this measure, the method employed by Floyd[15] will be used. This method is based on the fact, stated earlier, that the algorithm attempts to produce an estimate of the primary image that will generate the observed image when subjected to the physical processes expressed in the imaging model. It is apparent, then, that measuring the RMS difference between these two quantities should provide an indication of the convergence of the algorithm. This measure, denoted the L^2 norm, is stated as

$$\left| L^2 \right| = \sqrt{\frac{1}{N} \sum_i \left[I_i - estimated_i \right]} \quad . \quad (4)$$

In Eq. (4), $estimated_i$ is the current estimate of the observed image as discussed earlier. If the algorithm were able to find an estimate of the probability distribution p_j that exactly produced the observed image, the L^2 norm would vanish. In reality, limitations in the model will prevent this from happening, and the L^2 norm will decrease very slowly after a few iterations. An example of this behavior is shown in Fig. 8.

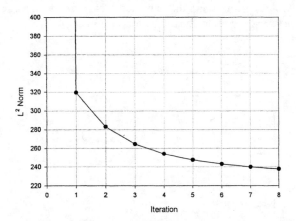

Fig. 8: The L^2 norm is a measure of the convergence of the algorithm. The value calculated before the first iteration is >4700.

The algorithm convergence may also be examined by considering the behavior of the pixel values in the phantoms step wedge. With the known attenuation properties of the acrylic and incident x-ray intensity, it is possible to calculate the expected scatter-free mean pixel intensity in each of the regions in the step wedge. This allows a comparison between the actual pixel intensity and the scatter free intensity in each step as a function of iteration.

Fig. 9 shows the pixel intensities in several selected regions as a function of iteration. These intensities are expressed as a percentage of the scatter-free intensity for each region. This graph shows that all regions initially have a substantial scatter component, with scatter fractions ranging from about 45% in step 1 to slightly more than 70% in step 9. This graph also shows that the majority of the scatter removal occurs in the first iteration of the algorithm, and in fact the pixel intensities 'overshoot' the final values and then slowly increase as they converge.

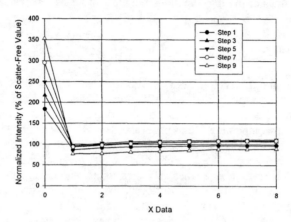

Fig. 9: The intensity in several regions relative to the scatter-free intensity in those regions, expressed as a percentage.

The convergence of the algorithm is shown another way in Fig. 10. In this figure, the top trace shows the mean pixel intensity in each step. The bottom two traces represent the scatter-free pixel intensities (dotted line) and the actual pixel intensities after 8 iterations of the EM algorithm. It can be seen in this graph that for the areas of highest attenuation (regions 1 and 2) and the region of lowest attenuation (region 10) the final pixel intensities are lower than the calculated scatter-free values. In other words, this algorithm over compensates (removes too much scatter) in these regions. The remainder of the regions have final values greater than the expected scatter-free values, and so are under compensated. These discrepancies show that the scatter generation function does not precisely predict the amount of detected scatter that is generated as a function of material thickness.

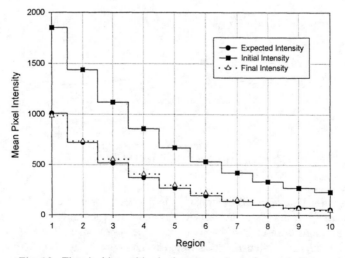

Fig. 10: The pixel intensities in the step wedge before and after processing.

4.3 Scatter Reduction and Contrast Enhancement

Fig. 11 shows the percentage of the initial scatter in region that is remaining after processing by the EM algorithm. A negative value means that there was too much signal removed, a positive value means not enough signal was removed. This plot clearly shows the trend mentioned in the previous paragraph. It is clear that a linear scatter generation function will not accurately correct for the scatter in all thicknesses of material. Fig. 11 is essentially a qualitative plot showing the difference between the linear model and a more accurate nonlinear model. Changing the scatter generation model would require that a new algorithm be derived and this has been done for a quadratic scatter model. The quadratic model has the additional complexity in that there are two results returned for the new estimate of the transmission probability, and the algorithm must select the correct root.

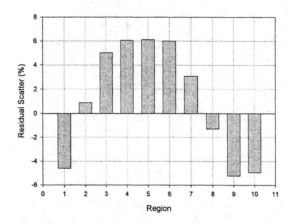

Fig. 11: Percent of the initial scatter radiation remaining.

Contrast is measured as the difference in the mean pixel intensity between adjacent regions relative to the average of the intensity in each region. This quantity is expressed as a percentage. Fig. 12 shows the contrast for selected sets of adjacent regions as a function of iteration of the EM algorithm. As before, it is clear that the greatest change in contrast occurs after the first iteration of the algorithm. After the first iteration, the contrast levels are relatively constant.

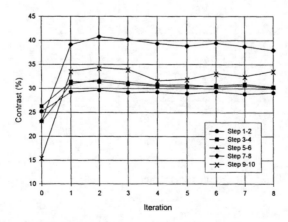

Fig. 12: Contrast between adjacent steps as a function of algorithm iteration.

Fig. 13 shows the final percent increase in contrast between adjacent steps after processing. In regions of low attenuation with correspondingly low initial scatter fractions, the change in contrast is relatively small. The more dense regions show a much greater increase in contrast.

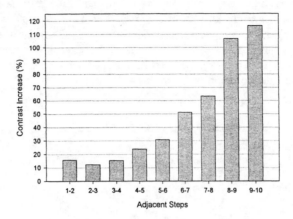

Fig. 13: The percent increase in contrast between adjacent steps after processing.

Noise enhancement is well known in this type of algorithm and is one of the reasons researchers have explored more sophisticated algorithms, such as Bayesian image processing. One of the features of these algorithms is the ability to constrain the noise in the image. Fig. 14 shows the noise enhancement in the current algorithm. The noise does decrease at the first iteration, and this is noticeable in the image as a smoothed appearance. It is difficult to accurately measure the noise with further iteration of the algorithm, however, since there is also an edge enhancing effect that causes "cupping" of the pixel intensity across the steps. This introduces a trend to the pixel values that will increase the standard deviation of pixel values in an ROI placed on a given step. This effect can be seen in Fig. 15.

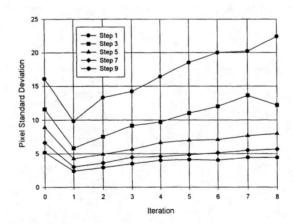

Fig. 14: Noise in selected steps.

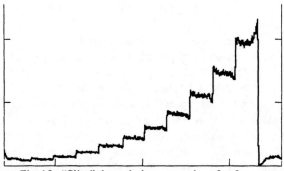

Fig. 15: "Slice" through the step wedge after 8
iterations showing the edge enhancement.

The contrast to noise ratio shows behavior that is generally governed by the behavior of the noise, since the contrast is generally constant after the first iteration of the algorithm. Fig. 16 shows the CNR for selected adjacent steps as a function of iteration of the algorithm. In regions in which the initial increase in contrast is great, the increasing noise

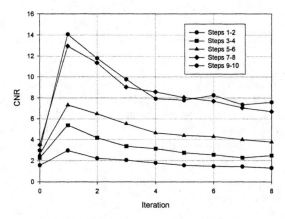

Fig. 16: The CNR ratio as a function of iteration.

does not reduce the final CNR level below the initial level. In the most transmissive regions, the change in CNR is small enough that the increased noise will reduce the CNR below the initial value. The final change in CNR is shown in Fig. 17.

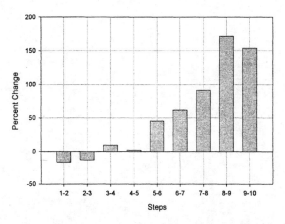

Fig. 17: Final change in CNR after processing by the
EM algorithm.

5. DISCUSSION

The goal of this work was to develop and implement a new EM algorithm that provides a numerically accurate reduction in detected scatter radiation. The algorithm shows good performance in reducing scatter, with a large percentage of the scatter being removed after 8 iterations. The linear model for the scatter generation function could obviously be improved upon, which should allow more accurate scatter removal over the range of densities in the phantom used. A quadratic model for scatter generation has been applied and an EM algorithm derived. This scatter model was of the form $s(p_j) = \alpha\, p_j(1 - p_j)$. This form was chosen so that when the transmission was zero (infinitely thick object) the amount of scatter generated was zero, and when the transmission was unity (raw x-ray beam) the amount of scatter generated was also zero. This model also has the advantage of requiring a single free parameter. It proved impossible, however, to find a value for this parameter so that this model performed better than the linear scatter model. It is postulated that a more general quadratic scatter model could perform as well or better than the linear model.

The noise in the image is generally enhanced after several iterations of the algorithm. Some of the 'noise' increase is due to the edge enhancement seen in Fig. 15. It is thought that this edge enhancement is due to the scatter radiation 'leaking' from the regions of lower transmission (thicker material) into adjacent higher transmission regions. This causes the assumption of a spatially invariant scatter response to be inaccurate near edges such as this. The algorithm then over-compensates on one side of the edge and under-compensates on the other side, leading to the edge enhancement. This effect has also prevented an accurate assessment of the algorithms ability to undue the effect of the system PSF, since the edge enhancing effect far outweighs the corrections that are expected from 'de-blurring' and image.

An improved version of this algorithm is one in which the scatter model was modified to more accurately remove scatter over the range of material thickness. The scatter generation parameters could then be adjusted such that accurate removal of the scatter occurred on the first iteration of the algorithm. This would also avoid the edge enhancing effect that is seen when the algorithm is iterated multiple times. Although this would no longer technically be an EM algorithm, it could provide improvement in CNR in clinical radiography, which could be most useful in exams where there is naturally a large scatter fraction, such as portable chest radiographs acquired with no grid.

[1] L.A. Shepp and Y. Vardi, "Maximum Likelihood Reconstruction for Emission Tomography," IEEE Transactions on Medical Imaging **MI-1**, pp. 113-122, 1982.

[2] T. Hebert and S. Gopal, "Maximum Likelihood Preprocessing for Improved Filtered Back-Projection Reconstructions," Journal of Computer Assisted Tomography **18**, pp. 283-291, 1994.

[3] M. Miller, T. Schaewe, C. Bosch and J. Ackerman, "Model-Based Maximum-Likelihood Estimation for Phase- and Frequency-Encoded Magnetic-Resonance-Imaging Data," Journal of Magnetic Resonance, **Series B 107**, pp. 210-221, 1995.

[4] G. Zeng and G. Gullberg, "A Study Of The Reconstruction Artifacts In Cone Beam Tomography Using Filtered Backprojection And Iterative EM Algorithms," IEEE Transactions on Nuclear Science **37**, pp. 759-767, 1990.

[5] B. Frieden, "Restoring With Maximum Likelihood And Maximum Entropy," Journal of the Optical Society of America **62**, pp. 511-518, 1972.

[6] T. Holmes, "Maximum-Likelihood Image Restoration Adapted for Noncoherent Optical Imaging," Journal of the Optical Society of America **5**, pp. 666-673, 1988.

[7] J.C. Brailean et al, "Application of the EM Algorithm to Radiographic Images" Medical Physics **19**, pp. 1175-1182, 1992.

[8] A.P. Dempster, N.M. Laird and D.B. Rubin, "Maximum Likelihood from Incomplete Data via the EM Algorithm," Journal of the Royal Statistical Society **39**, pp. 1-38, 1977.

[9] Z. Liang, R. Jaszczak and H. Hart, "Study and Performance Evaluation of Statistical Methods in Image Processing," Comput. Biol. Med. **18**, pp. 395-408, 1988.

[10] T. Miller and J. Wallis, "Fast Maximum-Likelihood Reconstruction," The Journal of Nuclear Medicine **33**, pp. 1710-1711, 1992.

[11] A. Baydush, J. Bowsher, J. Laading and C. Floyd, Jr., "Improved Bayesian Image Estimation for Digital Chest Radiography," Medical Physics **24**, pp. 539-545, 1997.

[12] W. Richardson, "Bayesian-Based Iterative Method of Image Restoration," Journal of the Optical Society of America **62**, pp. 55-59 1972.

[13] S. Kawata and O. Nalcioglu, "Constrained Iterative Reconstruction by the Conjugate Gradient Method," IEEE Transactions on Medical Imaging **MI-4**, pp. 65-71, 1985.

[14] CW Helstrom, "Image Restoration by the Method of Least Squares," Journal of the Optical Society of America **57**, pp. 297-304 1967.

[15] C.E. Floyd et al, "Scatter Compensation for Digital Chest Radiography Using Maximum Likelihood Expectation Maximization," Investigative Radiology **28**, pp. 427-433, 1993.

[16] K. Ogden, "Maximum Likelihood Estimation in Dual-Energy Digital Chest Radiography: Simultaneous Correction of Scatter Radiation and Resolution Degradation Via the Expectation Maximization Algorithm", Doctoral Dissertation, Medical College of Wisconsin, Milwaukee, WI, Appendix A, 1999.

[17] Granfors PR, "Performance characteristics of an amorphous silicon flat panel x-ray imaging detector," SPIE **3659**, pp. 480-490, 1999.

Effective Dose Reduction in Dual-Energy Flat Panel X-Ray Imaging: Technique and Clinical Evaluation

Gopal B. Avinash[a], Kadri N. Jabri[a], Renuka Uppaluri[a], Amber Rader[a], Frank Fischbach[b], Jens Ricke[b], and Ulf Teichgräber[b]

[a]General Electric Medical Systems, Waukesha, WI 53188
[b]Charite Campus Virchow-Klinikum, 13353 Berlin, Germany

ABSTRACT

Dual-energy (DE) chest radiography with a digital flat panel (DFP) shows significant potential for increased sensitivity and specificity of pulmonary nodule detection. DFP-based DE produces significantly better image quality compared to Computed Radiography (CR) due to high detective quantum efficiency (DQE) and wide energy separation. We developed novel noise reduction filtering that significantly improves image quality at a given dose level, thereby allowing considerable additional dose reduction compared to CR. The algorithm segments images into *structures*, which are processed using anisotropic smoothing and sharpening, and *non-structures*, which are processed using isotropic smoothing. A fraction of the original image is blended with the processed image to obtain an image with improved noise characteristics. DE decomposed radiographs were obtained at film equivalent of 400 speed chest exam dose for 12 patients (set A) and at twice the dose for 7 other patients (set C). Images from set A were filtered using our algorithm to form set B. Images were evaluated by four radiologists using a noise rating scale. A two-sample t-test showed no significant difference in ratings between B and C, while significant differences were found between A and B, and A and C. Therefore, our algorithm enables effective patient dose reduction while maintaining perceptual image quality.

Keywords: dual energy, X-ray, chest radiography, noise reduction filtering, dose reduction

1. INTRODUCTION

Lung cancer is currently the leading cause of cancer death in the United States, estimated to have caused 156,900 deaths in 2000[1], and is a growing cause of death worldwide. Although conventional chest radiography is low cost, low dose, and widely available, it has been shown to have relatively low sensitivity for detection of pulmonary nodules. This poor sensitivity for chest radiography precludes its use as an effective screening modality. Samei *et al* have shown that nodule detection in chest radiography is primarily limited by anatomic or structural noise, as opposed to radiographic or quantum noise[2]. If the anatomic noise in the chest radiograph could be reduced or eliminated, the sensitivity of chest radiography would be significantly increased.

1.1 Dual-energy radiography
Dual-energy imaging has been investigated as a means of reducing the impact of anatomic noise on pathology detection in chest radiography. Dual-energy radiography involves taking two exposures of the patient using different-energy x-ray beams. By exploiting the difference in the energy dependence of attenuation between bone and soft-tissue, the high-energy and low-energy images can be "energy-subtracted" or decomposed in order to create a soft-tissue image and a bone image.[3] The contrast of the bone (ribs and spine) is eliminated in the soft-tissue image, and the contrast of the soft-tissue is reduced in the bone image (Figure 1). Early development of such a system was hindered by the lack of a suitable detector. Computed tomography (CT) scanners were used in scout-view mode,[4] and even film has been proposed as a dual-energy receptor.[5] Recent CR systems have been hampered by poor subtraction (tissue

Medical Imaging 2002: Image Processing, Milan Sonka, J. Michael Fitzpatrick, Editors, Proceedings of SPIE Vol. 4684 (2002) © 2002 SPIE · 1605-7422/02/$15.00

contrast cancellation), workflow inconveniences, and DQE limitations. Despite these limitations, dual-energy CR has been shown to significantly increase the detection of lung cancer.[6]

GE Medical Systems has developed a digital flat-panel (DFP) imaging system based on a CsI:Tl scintillator coupled to an amorphous silicon TFT array.[7] For radiographic applications the panel has a size of 41 cm × 41 cm, 2048 × 2048 × 200 μm pitch. The key enabler for dual-exposure, dual-energy imaging is the ability to rapidly read the image data off of the commercially available detector.[8] The GE *Revolution XR/d* system currently offers dual-energy imaging capability with an inter-exposure time of less than 200 ms.

Energy separation between the two exposures is critical for effective tissue cancellation and good contrast-to-noise ratio in the subtracted image.[9,10] Sabol *et al.*[11] showed that the DFP-based, dual-exposure technique resulted in generally doubling the energy separation between the two images. Furthermore, DFP dual-energy had much better noise performance due to its higher detective quantum efficiency (DQE), and thus allowed for significant improvement in image quality and reduction in patient dose as compared to CR dual-energy systems.

In general, the improved tissue discrimination possible with dual-energy imaging comes at the cost of increased noise. To combat the concomitant increased stochastic noise and regain the benefits of reducing anatomical noise, noise reduction strategies are often employed in dual-energy imaging.[12, 13, 14, 15-23] In this study, we describe a novel noise reduction technique that significantly improves image quality at a given dose level, thereby allowing considerable additional dose reduction compared to CR.

1.2 Dose reduction through noise reduction filtering
Dual-energy imaging on DFP has better DQE and consequently less noise compared to CR. Noise levels in decomposed (soft-tissue and bone) images, however, are higher than in standard radiographs as a result of the decomposition process. Therefore, applying sophisticated noise reduction filtering techniques such as the one developed in this work can significantly improve noise characteristics while retaining diagnostically relevant image detail.

Noise reduction filtering can be used in one of two ways, either to improve image quality at a fixed dose, or to reduce dose at an equivalent image quality. For example, we can potentially lower patient dose by acquiring radiographs at a lower exposure than that used conventionally, and subsequently filter to regain the anticipated image quality. This concept is illustrated in Figure 2. Although we develop the filtering algorithm below as a dose reduction technique, its application is certainly not limited only for such purpose, and its power lies in giving the clinician a general method for improving diagnosis.

1.3 Previous work on noise reduction
The most fundamental noise reduction strategy, both computationally and theoretically, is the application of a simple smoothing filter. In the early days of dual-energy CT, Rutherford[24] first suggested using a 5x5 boxcar low-pass filter to smooth the noisy reconstructed images. Johns[25] extended the idea to smooth only the high-energy image to avoid blurring calcified structures. Driven by the use of dual-energy in CR, noise reduction strategies in the late 1980s and 1990s focused on more sophisticated algorithms. Kalender[18] developed an algorithm called correlated noise reduction (KCNR) that used knowledge about the anti-correlation in noise between the bone and tissue images. Kalender[18] and Ergun[20] proposed methods to improve performance of KCNR at sharp tissue edges. McCollough[17] showed that the algorithm of Kalender[18] was analytically related to measurement-dependent filtering methods of Macovski.[15-17] Kido[26] proposed an iterative noise reduction method to improve the noise magnitude, edges, and sharpness. Several other methods were also introduced focusing on improving the sharpness and noise texture, including noise forcing and noise clipping developed by Dobbins *et al.*[21-23]

In the image processing literature, many algorithms use multi-resolution decomposition (e.g., wavelet based techniques), which decompose the image into various frequency bands, process each band separately and the regroup all the frequency bands together to reconstitute the image. This class of techniques has the advantage of modifying a specific spatial frequency band of the image. A well-known corollary of these techniques in image compression is that substantially all the redundancies at a given scale are exploited to achieve high compression ratios without sacrificing the compression quality in these images. Another class of filters is segmentation-based. This class of techniques decomposes the image based on structures and non-structures, processes structures and non-structures separately and then recombine the processed structures and non-structures to form the final filtered image.[27,28] Unlike in the multi-resolution case, this class of methods exploits the spatial connectedness of structures to substantially perform different operations on structures and non-structures.

2. METHODS

The current algorithm differs from prior work in several significant ways. Noise reduction is performed after dual-energy decomposition on soft-tissue and bone images. The novel concept of the proposed technique involves combining the redundancy exploitation of multi-resolution-based techniques with the spatial connectedness of the segmentation-based techniques to obtain a robust noise reduction with computationally efficient implementation. Furthermore, this algorithm requires two images, one being a decomposed image (a soft tissue or bone image) and the other being the high-energy image.

In the proposed algorithm (Figure 3), the input image (I_1) and high-energy image (I_H) are first shrunk by a pre-specified factor x to form an intermediate image I_2 and I_{2H}. Image I_2 is filtered with a segmentation-based noise reduction filter, which uses two images to compute gradient and intensity thresholds to obtain the filtered image I_3. Next, I_3 is expanded by the same factor x to form I_4 using a suitable interpolation function. Finally, I_4 is blended with I_1 to form the final filtered output I_5.

2.1 Filtering algorithm
Input to the algorithm is either the decomposed soft tissue image, or the bone image (I_1), and the high-energy image (I_H). Major steps are described below.

2.1.1 Shrinking
The image I_1 is shrunk to obtain an image I_2 by neighborhood averaging. The size of the image is augmented to prevent loss of data, while images are shrunk. The amount of shrinking is set by a pre-specified factor x. The value of x was set to 4 in this study.

2.1.2 Segmentation
A robust method to determine structures and non-structures is described in detail elsewhere.[28] Here, we describe its salient aspects.

The segmentation algorithm essentially uses gradient magnitude and gradient direction to automatically arrive at a segmentation mask for a class of images. It uses the gradient direction to obtain the initial mask. However, most of the salient edges are broken up because of the noisiness of the direction metric. A connectivity analysis is used to eliminate "islands" in the mask and the total number of remaining edge points are used to select the gradient-based threshold (GBT). Gradient following can be used to further improve the robustness of GBT. Additionally, an intensity-based threshold (IBT) is derived for excluding highly attenuated regions in the high-energy image I_{2H}. Intensity threshold is obtained by multiplying the average intensity of the high-energy image by a scale factor. Next, a binary mask image is created such that the pixels are set to 1 if the corresponding pixels in the gradient image are higher than GBT and pixels in I_{2H} greater than IBT; otherwise the mask is set to 0. Isolated small segments are eliminated using a four-connected connectivity approach. Following this process, an initial mask corresponding to an initial classification of pixels is obtained. Finally, the final mask that describes *structure* and *non-structure* is obtained using a binary rank-order processing.

2.1.3 Anisotropic smoothing
Regions designated as *structures* are filtered to extract dominant orientation. Our method involves iteratively filtering the structure by a 3×1-smoothing kernel along the dominant direction in a given neighborhood, which would be the direction of majority of the local minimum variances in that neighborhood. This process has the tendency to bridge gaps and the amount is controlled by a parameter. The iterations are done for a set number of times (e.g., 3). Each iteration is accomplished using the following steps: First the structure region is scanned and a local orientation map is obtained by assigning one of the four orientation numbers, i.e., 1 for 45°, 2 for 135°, 3 for 90°, and 4 for 0°. The structure region is scanned again and the dominant orientation at any point is determined by counting the number of

different orientations in a neighborhood. The orientation getting the maximum number of counts is the dominant orientation. As a further refinement, we use the both dominant direction and its orthogonal direction to make a consistency decision. Pixel-averaging using a 3×1 kernel is performed along the direction which gets the most number of counts in that neighborhood.

2.1.4 Sharpening
This function is performed only on anisotropically smoothed structure pixels, which have gradients that are above a pre-specified limit (e.g., $2 \times$ FGT). The specific steps are the following:

i)   Obtain maximum directional edge strength image:
     a)   The 1-D Laplacian of the image at every pixel in each of the 4 directions mentioned before is obtained using the equation below,
$$E(k) = 2I(k) - I(k\text{-}1) - I(k\text{+}1)$$
        where the index ''k'' refers to the current location along a given direction, $E(k)$ is the edge strength and $I(k)$ is the intensity value at the pixel.
     b)   After computing all the four edge-strengths at a given pixel, determine the maximum directional edge strength and use it for the subsequent steps as the edge strength $E(x,y)$ at that location.
     c)   Continue this process for all the pixels in the image. Note that the border pixels in a given image have to be treated differently and we set them equal to zero for the subsequent steps.
ii)   Apply the sharpening equation,
$$I(x,y) = I(x,y) + T[\gamma(E(x,y))],$$
where γ is a weighting factor and T is a threshold on $E(x,y)$.

2.1.5 Isotropic smoothing
The homogenizing smoothing step consists of iteratively low-pass filtering the non-structure region with a 3×3 kernel. The iterations are done for a set number of times so that there is no structural information left and only the gradual intensity variations remain.

2.1.6 Expanding
Independently processed *structure* and *non-structure* regions are combined to produce I_3. Image I_3 is bicubically interpolated to obtain the image $I_4(x,y)$ to its original size. Bicubic interpolation is chosen because it provides a good compromise between computational efficiency and interpolated image quality.

2.1.7 Blending
The interpolated, filtered image $I_4(x,y)$ and the pre-filtration image $I_1(x,y)$ are blended using the equation to obtain the final result: $I_5(x,y) = \alpha *(I_4(x,y) - I_1(x,y)) + I_1(x,y)$; where $0 < \alpha < 1$.

2.2 Clinical evaluation
For the purpose of this study, 19 posterio-anterior dual-energy (soft-tissue and bone) chest exam films were reviewed by four radiologists. Twelve exams (set A) were done using a lower patient dose (equivalent to 400 film speed setting), and 7 other exams (set C) were done using a higher (factor of 2) dose. Noise level decreases with a higher dose and this allows us to evaluate the filter effectiveness over a range of clinical dose setting. Images from sets A and C were filtered using our algorithm to form sets B and D, respectively. All images were given a rating of 1 to 10, with a higher rating indicating better image quality.

3. RESULTS

Selected regions-of-interest from soft-tissue and bone images before and after filtering are shown in Figures 4 and 5. In both soft-tissue and bone images, noise was significantly reduced by filtering, and image quality was visibly improved. Quantitative evaluation of diagnostic image quality improvement is given below.

3.1 Soft-tissue image evaluation
Mean radiologist ratings for the lower dose and higher dose soft tissue images, with and without filtering are shown in Figure 6(a). Average ratings for sets A, B, C, and D are 6.33, 7.52, 7.53, and 8.03

respectively. Therefore, average improvements due to filtering are 23% and 8% for lower and higher dose acquisitions, respectively.

Paired t-tests show a significant effect of filtering on both lower dose and higher dose ratings ($p < 0.05$). A two-sample t-test performed on lower dose data with filtering (set B) versus higher dose data without filtering (set C) shows no significant difference ($p > 0.05$). A two-sample t-test performed on lower dose data with filtering (set B) versus higher dose data with filtering (set D) shows a significant difference ($p < 0.05$).

3.2 Bone image evaluation

Mean radiologist ratings for the lower dose and higher dose soft tissue images, with and without filtering are shown in Figure 6(b). Average ratings for sets A, B, C, and D are 4.72, 6.2, 5.64, and 7.28 respectively. Therefore, average improvements due to filtering are 39% and 40% for lower and higher dose acquisitions, respectively.

Paired t-tests show a significant effect of filtering on both lower dose and higher dose ratings ($p < 0.05$). A two-sample t-test performed on lower dose data with filtering (set B) versus higher dose data without filtering (set C) shows no significant difference ($p > 0.05$). A two-sample t-test performed on lower dose data with filtering (set B) versus higher dose data with filtering (set D) shows a significant difference ($p < 0.05$).

4. DISCUSSION AND CONCLUSIONS

Digital flat-panel-based dual-energy radiography produces significantly better image quality compared to CR due to high DQE and wide energy separation. In this study, we described a novel noise-reduction technique that significantly improves image quality at a given dose level, thereby allowing considerable additional dose reduction compared to CR. Our noise-reduction filtering makes use of spatial features and exploits information redundancies in an image. This has an efficient implementation, which can be used to effectively reduce patient dose by reducing image noise without blurring diagnostically relevant detail.

The average improvements in ratings for soft-tissue and bone (lower dose, higher dose) are 23% (8%) and 39% (40%), respectively. The higher improvements in bone image ratings compared to those for soft-tissue are likely due to the relatively higher noise content in the bone images. Nevertheless, comparable ratings for filtered lower dose images and unfiltered higher (double) dose images suggest that we can lower the dose by about 50% and still maintain equivalent perceptual image quality. Finally, the proposed filter gives the clinician the ability to control and vary dose according to application, without sacrificing image quality.

5. ACKNOWLEDGEMENTS

The authors would like to thank Dr. Heber McMahon (Univ. of Chicago) for his invaluable clinical and design input.

6. REFERENCES

1. American Cancer Society, *Cancer Facts and Figures 2000*, http://www3.cancer.org/cancerinfo/
2. E. Samei, MJ Flynn, and WR Eyler. "Detection of Subtle Lung Nodules: Relative Influence of Quantum and Anatomic Noise on Chest Radiographs", *Radiology* **213** pp. 727 - 734, 1999.
3. W. R. Brody, G. Butt, A. Hall, and A. Macovski, "A method for selective tissue and bone visualization using dual-energy scanned projection radiography" *Med. Phys.* **8** pp. 353-357, 1981.
4. LA Lehmann, RE Alvarez, A Macovski, WR Brody, NJ Pelc, SJ Riederer, AL Hall, " Generalized image combinations in dual KVP digital radiography ", *Med Phys.* **8** 659 - 667, 1981
5. RA Kruger, JD Armstrong, JA Sorenson, LT Niklason, "Dual energy film subtraction technique for detecting calcification in solitary pulmonary nodules", *Radiology* **140** pp. 213 - 219, 1981.

6. W. Ito, K. Shimura, N. Nakajima, M. Ishida, and H. Kato. "Improvement of detection in computed radiography by new single-exposure dual-energy subtraction", *J of Dig. Img.*, **6** pp. 42-47, 1993.

7. P.R. Granfors and R. Aufrichtig, "Performance of a 41 x 41-cm² amorphous silicon flat panel x-ray detector for radiographic imaging applications" *Med. Phys.* **27** pp. 1324-1331, 2000.

8. K. Kump, "Fast Imaging of a 41cm amorphous silicon flat-panel detector for radiographic applications", *Proc. SPIE* **4320**, 2001.

9. C. G. Shaw and D. Gur, "Comparison of three different schemes for dual-energy subtraction imaging in digital radiography: A signal-to-noise analysis" *Proc. SPIE* **1651** pp. 116-125, 1992.

10. D.M. Gauntt and G.T. Barnes, "X-ray tube potential, filtration and detector considerations in dual-energy chest radiography" *Med. Phys.* **21** pp. 203-218, 1994.

11. J.M. Sabol, G.B. Avinash, F. Nicolas, B. Claus, J. Zhao, and J.T. Dobbins, III, "Development and characterization of a dual-energy subtraction imaging system for chest radiography based on CsI:Tl amorphous silicon flat-panel technology" *Proc. SPIE* **4320** pp. 399-408, 2001.

12. S. Kido, J. Ikezoe, H. Naito, S. Tamura, T. Kozuka, W. Ito, K. Shimura, and H. Kato, "Single-exposure dual-energy chest images with computed radiography: Evaluation with simulated pulmonary nodules," Invest. Radiol. **28**, 482-487 (1993).

13. F. Kelcz, F. E. Zink, W. W. Peppler, D. G. Kruger, D. L. Ergun, and C. A. Mistretta, "Conventional chest radiography vs dual-energy computed radiography in the detection and characterization of pulmonary nodules," Am. J. Roentgenol. **162**, 271-278 (1994).

14. B. K. Stewart and H. K. Huang, "Single-exposure dual-energy computed radiography," Med. Phys. **17**, 866-875 (1990).

15. A. Macovski, D. G. Nishimura, A. Doost-Hoseini, and W. R. Brody, "Measurement-dependent filtering: A novel approach to improved SNR," IEEE Trans. on Med. Imaging **MI-2**, 122-127 (1983).

16. D. G. Nishimura, A. Macovski, and W. R. Brody, "Noise reduction methods for hybrid subtraction," Med. Phys. **11**, 259-265 (1984).

17. Q. Cao, T. Brosnan, A. Macovski, and D. Nishimura, "Least squares approach in measurement-dependent filtering for selective medical images," IEEE Trans. On Med. Imaging **7**, 154-160 (1988).

18. W. A. Kalender, E. Klotz, and L. Kostaridou, "An algorithm for noise suppression in dual energy CT material density images," IEEE Trans. on Med. Imaging **7**, 218-224 (1988).

19. C. H. McCollough, M. S. Van Lysel, W. W. Peppler, and C. A. Mistretta, "A correlated noise reduction algorithm for dual-energy digital subtraction angiography," Med. Phys. **16**, 873-880 (1989).

20. D. L. Ergun, C. A. Mistretta, D. E. Brown, R. T. Bystrianyk, W. K. Sze, F. Kelcz, and D. P. Naidich, "Single-exposure dual-energy computed radiography: Improved detection and processing," Radiology **174**, 243-249 (1990).

21. D. A. Hinshaw and J. T. Dobbins, III, "Recent progress in noise reduction and scatter correction in dual-energy imaging," Proc. SPIE **2432**, 134-142 (1995).

22. J. T. Dobbins, III, "Correlated polarity noise reduction for dual-energy imaging," RSNA, 220 (1996).

23. D. L. Ergun, W. W. Peppler, J. T. Dobbins, III, F. E. Zink, D. G. Kruger, F. Kelcz, F. J. de Bruijn, E. W. Bellers, Y. Wang, R. J. Althof, and M. G. J. Wind, "Dual-energy computed radiography: Improvements in processing," Proc. SPIE **2167**, 663-671 (1994).

24. R. Rutherford, B. Pullan, and I. Isherwoord, "Measurement of effective atomic number and electron density using an EMI scanner," Neuroradiology **11**, 15-21 (1976).

25. P. C. Johns and M. J. Yaffe, "Theoretical optimization of dual-energy x-ray imaging with application to mammography," Med. Phys. **12**, 289-296 (1985).

26. S. Kido, J. Ikezoe, H. Naito, J. Arisawa, S. Tamura, T. Kozuka, W. Ito, K. Shimura, and H. Kato, "Clinical evaluation of pulmonary nodules with single-exposure dual-energy subtraction chest radiography with an iterative noise-reduction algorithm," Radiology **194**, 407-412 (1995).

27. G.B. Avinash, "Method and apparatus for enhancing discrete pixel images," US Patent 6208763 (2001).

28. G.B. Avinash, "Method and apparatus for analyzing image structures," US Patent 6173083 (2001).

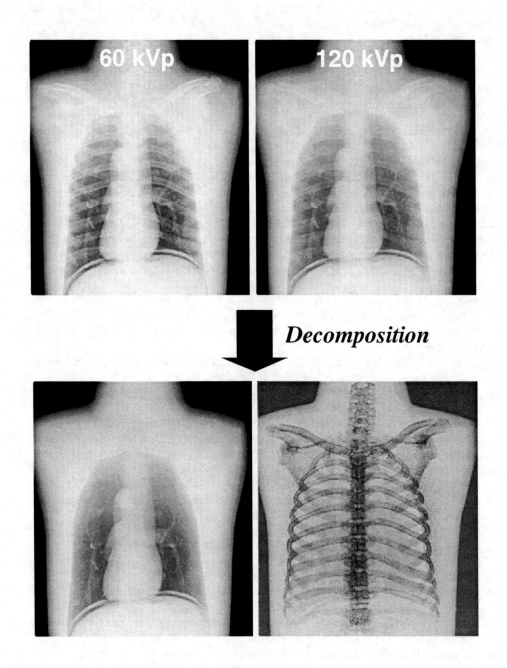

Figure 1: In dual-exposure dual-energy imaging using a flat panel, two images are acquired at different energies within a short time frame (<200ms), and are decomposed into *Soft-Tissue* and *Bone* images.

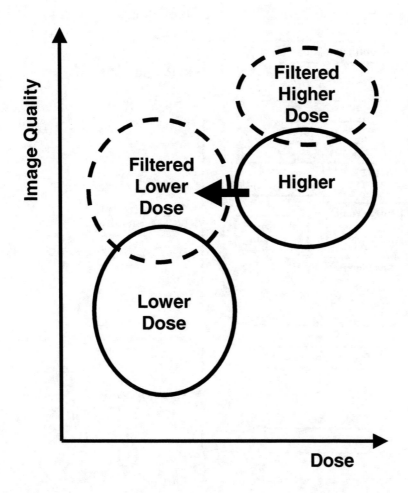

Figure 2: Schematic showing the concept of dose reduction through noise reduction filtering (Arrow indicates effective dose reduction through filtering).

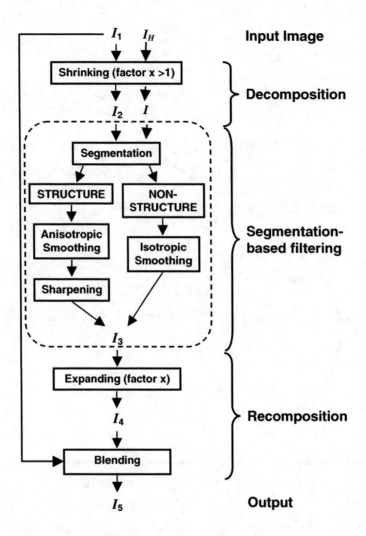

Figure 3: Schematic showing the main steps of the filtering algorithm.

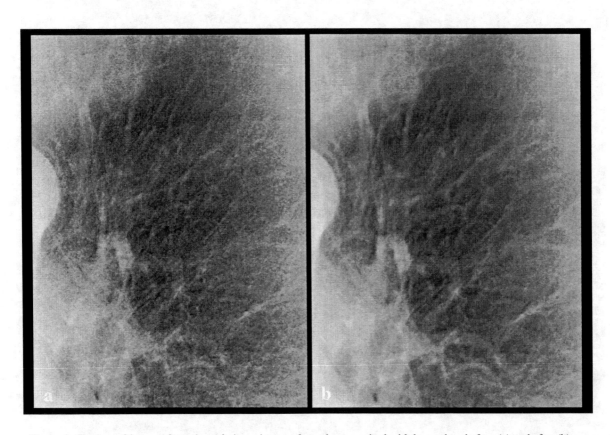

Figure 4: Region-of-interest from the soft tissue image of a patient acquired with lower dose before (a) and after (b) filtering.

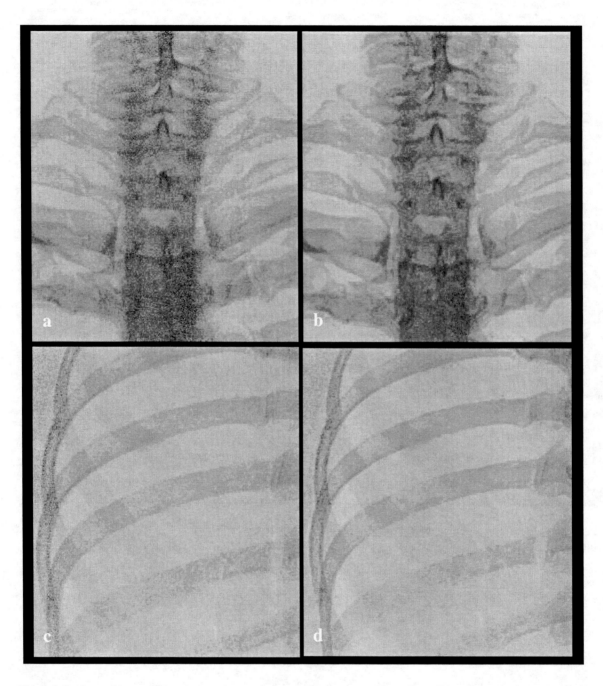

Figure 5: Regions-of-interest from the bone image of a patient acquired with lower dose before (a and c) and after (b and d) filtering.

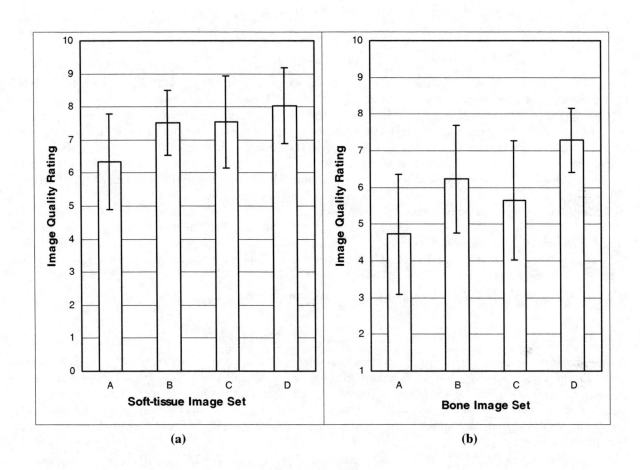

(a)   (b)

Figure 6: Mean radiologist ratings of soft tissue (a) and bone (b) images. Set A consists of images acquired at a lower dose without filtering. Set B consists of the same images in set A with filtering. Set C consists of higher dose (factor of 2) images without filtering. Set D consists of the same images in set C with filtering.

Additional Processing For Phase Unwrapping of Magnetic Resonance Thermometry Imaging

Suprijanto[a], F.M. Vos[a], M.W. Vogel[b], A.M. Vossepoel[a], H.A. Vrooman[b]

[a]Pattern Recognition Group, Department of Applied Physics,
Delft University of Technology 2628 CJ Delft, Netherlands
[b]Department of Radiology, Erasmus University Medical Center,
P.O. Box. 1738, 3000 DR Rotterdam, The Netherlands

ABSTRACT

Magnetic Resonance Thermometry imaging is a non-invasive method for temperature monitoring in hyperthermia treatment. The temperature can be determined from the phase shift in a gradient-echo sequence. Due to large temperature variations, the phase shift may exceed the $(-\pi, \pi)$ radians interval. The phase value beyond this interval will be wrapped. Unfortunately, the temperature is only proportional to the absolute phase change. Therefore, phase unwrapping (PU) is required to recover the absolute phase from the wrapped representation. While the phase may contain spurious discontinuities, the algorithm must distinguish them from true phase discontinuities. We propose additional processing to support PU in order to improve the algorithm for recovery of the best estimation of absolute phase. The Minimum Weight Discontinuity (MWD) algorithm was used for PU. The steps to be taken on additional processing consist of applying a Gaussian filter to the raw complex MRI images, deriving the weights of a quality map, and segmenting unreliable regions using the "magnitude" image. The raw wrapped phase images, acquired from a phantom and from a porcine liver (acquired under laser irradiation), were used to test the effect of additional processing. The effect was compared with the conventional approach (i.e. mere unwrapping with the MWD algorithm).

Keywords: Magnetic Resonance Thermometry Imaging, Phase Unwrapping

1. INTRODUCTION

During the past few years hyperthermia treatment has emerged as an alternative therapy for cancer. In conventional hyperthermia, relatively low temperatures in the range of 43°-50° Celcius are applied for several minutes to kill malignant cells. Spatial variations in tissue properties, e.g. perfusion and heat absorption rates, complicate such treatment by causing non-uniform temperature distribution. To ensure sufficient exposure of the tumor and also to spare healthy tissue, continuous monitoring both spatially and temporally of the temperature is required[1].

In practice both invasive and non-invasive approaches are applied to measure the temperature distribution. While invasive thermometry is locally quite accurate, the spatial sampling density is generally limited to minimize damage. A specific problem presents the case of a large deep-seated target volume. Here, a good representation of the temperature distribution cannot be obtained and quantitative assessment of thermal dose delivery is difficult to determine.

Magnetic Resonance Imaging (MRI) has been favored for monitoring local hyperthermia therapy, since it offers both target visualization and temperature sensitivity. Applying MRI for monitoring temperature is called Magnetic Resonance Thermometry Imaging(MRTI).

The temperature can be determined from the phase shift in a gradient-echo sequence. Due to large temperature variations, the phase shift may exceed the $(-\pi, \pi)$ radians interval. The phase value beyond this interval will be wrapped. Unfortunately, the temperature is only proportional to the absolute phase (unwrapped phase)

Further author information: (Send correspondence to Suprijanto : E-mail: supri@ph.tn.tudelft.nl

change. To solve this problem, the absolute phase must be reconstructed from the obtained wrapped data. The process of retrieving the absolute phase from a wrapped representation is called phase unwrapping(PU).

Phase unwrapping is essentially the process of recovering the integer multiple $c_{m,n}$ of 2π to be added to each pixel of the wrapped phase data $\psi_{m,n}$ in order to obtain the absolute phase $\phi_{m,n}$:

$$\phi_{m,n} = \psi_{m,n} + 2\pi c_{m,n}. \tag{1}$$

The integer multiples $c_{m,n}$ are called the *wrap counts*. Each wrap count is determined by how many *fringe lines* lie between a pixel under investigation and a reference pixel. A fringe line is the curve that marks the phase transitions from $-\pi$ to $+\pi$.

The raw wrapped phase contains noise and artifacts due to the imaging methods. Consequently, the raw wrapped phase may contain spurious phase discontinuities. To get the best estimation of absolute phase, the algorithm must distinguish such artifacts from true phase discontinuities.

In this paper, we propose additional processing to support PU in order to improve the Minimum Weighted Discontinuities (MWD)[2] algorithm for recovery of the absolute phase. The steps to be taken in additional processing (before PU) consist of applying a Gaussian filter to the raw complex MRI images, deriving the weights of a quality map (to distinguish true from spurious phase discontinuities) and segmenting unreliable regions using the "magnitude" image. After the Gaussian filter has been applied, the weight values of a quality map are derived by local frequency estimates. The quality map is derived from complex images rather than from the phase data alone, such as using pseudocorrelation and phase derivative variance[3]. For segmenting unreliable regions, a threshold is applied to the magnitude image, followed by some simple morphological operations.

We use two approaches for the evaluation of the PU solution. The first approach is to evaluate the number of remaining discontinuities in the absolute phase as a measure of success. We will also explore the proportional relation between absolute phase shift and temperature change, to evaluate the results of PU.

This paper is organized as follows. Section 2 describes the fundamentals of the MWD algorithm. In this section we will also elaborate on the concept of quality maps and complex image filtering. Section 3 describes experiments using the raw wrapped phase images acquired from a phantom and from a porcine liver (acquired under heating). In the experiments, the effect of additional processing to support PU was compared with the conventional approach (i.e. mere unwrapping with the MWD algorithm). Finally, conclusions will be given in section 4.

2. METHODS

2.1. The Minimum Weight Discontinuity

The unwrapping algorithm utilizes a tree-growing approach that traces paths of dicontinuities. If it is detected that such a path forms a loop, a multiple of 2π is added to the enclosed values. Thus, the number of phase discontinuities is reduced. A discontinuity is defined by a pair of adjacent(side-connected) pixels whose difference exceeds π in magnitude, oriented vertically or horizontally, called the *vertical* and *horizontal* phase jumps. For notation, we use $(v_{m,n})$ and $(z_{m,n})$ to represent the *vertical* and *horizontal* jump counts, defined by the equation Eq.-2 and Eq.-3,

$$v_{m,m} = Int(\frac{\phi_{m,n} - \phi_{m+1,n}}{2\pi}) \tag{2}$$

$$z_{m,m} = Int(\frac{\phi_{m,n} - \phi_{m,n+1}}{2\pi}) \tag{3}$$

where $Int(.)$ is the function that rounds to the nearest integer. Figure 1-b shows (for illustration)the jump counts computed from the wrapped phase image in Figure 1-a.

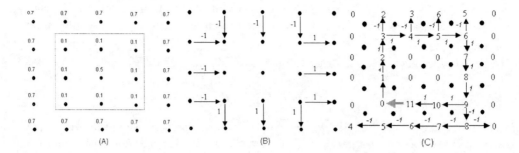

Figure 1. Illustration of the MWD Algorithm. (a) The *dots* represent pixels next to which the wrapped phase is given (scaled to range 0-1). The dashed lines shows a fringe curve. (b) The arrows indicate a nonnegative jump count (here defined by a phase transition larger than 0.5). (c) The set of trees during path extension represents one step before the loop is found (*each arrow represents an edge*).

The minimum weight discontinuity (MWD) criterion means that the solution of unwrapped phase is designed to yield a minimum over all choices of c (wrap counts, see Eq.-1). The criterion to be minimized is defined by:

$$E(c; \phi) = \sum w_{mn}|v_{m,n}| + \sum w_{mn}|z_{m,n}|, \tag{4}$$

where w_{mn} is an array of nonnegative integer coefficients defining the a quality map.

The algorithm generates a tree consisting of nodes and edges. A *node* is the point where 4 phase pixels intersect and an *edge* connects a pair of adjacent nodes. A leftward (resp. *rightward*) edge indicates an increment(*decrement*) of a vertical jump count; likewise, a downward(*upward*) edge indicates an increment (*decrement*) of a horizontal jump count. The value of an edge from the node *(m,n)* to the node *(m',n')*, will be denoted by $\delta V(m, n, m', n')$. δV is defined to be 1 if the edge induces a decrease in the magnitude of the jump count and -1 if it induces an increase.

The MWD algorithm creates a tree of nodes with the edges as the links. If the sequence of nodes (m_o, n_o), $(m_1, n_1), .., (m_L, n_L)$ defines the path from the root (m_o, n_o) to a node $(m_L, n_L) = $(m,n), then the value of the node is defined by

$$value(m, n) = \sum_{k=0}^{L-1} w_{mn}\delta V(m_k, n_k, m_{k+1}, n_{k+1}), \tag{5}$$

where $\delta V(m_k, n_k, m_{k+1}, n_{k+1})$ is the value of the edge that leads from node (m_k, n_k) to (m_{k+1}, n_{k+1}). Roots and isolated nodes both have the value 0. The addition of an edge from the node *(m,n)* to the node *(m',n')* resulting in *value(m',n')* will be tested by first calculating:

$$dval = value(m, n) + w_{mn}\delta V(m, n, m', n') - value(m', n'). \tag{6}$$

If *dval* is negative the edge is not added. If, however, *dval* is positive then the edge is added and *value(m',n')* is increased by *dval*. If the node *(m',n')* has a subtree (if three edges are leading from it to other nodes), then *dval* is also added to all the nodes in the subtree. Any existing edge connected to *(m',n')* is removed. After the addition of the new edge, the trees are searched for a loop. If there is already a path from *(m',n')* to *(m,n)*, then the new edge completes a loop. Figure 1-c. shows an example of a set of trees, one step before the loop is found. The large numbers represent the nodes and their value, the arrows represent the edges, and the small numbers specify the values of the edges. The large, shaded arrow indicates the new edge that can be added, so that the loop can be completed.

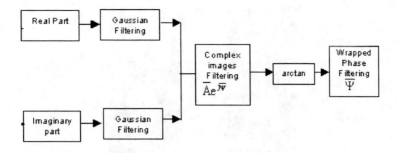

Figure 2: The flow chart of filtering on the MRI complex image

2.2. Complex Filtering

Magnetic Resonance Thermometry images often show poor signal to noise ratio (SNR). Noise can cause spurious phase discontinuities to arise on a raw wrapped phase. Because the phase is an aspect of a signal, filtering should be applied to the signal itself. The raw wrapped phase is obtained from an arctan operation on the complex signal. The complex signal is expressed by

$$z(l,m) = (Re[l,m] + n_{Re}[l,m]) + i(Im[l,m] + n_{Im}[l,m]) \tag{7}$$

where $Re[l,m]$ and $Im[l,m]$ denote the real and imaginary signal part respectively and $n_{Re}[i,j]$ and $n_{Im}[i,j]$ denote noise.

The noise contributions arising from the MRI scanner electronics are additive, and they are assumed to be uncorrelated, and characterized by a zero mean Gaussian probability density function. Before constructing the wrapped phase images, it is important to de-noise the complex signal. The flow chart for filtering the complex MRI image is shown in Figure-2. As we mentioned above, the filtered "magnitude" image is used to segment unrealible regions in a wrapped phase image. A threshold was applied to the magnitude images, followed by some simple morphological operations(such as opening and closing). The unrealible region consists of air, and it is not used to determine the absolute phase in the object.

2.3. Quality Maps Using Local Frequency Estimates

Although filtering was applied, still some erroneous regions remain. To obtain the best estimate of the absolute phase, the PU algorithm must distinguish true phase discontinuities from a spurious ones. Quality maps are arrays of values that each define the quality of a pixel value. The quality map will mark spurious phase discontinuities with a low weight value which are will be ignored during PU.

Commonly, the quality maps are derived from wrapped phase data alone[3]. We define our quality map by the local frequency estimates, that are suggested to replace the wrapped phase difference [4]. The quality map is derived from the complex filtered signal. The local frequency estimate is defined by equation 9.

$$\hat{Z}(l,m) = (\sum[z(l+1,m)z^*(l,m)]) + (\sum[z(l,m+1)z^*(l,m)]) \tag{8}$$

$$\hat{f}(l,m) = arctan[\hat{Z}(l,m)] \tag{9}$$

where $z(l,m)$ is a complex MRI signal and $z(l,m)^*$ is its conjugate and $\hat{f}(l,m)$ is a local frequency estimate. To obtain a weight array that is suitable to apply on the MWD algorithm, the results from $\hat{f}(l,m)$ are processed by the following steps; first, select the maximum value from n x n windows of $\hat{f}(i,j)$ and negate this value to give the lowest weight value to the bad pixels; second apply a threshold on the result, so that it can assume only two values: 0 or 1. The threshold value is chosen from a histogram of the image using the isodata algorithm[5]. Fig-3-a shows the results of the local frequency estimate of a porcine liver image. The weight values applied in the MWD algorithm are shown in Fig-3-b.

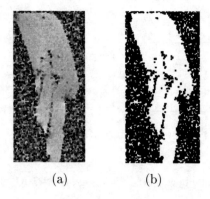

(a) (b)

Figure 3: The results of local frequency estimation from liver porcine image, after processing step-1(a) and step-2(b)

3. RESULTS

The effect of additional processing to support PU was compared with the conventional approach (i.e. mere unwrapping with the MWD algorithm). The raw wrapped phase images were created from a phantom that contained fat and water, and from an ex-vivo porcine liver taken under laser irradiation.

3.1. Study-1 : The Phantom Images

We evaluated the effect of our approach on phantom images that contain fat and water. The raw magnitude and phase images are shown in figure-4-a and 4-b. The phantom images were created with a gradient echo sequence using a short echo time. For that reason, the resulting a raw wrapped phase image contained many fringe lines.

In the first experiment, only the MWD algorithm was applied to recover the wrapped phase. In Fig. 5-a the absolute phase variation along the middle row of the image array is shown. The absolute phase produced an erroneous value that is marked with an arrow.

In the second experiment, we applied the proposed approach. In Fig. 5-b the result along the middle row is shown. We can see here that the correct absolute phase profile in the object is recovered. Evaluation based on the number of remaining discontinuities in the absolute phase shows that its number is reduced from 21.1%(conventional) to 1.7%(proposed approach) both of 16384 pixels .

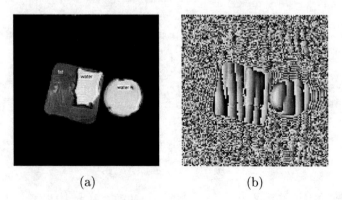

(a) (b)

Figure 4: The phantom images: (a) Magnitude and (b) Raw wrapped phase

3.2. Study-2 : The Porcine Liver Images Under Laser Irradiation

In this section we apply the proposed approach to the image of an object under heating. A porcine liver was placed in a waterbath at ambient temperature inside the MR scanner (Signa CV/i 1.5 T; General Electric, Milwaukee, WI). We used a Laser(Nd:YAG,20W), as heat source and, for delivering energy, a laser fiber with a

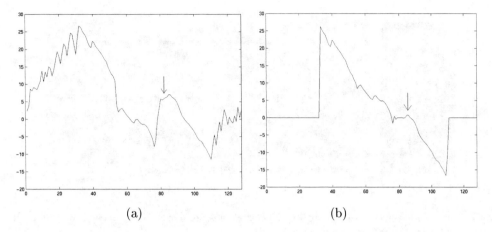

(a)   (b)

Figure 5. Plots of the absolute phase variation along the middle row that produced by PU with conventional (a) and proposed approach (b).

diffusing tip (0.600 mm, 2cm diffuser length) was inserted on the liver. A cooling laser catheter was installed to keep the surrounding tissue on ambient temperature. Only the diffusing tip gave a contribution to the heating. The target region is shown in Fig. 6-a(marked by the white square).

The gradient echo sequence was applied to maximize temperature sensitivity of the phase images. The liver was irradiated for 19 minutes under continuous monitoring with MRTI. The image acquired at t= 0 min (before the laser was applied), was used as initial image. An image was acquired each 1 minutes to be evaluated. Fig. 6-b shows the raw phase image at t=0 min. The effect of increasing duration of laser irradiation at t=5 min, t=6 min and t=19 min on the raw phase images is shown in Fig. 6 c,d and e.

In experiment-1, we recovered the absolute phase images with the conventional approach, and then the phase shift caused by laser irradiation was computed from each image(at t= 1 min until t=19 min) by subtracting the initial image. We computed the average phase shift in the target region(with the area as defined in Fig. 6-a), to evaluate the proportional phase shift due to increased duration of irradiation. In Fig. 7-b. the results are presented. Here, we found large phase shifts in the subtracted images at t=5 min, t=8 min, t=17 min and t=18 min. These results are not correct, because the phase shift per degree celcius is approximately 0.02 radian at an echo time of 20 ms [6]. For clarity, the plot of absolute phase variation along the center of the target area from experiment-1 is shown in Fig. 8-b. The absolute phase at t=5 min has a higher value than the absolute phase at t=6 min, with an error offset around 2π.

In experiment-2, the absolute phase was recovered by the proposed approach and then again a phase shift due to laser irradiation was computed. A plot of the phase shift as a function of duration of irradiation is shown in Fig. 7-c . With this approach, acceptable phase shift values can be obtained. In Fig. 8-c a plot of the the absolute phase variation along the center of target area is shown. In this plot one can see that the erroneous offset value of the absolute phase is avoided.

Finally, we also evaluate the number of remaining discontinuities in absolute phase of the porcine liver (see Table-1). The values were computed from average remaining discontinuities from images taken duration irradiation on t=0 min until t=19 min. Comparing with the results from experiment-1, the remaining number of discontinutities is significant reduced in experiment-2.

Table 1: The number of remaining discontinuities in absolute phase the porcine liver from experiment 1 and 2

Experiment-1	Experiment-2
12.2% of 32768 pixels	2.04% of 32768 pixels

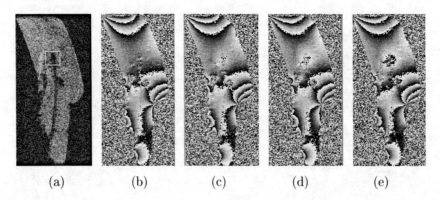

(a)   (b)   (c)   (d)   (e)

Figure 6. (a) The magnitude temperature image,(b) The raw phase under laser irradiation at t=0 minutes, (c) at t=5 minutes, (d) at t=6 minutes, (e) at t=19 minutes

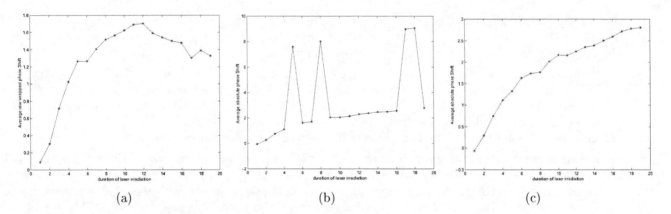

Figure 7. (a) Plot of average of raw wrapped phase shift, (b) Plot of average of absolute phase shift from experiment-1 with duration of laser irradiation and (c) Plot of average of absolute phase shift from experiment-2 with duration of laser irradiation

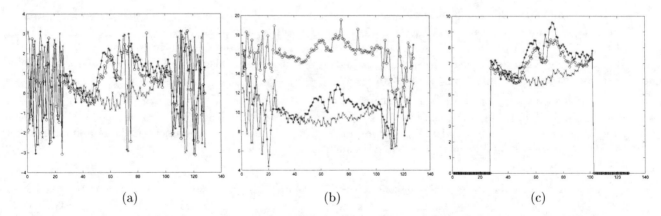

Figure 8. (a) Plot of phase variation along the center of the target area from the raw wrapped phase, (b) The absolute phase from experiment-1 and (c) the absolute phase from experiment-2. (note : 'x' for image at 0 minute , 'o' for image at t=5 min and '*' for image at t=6 min

4. CONCLUSIONS

The paper proposes additional processing to support a phase unwrapping algorithm. The additional processing consists of complex filtering, derivation of a quality map and segmentation of unreliable regions from magnitude images.

The proposed approach was tested on two studies. In study-1, we showed the advantage of our approach in recovering the absolute phase in a fat and water phantom. In study-2, the absolute phase shift due to laser irradiation is evaluated. While the PU algorithm alone produced erroneous phase shifts during irradiation, this problem has been solved with the proposed approach.

From the three additional processing components, the quality map and complex filtering provide a significant contribution to the correct solution. Segmenting the noisy region in the wrapped phase is less effective in the PU algorithm, particularly if the noisy region is not completely removed. Development of more advanced methods for segmenting noisy regions in wrapped phase images is still necessary.

ACKNOWLEDGMENTS

This research is part of the MISIT (Minimally Invasive Surgery and Interventional Techniques) programme of the Delft Interfaculty Research Center on Medical Engineering (DIOC-9).

REFERENCES

1. J. MacFall, D. Prescott, H. Charles, and T. Samulski, "H^1 mri phase thermometry in vivo canine brain, muscle, and tumor tissue," *Medical Physics* **23**, pp. 1775–1782, October 1996.

2. T.J. Flynn, "Two-dimensional phase unwrapping with minimum weighted discontinuity," *Journal of Optical Society of America A* **14**, pp. 2692–2701, 1997.

3. D. C. Ghiglia and M. D. Pritt, *Two-Dimensional Phase Unwraping, Theory, Algorithms and Software*, John Willey and Sons, Inc, New York, 1998.

4. E. Trouve, J. Nicolas, and H. Maitre., "Improving phase unwrapping techniques by the use of local frequency estimates," *IEEE Transcations on Geoscience and Remote Sensing* **36**, pp. 1963–1972, 1998.

5. I.T. Young, J.J. Gerbrands, and L.J. Van Vliet, *Fundamentals of Image Processing*, Delft University of Technology, Netherlands, 1995.

6. M.W. Vogel, Suprijanto, F.M. Vos, H.A. Vrooman, A.M. Vossepoel, and P.M.T. Pattynama, "Towards motion-robust magnetic resonance thermometry," in *MICCAI 2001 Proceedings:LNCS Vol 2208, Springer-Verlag ,Berlin*, pp. 401–408, 2001.

A Sequential Approach to Three-Dimensional Geometric Image Correction

Frank Crosby*, A. Patricia Nelson[+]

*Naval Surface Warfare Center, Coastal Systems Station, Panama City FL 32407

[+]Nelson Medical Associates, San Diego, CA 92126

ABSTRACT

This paper presents a new and comprehensive approach for correcting magnetic-resonance images that are subject to three-dimensional geometric distortion. Distortion in such images is typically caused by variations in the magnetic-field gradient in each of the three spatial dimensions. The new approach sequentially applies one-dimensional and two-dimensional correction techniques to achieve a complete three-dimensional geometric correction. It thus avoids many theoretical complications and computational inefficiencies that are inherently associated with direct (non-sequential) three-dimensional correction techniques.

Keywords: Three-dimensional Geometric Correction, Image Warping.

1. INTRODUCTION

The deviation of image points from their position in a true representation of an object is called *geometric distortion*. Almost all magnetic resonance images are subject to some three-dimensional geometric distortion. A major cause is that the actual magnetic field within the material being imaged does not match its assumed behavior. Over the volume to be imaged, V, most magnetic-resonance imaging systems are based upon the assumptions: (1) the direction of the magnetic field is constant, and (2) the magnitude of the magnetic field varies linearly over V, i.e., the three components of the magnetic-field gradient are constants. However, the second assumption is usually valid only over a small volume, v, near the center of V. Thus, the volume v becomes smaller as V is decreased, and vice versa.

The volume used for magnetic resonance imaging of the human head is relatively small because the human head is relatively small. Because of the small size, head images are particularly susceptible to geometric distortion, yet they are becoming more popular due to their use in functional magnetic-resonance imaging. Geometric image correction techniques can be used to modify distorted images. In particular, they can be used to correct for distortion arising from non-linear magnetic field variation in magnetic resonance imaging systems.

The approach presented here is based on correction in the spatial domain. The spatial domain is the set of pixel coordinates that make up an image. Spatial domain procedures are those that operate directly on the pixel coordinates. Image processing functions in the spatial domain may be expressed as $g(\mathbf{z}) = I(F^{-1}(\mathbf{z}))$, where I is the original image, g is the resultant image, and $\mathbf{z}$ is an element of the domain of the image. The function F maps the location of a pixel A to the location of another pixel B. (The location of B will be the same as that of A when there is no distortion to be corrected at the location of A.) The functions I and g assign intensities to the pixels at the locations $\mathbf{z}$ in the spatial domain. The relationship is depicted in Figure 1. The spatial correction may also be constructed as $g(F(\mathbf{z})) = I(\mathbf{z})$. It is this latter form that will be employed.

Medical Imaging 2002: Image Processing, Milan Sonka, J. Michael Fitzpatrick, Editors, Proceedings of SPIE Vol. 4684 (2002) © 2002 SPIE · 1605-7422/02/$15.00

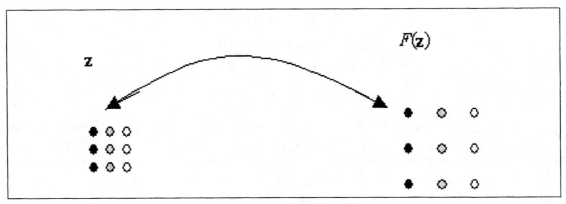

Figure 1: Image correction function

Geometric correction must be done in three dimensions to obtain a true representation of an imaged object. The problem to be solved is to find a function, $F : \Re^3 \to \Re^3$, such that F unwarps an image to give a better representation of an object. Once the function is determined, it may be used to correct any image that is subject to identical distortions.

Although the function corrects the entire image, it is determined using a subset of image points. These points are chosen from the image of a phantom (a test object) with known dimensions and will be called *control points*. Since the test object has known dimensions, the amount of geometric distortion may be measured precisely at these points allowing the points to be matched with their accurate locations.

There are two main issues involved in this approach to three-dimensional geometric image correction. One is the selection of the control points. Determining the three-dimensional coordinates of image points presents several challenges when performed either manually or automatically. The second is the choice of an interpolating function that defines F between the control points. There is currently very little development of vector-valued interpolation functions defined on $\Re^3$. Thus, the proper choice of a vector-valued interpolating function for this type of approach is not obvious.

The correction function F is constructed from functions defined in two dimensions. The next section shows this construction and how sequential application may be used to achieve a three dimensional correction. The correction function will unwarp the entire image, removing the nonlinear gradient effects. The selection of the control points that are used to determine the correction function is addressed in section 3. In section 5 some practical aspects of resampling the image are resolved.

2. THE SEQUENTIAL APPROACH

To avoid the difficulties associated with vector-valued interpolation functions, the approach presented here uses a pairing or grouping of standard interpolating functions which have the form $f : \Re^n \to \Re$. The desired function, F, may then be formed as,

$$F(x, y, z) \equiv [f_x(x, y, z), f_y(x, y, z), f_z(x, y, z)]$$

where $f_x, f_y, f_z : \Re^3 \to \Re$. (Not all interpolating functions are well behaved when combined in this way, as we will later demonstrate.) The function F could also have been written as a composition of functions. That is

$$F(x, y, z) \equiv (F_x \circ F_y \circ F_z)(x, y, z)$$

where

$$F_x(x, y, z) = [f_x(x, y, z), y, z]$$
$$F_y(x, y, z) = [x, f_y(x, y, z), z]$$
$$F_z(x, y, z) = [x, y, f_z(x, y, z)]$$

Each of these functions, F_x, F_y, and F_z acts as the identity function on two coordinates.

It can be easily seen that the composition of the three coordinate correction functions is commutative. When employing such a method of interpolation, the dimensions may be corrected in any order. Furthermore, the form of F shows that the correction in each dimension is independent of the others. A sequential correction of the dimensions is therefore justified.

Spatial domain image correction techniques usually treat images as discrete functions. Thus, a correction of the type $F(x, y, z) = [f_x(x, y, z), f_y(x, y, z), f_z(x, y, z)]$ may be implemented iteratively. To see this, let $\mathbf{Z}$ represent the integers. Suppose that the image is given by $I : \mathbf{X} \to \Re$ where $\mathbf{X} \in \mathbf{Z}^3$. If $\mathbf{X} = [0, 12] \times [0, 10] \times [0, 10]$, then applying F to $\mathbf{X}$ is equivalent to successive application of F to $i \times [0, 10] \times [0, 10]$, $i = 0, 1, \ldots, 12$.

A yz-plane correction, $F(x, y, z) = [x, f_y(x, y, z), f_z(x, y, z)]$, applied iteratively to $i \times [0, 10] \times [0, 10]$ treats the first coordinate as a constant. By allowing each plane to be corrected independently, the coordinate functions, f_y and f_z, may also treat the first coordinate as a constant. This reduces them to functions of two variables. The corresponding correction function can be defined by $\widehat{F}(x, y, z) = [x, \widehat{f}_y(y, z), \widehat{f}_z(y, z)]$. Thus, the collection of potential interpolation functions may be widened to include not only those defined on $\Re^3$, but also those defined on $\Re^2$. The focus of the methods that are presented here is functions $f : \Re^2 \to \Re$.

The equation $g(\mathbf{z}) = I[F^{-1}(\mathbf{z})]$ makes it evident that we need only consider the domain of I. The resulting image g is not defined outside of the range of F, so it is not necessary to map points outside of $\mathbf{X}$.

3. DISTORTION ASSESSMENT

A cylindrical phantom with an interior composed of a three-dimensional grid was imaged. A total of 67 axial slices was acquired. The image matrix was $128 \times 128 \times 67$ which corresponded to a field of view in centimeters of $30.0 \times 30.0 \times 26.8$

The independence of the coordinate corrections, along with an iterative application of the interpolation functions, makes for a simple determination of the control points and their desired locations. The most readily identified points in the image of the phantom are the grid intersections. These points were used as the control points.

If a vector valued interpolation function defined on $\Re^3$ were used for the correction then the three-dimensional spatial coordinates of the control points throughout the volume would have to be determined. It is very difficult for an observer to determine a three-dimensional coordinate when limited to viewing a two-dimensional display. The locations would therefore have to be determined using a three-dimensional pattern recognition algorithm (the pattern being the intersections). However, there are several obstacles in the development of a solution to this problem.

One is that the morphology of an intersection is different at different spatial locations throughout the image. Near the center of the volume, which corresponds to the center of the field of view, the lines that define an intersection meet at right angles. Near the edge of the volume, which corresponds to the edge of the field of view, the lines meet at other degree angles. The degree depends on the amount of distortion at a particular location. Second, there is a significant loss of signal in certain parts of the volume.

An iterative application of the interpolation function allows for control points to be determined for each plane and so the control points may be determined manually. The independence of the coordinate corrections assures that, for example, if a point in a plane parallel to the xy-plane is selected as a control point, the value of the point's z coordinate is immaterial.

Additionally, if all three dimensions were to be corrected simultaneously, then the interpolation functions would have a large number of terms. Hence, the application of the interpolating function to the image could present possible data storage problems.

The image of our phantom was divided into slices parallel to the xy-plane. The grid intersections were determined. Next, the volume was divided into slices which were parallel to the xz-plane. Where there was not enough information to be able to determine an intersection, a best guess was made. No correspondence between the set of points in the xy-planes and the set of points in the xz-planes was assumed.

Although the coordinate corrections are independent of each other, the determination of the control points is not. To exhibit this dependence, suppose that all control points are found. The correction then proceeds in slices. If $(x_i . y_i)$ is a control point and the xz-planes are corrected, then the point (x_i, y_i) has been moved to say $(\overline{x}_i, y_i)$. This indicates that if xz-planes are corrected first, then the map f_x must be inverted so that the point $(\overline{x}_i, y_i)$ is correctly identified with $(x_i . y_i)$ from the original image.

An alternative method is to use the control points in the xy-planes to correct the image, then find the control points in the xz-planes. In this procedure, the point $(\overline{x}_i . y_i)$ is a control point. However, each subsequent image that is unwarped, must be unwarped in the same sequence that was used in the determination of the control points. We employed this latter method.

Since information from each set of slices can be used to correct the image in two dimensions, one dimension could be mapped twice. While there may not be a significant error introduced by this over correction, we chose to only do a correction in one dimension with the second set of slices. Thus, the correction, as implemented, had the form

$$F \equiv (F_x, F_{yz})$$

where $F_{yz} \equiv (F_y \circ F_z)$.

Investigator error is certainly a factor in the manual selection of control points. In order to address this error, a smoothing spline was fitted to a sequence of points through the volume. A cubic spline was chosen because we had no information about the analytic form of the curve which was determined by the points to be fitted. A draw back to using a spline is that the functional value is zero outside of the interval where the interpolation points are defined. Hence, they are not useful for any extrapolation that may need to be done due to the size of the phantom or the selected field of view. A smoothing spline is a variant of an interpolating spline which allows for a reduction in the random error which may be contained in a measured set of data.

The smoothing spline was developed by Reinsch and has the following characteristics[1]. Let $x_i, \quad i = 1, 2, \ldots, n$ be an increasing sequence of abscissae, and $y_i, \quad i = 1, 2, \ldots, n$ the associated ordinates. The smoothing function $S(x)$, to be determined minimizes $\sum_{i=1}^{n-1} (h'')^2$ among all functions, h, with two continuous derivatives such that

$\sum (h(x_i) - y_i)/d_i \leq s$. The numbers d_i must be nonnegative and are called observation weights. A recommended value is an approximation to the standard deviation of error of the values y_i. The value s is nonnegative and controls the smoothing. If it is set equal to zero, then the function S interpolates the values y_i, $i = 1, 2, ..., n$. It can be shown that the function, $S(x)$, which solves this optimization problem is a cubic polynomial on each subinterval $[x_i, x_{i+1}]$.

If the numbers d_i are as recommended above, then a recommended value for s is n. However, by inspection we chose a much smaller value.

There is more than one choice for which points to fit to the spline. For example, there are lines in each slice which may be fit. So, if a grid is 10x15 one could construct 10 lines fit to 15 points. On the other hand if there were 20 slices, one could fit the spline through the slices. That is fit 150 lines through 20 points. We chose to fit through slices, 150 lines through 20 points. In this manner, we would also have a measure of the intra-slice distortion. The measure of intra-slice distortion is used to correct future slices which may not correspond exactly to those which were used in the determination of the control points.

4. INTERPOLATION

There are several considerations to be made when choosing an interpolating function that maps $\mathfrak{R}^2$ to $\mathfrak{R}$. One is that the particular form of the functions are chosen so that there is no implied condition on the location of the control points. For example, bilinear interpolation assumes that the control points are located on a grid. Another consideration in the choice of an algorithm is how well the function formed by pairing the interpolation function preserves the character of the two-dimensional data.

Several interpolation schemes will not give satisfactory results when used as mappings from $F : \mathfrak{R}^2 \rightarrow \mathfrak{R}^2$. The Hardy multiquadric methods allow us to demonstrate the extremes which are possible. The Hardy multiquadric methods are a global basis function type method of interpolation[2]. The development of this form of interpolating function is based on solving the problem of approximating smooth surfaces with the summation of regular basis surfaces, particularly quadric forms. Each basis surface is associated with a control point. The Hardy multiquadrics have the form,

$$F(x, y) = \sum_{k=1}^{n} a_k B_k(x, y)$$

The B_k's are the basis functions and the a_ks are coefficients determined so as to meet the interpolating conditions. The B_ks are quadric functions with the form $B_k(x, y) = (d_k^2 + R^2)^q$, where $d_k = \sqrt{(x - x_k)^2 + (y - y_k)^2}$.

The numbers R and q are user specified parameters. By varying their values we can see some of the various possibilities that paired functions are capable of producing. Figure 2 shows a distorted axial slice of the cylindrical phantom. The image has been enhanced by histogram equalization to aid in viewing. The slice is near the edge of the field of view and consequently shows the most distortion and some signal loss appearing as a dark ring. Ideally the phantom would appear circular as in Figure 3. Figure 3 is also an axial slice, but it is close to the center of the field of view so it has only minor distortion around the edge of the phantom. This image is for comparison to Figure 2.

Figure 4 shows the result of applying a pair of multiquadric functions. This image has been reversed for clarity. Notice that the control points are mapped to their desired locations. However, all other points from the original image are clustered in the upper left of new the image.

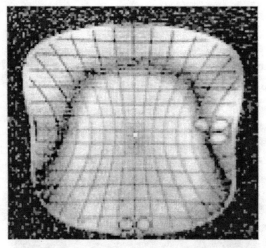

Figure 2: An axial slice of the phantom.

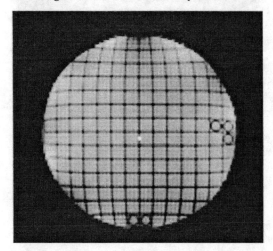

Figure 3: An axial slice of the phantom.

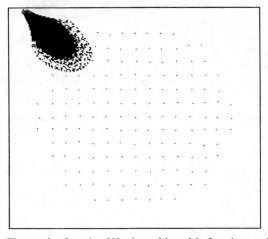

Figure 4: The result of a pair of Hardy multiquadric functions on Figure 1.

A similar global basis function method is the thin plate spline method. In this case, we take

$$B_k(x, y) = d_k^2 \log d_k$$

This method does preserve the character of the image when used in a paired mapping. The results for this method were similar to the multiquadric methods with certain values of R and q. Further, the absence of user specified parameters facilitated automatic implementation. Figure 5 shows the results of applying a pair of thin plate splines to the distorted image in Figure 5. Notice that the character of the image is preserved.

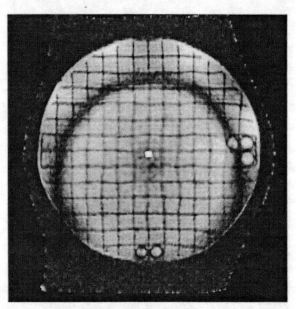

Figure 5: The result of a pair of thin plate spline interpolants on Figure 1.

5. RESAMPLING

After the construction of the mapping to transform the image, the image is converted from a discrete image to a continuous one. The application of the mapping to a continuous image results in no loss of information. Further, a continuous image may be resampled anywhere and thus, prevent drop out in the final result. The construction of a continuous image requires another interpolation problem to be solved. Again we need to consider only those interpolation routines which allow for irregularly distributed points. In addition, the storage requirements and speed of the interpolation algorithm are important factors. Where as previously we had to be concerned with the effects of pairing and interpolating function, there is no such pairing in this situation. We eliminated both the Hardy multiquadric and the thin plate spline method because of their storage requirements. The algorithms are moderate in terms of computational speed. However, they require storage on the order of n^2, which is prohibitive for even a moderately sized image of 128 × 128.

We created a continuous image by using a modified quadratic shepard routine[3]. The function Q is defined as

$$Q(w_1 q_1 + w_2 q_2 + \cdots + w_n q_n) / (w_1 + w_2 + \cdots + w_n),$$

where

$$q_k = a_{1,k}(x - x_k)^2 + a_{2,k}(x - x_k)(y - y_k) + a_{3,k}(x - x_k)(y - y_k)^2 + a_{4,k}(x - x_k) + a_{5,k}(y - y_k) + f_k$$

Thus, q_k is a quadratic function which interpolates the data at a point (x_k, y_k). Its coefficients, $a_{\star,k}$, are obtained by a weighted least squares fit to the data points in a user specified neighborhood. The weights, w_i, are taken to be

$$w_k(x, y) = (R_k - d_k)_+ / (R_k d_k)$$

where

$$(R_k - d_k)_+ = \begin{cases} R_k - d_k & \text{if } R_k > d_k \\ 0 & \text{otherwise} \end{cases}$$

and R is user specified.

This method is not particularly fast, but it does offer one of the lowest storage requirements of most two-dimensional interpolation algorithms[4]. Its storage requirement is on the order of $5n$.

6. ADDITIONAL RESULTS

The results presented in Figure 5 shows the correction that was obtained for an axial image. The correction removed the distortion in two of the three dimensions. Figure 6 is a coronal slice of the phantom. Most of the remaining distortion is in the vertical dimension. The dipping of the line at the top of the phantom shows the one-dimension that is still uncorrected. The horizontal variations remain after correction because of the interpolated area between control points. Horizontal distortion can be corrected again. However, the one-dimensional correction that is shown in Figure 7 demonstrates that the additional computations are unnecessary.

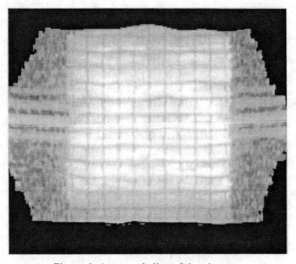

Figure 6: A coronal slice of the phantom

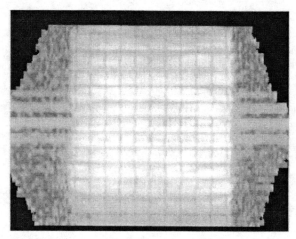

Figure 7: A corrected coronal slice of the phantom

7. CONCLUSION

Geometric image correction techniques can be used to modify distorted images. The approach presented here is based on correction in the spatial domain. Image processing functions in the spatial domain may be expressed as

$g(\mathbf{z}) = I(F^{-1}(\mathbf{z}))$, where I is the original image, g is the resultant image, and $\mathbf{z}$ is an element of the domain of the image. The function F maps the location of a pixel A to the location of another pixel B.

An iterative application of the interpolation function allows for control points to be determined independently for each plane and so the control points may be determined manually. The independence of the coordinate corrections assures that, for example, if a point in a plane parallel to the xy-plane is selected as a control point, the value of the point's z coordinate is immaterial.

Additionally, if all three dimensions were to be corrected simultaneously, then the interpolation functions would have a large number of terms. Hence, the application of the interpolating function to the image could present possible data storage problems.

This paper has shown how two-dimensional geometrical correction techniques can be used to achieve a three-dimensional geometric correction. The use of two-dimensional techniques allows for the simple selection of control points. These control points are then used with a paired interpolation function to give a two-dimensional correction. It was shown that not all interpolation functions give satisfactory results when used as paired mappings. Finally, aspects of resampling the image after the correction were addressed.

REFERENCES

[1] C. H. Reinsch, "Smoothing by Spline Functions", Numerische Mathematik **10**. 1963.

[2] Hardy, R. "Multiquadric Equations of Topology and other Irregular Surfaces", *Journal of Geophysics* **76,** pp.1905-1915, 1971.

[3] Barnhill, R.E.,"Representation and Approximation of Surfaces", *Mathematical Software* III, pp.117, 1977.

[4] Franke, R. "Scattered Data Interpolation: Tests of Some Methods", *Mathematics of Computations* **38** pp. 181-200, 1982

De-noising of Cone Beam CT Image Using Wavelet Transform

Yi-Qiang Yang[a], Nobuyuki Nakamori[a], Yasuo Yoshida[a],
Takanori Tsunoo[b], Masahiro Endo[b], and Kazumasa Sato[c]

[a]Kyoto Inst. of Tech., Matsugasaki, Sakyo-ku, Kyoto 606-8585, Japan
[b]National Inst. of Radiological Sci., Anagawa, Inage-ku, Chiba 263-8555, Japan
[c]Sony Corp., Kitashinagawa, Shinagawa-ku, Tokyo 141-0001, Japan

ABSTRACT

We have developed a method to remove the noise from the cone beam CT image and consider the reduction of a patient's dose. In diagnostic medicine, cone beam CT increases a patient' exposure dose. The X-ray CT image is degraded by the noise that is called quantum mottle, and the noise becomes so remarkable with decreasing patient' dose. It is known that the image signal can be separated from the noise by measuring the Lipschitz exponents of the image singularities from the evolution of wavelet transform modulus maxima across scales. We identify the singularities of 2-D projections by computing the wavelet transform modulus sum (WTMS) in the direction which is indicated by the phase of wavelet transform. Our preliminary results show the validity of the method based on 2-D WTMS for removing quantum mottle from 2-D projection. And it shows the possibility that the patient's dose can be reduced by this method.

Keywords: cone beam, computed tomography (CT), quantum mottle, wavelet transform, patient' dose, noise reduction

1. INTRODUCTION

Cone-beam computed tomography has been a very important modality to give doctors the information about internal organs of patient without any surgical treatments. Recent years, the developed CT techniques such as spiral CT and multi-slice CT have been used in hospitals to perform diagnostic studies due to visualizing the fine structures of the body in shorter scan time. In spite of these merits, all these CT scanners face the radiation exposure problem to patients. It has been also reported by FDA of U.S Department of Health and Human Services that many people receive the high radiation exposure from CT scanners every year. But if we reduce the radiation exposure, the noise in CT image will become remarkable and will have bad influence on medical diagnosis. Therefore, it becomes very necessary to remove the noise to improve quality of CT image.

Recently, wavelets have been widely used to analyze the characteristics of a signal with irregular structure. Biomedical images are often with irregular structures. It is very reasonable to analyze these signals using wavelets.[1] Many important properties of wavelets have been used in noise reduction.[2] Donoho et al developed a theoretical discrete wavelet transform (DWT) framework for the estimation of signals degraded by additive noise, and proposed wavelet shrinkage (WS) method.[3] This method is used to denoise due to its simplicity and effectiveness. It has been studied by some researchers in tomography reconstruction.[4] But to estimate a proper threshold is often not easy. One has to have a priori knowledge of the noise intensity to determine the optimal threshold. Furthermore, edge information of the signal maybe be removed in this denoising process. In 1992, Mallat et al introduced a denoising technique by virtue of wavelet transform modulus maxima (WTMM).[5] The WTMM representation of a signal records the values and locations of local maxima of its wavelet transform modulus (WTM). Mallat et al proved that the local Lipschitz exponent of a signal can be estimated by tracing the evolution of its WTMM across scales. The Lipschitz exponent is usually used to measure the singularity of function in mathematics. The interscale information is included in WTMM. Hsung et al developed a new

---

Further author information: (Send correspondence to N.N.)
N.N.: E-mail: yang@djedu.kit.ac.jp, Telephone: +81-(0)75-724-7483

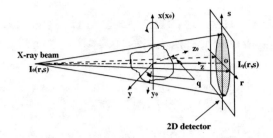

Figure 1: The diagram of cone beam CT scanner.

method[6] based on the theory proposed by Mallat et al. This method is only by computing the wavelet transform modulus sum (WTMS) to obtain denoised WTMM. In our previous study, we have applied the 1-D WTMS to remove the noise from the 1-D projection data. The results show that the denoised images are with better visual quality than those denoised by using wavelet shrinkage. They also show that it is possible to reduce a patient' dose to 1/10.

In this study, we have developed a method to denoise the 2-D filtered projection by extending the 2-D WTMS. This method requires very little priori information of the signal or noise. We have investigated the relation between the number of the X-ray photons and the quality of the denoised CT images.

2. THE PROJECTION OF CONE BEAM CT

In this section, firstly, we introduce the 2-D projection model degraded by quantum mottle. It is usually considered that there are two types of noise in CT images.[7] One is a continuously varying error due to electrical noise or roundoff errors, and the other is a discretely varying error due to X-ray photon fluctuation. Because our ultimate purpose of the study is to reduce the dose of the patient, we assume that the electrical noise is little enough to be negligible, and consider the quantum mottle only, which is caused by X-ray photon fluctuation.

In Fig.1, an object is illuminated by cone typed X-ray beam at the angle θ. We denote the intensity of incident X-rays by $I_0(r,s)$ and the intensity of X-rays passed through the object at the location (r,s) by $I_\theta(r,s)$. The projection data $P_\theta(r,s)$ can be calculated by

$$P_\theta(r,s) = \ln \frac{I_0(r,s)}{I_\theta(r,s)}. \tag{1}$$

We assume that the incident X-ray flux is large enough so that $I_0(r,s)$ may be considered to be with negligible error. The randomness of $I_\theta(r_0,s_0)$ at the location (r_0,s_0) is statistically described by the Poisson probability function given by

$$p\{I_\theta(r_0,s_0)\} = \frac{[\bar{I}_\theta(r_0,s_0)^{I_\theta(r_0,s_0)}]}{I_\theta(r_0,s_0)!} e^{-\bar{I}_\theta(r_0,s_0)}, \tag{2}$$

where $p\{.\}$ denotes the probability and $\bar{I}_\theta(r_0,s_0)$ denotes the expected value of the measurement. And $\bar{I}_\theta(r_0,s_0) = E\{I_\theta(r_0,s_0)\}$, where $E\{.\}$ denotes statistical expectation. Because of the randomness in I_θ, the measured projection $P_\theta(r,s)$ differs from its true value. The error is the noise which is based on X-ray photon fluctuation. We can obtain the 3-D CT image degraded by quantum mottle from the projection $P_\theta(r,s)$ by using 3-D CT reconstruction algorithm.

3. 2-D WAVELET TRANSFORM AND NOISE REMOVAL

Wavelet theory has been extensively studied in recent years as a promising tool in noise reduction. In this study, we use the 2-D fast discrete wavelet algorithm.[8] The 2-D dyadic wavelet transform of the projection is described as follows.

Throughout the paper, the function $f(x,y)$ is defined as 2-D filtered projection. Furthermore, we define the smooth and detail components of $f(x,y)$ as $S_s f(x,y)$, $W_s^1 f(x,y)$, and $W_s^2 f(x,y)$ respectively. The scale s varies only along the dyadic sequence $(2^j)_{j \in [1,J], J \in Z}$, Z is the set of all integers. The wavelet transform components can be obtained by the convolutions of $f(x,y)$ with the scaling function $\phi_{2^j}(x,y)$ and wavelet functions $\psi_{2^j}^1(x,y)$ and $\psi_{2^j}^2(x,y)$. The wavelets are the partial derivatives of a smooth function $\Phi(x,y)$[5] along the x and y, respectively. That is, $\psi_{2^j}^1(x,y) = \partial\Phi(x,y)/\partial x$, $\psi_{2^j}^2(x,y) = \partial\Phi(x,y)/\partial y$. Then, $f(x,y)$ can be decomposed by

$$f(x,y) = \sum_{j=1}^{J} (W_{2^j}^1 f(x,y) + W_{2^j}^2 f(x,y)) + S_{2^J} f(x,y), \tag{3}$$

$$\left. \begin{array}{l} W_{2^j}^1 f(x,y) = f(x,y) * \psi_{2^j}^1(x,y) \\ W_{2^j}^2 f(x,y) = f(x,y) * \psi_{2^j}^2(x,y) \\ S_{2^j} f(x,y) = f(x,y) * \phi_{2^j}(x,y) \end{array} \right\}. \tag{4}$$

In addition, the magnitude and orientation of the gradient vector of the wavelet coefficients at a particular point (x,y) are defined as

$$M_{2^j} f(x,y) = \sqrt{|W_{2^j}^1 f(x,y)|^2 + |W_{2^j}^2 f(x,y)|^2}, \tag{5}$$

$$A_{2^j} f(x,y) = \arctan(W_{2^j}^2 f(x,y)/W_{2^j}^1 f(x,y)), \tag{6}$$

respectively. Because the Eq.(6) indicates the direction of the maximum local variation of a signal, we can identify the singularity of the signal only by measuring the Lipschitz exponent in that direction.

The local Lipschitz exponent α at a particular point of the signal singularities can be estimated by tracing the maxima curves inside the corresponding "directional cone of influence" (DCOI) in scale space. We can process the maxima curves in scale space to obtain the denoised WTMM according to Mallat' theory. But there may be many errors and ambiguities. Besides, in WTMM processing the wavelet reconstruction process is complicated due to the irregularly located maxima.[9] To avoid these demerits, Hsung et al proposed a simplified method to estimate the regularity of a signal from the evolution of its wavelet transform coefficients across scales and obtain the denoised WTMM. It is only by computing the WTMS inside DCOI in scale space. The WTMS of the 2-D filtered projection at the point (x_0, y_0) is computed by

$$N_s f(x_0, y_0) = \int_{(x,y) \in D_s} |M_s f(x,y)| dx dy, \tag{7}$$

$$D_s : \left\{ \begin{array}{l} (x - x_0)^2 + (y - y_0)^2 \leq K s^2 \\ (y - y_0)/(x - x_0) = \tan(A_s f(x_0, y_0)) \end{array} \right\}, \tag{8}$$

where K is the support of mother wavelet and s is wavelet scale, $s = \{2^j\}_{j \in Z}$. If the point (x_0, y_0) corresponds to signal edge or regular signal, it is known that the Lipschitz exponent α at this point is no less than 0. Inversely, it is the noise or irregular signal if α at the point is less than 0. Through easily measuring the 2-D interscale ratio, we can estimate Lipschitz exponent α at the point (x_0, y_0) corresponding to the edge or the regular part of the function f by

$$\frac{N_{2^{j+1}} f(x_0, y_0)}{N_{2^j} f(x_0, y_0)} = 2^{\alpha+1} \geq 2, \quad for \ 1 \leq j < J. \tag{9}$$

Then we can select the wavelet coefficients at the scale of j by

$$\hat{W}_{2^j}^{(1,2)} f(x_0, y_0) = \left\{ \begin{array}{ll} W_{2^j}^{(1,2)}(x_0, y_0) & if \ \alpha \geq 0 \\ 0 & if \ \alpha < 0, \end{array} \right. \tag{10}$$

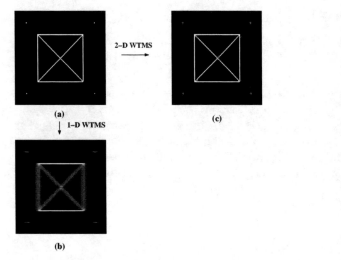

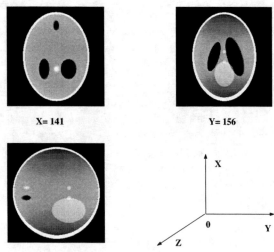

X= 141

Y= 156

Z= 125

Figure 2. The comparisons of the 1-D WTMS and the 2-D WTMS. (a)Sample image. (b)The result image processed by 1-D WTMS. (c)The result image processed by 2-D WTMS.

Figure 3. Ideal sectional cone beam CT images in three coordinate directions. 256×256 pixels.

where $1 \leq j < J, j \in Z$. The denoised filtered projection $\hat{f}(x,y)$ can be recovered from these new denoised components by

$$\hat{f}(x,y) = \sum_{j=1}^{J} (\hat{W}_{2^j}^1 f(x,y) + \hat{W}_{2^j}^2 f(x,y)) + \hat{S}_{2^J} f(x,y).$$ (11)

We repeat the denoising process until all the 2-D projection data have been processed. Finally, we can obtain denoised 3-D CT image reconstructed from these denoised filtered projection.

4. RESULTS AND DISCUSSION

In our previous study, we have shown that the noise in 1-D filtered projection can be removed using 1-D WTMS. The singularities of 1-D projection are smoothed with noise removal. We have to consider to preserve the signal singularities in 1-D filtered projection case. We show a simple example in Fig.2 that indicates the 2-D WTMS method can remove noise with edges preserved. In Fig.2(a), there are four noise points around the square signal. The edges in Fig.2(c) are well preserved with noise points removed. Vice versa, the horizontal lines only are preserved in Fig.2(b). The orientation component used is the main difference between one and two-dimensional WTMS. We can know that the edges of the signal can be measured and kept according to the directional information of edges.

For Shepp-Logan 3-D phantom, we have the simulation to evaluate the performance of the denoising method. The Shepp-Logan 3-D head phantom is used as the experimental phantom. This phantom is composed of 12 ellipsoids.[10] The matrix size of 2-D projections is 256×256 pixels. 360 projection data can be collected at every angle from 0° to 360°. The reconstruction algorithm we used is the extended filtered back projection (FBP) reconstruction algorithm[11] by Feldkamp. In Fig3, we show the ideal sectional CT images from three coordinate directions.

For Shepp-Logan 3-D phantom, we have little interest in the region out of the head phantom and there usually exists much noise which is hard to be removed in the region. Therefore, in this study we only compute the SNR value in the regions of interest (ROI) of Shepp-Logan 3-D phantom to evaluate the result. We compute the SNR in ROI using the equation denoted by

$$SNR = 10 \log_{10} \frac{\sum_{z=64}^{192} \sum_{y=64}^{192} \sum_{x=64}^{192} (f_0(x,y,z))^2}{\sum_{z=64}^{192} \sum_{y=64}^{192} \sum_{x=64}^{192} (f_r(x,y,z) - f_0(x,y,z))^2},$$ (12)

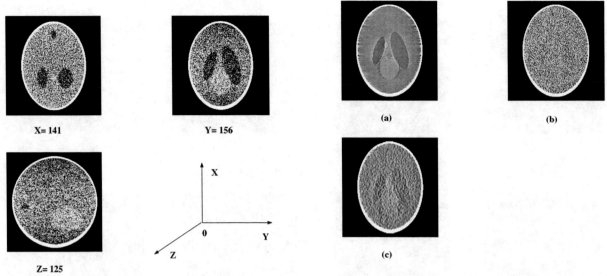

X= 141   Y= 156

Z= 125

Figure 4. Noisy sectional cone beam CT images in three coordinate directions. $N_{in} = 10^5$, 256×256 pixels.

Figure 5. The 2-D filtered projection Data. (a)The noiseless filtered projection, (b)The noisy filtered projection. (c)The denoised filtered projection. The rotation angle $\theta = 90^\circ$, $N_{in} = 10^5$, 256×256 pixels.

where f_r is the reconstructed phantom image, f_0 is ideal phantom image.

We give an example of process when the number of incident X-ray photons N_{in} is 10^5. We show the noisy sectional CT images from three coordinate directions in Fig.4. Comparing with Fig.3, it is easily known that there exists much noise in the phantom with $N_{in} = 10^5$, and it is not easy to discriminate the interior structures. Before the cone beam CT image is reconstructed, the noisy projection is considered to be denoised for obtaining good visual quality CT 3-D image. Fig.5(a) and (b) show the 2-D noiseless and noisy filtered projection at the rotation angle $\theta = 90$. The denoised filtered projection is shown in Fig.5(c). Fig.6(a) and (b) are the wavelet horizontal and vertical components of the Fig.5(b), respectively. Fig.6(c) and (d) are the modulus of the wavelet transform at scale 1 and scale 2, respectively. Fig.6(e) is orientation component at scale 2. It indicates the direction of the WTM of a signal. Fig.6(f) shows the binary image of interscale ratio of WTMS by using Eq.(9). The denoised wavelet horizontal and vertical components are shown in Fig.6(g) and (h). We can identify the signal singularities and obtain the denoised WTMM only by computing the integral of the WTM and using the 2-D interscale ratio condition. That is, according to Eq.(7) and Eq.(9), Firstly, from the modulus of wavelet transform at the two scales which are shown in Fig.6(c) and (d), the wavelet transform modulus sum (WTMS) in the direction shown in Fig.6(e) inside the COI can be computed. After the interscale ratio of WTMS is processed with a threshold by using Eq.(9), we can obtain the binary image Fig.6(f). The binary image shows that the white region of edge is preserved and the black region with noise is processed. Then, the wavelet components shown in Fig.6(a) and (b) can be processed in the same region shown in the binary image. The denoised wavelet components are shown in Fig.6(g) and (h). We can recover the filtered projection using these denoised components. Then, the 2-D filtered projection data measured with the rotational angle from 0° to 360° are denoised by the same method as the one above. Finally, the denoised cone-beam CT image can be reconstructed from these denoised filtered projection data. The denoised sectional images from three coordinates directions are shown in Fig.7. The most noise in Fig.7 has been removed in comparison with Fig.4.

The comparisons of the signal to noise ratio (SNR) of the denoised 3-D CT phantoms are shown in Fig8. According to Fig.8, we can know that the denoised result has more than 10dB up better than the noisy one inside the ROI of Shepp-Logan phantom when N_{in} is 10^4 and 10^5.

The quality of CT images will be better with the increment of the number of incident X-ray photons N_{in}. That is confirmed in the top row of Fig.9. We reconstruct cone beam CT image when the number of the

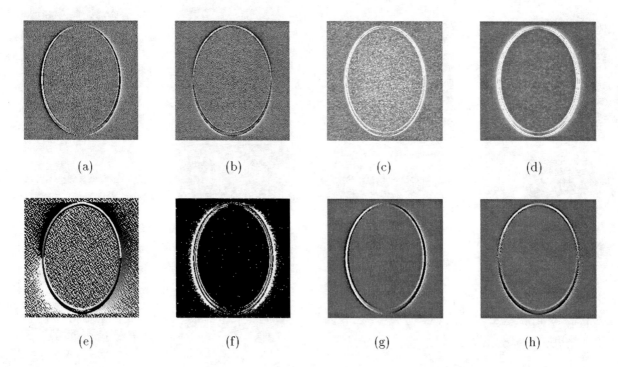

Figure 6. The wavelet transform components (WTC) of the 2-D filtered projection. All images are with 256×256 pixels. (a)The horizontal WTC of the 2-D projection with noise. (b)The vertical WTC of the 2-D projection with noise. (c)The modulus of the wavelet transform at the scale 1. (d)The modulus of the wavelet transform at the scale 2. (e)The orientation component between horizontal and vertical components at the scale 2. (f)The binary imageof interscale ratio($\alpha \geq 0 : white, \alpha < 0 : black$). (g)The horizontal WTC of the 2-D denoised projection. (h)The vertical WTC of the 2-D denoised projection.

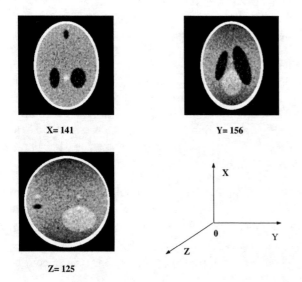

Figure 7. Denoised sectional cone beam CT images in three coordinate directions. $N_{in} = 10^5$, 256×256 pixels.

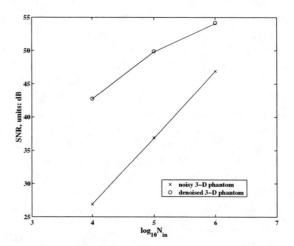

Figure 8. Numerical comparisons of 3-D CT phantom with the different N_{in}.

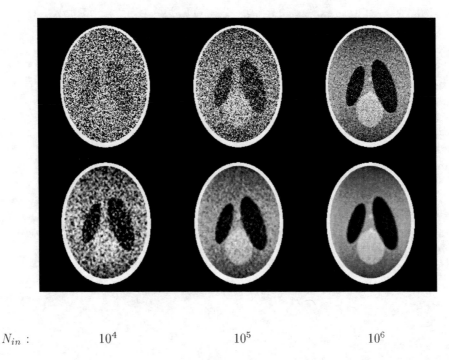

N_{in} :　　　　　10^4　　　　　　　10^5　　　　　　　10^6

Figure 9. The comparison of results with the different N_{in}. The top row shows sectional noisy images; the bottom row shows sectional denoised images. The N_{in} increases from left to right. All sectional images are at $y = 156$, with 256×256 pixels.

incident X-ray photons N_{in} varies and investigate their dependent relation. Our denoised results are shown in the bottom row of Fig.9. ¿From Fig.9, we can distinguish the structures of head phantom which are not easy to do in the noisy images when N_{in} is 10^4 and 10^5. In our previous study, we have shown that the noise in 1-D filtered projection can be removed using 1-D WTMS. The results show good visual quality in the interior structures of CT image and better SNR values than using wavelet shrinkage. It shows the possibility that the patient' dose can be reduced to 1/10. In this study, the most noise in 2-D projection can be removed with the edges well-preserved. The results by using 2-D WTMS for 2-D projection have better SNR gain than using 1-D WTMS for 1-D projection. Our results in this study also show the possibility that the patient' dose can be reduced to less than 1/10 for 3-D CT or real-time 3-D CT.

5. CONCLUSION

After wavelet transform with the increment of scale, the WTMM of the regularities in a signal will not decrease, inversely, the one of signal singularities will decrease fast. In the study, the 2-D WTMS method based on this interscale information has been used to remove the noise from 2-D projection for cone beam CT. The results show that the structures in the images reconstructed from the denoised 2-D projection can be distinguished in comparison with noisy ones. We have confirmed the validity of 2-D WTMS method applied in denoising of cone beam CT. Furthermore, we investigate the relation between the X-ray photons and quantum mottle in cone beam CT. The result shows it is possible to reduce patient' dose to less than 1/10 for 3-D CT.

REFERENCES

1. U. Michael and A. Akram, "A review of wavelets in biomedical application," *Proc. IEEE* **84**, pp. 626–637, 1996.
2. W. Tsukamoto, N. Nakamori, T. Tsunoo, and Y. Yoshida, "The effect to cone beam ct image and image improvement," *J. Medical Image Info.* **16**, pp. 20–28, 1999.

3. D. L. Donoho and I. M. Johnstone, *Ideal Spatial Adaptation by Wavelet Shrinkage*, Dept.of Stat. Stanford University, Tech. Report, Stanford, 1992.

4. E. Kolaczyk, "A wavelet shrinkage approach to tomographic image reconstruction," *J. of Amer. Stat. Assoc.* **91**, pp. 1079–1090, 1996.

5. S. Mallat and W. L. Hwang, "Singularity detection and processing with wavelets," *IEEE Trans. Info. theory* **38**, pp. 617–643, 1992.

6. T. C. Hsung, D. P. K. Lun, and W. C. Siu, "Denoising by singularity detection," *IEEE Trans. Signal Processing* **47**, pp. 3139–3144, 1999.

7. A. C. Kak and M. Slaney, *Principles of Computerized Tomographic Imaging*, IEEE Press, New York, 1988.

8. S. Mallat and S. Zhong, "Characterization of signals from multiscale edges," *IEEE Trans. Pattern Anal. Machine Intell.* **14**, pp. 710–732, 1992.

9. A. Liew and D. T. Nguyen, "Uniqueness issue of wavelet transform modulus maxima representation and a least squares reconstruction algorithm," *Electron. Lett.* **31**, pp. 1735–1736, 1995.

10. S. Zhao and G. Wang, "Feldkamp-type cone-beam tomography in the wavelet framework," *IEEE Trans. Medical Imaging* **19**, pp. 922–929, 2000.

11. K. A. Feldkamp, L. C. Davis, and W. Kress, "Practical cone-beam algorithm," *J. Opt. Soc. Am.* **1**, pp. 612–619, 1984.

Tree structured wavelet transform signature for classification of melanoma.

Sachin V. Patwardhan[a], Atam P. Dhawan*[a] and Patricia A. Relue[b].

[a] Department of Electrical & Computer Engineering, New Jersey Institute of Technology,
[b] Department of Bioengineering, The University of Toledo.

ABSTRACT

The purpose of this work is to evaluate the use of a wavelet transform based tree structure in classifying skin lesion images into melanoma and dysplastic nevus classes based on the spatial/frequency information. The classification is done using the wavelet transform tree structure analysis. Development of the tree structure in the proposed method uses energy ratio thresholds obtained from a statistical analysis of the coefficients in the wavelet domain. The method is used to obtain a tree structure signature of melanoma and dysplastic nevus, which is then used to classify the data set into the two classes. Images are classified by using a semantic comparison of the wavelet transform tree structure signatures. Results show that the proposed method is effective and simple for classification based on spatial/frequency information, which also includes the textural information.

Key words: Melanoma, Dysplastic Nevus, Tree Structured Wavelet Transform, and Nevoscope.

1. INTRODUCTION

Abnormal cell division of melanocytes may give rise to malignant melanoma. Malignant melanoma is a disease of the skin in which melanocytes become cancerous. Melanoma tends to spread out within the epidermis before moving into the deeper layer of the skin (the dermis). The level of spread of melanoma within the epidermis and then the dermis is determined as the Clark level, which indicates the stage (i.e. the severity) of the spread of melanoma. Melanoma is distinguished from dysplastic nevus by a physician by observing: i) change in color, especially multiple shades of dark brown or black; ii) change or spreading of color from the edge of the mole into surrounding skin; iii) change in size, especially sudden or continuous enlargement, or change in shape, especially development of irregular margins or border; iv) change in elevation, especially sudden elevation of a previously flat mole; v) change in the surface characteristics of a mole, especially scaliness, erosion, oozing, crusting, ulceration, or bleeding; vi) change in the surrounding skin, especially redness, swelling, or new moles; and vii) change in sensation, especially itching, tenderness, or pain.

In the early stages of melanoma these differences are hardly visible and may lead to a false diagnosis. Most of the above features suggest that there will be a change in the surface characteristics of the nevus as it progresses towards melanoma. The purpose of this work is to classify epiluminesence images of the skin lesions obtained using the Nevoscope [1], [2] as melanoma or dysplastic nevus. This classification is based on the spatial/frequency information, including textural information, derived from a tree structure wavelet transform analysis of the images.

A texture provides important characteristics for surface and object identification and finds many applications in biomedical image processing and industrial monitoring. Among the different methods used for texture analysis, the Gaussian Markov random field [3], [4], [5] and Gibbs distribution texture model [6], [7] characterize the gray levels between nearest neighboring pixels by a certain stochastic relationship. The weakness is, they focus on the coupling between image pixels on a single scale and fail to characterize different scales of texture effectively. Wavelet transform [8], [9], [10], [11], Gabor transforms and Wigner distribution [12], [13], [14] provides good multi-resolution analytical tools and help to overcome this difficulty. The filtering-based methods such as Laws and Gabor filters use a fixed number of filter masks with predetermined frequencies and bandwidths. The set of filter masks is determined by extensive experiments and may vary for different textures. In contrast, tree-structured wavelet decomposition determines important frequency channels dynamically according to energy calculations and can be viewed as an adaptive multi-channel method [16].

2. TREE STRUCTURE WAVELET TRANSFORM ANALYSIS

The pyramid-structured wavelet transform decomposes a signal into a set of frequency channels that have narrower bandwidths in the lower frequency region. The transform is suitable for signals consisting primarily of smooth components so that their information is concentrated in the low frequency regions, but is not suitable for quasi-periodic signals whose dominant frequency channels are located in the middle frequency region. The most significant spatial/frequency information often appears in the middle frequency region. Thus, decomposition just in the lower frequency region, as the conventional wavelet transform does, may not help much for the purpose of classification. To analyze signals of this type, tree-structured wavelet transform or wavelet packets are used [15]. In tree structure wavelet transform analysis the decomposition is no longer applied to the low frequency channels recursively but it can be applied to the output of any channels, H_{ll}, H_{lh}, H_{hl} or H_{hh}, where the subscripts l and h denote the low-pass and high-pass filtering characteristics in the x and y directions, respectively.

2.1 Development of the tree structure

The decomposition of a particular channel is decided using the averaged l_1 norm in order to obtain the tree structure and the energy map of dominant frequency channels for the image. The given image is decomposed with a two-dimensional wavelet transform into four sub-images at each scale. The energy of a sub-image (or channel) x(m, n) is

$$e = \frac{1}{MN} \sum_{m=1}^{M} \sum_{n=1}^{N} | x(m, n) | \tag{1}$$

where M and N are the sub-image dimensions and $1 \leq m \leq M$ and $1 \leq n \leq N$. Further decomposition of the sub-image is decided by comparing the energy e of the sub-image with the largest energy value e_{max} in the same scale. Decomposition of the sub-image is stopped if $e < C\, e_{max}$, where C is a threshold constant less than 1. The number of decomposition levels used in the tree structure depends on the resolution of the sub-images.

2.2. Classification using the tree structure

Once the tree structure is developed, energy in the leaves of the tree defines an energy function in the spatial-frequency domain called the energy map. This energy map is used in the texture analysis and classification of the images, where each leaf of the tree corresponds to a feature.

The candidate image is decomposed to obtain its tree structure and the energy map using the same algorithm. The distance between the features of the unknown texture and the corresponding features of the known set of textures is used to classify the candidate image to a texture class. A progressive classification algorithm is used when the textures have no significant dominant frequency channels, such as random textures or when multiple textures have similar dominant frequency channels. Here, we start with one feature, which eliminates the most unlikely candidates, and then another feature is added for further elimination. The procedure is repeated until there is only one texture left in the candidate list [16].

2.3. Major issues with the tree structure analysis

Tree structure analysis has two main drawbacks. First, selecting a different threshold value may generate an all-together different tree structure and hence a different set of dominant frequency channel features. In addition there is no fixed criterion for selection of the threshold constant. Although the energy ratios within the decomposed channels may change considerably at the different levels of decomposition, the same threshold value is used throughout the tree structure development. Second, this method assumes that high energy means better discriminability. Only the dominant frequency channels based on the maximum energy criterion are decomposed further in the tree structure development. If the image textures are very close to each other, this method can lead to almost identical tree structures and energy maps for all the textures. Classification in this case would be highly dependent on the number of features used, but it is difficult to determine the number of features required for classification a priori.

3. PROPOSED METHOD

Instead of selecting a threshold constant randomly, statistical analysis was used for finding an energy ratio threshold for every channel used in the development of the tree structure. This statistical method was applied to obtaining wavelet transform tree structure signatures of melanoma and dysplastic nevus. These signatures were then used in classifying the data set into melanoma and dysplastic nevus classes using a semantic comparison.

3.1. Learning phase

During the learning phase a known set of melanoma and dysplastic nevus images were used. All images were decomposed up to 4 levels in Matlab using the db3 wavelet. The thresholds for channel decomposition were obtained by performing a statistical analysis over the channel energies as explained below. These threshold values were then used in obtaining the wavelet transform tree structure signatures for the two image classes, melanoma and dysplastic nevus.

3.1.1. Threshold selection

During the learning phase, the features used in the statistical analysis for finding the threshold values were various channel energies and ratios of channel energies for a given decomposition level. For example, an image is decomposed into four sub-images $a(m,n)$, $b(m,n)$, $c(m,n)$ and $d(m,n)$. The mean channel energies of each of the sub-images are used as features. If image $c(m,n)$ has the maximum channel energy of the four sub-images, the ratios of channel energies of images $a(m,n)$, $b(m,n)$ and $d(m,n)$ with image $c(m,n)$ are also used as features. In addition, the ratio of channel energy for each sub-image to the sum of the remaining three channel energies, such as the ratio of channel energies for image $a(m,n)$ to the sum for images $b(m,n)$, $c(m,n)$ and $d(m,n)$, are also used as features. These energies and energy ratios generate a set of 11 features for the first level of decomposition, 44 features for the second level of decomposition, and 176 features for the third level of decomposition. In other words, 11 features per channel are generated. For reference, the main image is numbered as 0, and its low-low, low-high, high-low and high-high filter channels for the first level of decomposition are numbered 1, 2, 3 and 4, respectively,. The channels for the second level of decomposition for channel 1 are numbered 1.1, 1.2, 1.3 and 1.4, and so on for the other channels and further levels of decomposition in this analysis.

For each individual feature, clusters were formed for the two texture classes, melanoma and dysplastic nevus. All the features that generated unimodal distributions were rejected, and thresholds were found for all the features that generated bimodal distributions. The means of the feature values for the two classes and their variance were used in determining if a feature generated a unimodal or a bimodal distribution. If more than one feature for a particular channel gave a bimodal distribution, then the feature with the maximum mean separation and smallest variance was used in the analysis. For all features that generated linearly separable pure clusters for the two classes, energy ratio thresholds were obtained by averaging the upper bound of the lower cluster and the lower bound of the upper cluster. Channel 2.1, 3.1 and 2.1.4 produced linearly separable pure clusters. Clusters and thresholds obtained for these channels are shown in Figure 1 where the feature values are plotted against the subject number for clarity, as the actual clusters are only one-dimensional. For bimodal clusters that were not linearly separable, it was assumed that the features have a bimodal Gaussian distribution and that the two texture classes have an equal probability of occurrence. The optimal threshold with a minimal classification error is then equal to the average of the means of the two classes [17]. Channels 2 and 3 had bimodal features of this type. Thresholds were obtained for these channels by taking the average of the feature means for the two classes. For channel 2, a threshold value of 0.0366 was obtained for the ratio of channel 2 and channel 1 energies, and for channel 3, a threshold value of 0.043 was obtained for the ratio of channel 3 and channel 1 energies.

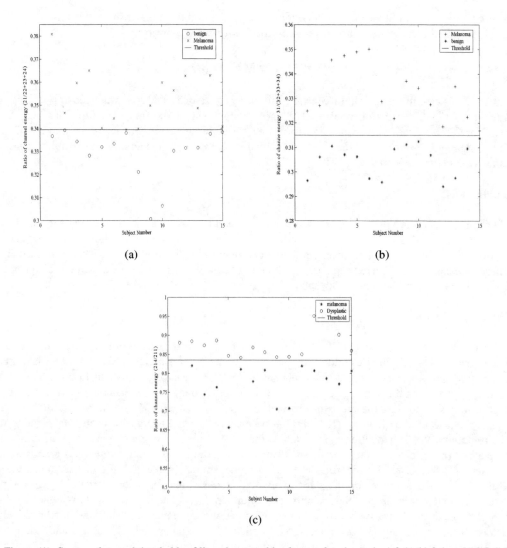

(a)

(b)

(c)

Figure (1): Scatter plots and thresholds of linearly separable clusters for channel: a) 2.1, (b) 3.1 and (c) 2.1.4.

3.1.2. Development of the tree structure signatures

Based on the thresholds selected above, the image decomposition algorithm was developed for obtaining the tree structure. For any channel whose features were all unimodally distributed, decomposition was stopped. Since all the features of channels 1 and 4 had unimodal distributions, further decomposition of these channels was stopped. The remaining channels, having at least one bimodally distributed feature, were decomposed further if the features satisfied the corresponding energy ratio threshold. Thresholds were selected to separate the melanoma images from the dysplastic nevus images. With reference to Figure 1, channel 2.1 will only be decomposed further if the mean channel energy of 2.1 ratioed to the sum of the mean channel energy of 2.2, 2.3 and 2.4 is greater than the threshold value of 0.34. For channel 3.1 to be decomposed further, the mean channel energy of 3.1 ratioed to the sum of the mean channel energy of 3.2, 3.3 and 3.4 must be greater than 0.315. Channel 2.1.4 will be decomposed further only if the mean channel energy ratio of 2.1.4 to 2.1.1 is less than 0.837. Similarly, decomposition of channels 2 and 3 was based on the thresholds given in section 3.1.1. The resulting tree structure signature of melanoma is shown in Figure 2a. Note that only channels 0, 2, 3, 2.1, 3.1 and 2.1.4 were decomposed further and the decomposition of all other channels was stopped since all of their features produced unimodal distributions. Also note that due to the definition of these thresholds, the algorithm will not decompose dysplastic nevus images beyond the first level. A dysplastic nevus will thus generate a tree structure as shown in Figure 2b.

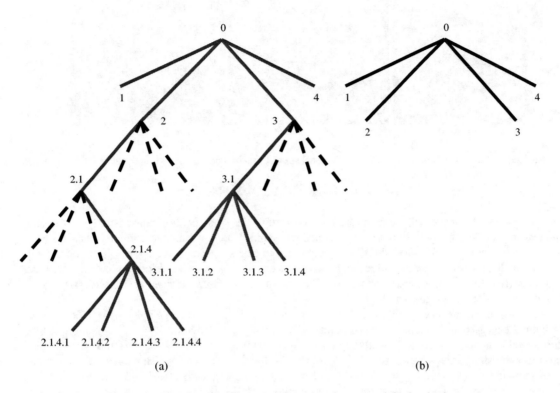

Figure (2): Tree Structure Signatures for: (a) melanoma and (b) dysplastic nevus.

3.2. Classification phase

During the classification phase the tree structure of the candidate image obtained using the same decomposition algorithm is semantically compared with the tree structure signature of melanoma and the dysplastic nevus. A classification variable CV is set to a value of 1 when the main image is decomposed. The value of CV is incremented by one for all subsequent decompositions of the channels. If the algorithm decomposes all the channels for which thresholds were obtained (0, 2, 3, 2.1, 3.1 and 2.1.4), CV has a value of 6. When the algorithm decomposes a dysplastic nevus image, only channel 0 should be decomposed, so CV has a value of 1. Hence, when the algorithm decomposes the candidate image, if the value of CV is 1, the image is assigned to the dysplastic nevus class. If CV has a value greater than 1, it is assigned to the melanoma class.

3.3 Data

Epiluminesence images of skin lesions from individuals of various age groups and genders were used for this analysis. The images were collected using the Nevoscope by scanning 173 individuals with suspicious melanoma under the observation of a dermatologist/cancer specialist over a period of one year. In all, 15 images of melanoma and 15 images of dysplastic nevus were used during the learning phase and 7 images of melanoma and 20 images of dysplastic nevus were used in the classification phase of this work. The cases of melanoma were confirmed by histology. All images were 1024 X 768 pixels in size. Samples of images from the data set are shown in Figure 3 along with an epiluminesence image of normal skin.

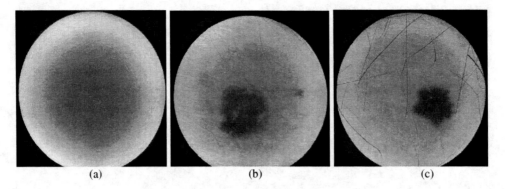

(a)   (b)   (c)

Figure 3: Sample epiluminesence images of (a) normal skin, (b) malignant nevus, and (c) dysplastic nevus.

4. RESULTS & DISCUSSION

Out of the 27 images of the skin lesions used during the classification phase, the tree structure wavelet transform algorithm with statistically obtained threshold values was able to correctly classify the 7 images to the melanoma nevus class which were confirmed to be melanoma from the histology reports. Of the remaining 20 images, 18 were correctly classified to the dysplastic nevus class and 2 images were wrongly classified to the melanoma nevus class. The true positive value obtained for this classifier was 100% and the false positive value was 10%.

The mean channel energy ratio of channel 2 to channel 1 has an average value of 0.0366 and the mean channel energy ratio of channel 3 and channel 1 has an average value of 0.043. The method of tree structure development by randomly selecting a threshold constant thus reverts to the pyramid type wavelet transform for threshold values higher than 0.043 as only the low-low frequency channels are decomposed. The tree structure and the energy maps developed are highly sensitive to changes in the value of the threshold constant below 0.043. Hence, an adaptive method of selecting this threshold value would be a better approach than randomly selecting a value with no criterion. Obtaining the threshold values from a statistical analysis of the channel energies and their energy ratios provides the required adaptivity to the tree structure development. Statistical selection of threshold values also makes the wavelet tree structure more robust and hence a good candidate for surface characterization and texture representation. It should be noted that since the thresholds were obtained from bimodal distributions, reversing the thresholds would reverse the tree structure signature for the two classes. The dysplastic nevus was a logical choice instead of the melanoma as a basis for classification since more dysplastic nevus data are available.

The two images of dysplastic nevi that were wrongly classified as melanoma were decomposed beyond the first level. For both of these images, channel 2 was decomposed further. Decomposition for both the images stopped after the second level. These images were classified to the melanoma nevus class since for them the classification variable CV was 2. It should be noted that the tree structures for these two images is different from the tree structure signature of melanoma since channels 2.1, 3, 3.1 and 2.1.4 were not decomposed. This difference in decomposition could be truly misclassification, or could signify that these two nevi are in the early stages of melanoma progression but are not showing features visible to a physician to be identified as melanoma. Further investigation of this phenomenon is needed before any conclusions can be made.

The proposed method is especially effective and fast as compared to the progressive classification algorithm [16], explained in section 2.2, when images having different surface characteristics but similar dominant frequency channels are to be classified.. These images can now be classified by using a semantic comparison of the wavelet transform tree structure signature. This method eliminates the distance measurement between the features and iteratively adding new features in the classification process, thus making the classification process simpler. Although the statistical method proposed in this work is used in categorizing the images into two classes based on the spatial/frequency information, it can be easily adapted to classify images into more classes. However, the learning phase, especially obtaining the threshold values, may become tedious with an increase in the number of classes in the data set. Instead of using a single threshold value, multiple thresholds will have to be obtained depending upon the number of classes.

5. CONCLUSIONS

Results show that the proposed statistical method for selection of thresholds between classes is effective and simple for classification of the images based on their spatial/frequency information. This work also shows a promising use of epiluminesence images of skin lesions obtained using the Nevoscope in the early diagnosis of melanoma.

ACKNOWLEDGEMENTS

The authors would like to thank all the patients who participated in this study. We would also like to thank The Medical College of Ohio, Toledo, OH and Dr. Prabhir Chaudhuri for the contribution in the data collection. We would also like to thank the Whitaker Foundation for providing partial funding for this research under the Whitaker Foundation Research Grant RG-99-0127.

REFERENCES

1. A.P. Dhawan, "Early detection of cutaneous malignant melanoma by three dimensional nevoscopy," *Computer Methods and Programs in Biomedicine*, vol. **21**, pp. 59-68, 1985.
2. A.P. Dhawan, R. Gordon and R.M. Rangayyan, "Nevoscopy: three-dimensional computed tomography of nevi and melanomas in situ by transillumination," *IEEE Trans. Med. Imag.*, vol. **3(2)**, pp. 54-61, June 1984.
3. R. Chellappa, "Two dimensional discrete Gaussian Markov random field models for image processing," *Pattern Recognition*, vol. **2**, pp. 79-122, 1985.
4. G.R. Cross and A.K. Jain, "Markov random field texture models," *IEEE Trans. Pattern Anal. And Machine Intell.*, vol. **5**, pp. 25-39, Jan. 1983.
5. J.W. Woods, S. Dravida and R. Mediavilla, " Image estimation using doubly stochastic Gaussian random field models," *IEEE Trans. Pattern Anal. And Machine Intell.*, vol. **9**, pp. 245-253, Mar. 1987.
6. H. Derin, "Segmentation of textured images using Gibbs random fields," *Computer, Vision, Graphics and Image Processing*, vol. **35**, pp. 72-98, 1986.
7. H. Derin and H. Elliott, "Modeling and segmentation of noisy and textured images using Gibbs random fields," *IEEE Trans. Pattern Anal. And Machine Intell.*, vol. **9**, pp. 39-55, Jan. 1987.
8. I. Daubechies, "Orthonormal bases of compactly supported wavelets," *Communications on Pure and Applied Mathematics*, vol. **41**, pp. 909-996, Nov. 1988.
9. I. Daubechies, " The wavelet transform, time-frequency localization and signal analysis," *IEEE Trans. Info. Theory*, vol. **36**, pp. 961-1005, Sept. 1990.
10. C.E. Heil and D.F. Walnut, "Continuous and discrete wavelet transforms," *SIAM Review*, vol. **31**, pp. 628-666, Dec. 1989.
11. S.G Mallat, "A theory for multi-resolution signal decomposition: the wavelet representation," IEEE *Trans. Pattern Anal. And Machine Intell.*, vol. **11**, pp.674-693, July 1989.
12. T.R. Reed and H. Wechsler, "Segmentation of textured images and Gestalt organization using spatial/spatial-frequency representations," *IEEE Trans. Pattern Anal. And Machine Intell.*, vol. **12**, pp. 1-12, Jan. 1990.
13. A.C. Bovik, "Analysis of multi-channel narrow band filters for image texture segmentation," *IEEE Trans. Signal Processing*, vol. **39**, pp. 2025-2043, Sept. 1991.
14. A.C. Bovik, M. Clark and W.S. Geisler, "Multi-channel texture analysis using localized spatial filters," *IEEE Trans. Pattern Anal. And Machine Intell.*, vol. **12**, Jan. 1990.
15. R.R. Coifman and M.V. Wickerhauser, "Entropy based algorithms for best basis selection," *IEEE Trans. Info. Theory*, vol. **38**, pp. 713-718, Mar. 1992.
16. Tianhorng Chang and C.C. Jay Kuo, "Texture analysis and classification with tree-structured wavelet transform," *IEEE Trans. Image processing*, vol. **2**, No. 4, pp. 429-441, Oct. 1993.
17. R.C. Gonzalez and R.E. Woods, *Digital image processing*, pp.443-458, Addison-Wesley publishing company, 1992.

* dhawan@adm.njit.edu; phone 973-596-3524; fax 973-596-5680; http://www.njit.edu/ECE/dhawan; Department of Electrical & Computer Engineering, New Jersey Institute of Technology, University Heights, Newark, NJ 07102.

Line Vector Quantization Using Non-Integer Subsampled Wavelet Pyramids and its Application in Medical Imaging

Vadim Kustov*, Andrew Zador**

Finline Technologies Ltd., Impress Research Division

ABSTRACT

We have developed two novel techniques that can improve quality and speed for wavelet based compression algorithms without major modification of the latter. We show that replacing traditional block-shaped vectors with line vectors of the same dimension (defined along a row or column of an image or its transform), significantly reduces the distortion in the reconstructed image, while accelerating coding and decoding times. To improve the performance of the clustering algorithm, we introduce a non-integer-sub-sampled wavelet pyramid. This new type of wavelet decomposition possesses certain shift-invariant properties not found in classical wavelet pyramid structures. Unlike frames and other types of mapping that introduce data redundancy into the transform in order to induce shift-invariance, our new pyramid does not introduce any data redundancy. A fast method for implementing this new pyramid is introduced. It is shown that the resulting zerotree structure is both sparser, and more efficiently coded due to the non-integer sub-sampling process. Experimental data is provided, demonstrating the performance of our proposed architecture employing line vectors. Our data also indicates that replacing the classical pyramid with this new pyramid can significantly improve performance for a wide range of quantizer designs.

Keywords: Vector Quantization, wavelet pyramid, shift-invariance, zerotree

1. INTRODUCTION

During the last several years a number of medical establishments have transitioned from film to digital radiological imaging. Recent surveys have shown that this transition has had a significant positive effect[1]. The number of lost and mislabeled images has been reduced, the average image-retrieval time using picture archiving and communication systems (PACS) has been decreased as well. As a result, doctors have been able to better use the extra time on their patients, which had previously been spent waiting for film images in process or transit.

However, the transition from film to digital radiology has brought up some problems as well. Uncompressed images take up large amounts of space on storage media. Taking into account that radiological images are typically large, high-resolution images with more than eight bits per pixel, and that many such images are acquired on a daily basis, the problem of having insufficient storage media for image archival is an acute one.

One solution to the problem is to compress images, so that they take up less storage space than the original uncompressed data. Lossless compression (i.e. the type of compression where the original image can be completely recovered without distortion), typically results in up to 3:1 compression ratios, depending on the image content. Compressions of up to 18:1 can be achieved if the image is segmented prior to compression, with only the region of interest compressed losslessly[2]. Lossy compression algorithms, (those algorithms that permit information to be lost gradually), have been reported to produce visually acceptable reconstructed images with compression ratios up to 100:1[3]. While lossy compression is not allowed for diagnostic images in current use, it is allowed for archiving images that have not been in use for a significant period of time. In lossy compression the goal is to introduce the least amount of distortion at a given compression ratio or to achieve the highest compression ratio achieving a predetermined quality level. Algorithms, which introduce the least distortion at high compression ratios often use vector quantization (VQ), as opposed to scalar quantization (SQ). VQ-based algorithms, although superior to SQ-based algorithms at preserving image quality at high compression ratios, have several drawbacks, one of which is a long encoding time. In this paper we present two techniques which, when combined together, can decrease the execution time of existing VQ-based

*z1m01@ttacs.ttu.edu; ** amzador@golden.net; phone 1 519 746-1023; fax 1 519 746-1131; http://www.finline.com;

Finline Technologies Ltd., 180 Frobisher Drive, Unit 1-C, Waterloo, Ontario, Canada, N2V 2A2

Medical Imaging 2002: Image Processing, Milan Sonka, J. Michael Fitzpatrick, Editors, Proceedings of SPIE Vol. 4684 (2002) © 2002 SPIE · 1605-7422/02/$15.00

algorithms without requiring a major modification of the algorithms themselves. In addition these techniques can be used to improve the fidelity of the reconstructed images, specifically by being able to better preserve edge information, which plays a very important role in the analysis of radiological images.

2. LINE VECTOR QUANTIZATION

According to one of the fundamental theorems of signal compression, the optimal vector quantizer introduces an equal or smaller amount of statistical distortion than does the optimal scalar quantizer under the same entropy contraints[4]. This is due to the fact that VQ exploits the existing data dependency among the elements of the data set. If there is no data dependency, the optimal VQ performance is equal to that of the optimal SQ. For example, applying VQ to white noise does not result in a better performance over SQ. It is important to note here, that perceptual issues would further complicate this comparison. Employing sparse block vectors to represent white noise may achieve identical statistical quality compared with SQ. However the human visual system is capable of discerning small adjacent identical blocks of quantized noise, and repetitions of such blocks may give the false impression of patterns, so that in this example SQ would outperform VQ visually. Compression gained from applying VQ depends, among other factors, on the type of original signal, the transform performed on the signal (if the quantization takes place in the transform domain), and the shape of the vectors used if the input signal is multidimensional. To avoid confusion the word "dimension" is used in this paper to denote the physical dimensions of a signal, while the word "length" is used to denote the number of elements in a vector. It is a common practice in VQ-based image compression algorithms to use vectors sampled on a rectangular or square grid, i.e. vectors of lengths L represent $\sqrt{L}$ by $\sqrt{L}$ ($\sqrt{L} \in Z$) blocks of elements in the original image or transform domain, and are consequently called block vectors in this paper. Block vectors are usually symmetric with respect to their horizontal and vertical dimensions (i.e. square), which is an attractive feature when there are no significant statistical differences between the horizontal and vertical dimensions. This is often the case for large areas in the majority of natural images (as distinguished from synthesized images). The situation may change if the vectors are sampled from a transform of an image. Transforms may be performed in one dimension only, and therefore their statistics may exhibit highly anisotropic properties. For example, statistical properties of a horizontal high-pass band of a symmetric image are typically different in the horizontal and the vertical directions. The problem of finding the optimal shape of a vector, i.e. the shape that will result in the smallest amount of distortion under the same entropy constraints, will have a different solution depending on the image content, the transform performed, its geometry, etc. Here we propose to use line vectors, i.e. 1 by L (1 by L) vectors defined along a row (column) of an image's or its transform's matrix. Their directionality, geometry and the fact that different vectors can represent areas one element apart in the image/transform space is exploited in the wavelet transform space to develop a new technique, which cannot be implemented for block vectors.

In order to see potential advantages of line vectors over block vectors, let us analyze and compare one of the important statistical characteristics of block and line vectors – the correlation between adjacent vectors in wavelet space.

To make a meaningful comparison, let us assume that the block and line vectors are of equal length L, and that $L \geq 4$ ($L = 1$ is a scalar case, and $\sqrt{L} \notin Z$ for $L = 2, 3$). Using a common model for the wavelet coefficients' autocorrelation functions for unsubsampled HH subbands[5]: $r_{m,n} = r_{00} \gamma^{-(|m|+|n|)}$ (here m and n are the spatial distances in the vertical and horizontal directions, γ is some real constant greater than one, and r_{00} is the variance), it can be shown that the average correlation between adjacent vectors is higher for line vectors than for block vectors. Let us assume that the size of the subband is N by N, and denote $K = N/L$. The average correlation between the closest neighbor block vectors $\bar{r}_{BL}$ can be expressed as: $\bar{r}_{BL} = \dfrac{N^2}{L} r_{00} \gamma^{-\sqrt{L}} / (N^2 / L)$, i.e. all N^2 / L block vectors have their closest spatial neighbors at a spatial distance $\sqrt{L}$, while $N^2 / L - (N/L - 1)$ line vectors have their closest spatial neighbors at a spatial distance of one, and the remaining $(N/L-1)$ vectors are at a spatial distance L. Consequently, the average correlation between the adjacent neighbor line vectors $\bar{r}_{LN}$ can be expressed as follows:

$$\bar{r}_{LN} = [(\frac{N^2}{L} - (\frac{N}{L}-1))r_{00}\gamma^{-1} + (\frac{N}{L}-1)r_{00}\gamma^{-L}]/(N^2/L). \tag{2.1}$$

Now we will show that $\bar{r}_{LN} > \bar{r}_{BL}$. Obviously that is the case for $K=1$, since $\gamma^{-1} > \gamma^{\sqrt{L}}$. Let us show that this is also true for the case of $K \geq 2$:

$$\frac{N^2}{L}r_{00}\gamma^{-1} - (\frac{N}{L}-1)r_{00}\gamma^{-1} + (\frac{N}{L}-1)r_{00}\gamma^{-L} > \frac{N^2}{L}r_{00}\gamma^{-\sqrt{L}}, \tag{2.2}$$

dividing both sides of (2.2) by $\frac{N^2}{L}r_{00}\gamma^{-\sqrt{L}}$ and recalling that $K = N/L$ we obtain:

$$\gamma^{\sqrt{L}-1} - 1 > \frac{K-1}{K^2L}(\gamma^{\sqrt{L}-1} - 1) + \frac{K-1}{K^2L}(1 - \gamma^{\sqrt{L}-L}), \tag{2.3}$$

and dividing both sides of (2.3) by $\gamma^{\sqrt{L}-1} - 1$ we arrive at:

$$1 > \frac{K-1}{K^2L} + \frac{K-1}{K^2L}\frac{(1-\gamma^{\sqrt{L}-L})}{(\gamma^{\sqrt{L}-1}-1)}$$

Now we consider the factor $\dfrac{(1-\gamma^{\sqrt{L}-L})}{(\gamma^{\sqrt{L}-1}-1)}$ on the interval of interest of γ, i.e.: $(1,\infty)$. As γ increases, the factor monotonically decreases, and therefore has a maximum when γ approaches one.

$$\lim_{\gamma \to 1}\frac{(1-\gamma^{\sqrt{L}-L})}{(\gamma^{\sqrt{L}-1}-1)} = \frac{L-\sqrt{L}}{\sqrt{L}-1} \tag{2.4}$$

Now we have to prove that: $1 > \dfrac{K-1}{K^2L} + \dfrac{K-1}{K^2L}\dfrac{L-\sqrt{L}}{\sqrt{L}-1}$

$$\frac{K-1}{K^2L} + \frac{K-1}{K^2}(\frac{1}{\sqrt{L}-1} - \frac{1}{L-\sqrt{L}}) > \frac{K-1}{K^2L} + \frac{K-1}{K^2}\frac{1}{\sqrt{L}-1} \tag{2.5}$$

The right hand side of (2.5) achieves its maximum when both K and L have the smallest values, which are two and four respectively. Plugging in the numbers we find:

$$\frac{K-1}{K^2 L} + \frac{K-1}{K^2}\frac{1}{\sqrt{L}-1} \le \frac{5}{16} < 1 \qquad (2.6)$$

The left-hand side of (2.6) is less than one, and consequently $\overline{r}_{LN} > \overline{r}_{BL}$. We have used the assumption of a square subband (N by N). If the subband is not square, line vectors can be aligned along the greater dimension of the subband, decreasing K, and consequently increasing the correlation. Thus, the square-shaped subband, for which we have shown that $\overline{r}_{LN} > \overline{r}_{BL}$, has the smallest $\overline{r}_{LN}$, and (2.6) is true for rectangular subbands. It can also be easily shown that the HH subband is the worst case for $\overline{r}_{LN}$. By exploiting directionality of line vectors in the H, HL, LH, etc. subbands $\overline{r}_{LN} - \overline{r}_{BL}$ is the smallest in the HH subband.

The fact that on average there is a greater correlation between adjacent neighboring line vectors than between block vectors does not indicate that the distances between line vectors are smaller than the distances between block vectors in their respective spaces. Simply replacing block vectors with line vectors does not lead to lower distortion under the same entropy constraints. However the greater degree of correlation between spatially adjacent line vectors along with their geometry can be advantageous.

Our experimental data shows that the most common type of dependencies between adjacent line vectors in unsubsampled high-pass subbands is a shift type dependency. No predominant transformation, which can account for dependencies between adjacent block vectors has been found. Figure 2.1. shows line and block vectors taken from the same area of the horizontal H subband of the "Lena's shoulder" (an area of the standard "Lena" image). The shift type relationship between the vectors is obvious. This relationship among some of the block vectors is barely noticeable.

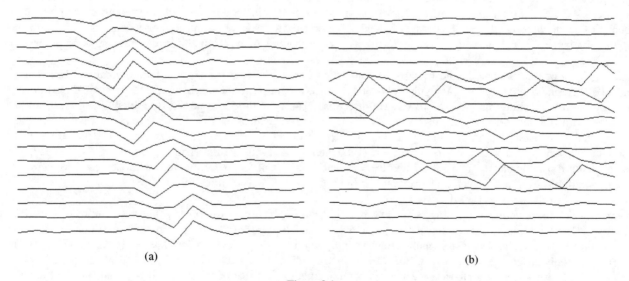

(a)   (b)

Figure 2.1
Line vectors (a) and block vectors (b), from the horizontal (unsubsampled) high-pass subband of "Lena's" shoulder.

These shift-type dependencies and the geometry of line vectors can be exploited, if some algorithm can compensate for the shifts. In that case, the average clustering distance of the vector set will be reduced by the parts of the distances due to the shifts.

A method of unambiguously indexing a line vector ("shift-compensating"), in a graphically optimal manner from within a zerotree, shall now be described. For a given instance of transform-based line vector, the most important distinguishing feature is its maximum value of either polarity (or alternatively, the zero-crossing between opponent polarities having the largest separation), as this feature's amplitude approximately represents the local maximum contrast, while the location of the maximum is very near to the zero-crossing of the edge being represented. In the zerotree vector addressing system, the line vector can be pointed-to using this maximum. Similar line vectors in a codebook can then be delta-coded, aligned to the maximum of the nearest-neighbor representative already in the codebook. To eliminate the possibility of ambiguity due to multiple identical maxima, one may arbitrarily declare the left-most occurrence within the line vector to be the relevant feature, and use sufficiently short line vectors. Even in the event of loss of the codebook, the zerotree now clearly represents a sketch of the image. By comparison, pointing to the leading edge of a line vector would specifically not indicate the most visible feature location, and would be dependent upon the support-length of the filter and the size of transform dead-band. To minimize codebook entropy for the latter case, given all possible variations of each prototype line vector, all present shifts and differences would have to be encoded, which would be inefficient. Given a two-dimensional block vector of the same length, there is no analogous method to point to a single most-significant feature (e.g. there is a higher probability of a line traversing the block over multiple rows or columns). Allowing for all possible variations of block vector can lead to a very high codebook entropy. Maximum-feature position-indexed line vectors can therefore represent successive scan-line crossings of an extended image feature within a region more effectively than block vectors covering the same region.

So far we have considered unsubsampled subbands, which are shift invariant. If a subband is subsampled, shift-invariance is lost, i.e. adjacent vectors that were shifted versions of each other in the unsubsampled band, might no longer resemble each other, and no longer belong to the same Voronoi region. Although algorithms can be designed to alleviate the problem, we partially solve the problem by using a special wavelet pyramid, which possesses some shift-invariant properties not found in the classical dyadic wavelet pyramid.

3. NON-INTEGER SUBSAMPLED PYRAMIDS

The classical dyadic pyramid is by far the most commonly used type of wavelet decomposition in image compression. It possesses some useful features for image compression. For example: the total number of coefficients in the pyramid is equal to that of the original image (no data redundancy), and the next level of the pyramid contains one fourth the number of elements in the previous level and represents coarser features in the original image (multiresolution property).

The first level of the classical dyadic wavelet decomposition consists of four subbands commonly called LL, LH, HL, and HH subbands, produced by applying low- and high-pass filters in the horizontal and vertical direction and subsampling the resulting outputs by two in each direction. The procedure is repeated iteratively using the resulting LL subband as the input, to produce higher levels of the transform, which together form the dyadic wavelet pyramid. The procedure is symmetric in the horizontal and the vertical directions. If the decomposition filters that are used to build the pyramid form a perfect reconstruction (PR) filter bank (with another pair of filters or themselves), the decomposition is completely reversible, i.e. the original image can be reconstructed without any loss of data. The pyramid, however, is shift-variant because it is subsampled by two in each direction at each iteration.

It can be easily observed that avoiding both subsampling the H subband and filtering in the second dimension neither destroys PR, nor introduces data redundancy into the transform. The next level still contains one fourth of the elements of the previous level, and thus the multiresolution property is not affected either. The H band, however, being subsampled only in one dimension is shift-invariant in the other. The invariance is destroyed at the next level of transform, but the degree of shift-variance for this band is smaller than that of the classical pyramid; the next level is subsampled by two as opposed to being subsampled by four (with respect to the original image) in the case of the classical transform. This reduced shift variance propagates to the higher levels of the transform, resulting in the total reduction of shift-variance. The resulting subbands are depicted in Figure 3.1 (a). This shift-variance reduction approach can be improved upon if the number of the coefficients in the unsubsampled subband (in one direction) is increased. This means that this subband has to be subsampled in the opposite direction by a non-integer factor. Figure 3.1 (b) illustrates the shapes and sizes of the subbands of a pyramid which contains a subband that has not been subsampled in the vertical direction and has effectively been subsampled by one and a half in the opposite direction.

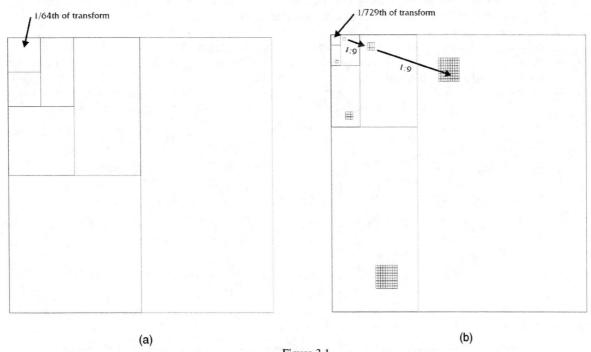

Figure 3.1
The resulting subbands of the dyadic pyramid with shift-invariance reduction (a),
and non-integer subsampled pyramid with the same property (b).

A method for creating non-integer subsampled pyramids (NISUMP) was previously reported in [6]. The forward transform was based on applying the decomposition filters of a 3-channel PR filter bank and subsampling by 3 in that dimension, then merging the two resulting higher frequency subbands into one double-width subband using the reconstruction filters of a 2-channel PR bank. The procedure was repeated in the other dimension on the low-pass band produced by the low-pass filter of the 3-channel filter bank, resulting in an LL subband occupying 1/9th of the original image. The entire procedure was iterated on each LL subband to produce the next level of the transform. The inverse transform consisted of repeatedly splitting the current high frequency subband in two by applying the decomposition filters of the 2-channel bank and performing the inverse 3-channel transform on the resulting two high-pass subbands and the low-pass subband.

The described procedure is slow due to repeated merging and splitting operations. To introduce a fast procedure for NISUMP, let us consider the role of the 2-band reconstruction filters in creating one double-width band. Let us denote by $F_0(z)$ and $F_1(z)$ the z-transform of the low- and high-pass 2-channel bank reconstruction filters respectively, and by $X_1(z)$ and $X_2(z)$ the z-transform of the mid- and high-frequency subbands of a three channel decomposition. Then the z-transform of the combined band $X_{12}(z)$ can be expressed as:

$$X_{12}(z) = F_0(z^2)X_1(z^2) + F_1(z^2)X_2(z^2) \qquad (3.1)$$

As can be seen from (3.1) no spectral component exchange is taking place between the mid- and the high-frequency subbands when there are being merged into one double-width subband. The corresponding coefficients of the mid- and high-frequency subbands become even/odd (neighboring coefficients) of the new combined non-integer subsampled subband. The even and odd components of the new double-width subband represent different spectral components that have different visual importance. In order to apply a uniform quantizer to such a subband, the spectra of even and odd components should be appropriately weighted to result in a more homogeneous set of coefficients in the combined subband. The role of the 2-band filters is to attach appropriate weights to the spectral components of the mid- and high-frequency subband spectra to form a more spectrally homogeneous double-width subband. This process is illustrated in Figure 3.2 (a) and (b). The spectra of the original mid- and high-pass filters Figure 3.2 (a) are "shifted" towards each other in Figure 3.3 (b). No actual spectral shift takes place; the effect is due to weighting, and is desired if a uniform quantizer is to be applied to the entire combined subband.

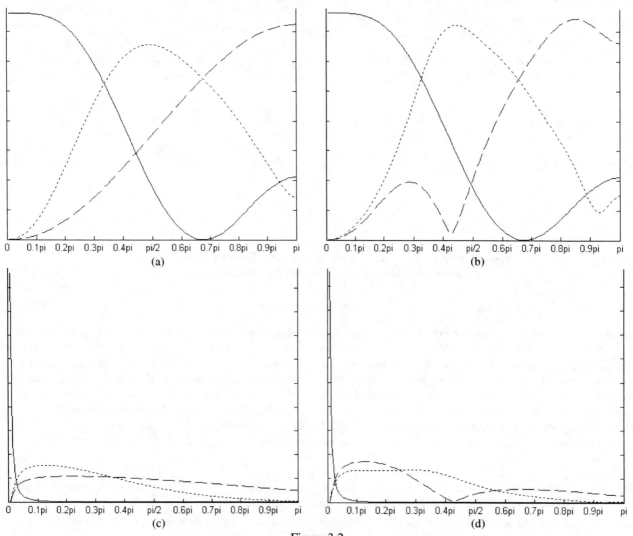

Figure 3.2
Original spectrum of a 3-channel bank (a). Its weighted spectrum (b).
(c) shows the input image's spectra passed by the bank in (a), while
(d) shows the input image's spectra passed by the bank in (b),

The effect of the weighting is readily visible in Figure 3.2 (c) and (d), which show the input image spectrum distribution among the three subbands. In Figure 3.2 (c) the output from the mid-frequency filter dominates the output from the high-frequency filter up to about 0.35π. They switch their dominances from 0.35π to π. This type of spectral relationship between the mid- and high-frequency subbands is undesirable because neighboring coefficients represent different spectral components of the input image. In Figure 3.2 (d) the outputs from the mid- and high-frequency subbands are convoluted up to around 0.6π. The resulting neighboring components of the combined subband are more homogeneous in the frequency space, and applying a uniform quantizer to the entire band results in lower distortion.

As was stated above, merging the mid- and high-frequency subbands using a 2-band PR filter is equivalent to applying a 3-channel PR bank with frequency weighted mid- and high-pass filters. The explicit operation of convolving the mid and high frequency subbands with 2-channel bank filters can be avoided. If we denote by T_3 the decomposition matrix of a 3-channel PR bank whose upper rows consist of the shifted low-pass filter, and by T_2 a matrix whose upper third rows have ones on the main diagonal, and the lower two-thirds rows are the reconstruction matrix of a 2-channel bank, then multiplying the image matrix by $T_3 T_2^t$ is equivalent to performing a 3-channel decomposition and merging the mid- and high-frequency subbands using the 2-channel bank. The rows of $T_3 T_2^t$ are now the new (shifted) 3-channel filters with weighted spectra (by the 2-channel bank).

The question may arise: why use spectral weighting to produce homogeneity in the combined band instead of designing the mid and high-pass filters with heavily overlapping (extremely aliased) spectra? The answer lies in the fact that filters in a PR bank "rely" on each other for aliasing cancellation. Thus, the same amount of quantization results in higher aliasing distortion when applying filters with heavily overlapping spectra.

4. RESULTS AND DISCUSSION

As was expected, the computation of NISUMP is a faster procedure compared to the computation of the classical dyadic wavelet transform: first, because an extra filtering operation is avoided at each level, secondly because the desired size of the LL band is achieved at a lower transform level. The decrease in the execution time, however, is greater than what one would expect by analyzing the decrease in the number of additions and multiplications needed. The extra gain in speed is due to the reduction in the data access time. Sequential elements in two-dimensional arrays (such as images) typically occupy sequential physical memory locations only in one dimension. In this dimension the average data element access time is small. In the second dimension sequential elements of an array are stored far apart in the physical memory. Accessing subsequent pixels in this orientation requires many clock cycles. By not having to access the data in the second dimension for two-thirds of the data set, and avoiding one extra second dimension processing for the higher level subbands, a further reduction in the execution time is achieved.

For the same reason, a reduction in the data access time is achieved for line vectors over block vectors: all L elements of a vector stored in adjacent physical memory locations. In the case of block vectors, each time after accessing $\sqrt{L}$ adjacent memory location, a different area of memory has to be accessed.

The final reduction in the execution time comes from the fact that by using our shift-compensating algorithm on line vectors, the same quality of reconstructed image can be achieved using fewer centroids. Figure 4.1 shows a typical x-ray image reconstructed from a quantized two-level NISUMP. The high frequency bands were quantized by a total of 32 vectors of length 9 using either regular block vectors or line vectors with the shift-compensating algorithm.

Figure 4.1
Original 512x512 8-bit X-ray image (a). Reconstructed image
from 32 block vectors representing the high-frequency bands of a
two level NISUMP (b). Reconstructed image from 32 line
vectors with shift-compensating algorithm representing the same
high-frequency bands of a two level NISUMP (c). Significant
blurring of edges is apparent in (b), while edge distortion in (c) is
barely noticeable.

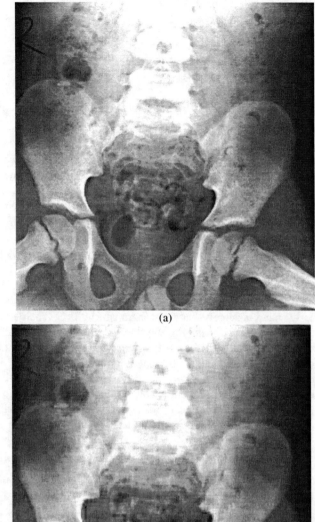

(a)

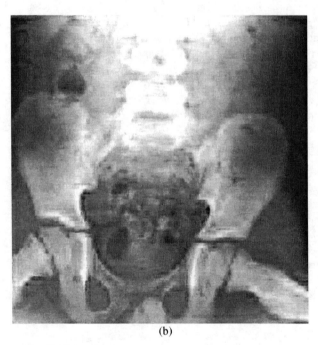

(b)

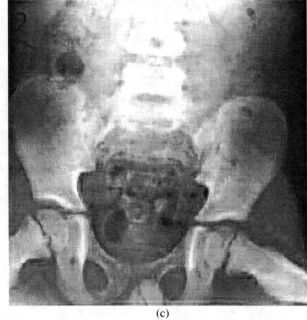

(c)

Figure 4.2 shows the reconstructed standard Barbara image. Identical quantization procedures to those used for the x-ray image were performed.

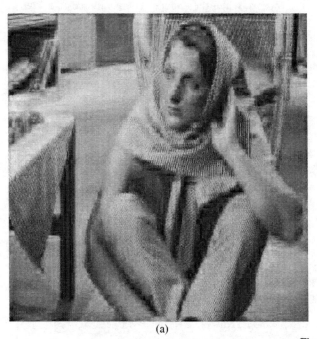
(a)
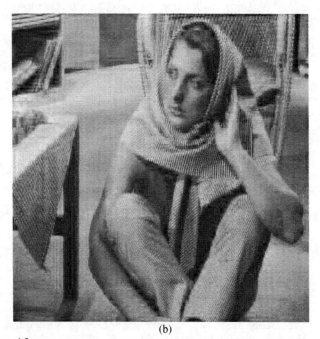
(b)

Figure 4.2
Standard 512x512 Barbara image reconstructed from a 2-level NISUMP using 32 block vectors (a),
and 32 line vectors with shift-compensating algorithm (b), to represent all the high-frequency bands.

The standard Barbara image contains a large number of edges. A significant improvement achieved for the Barbara image demonstrates a superior edge preserving capability of line vector quantization with the shift-compensating algorithm. Table 1 contains the mean squared error (MSE) and peak signal-to-noise ration (PSNR) figures for the reconstructed images of Figure 4.1 and 4.2.

Table 1. Reconstruction using 32 centroids: block vs. line vectors with shift compensating algorithm

	MSE		PSNR	
Image	Block	Line	Block	Line
Barbara	132.36	58.07	26.91	30.49
X-ray	72.99	43.87	29.50	31.71

Table 1 shows that greater than 2dB improvement was achieved for a typical x-ray image, and more than 3dB improvement obtained for the standard Barbara image, which contains a large number of edges. Table 2 contains MSE and PSNR values for the same images when the number of centroids was quadrupled for the block vector quantizer.

Table 2. Reconstruction using 128 centroids for block vectors only

Image	MSE	PSNR
Barbara	87.01	28.73
X-ray	49.96	31.14

As can be observed, the block vector quantizer even with a quadrupled number of centroids is still outperformed by the line vector quantizer using the shift-compensating algorithm. Increasing the number of centroids (as was necessary for the block VQ case), not only results in less compression for a given quality, but also in increased execution time.

5. CONCLUSION

We have demonstrated two novel approaches that can be used in image/video compression to decrease the coding/decoding time and/or improve the quality of the reconstructed images, when the encoder is constrained to a low bit budget. The processes employing these approaches do not require major modifications to existing VQ-based compression algorithms. Specifically, applied to a standard zerotree process, the basic algorithmic changes in replacing the classical dyadic pyramid with the non-integer subsampled wavelet pyramid include removing the diagonal branch of the zero-tree and redistributing the bit budget among the different levels of the transform. In this paper we have used 3- and 2-channel filter banks to construct a non-integer subsampled wavelet pyramid. The resulting pyramid is a close approximation to the multiresolution features found in the human visual system, which does not exhibit dyadic behavior. The extension of this technique to using other than 3- and 2-channel filter banks for various signal processing purposes is straightforward.

REFERENCES

1. Eliot L. Siegel, "The Changing Face of Clinical Practice: the Digital Revolution", *Keynote Address, Proceedings from 14th IEEE Symposium on Computer-Based Medical Systems*, published by the IEEE Computer Society, Bethesda MD., 2001.

2. B. Grinstad, H. Sari-Sarraf, S. Gleason, and S. Mitra "Content-Based Compression for Telecommunication and Archiving", *Proceedings from 13th IEEE Symposium on Computer-Based Medical Systems*, pp. 37-42, published by the IEEE Computer Society, Houston, TX., 2000.

3. S. Mitra, Shu-Yu Yang, and V. Kustov "Wavelet-Based Vector Quantization for High Fidelity Compression and Fast Transmission of Medical Images ", *Journal of Digital Imaging, Vol.11, No. 4*, pp. 24-30, 1998.

4. Allen Gersho and Robert M. Gray *"Vector Quantization and Signal Compression"*, Kluwer Academic Publishers, Norwell, Massachusetts, Third Printing, 1993.

5. H. Zhang, A. Nostratina, and R. Wells, Jr., "Image Denoising via Wavelet-Domain Spatially Adaptive FIR Wiener Filtering", *IEEE Proceedings from the International Conference on Acoustics, Speech and Signal Processing,* Istanbul, Turkey, 2000.

6. A. Zador and V. Kustov "New Low-Pass Spit Wavelet Pyramids and Their Application to Efficient Zero-Tree Coding of Medical Images ", *Proceedings from 14th IEEE Symposium on Computer-Based Medical Systems*, pp. 521-526, published by the IEEE Computer Society, Bethesda, MD., 2001.

A Scale-Based Method for Correcting Background Intensity Variation in Acquired Images

Ying Zhuge, Jayaram K. Udupa, Jiamin Liu, Punam K. Saha, Tad Iwanaga
Department of Radiology - MIPG
423 Guardian Drive – 4th Floor Blockley Hall
University of Pennsylvania, Philadelphia, PA 19104

ABSTRACT

An automatic, acquisition-protocol-independent, entirely image-based strategy for correcting background intensity variation in medical images has been developed. Local scale – a fundamental image property that is derivable entirely from the image and that does not require any prior knowledge about the imaging protocol or object material property distributions – is used to obtain a set of homogeneous regions, no matter what each region is, and to fit a 2nd degree polynomial to the intensity variation within them. This polynomial is used to correct the intensity variation. The above procedure is repeated for the corrected image until the size of segmented homogeneous regions does not change significantly from that in the previous iteration. Intensity scale standardization is effected to make sure that the corrected images are not biased by the fitting strategy. The method has been tested on 1000 3D mathematical phantoms, which include 5 levels each of blurring and noise and 4 types of background variation – additive and multiplicative Gaussian and ramp. It has also been tested on 10 clinical MRI data sets of the brain. These tests, and a comparison with the method of homomorphic filtering, indicate the effectiveness of the method.

Keywords: MRI, RF field, inhomogeneity, image segmentation, image intensity scale, scale

1. INTRODUCTION

Background image intensity variations caused by imperfections in imaging devices pose major challenges for further processing, segmentation, and analysis of acquired images. In magnetic resonance imaging (MRI), such effects originating from imperfections in the radio frequency (RF) field are well known[1]. These effects are also known to exist in other imaging modalities. In MRI, a variety of techniques have been developed over the past 15 years to address this problem[1-9]. While many of these methods have provided an effective solution in MRI, there is room for improvement in the sense of developing a general method that fulfills many or all of the following requirements: (R1) application independent; (R2) imaging protocol (e.g., pulse sequences in the case of MRI) independent; (R3) imaging device independent; (R4) no need for user help especially on a per-scene basis; (R5) no need for prior segmentation of objects in the scene; (R6) no need for prior knowledge of the image intensity distributions for object classes (i.e., tissue classes in medical imaging).

It is clear that some object information is vital in order to estimate (and, therefore, to correct) the background variation component of the intensities in the scene. This, however, we argue, need not come in the form of explicit object segmentation. To liberate a solution to inhomogeneity correction from the vagaries of scene segmentation will be a good idea since the latter itself is a difficult problem which has defied a solution fulfilling (R1) - R6) (or even a subset of them) up till now. The object information need not come even less explicitly in the form of prior knowledge of object intensity distributions that lead to rough object segmentations because such a strategy will also suffer from not being able to fulfill (R1 – R6). What is needed is sample (nor necessarily complete) object regions constituting the *same* object material (tissue in medical imaging). If such information can be obtained from any image automatically, we are through. Our initial quest to find a solution to this problem was less modest than what is implied by (R1) – (R6). In our on-going applications, we deal with 15 different MRI protocols (under two brands of MRI scanners) at present. We were seeking a method that would work on scenes acquired under all these protocols. We present a significant body of evidence in this paper that this is indeed feasible through the use of a local scene concept called "scale", introduced in[10]. After developing such a method and observing its behavior, we have realized its more general characteristics.

Scale[10] at any image element v in a given scene is a number that represents the radius of the largest ball centered at v within which the scene intensities are homogeneous under an appropriate homogeneity criterion. We have demonstrated that this simple concept is very useful in segmentation[10-12], filtering[13], and registration[14] of scenes. Our method, described in Section 2, consists of first identifying regions (balls) corresponding to the largest scale values in the foreground of the scene, then thresholding the scene by using intensity intervals estimated from these regions, and then estimating and correcting for intensity variations by using the segmented region (which constitutes the sample regions mentioned earlier). The process is iteratively repeated on the resulting scenes. We demonstrate in Section 3 both qualitatively (on a variety of scenes) and quantitatively (by utilizing mathematical phantoms and clinically acquires scenes) the effectiveness of the method in correcting even severe inhomogeneities coming from surface coils. Although we cannot objectively claim that this method fulfills all of (R1) - (R6) (which requires a daunting evaluative process), we give ample evidences to indicate that this method goes in that direction. Our concluding remarks are stated in Section 4.

2. THE SCALE-BASED METHOD

2.1 Preamble

We refer to a volume image as a *scene* and represent it by a pair $\mathcal{C} = (C, f)$, where C, called the *scene domain*, is a rectangular array of cuboidal volume elements, usually referred to as *voxels*, and f is the scene *intensity function* which assigns to every voxel $v \in C$ an integer called the *intensity* of v in $\mathcal{C}$ in a range $[L, H]$. We will use the following notation throughout.

$\mathcal{C}$: a given scene corrupted by background variation (such as the one produced by an imaging device)

$\mathcal{C}_{bt} = (C, f_{bt})$: the true background variation component in $\mathcal{C}$.

$\mathcal{C}_u = (C, f_u)$: $\mathcal{C}$ without the background variation component $\mathcal{C}_{bt}$.

$\mathcal{C}_c = (C, f_c)$: the scene resulting from applying a correction algorithm α to $\mathcal{C}$ to suppress background variation in $\mathcal{C}$.

$\mathcal{C}_{be} = (C, f_{be})$: the background variation component in $\mathcal{C}$ estimated by the correction algorithm α.

$|C|$: the number of voxels in C.

We make the following assumptions in designing our method.

(A1) : f_{bt} is sufficiently slow varying such that there exist homogeneous regions in the foreground of $\mathcal{C}$ that represent the same object material.

(A2) : $\mathcal{C}$ with its background variation results from a known *invertible* operation between $\mathcal{C}_u$ and $\mathcal{C}_{bt}$.

(A1) reflects the core spirit of our approach. It says that, even in the presence of background inhomogeneity, if homogeneous regions can be found in the foreground, then they must represent regions containing the same object material. Such sample homogeneous regions are enough for our method to estimate and correct for the background variation component. The background variation introduced by MRI scanners is generally considered to be a multiplicative phenomenon. Along with the background variation, any acquired scene $\mathcal{C}$ embodies several other artifacts including blurring, and statistical noise, and often (as in MRI) acquisition-to-acquisition image intensity gray scale variation [15]. The exact nature of these component artifacts and how they interact among themselves and with $\mathcal{C}_{bt}$ are not known, and there do not seem to have been any attempts to study these interactions. (A2) reflects the fact that, in the absence of such knowledge, we rely on $\mathcal{C}_{be}$ to correct for background variation, but in the process, not to significantly amplify the effects due to other artifacts. The influence of the effect of the validity/violation of (A2) on the output of a correction algorithm α cannot be ascertained theoretically at the present state of knowledge, but can be assessed through properly designed evaluation strategies. If α can achieve better homogeneity of scene intensity within the same object region without amplifying other artifacts, that is what matters.

2.2 Outline of the Method

The procedure for correcting background variation, which we name SBC (for Scale-Based Correction), consists of the following steps. The method has no parameters to be specified by the user. It is an iterative procedure, which proceeds until the changes found in two successive iterations is sufficiently small.

Procedure *SBC*

Input : A scene $\mathcal{C}$.

Output : Corrected scene $\mathcal{C}_c$.

begin

    *S*0. set $\mathcal{C}_c = \mathcal{C}$;

    *S*1. determine the scene $\mathcal{C}_F = (C, f_F)$ corresponding to the foreground of $\mathcal{C}_c$;

    *S*2. compute scale scene $\mathcal{C}_S = (C, f_S)$ for $\mathcal{C}_F$;

    *S*3. determine a binary scene $\mathcal{C}_B = (C, f_B)$ that constitutes regions of the same object material type in $\mathcal{C}_c$ by utilizing $\mathcal{C}_S$;

    *S*4. if $\mathcal{C}_B$ determined in the previous iteration is insignificantly ($< 5\%$) different from the current $\mathcal{C}_B$, stop;

    *S*5. else, estimate background variation in $\mathcal{C}_F$ as a scene $\mathcal{C}_{be}$, correct $\mathcal{C}_c$, replace $\mathcal{C}_c$ by the corrected scene, and go to *S*1;

    end

2.3 Description of Procedure *SBC*

Step S1. Foreground separation

This step has two purposes – to speed up *SBC* and to make it more effective and fail-safe. If *S*2 and *S*5 (especially *S*2) are carried out on the entire scene domain C of $\mathcal{C}_c$, the computation time increases considerably. The scene $\mathcal{C}_F$ corresponding to the foreground is obtained by the following simple criterion: for each $v \in C$,

$$f_F(v) = \begin{cases} f(v), & \text{if } \quad f(v) \geq \theta_m \\ \\ 0 \quad , & \text{otherwise,} \end{cases} \tag{1}$$

where

$$\theta_m = \frac{\sum\limits_{v \in C} f(v)}{|C|}.$$

(2)

Our aim here is a rough segmentation of the foreground. This simple scheme works remarkably well as determined by the separation of foreground in 100s of scenes in this and other applications[15]. Figure 1(a) shows a slice of a given scene $\mathcal{C}$, which is a proton density-weighted MR scene of the head of a human subject, and Figure 1(b) shows the corresponding slice of $\mathcal{C}_F$.

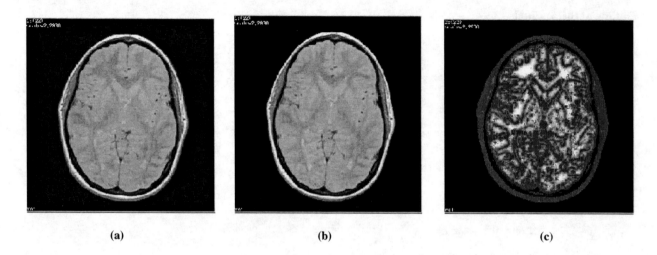

(a)   (b)   (c)

Figure 1: (a) A slice of a PD MR scene of a subject's head. The corresponding slices of the foreground scene (b) and the scale scene (c).

Step S2: Computation of scale

The *scale* at any voxel v in any scene $\mathcal{C}$ is the radius of the largest ball in $\mathcal{C}$ centered at v, which is such that the scene intensity within the ball is homogeneous under a certain definition of homogeneity. The scale value at v represents roughly the size of the structure containing v at v. An algorithm is presented in Ref[10] for computing the scale values of any given scene as another scene. "Homogeneity" is specified by one parameter, and Ref[10] describes how this parameter can be estimated automatically for any given scene. Since the computation of the scale scene is expensive and homogeneous regions in the background of a given scene are not useful for (and actually mislead) inhomogeneity estimation, we compute scale only for the foreground. The resulting scene is $\mathcal{C}_S = (C, f_S)$, where for any $v \in C$, $f_S(v) = 0$ if $f_F(v) = 0$, and $f_S(v) =$ the scale value at v if $f_F(v) > 0$. Figure 1(c) shows one slice of $\mathcal{C}_S$ corresponding to the slice of $\mathcal{C}_F$ displayed in Figure 1(b).

Step S3. Determining an object region

In this step, the largest scale value in $\mathcal{C}_S$ is determined and the union R_S of the balls centered at all voxels having this largest value is computed. The result for the scene $\mathcal{C}_S$ depicted in Figure 1(c) is sown in Figure 2(a). The mean μ_O and the standard deviation σ_O of the scene intensities $f_F(v)$ of all voxels v in R_S is then estimated, $\mathcal{C}$ is thresholded by using the interval $[\mu_o - \sigma_o, \mu_o + \sigma_o]$, and small connected components ($< 5\%$ of $|C|$) are discarded and the result is output as a binary scene $\mathcal{C}_B$. This output gives us sample object regions (although not with a perfect segmentation by any means) containing roughly the same object material. Figure 2(b) shows the corresponding slice of $\mathcal{C}_B$ for our running example.

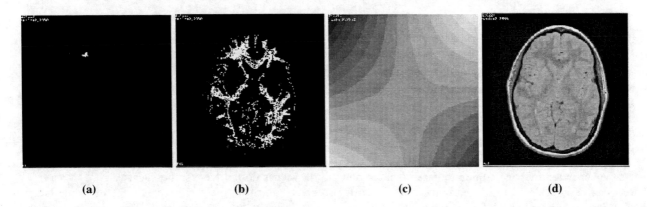

(a) **(b)** **(c)** **(d)**

Figure 2: The slice corresponding to that shown in Figure 1 for $\mathcal{C}_B$ (b), and $\mathcal{C}_{be}$ (c), and $\mathcal{C}_c$ (d). The region R_S corresponding to the largest scale value in $\mathcal{C}_S$ is depicted in (a).

Step S4. Stopping criterion

The basic premise of this method is that, as correction is effected, the largest scale region R_S, and therefore, subsequently, the object region represented in $\mathcal{C}_B$, will increase gradually. When this increase is insignificant, the iterative procedure stops.

Step S5. Correction

In this step, the background variation is estimated first and then corrected. Let O_S be the set of all 1-valued voxels in $\mathcal{C}_B$. The mean μ_{O_S} of scene intensities within O_S is determined by

$$\mu_{O_S} = \frac{\sum_{v \in O_S} f(v)}{|O_S|}. \tag{3}$$

The background variation is then estimated as a function $\beta_d(v)$ whose domain is O_S and whose functional values are defined by, for all $v \in O_S$,

$$\beta_d(v) = f(v) \; \tau^{-1} \; \mu_{O_S}, \tag{4}$$

where τ is the operation (mentioned in assumption (A2)) between $\mathcal{C}_u$ and $\mathcal{C}_{bt}$ that yields $\mathcal{C}$. We denote this by $\mathcal{C} = \mathcal{C}_u \; \tau \; \mathcal{C}_{bt}$. To the discrete function $\beta_d(v)$, a 2nd order polynomial $\beta(x)$ is fitted by minimizing $\sum_{v \in O_S} \left[\beta(v) - \beta_d(v) \right]^2$.

The estimated background variation scene $\mathcal{C}_{be}$ is then computed by, for all $v \in C$, $f_{be}(v) = \beta(v)$.

Since τ is invertible, $\mathcal{C}_u = \mathcal{C} \ \tau^{-1} \ \mathcal{C}_{bt}$, and therefore, by (A2),

$$\mathcal{C}_u \approx \mathcal{C}_c = \mathcal{C} \ \tau^{-1} \ \mathcal{C}_{be} . \tag{5}$$

In MRI, τ is generally considered to be a multiplication operation, and therefore, τ^{-1} becomes division. In general if τ is known and invertible, (i.e., τ^{-1} is known), then from Equation (5), we can determine $\mathcal{C}_c$. Note that, in procedure *SBC*, there is no assumption about its applicability to the characteristics of a particular imaging modality, or to a particular operation τ, or to any prior knowledge about object material intensity distribution. In Figures 2(c) and (d), we display $\mathcal{C}_{be}$ and $\mathcal{C}_c$ for the running example.

2.4 Standardization

As demonstrated in[15], in addition to background variation, MR scenes do not have scene intensity gray scales ([*L*, *H*]) that can be considered to be nearly the same, even for scenes obtained on the same scanner, for the same body region, using the same protocol, for the same subject. A method was proposed in[15] to overcome this problem. In consists of a one-time training phase, which, from a set of scenes (for the same body region and protocol) provided as input, estimates a set of parameters of a standardizing transformation. In the second (actual transformation) phase, each given scene is transformed so that the transformed scene intensities are on a standard gray scale. The process of background variation correction via *SBC* does not overcome the above non-standardness issue. Further, the process of estimating function $\beta(\mathrm{x})$ in Step S5 of *SBC* may introduce a further non-standardness. In order to overcome these effects, we apply the standardization procedure to all corrected scenes $\mathcal{C}_c$ output by *SBC* before they are utilized in any application.

3. RESULTS AND EVALUATION

In this section, to understand how effective *SBC* is in correcting background variation, we present a set of examples showing scenes before and after applying the correction procedure. We also present a quantitative evaluation based on mathematical phantoms with different types of background variations applied by using different operators τ, and based on clinical images.

3.1 Qualitative

In Figure 3, we present several examples involving different MRI protocols and scenes from different body regions. One slice from the original scene, and the same slice of the corrected scene are shown for each data set. Figure 4 demonstrates how *SBC* improves the correction effect gradually from iteration to iteration. These figures give a qualitative indication of the effectiveness of *SBC* in suppressing background variation. Note how even severe background variations are significantly overcome (Figures 3(e), (f) and 4).

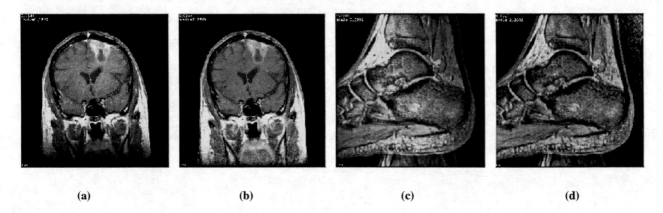

(a)	(b)	(c)	(d)

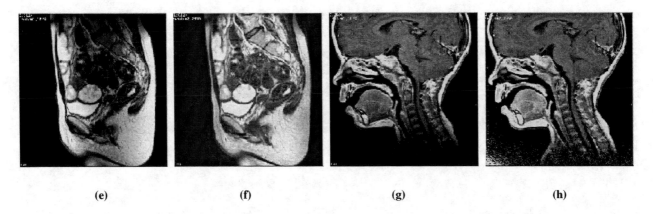

(e)   (f)   (g)   (h)

Figure 3: (a), (c), (e), (g). A slice of the MR scenes of different body regions acquired by using different MRI protocols. (b), (d), (f), (h). The corresponding slices of the scenes after correction.

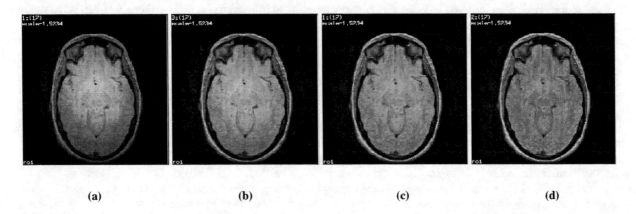

(a)   (b)   (c)   (d)

Figure 4: Illustration of how the iterative process of *SBC* improves correction. (a) Original scene, after two (b), four (c) and nine (d) iterations.

3.2 Quantitative

We created a set of 10 binary scenes by segmenting the white matter regions in 10 MR PD scenes of normal subjects by using a fuzzy connectedness algorithm and subsequently by making any necessary corrections to this segmentation. From these binary scenes, 10 gray-level scenes were created by assigning a constant value, equal to the mean white matter intensity in each original scene, to the white matter region in the corresponding segmented scene. Similarly, a constant gray matter background was given by using the mean intensity of the gray matter region. To each of these 10 scenes, 5 different levels each of blurring and noise was added, resulting in a set A of 250 scenes. To each scene in A, four types of background variation were applied: multiplicative and additive (τ) ramp and Gaussian functions. This yielded a total of 1000 scenes.

We also implemented a version of the homomorphic filtering (*HF*) method for comparison. Figure 5 shows one slice of one of these 1000 scenes and its corrected versions created by using *SBC* and by using homomorphic filtering. The root mean squared (*RMS*) value, over the 10 scenes for each level of blurring and noise, of the difference in scene intensities between a scene $\mathcal{C} \in A$ and its corrected scene $\mathcal{C}_c$ was computed for all types of background variations and for both methods *SBC* and *HF*. In all 100 cases (5 levels of blurring × 5 levels of noise × 4 types of background variation) the *RMS* value for the *SBC* method was 10-20 times smaller than for the *HF* method. We also observed that the improvement obtained for the multiplicative type of variation was better than for the additive type. Similarly, the correction obtained for the ramp variation was better than for the Gaussian variation.

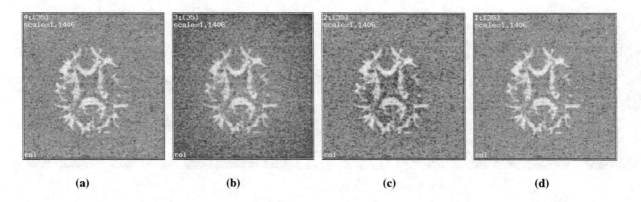

| (a) | (b) | (c) | (d) |

Figure 5: (a) A slice of the phantom scene corresponding to a medium level of blurring and noise. The corresponding slice of the corrected scene output by the *HF* (b) and *SBC* (c) methods.

Another comparison was made by examining the normalized standard deviation *NSD* of scene intensities (standard deviation/intensity range) in segmented white matter, gray matter, and *CSF* regions for 10 MR PD scenes of 10 normal subjects. Lower *NSD* values were obtained for all scenes and for all tissue regions after applying *SBC* than before applying any method and after applying the *HF* method.

4. CONCLUDING REMARKS

Background variation in scenes due to imperfections in imaging devices is a problem commonly encountered in image analysis in many areas, particularly in medical MR imaging. Although many solutions have been proposed in the past, they all had varying degrees of dependency on the particular protocol, body region, application domain, and the type of variation. In an attempt to liberate this dependency, we have devised a method that depends entirely on the information available in the given scene. It uses a local concept defined on scenes called scale for the correction process. The largest scale regions in the foreground of the scene give us information about object regions containing the same object material, which is utilized for estimating and correcting background variation. The method has no parameters whose values are to be determined or to be provided by the user or that need adjustment from one imaging device/protocol to another. Our qualitative and quantitative evaluation experiments indicate that its performance is effective. Its performance seems to be better on multiplicative than additive variations and on a ramp than on a Gaussian variation. The latter may be due to the fact that we use a 2nd degree polynomial to fit the variations.

As related to (A2), some comments are in order. There are basically the following three types of operations commonly done on MR images before further carrying out other image processing and analysis operations on them: correction of background variation, filtering to suppress noise, and intensity scale standardization. There is perhaps some interaction among the effects of these operations, which, to our knowledge, has not been studied. To what extent the order in which these operations are carried out influences the results is also unknown. Given the importance of these operations, obviously it is worthwhile to study the above issues carefully.

ACKNOWLEDGMENTS

The research reported here is supported by DHHS Grants AR 46902 and NS 37172. The authors are grateful to Mary A. Blue for typing the manuscript.

REFERENCES

[1]   L. Axel, J. Costantini and J. Listerud: "Intensity Corrections in Surface-Coil MR Imaging," *American Journal of Roentgenology*, 148:418-420, 1987.

[2]   M.W. Vannier, C.M. Speidel and D.L. Rickman: "Magnetic Resonance Imaging Multispectral tissue Classification," *News in Physiological Sciences*, 3:148-154, 1988.

[3]   J. Haselgrove and M. Prammer: "An Algorithm for compensation of Surface-Coil Images for Sensitivity of the Surface Coil," *Magnetic Resonance Imaging*, 4:469-472, 1986.

[4]   B.M. Dawant, A.P. Zjidenbos and R.A. Margolin, "Correction of Intensity Variations in MR Images for Computer-Aided Tissue Classification," *IEEE Transactions on Medical Imaging*, 12:770-781, 1993.

[5]   C.R. Meyer, P.H. Bland and J. Pipe: "Retrospective Correction of Intensity Inhomogeneities in MRI," *IEEE Transactions on Medical Imaging*, 14(1):36-41, 1995.

[6]   W.M. Wells, W.E.L. Grimson, R. Kikinis and F.A. Jolesz; "Adaptive Segmentation of MRI Data," *IEEE Transactions on Medical Imaging*, 15:429-443, 1996.

[7]   R. Guillemaud and M. Brady: "Estimating the Bias Field of MR Images," *IEEE Transaction on Medical Imaging*, 16:238-251, 1997.

[8]   J.G. Sled, A.P. Zijdenbos and A.C. Evans: "A Nonparametric Method for Automatic Correction of Intensity Nonuniformity in MRI Data," *IEEE Transactions on Medical Imaging*, 17:87-97, 1998.

[9]   M. Styner, C. Brechbühler, G. Székely and G. Gerig: "Parametric Estimate of Intensity Inhomogeneities Applied to MRI," *IEEE Transactions on Medical Imaging*, 19(3):153-165, 2000.

[10]   P.K. Saha and J.K. Udupa: "Scale-Based Fuzzy Connected Image Segmentation: Theory, Algorithms and Validation," *Computer Vision and Image Understanding*, 77(2):145-174, 2000.

[11]   T. Lei, J.K. Udupa, P.K. Saha and D. Odhner: "Artery-Vein Separation via MRA - An Image Processing Approach," *IEEE Transactions on Medical Imaging*, 20(8):689-703, 2001.

[12]   P.K. Saha and J.K. Udupa: "Optimum Image Thresholding via Class Uncertainty and Region Homogeneity," *IEEE Transactions on Pattern Analysis and Machine Intelligence*, 23(7):689-706, 2001.

[13]   P.K. Saha and J.K. Udupa: "Scale-Based Image Filtering Preserving Boundary Sharpness and Fine Structure" *IEEE Transactions on Medical Imaging*, 20(11):1140-1155, 2001.

[14]   L.G. Nyul, J.K. Udupa and P.K. Saha: "Task-Specific Comparison of 3D Image Registration Methods," *SPIE Proceedings*, 4322:1588-1598, 2001.

[15]   L.G. Nyul and J.K. Udupa: "On Standardizing the MR Image Intensity Scale," *Magnetic Resonance in Medicine*, 42:1072-1081, 1999.

Inter-Slice Interpolation of Anisotropic 3-D Images Using Multi-Resolution Contour Correlation

Jiann-Der Lee, Shu-Yen Wan*, and Cherng-Min Ma

Graduate Institute of Computer Science and Information Engineering

Department of Information Management, Chang Gung University, Taiwan, R.O.C.

*E-mail: sywan@mail.cgu.edu.tw

ABSTRACT

To visualize, manipulate and analyze the geometrical structure of anatomical changes, it is often required to perform three-dimensional (3-D) interpolation of the interested organ shape from a series of cross-sectional images obtained from various imaging modalities, such as ultrasound, computed tomography (CT), magnetic resonance imaging (MRI), etc. In this paper, a novel wavelet-based interpolation scheme, which consists of four algorithms are proposed to 3-D image reconstruction. The multi-resolution characteristics of wavelet transform (WT) is completely used in this approach, which consists of two stages, boundary extraction and contour interpolation. More specifically, a wavelet-based radial search method is first designed to extract the boundary of the target object. Next, the global information of the extracted boundary is analyzed for interpolation using WT with various bases and scales. By using six performance measures to evaluate the effectiveness of the proposed scheme, experimental results show that the performance of all proposed algorithms is superior to traditional contour-based methods, linear interpolation and B-spline interpolation. The satisfactory outcome of the proposed scheme provides its capability for serving as an essential part of image processing system developed for medical applications.

Keywords: Image reconstruction, Wavelet transform, Medical image processing

I. INTRODUCTION

3-D reconstruction from a series of cross-sectional images is becoming increasingly important in a variety of fields such as computer vision, medical imaging and image generation. The method aids in the comprehension of object's structure, and facilitates its automatic manipulation and analysis. A 3-D visualization of objects generally requires three steps in a computer-aided reconstruction process. First, the regions (or the contours) of interest in all the cross-sectional images are extracted to obtain lower-resolution data in the z direction. Second, the missing slice data are interpolated by the contours of successive slices. Finally, surfaces are formed by using shading techniques to visualize the interpolated object. There are no standard approaches for these three steps. In other words, researchers usually look for an algorithm that offers better results and lower computational cost. Therefore, to obtain the shapes of the desired region, or to interpolate the lost data between successive known slice data, an efficient and precise algorithm is needed. All of these tasks are to look for the maximum similarity between the 3-D reconstruction and the real object. If the object is not extracted or interpolated properly, discontinuity will exist when displaying the entire object. Ideally, 3-D image is formed by directly stacking a contiguous series of 2-D digital medical images. Unfortunately, common medical imaging modalities tend to have a gap between adjacent slices. Medical image like CT/MRI have lower resolution in the z direction than those in the x and y directions. Therefore, in the application of 3-D reconstruction, how to interpolate the missing slice to improve the resolution in z direction becomes an important issue.

In the past, many interpolation approaches based on various ideas[1-11] have been proposed to solve the 3-D reconstruction problem. These interpolation methods can be divided into two categories: scene based and object based. In scene–based approaches[1-3], the intensity value of interpolated image are derived from the intensity value of the source scene. On the other hand, for the object-based methods[4-7], interpolation is performed by directly using the object information obtained from the scene. According to the previous papers[6-9], the performances of the object-based methods are superior to the scene-based ones. Shape-based interpolation is one of the object-based methods. Since this method interpolates the binary image after segmentation, the calculating time is less than the previous methods, which use direct gray data. In addition, it is shown that the shape-based method gives more accurate results than the conventionally used linear gray-level interpolation after segmentation. The interpolation strategy of these mentioned methods belongs to the region-based methods, which interpolate the complete object in the scene. Generally, this kind of approach is time-consuming.

In some application, the task for image visualization is to reconstruct the surface data of the object from a series of slice images. In this case, it can significantly reduce the time for interpolation if only the contours of the object

Medical Imaging 2002: Image Processing, Milan Sonka, J. Michael Fitzpatrick, Editors, Proceedings of SPIE Vol. 4684 (2002) © 2002 SPIE · 1605-7422/02/$15.00

between the adjacent slice images are used. The typical example of this contour-based approach is the dynamic elastic interpolation, proposed by Lin et al.[10-11], which utilizes the "force field" on a contour to try to distort it toward another contour. The "force field" is determined by the displacement between a vertex and its nearest line segment in another contour. An iterative process is formulated to generate the intermediate contours from the initial contour to the goal contour. Ideally, the contour-based method can achieve satisfactory result. However, there exists one common shortcoming, the need of feature matching, for these methods in practical application. Feature matching is a time consuming process, especially for complex images. In addition, false feature matching will result in bad or even unacceptable reconstruction result. These shortcomings can be avoided if we perform the interpolation by using the whole contour instead of the feature points. For all interpolation schemes mentioned above, the local information of the contour is not carefully treated in both theoretical and practical, except for kriging interpolation. Therefore, in this paper, a wavelet-based scheme for three-dimensional object reconstruction from a series of cross-sectional images is proposed.

Since 1980's, wavelet analysis[12-20] has provided another choice for analyzing a one-dimensional or two-dimensional signal. Cohan and Kovacevic[15] introduced the main advantage of the wavelet decomposition process, and derived its multi-resolution property in the spatial-frequency domain from its mathematical background. Wavelet transform (WT) also provides fast computation scheme during decomposition and reconstruction process. Olivo[16] used WT to develop an automatic threshold selection scheme for image segmentation and then extract the desired object. Others developed features extraction algorithms with WT to carry out pattern recognition and data interpolation[17-19], and to compress the images during transmission[20].

In this paper, we first use WT to detect the edge of an object via radial search on its grayscale profile. Next, WT is employed to extract the features of 2-D planar curves[21-31], and to interpolate a series of boundary curves from the same organs. Although previous interpolation techniques, like B-Spline nonlinear interpolation or distance transform based interpolation, are widely used for image interpolation, the performance can be improved by using WT to reduce the computational cost. While it is important to compare the performance of interpolation schemes with the final visualization result, the objective comparison of interpolation is easily achieved by using the interpolated results. More specifically, the slice with the maximum difference between its adjacent slices is estimated by each interpolation method and compared to the original slice at the same location using various measures based on *area*, *curve length*, and *curve shift*.

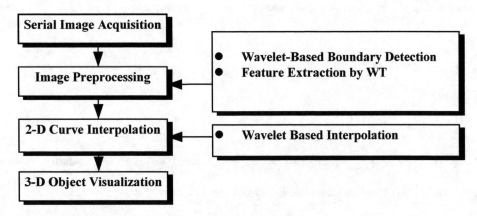

Fig. 1 The flowchart of the proposed approach.

The flowchart of the proposed algorithm is illustrated in Fig. 1. Three image sets are randomly selected from our medical image database. These image sets consist of CT chest images, CT head images, and MR head images. For example, in the set of CT chest images, the thickness of each slice and the inter-distance between adjacent slices are 1 mm and 5 mm, respectively. The regions of interest are the bronchi with branch structure on each CT chest image. WT is used to achieve boundary detection and feature extraction in the step of image pre-processing. Following, WT is utilized to 2-D curve interpolation and then achieve 3-D object reconstruction. At the end, shading techniques are used to visualize the reconstructed 3-D objects.

The paper is organized as follows. Section II gives a brief review of the WT. The concepts and property of WT are introduced. Section III presents the strategy for edge detection of a 2-D medical image and the algorithm for feature extraction of a planar curve. Section IV illustrates the detailed procedure of the proposed interpolation scheme with different attempts. The method to solve single tube and branch problem in a real medical image is also discussed in this section. The experimental results and visualization operation by using synthetic and medical images, and the performance comparison of various interpolation methods are illustrated in Section V. At last, conclusions and suggestions are included.

II. BRIEF REVIEW OF WAVELET TRANSFORM

In recent years, the wavelet transform became an active area of research for multi-resolution signal and image analysis. The detailed knowledge of the wavelet theory can be found in[14-20]. Here, the brief review of wavelet transform is summarized as below.

Let $(V_m)_{m \in Z}$ be a multi-resolution approximation of $L^2 (R)$, then there exists an unique function $\phi(t) \in L^2 (R)$, called a scaling function, such that its dilations and translations

$$\phi_n^m (t) = \frac{1}{\sqrt{2^m}} \phi(\frac{t}{\sqrt{2^m}} - n), \, m, n \in Z \tag{1}$$

constitute an orthonormal basis of V_m. Filter H with impulse response $h[n] = < \phi^{m-1}(k), \phi^m(k-n) >$ is the corresponding conjugate filter and $h[n]$ is a low-pass filter. A function $\psi (t)$, called mother wavelet function, can be determined such that its dilations and translations

$$\psi_n^m (t) = \frac{1}{\sqrt{2^m}} \psi(\frac{t}{\sqrt{2^m}} - n), \, m, n \in Z \tag{2}$$

also constitute an orthonormal basis of $L^2 (R)$. Similarly, a discrete filter G with impulse response $g[n] = < \psi^{m-1}(k), \psi^m(k-n) >$ is obtained and $g[n]$ is called mirror highpass filter for $h[n]$. Besides, there exists a dual function $\widetilde{\psi}(t)$ such that $\widetilde{\psi}_n^m (t)$, $m, n \in Z$, satisfies $<\psi_n^m, \widetilde{\psi}_{n'}^{m'}> = \delta_{m,m'}, \delta_{n,n'}$ and $\{\psi_n^m, \widetilde{\psi}_n^m\}_{m,n \in Z}$ is called a pair of biorthogonal Riesz bases. If $f(t) \in L^2 (R)$, then the wavelet coefficients q_n^m of $f(t)$ can be computed via

$$q_n^m = \int_{-\infty}^{\infty} f(t)\psi_n^m(t)dt \equiv \left\langle f, \psi_n^m \right\rangle \tag{3}$$

thus, we have

$$f(t) = \sum_{m,n=-\infty}^{\infty} q_n^m \widetilde{\psi}_n^m (t), \tag{4}$$

The bases $\{\psi_n^m (t)\}_{m,n}$ and $\{\widetilde{\psi}_n^m (t)\}_{m,n}$ are known as the biorthogonal wavelets. Particularly, if the mother wavelet $\psi(t)$ is equal to its dual $\widetilde{\psi}(t)$, they become the orthogonal wavelet. For $f(t) \in V_0$, we have

$$f(t) = \sum_{n=-\infty}^{\infty} p_n^0 \widetilde{\phi}_n^0 (t)$$

$$= \sum_{n=-\infty}^{\infty} p_n^M \widetilde{\phi}(t)_n^M + \sum_{m=1}^{M} \sum_{n=-\infty}^{\infty} q_n^m \widetilde{\psi}_n^m (t), \tag{5}$$

which is known as the finite scale biorthogonal wavelet expansion. More specifically, The successive (coarser) approximations of $f(t)$ are given by the projections $S_j f$ onto the subspaces V_j, $j \geq 1$, of $L^2 (R)$. The difference in information between two successive coarser approximations is given by the projections $U_j f$ onto the subspaces W_j, $j \geq 1$, of $L^2 (R)$. Since $V_j = V_{j+1} \oplus W_{j+1}$, where $\oplus$ is the direct sum, Eq. (5) can be rewritten as

$$f(t) = S_0 f(t) = S_{-j} f(t) + \sum_{k=-j}^{-1} U_k f(t) \tag{6}$$

Hence, the coefficients q_n^m and p_n^M can be computed from the coefficients p_n^0 by the following recursive formulas

$$p_n^{m+1} = \sum_u h_{u-2n} p_u^m$$

$$q_n^{m+1} = \sum_u g_{u-2n} p_u^m \; , m=0,1,\ldots,M\text{-}1 \tag{7}$$

On the other hand, one can obtain the coefficients q_n^m and p_n^M via the synthesis formulas

$$p_n^{m-1} = \sum_u (\tilde{h}_{n-2u} p_u^m + \tilde{g}_{n-2u} q_u^m) \; , m=\text{M,M-1},\ldots,2,1 \tag{8}$$

where $g_n = (-1)^{n+1} \tilde{h}_{-n+1}$, $\tilde{g}_n = (-1)^{n+1} h_{-n+1}$ and the filters h_n, $\tilde{h}_n$, g_n and $\tilde{g}_n$ are called the biorthogonal filter bank. In the orthogonal filter bank, we choose $h_n = \tilde{h}_n$, $g_n = \tilde{g}_n$ and $g_n = (-1)^{n+1} h_{-n+1}$. Eqs. (7) and (8) are called the forward and inverse wavelet transforms, respectively. These decomposition and reconstruction algorithms used in this approach are illustrated in the block diagram shown in Fig. 2. In this figure, (a) shows the decomposition block diagram (i.e., decomposition of a discrete approximation p_n^m into an approximation at a coarser resolution p_n^{m+1} and the signal detail q_n^{m+1}). Fig. 2(b) shows the reconstruction block diagram (i.e., reconstruction of a discrete approximation p_n^m from an approximation at a coarser resolution p_n^{m+1} and the detail q_n^{m+1}).

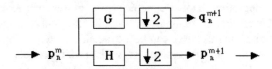

(a) Decomposition block diagram

(b) Reconstruction block diagram

Fig. 2. Decomposition and reconstruction block diagram.

III. BOUNDARY EXTRACTION USING RADIAL SEARCH WITH WAVELET ANALYSIS

Since a contour representation of objects can be useful for understanding of 2D and 3D images, boundary extraction becomes an essential step for further medical image analysis and pattern recognition. In particular, the accuracy of boundary extraction is a key factor to the performance of 3-D reconstruction from a series of cross-sectional images. In our case, it is essential to extract the contour of bronchus from a chest CT image before performing 3-D interpolation.

Usually, in order to detect the boundary of an object from a gray-level image, the previous approaches can be classified into three categories[21-24]. The first approach is to select a threshold manually[21] for the desired object, then proceed with morphology operation, and at last boundary tracing is performed. The second approach is to use the 'Deformable Model', which is more accurate because it derives the contour by energy minimum strategy based on optimization procedure. The third approach is to determine the maximum gradient[22-24] of the gray-level profile. These three approaches have some shortages. The first approach is inconvenient because the precise threshold is not easy to find. The second approach may result in undesired edges without a good initial contour. The third one will find an erroneous contour only if the local maximum gradient of the curve without its global property is considered.

In this approach, we adopt the 2nd derivative of Gaussian function as the basis function of the WT, and the locations of zero-crossings can then represent the violent variation of the original signal. In our case, the signal is a grayscale profile obtained from radial search. Because the locating ability is decreased at lower resolution, we have to perform the position adjustment from low-resolution scale to high-resolution scale. For the consideration of automatic boundary detection, we pre-select a decomposition level M. Usually, 8~10 levels is enough. Then, by using WT, we calculate the numbers of zero-crossings at each level m. Let m be ranged from 1 to M. The numbers of zero-crossing will be decreased as m increases. This is because the entire profile will be smoother as scale increases (i.e., resolution decreases). If the number of zero-crossing keeps unchanged for 3 scales successive, the process stops and we assume that it stops at level k. We call the process "*Forward computation*". Next, let m be ranged from the stopped level k to level 2 (because level 1 is very sensitive to slightly variation and noise, it is omitted here) with 1 level decreasing, and map the position of these zero-crossings to the ones in previous level with minimum position drift until level 2 is reached. We call this "*Backward mapping*". The boundary point occurs at the location with minimum drifting of each level. After using radial search for each scan line, the boundary of the object is obtained via connecting these detected boundary points with B-Spline function. The difference between our method and the traditional methods mentioned above is that our approach is more robust and accurate because multi-resolution profile analysis is fully used. More important, the range of scale is determined automatically without manual selection. This characteristic is necessary in practical application such as pattern recognition. However, this costs more computation time on the 'Forward computation' and 'Backward mapping' procedure. Once obtaining the boundary curve of the desired object in terms of Cartesian coordinates (x, y), the feature points on this curve can be extracted for later use in 3-D interpolation.

Here, features are the points, which are the positions of violate variation occurrence on the curve[25-31]. To extract the features of the boundary curve, we use the tangent angle $\theta(l)$ along the contour for curve representation, where l is the serial position of the total curve length L. In other words, this 1-D signal $\theta(l)$ derived from a test signal is expressed as

$$\theta(l) = \tan^{-1}(\frac{\Delta y}{\Delta x}) \tag{9}$$

Because the boundary points are discrete pixels in the image, the change of tangent direction may produce infinity. Thus, if we select a wider support to calculate the tangent angle, the influence caused by the discrete quantization error will be reduced. In Eq. (10), Δx and Δy are redefined as

$$\Delta x = (x_{l+i} - x_{l-i}) \tag{10}$$
$$\Delta y = (y_{l+i} - y_{l-i})$$

Substitute Eq. (10) to Eq. (9), we have

$$\theta(l) = \tan^{-1}(\frac{y_{l+i} - y_{l-i}}{x_{l+i} - x_{l-i}}) \tag{11}$$

The parameter i is the neighborhood along both side of the position l. In our case, the parameter i is chosen to be 3. By the function $\tan^{-1}$, the domain of $\theta(l)$ should be bounded in the region $\{-\pi \leq \theta \leq \pi\}$. Notice that discontinuity occurred at slope equal infinity, i.e., $\theta(l) = -\pi$ and $\theta(l) = \pi$. Thus, the profile should be compensated. The compensation is formulated as Eq. (12)

$$\theta_c(l) = \theta(l) + \text{sgn}(|\theta(l) - \theta(l-1)|) \times 2\pi \tag{12}$$

where sgn(x)=1 for $x\geq\pi$ and sgn(x)=0 for $x<\pi$.

Taking the θ_c (l) as the 1-D profile, the procedure of feature extraction is similar to boundary detection introduced above. That is, using "Forward computation" and "Backward mapping", all the violate variation occurrence of the profile are detected as the features and are reserved for 3-D interpolation, which will be introduced in the next section.

IV. 3-D RECONSTRUCTION ALGORITHM

Because the serial cross-sectional CT/MRI images are not contiguous, how to reconstruct the lost 3-D data from known slices becomes an important issue. The 3-D reconstruction provides doctors not only the information about the appearance of desired organ, but also its real location in the human body. It then offers the doctors a good suggestion when diagnosing patients or before performing an operation. The traditional technique with interpolation[11] is to use the coordinates of these 2-D curves directly, such as linear interpolation, and nonlinear interpolation with fitting function $f(s)$ where the order of $f(s)$ is two or higher.

Most of all, the methods performing interpolation for each boundary points don't concern about the global property of the entire boundary curves. They just solve the one-to-one interpolation problem, and cannot be applied to the contour interpolation with branch structure, as illustrated in Fig. 3. To deal with the branch problem, the proposed algorithm use the concept of "virtual connect" to merge two contour into ones gradually during the interpolation process. According to the experimental results, the performance of this procedure for solving branch structure is satisfied.

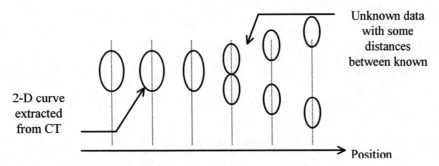

Fig. 3. Contour interpolation with branch structure.

In this paper, four wavelet–based methods for contour interpolation are proposed. They are linear wavelet interpolation (LWI), B-Spline wavelet interpolation (BSWI), hybrid wavelet interpolation (HWI), and B-Spline wavelet interpolation with matched segments using feature matching (BSWSI). All the advantages of wavelet transform, fast linear function and smooth B-Spline function[22] of nonlinear interpolation techniques are investigated. The novel algorithms based on wavelets are developed. Moreover, various measures are designed to test the efficiency of these methods such that the best one can be determined.

The BSWSI technique has the most complicated algorithms than others. Its detailed procedures are described as follows:

Step 1. Represent the boundary curves of the bronchus with (x,y) coordinates for each slice k, i.e.,

$$C_k(l) = \{x_k(l), y_k(l)\}, \quad 1 \leq l \leq L \tag{13}$$

Step 2. Determine the distance of adjacent boundary curves such that we can decide the number of interpolated slices.

$$N \text{ (interpolated slice number)} = \frac{D \text{ (distance of adjacent slices)}}{d \text{ (distance of pixels on screen)}} \tag{14}$$

Step 3. Perform the 1-D WT of $\theta(l)$ of the boundary curve. Pick the entire zero-crossings occurrence as the required features for segment matching.

Step 4. Match the features obtained in step 3 to obtain the matched segments.

Step 5. Normalize the two matched segments and perform WT to them at a selected scale K. More specifically, we obtain the wavelet coefficients by applying WT to the parameterized coordinates $x(l)$ and $y(l)$ of the matched segments of the object contours on adjacent slices. Here, for the simplicity of presentation, these coordinate are assumed to belong to the subspace V_0. However, the appropriate subspace V_k is needed to be chosen to provide sufficient approximation of the contours in practical applications. Even so, the proposed method can be applied to other similar applications. By using Eq. (5) to calculate the wavelet coefficients, we have

$$x(l) = \sum_{n=-\infty}^{\infty} Xp_n^M \tilde{\phi}(l)_n^M + \sum_{m=1}^{M} \sum_{n=-\infty}^{\infty} Xq_n^m \tilde{\psi}_n^m(l),$$

$$y(l) = \sum_{n=-\infty}^{\infty} Yp_n^M \tilde{\phi}(l)_n^M + \sum_{m=1}^{M} \sum_{n=-\infty}^{\infty} Yq_n^m \tilde{\psi}_n^m(l), \tag{15}$$

And we define

$$x_a^M(l) = \sum_n Xp_n^M \tilde{\phi}_n^M(l) \quad , y_a^M(l) = \sum_n Yp_n^M \tilde{\phi}_n^M(l), \tag{16}$$

are the approximation coefficients at scale M, and

$$x_d^m(t) = \sum_n Xq_n^m \tilde{\psi}_n^m(l) \quad , y_d^m(t) = \sum_n Yq_n^m \tilde{\psi}_n^m(l), \tag{17}$$

are the detail signal at scale m with $1 \le m \le M$. Therefore, the wavelet coefficients of $\hat{C}_k$ and $\hat{C}_{k+1}$ are described by $(Xp_n^M)_i, (Yp_n^M)_i, (Xq_n^m)_i, (Yq_n^m)_i$, $l=k, k+1$. For the simplicity of presentation, we use $W(\hat{C}_k)$ to these four coefficients of contour $\hat{C}_k$.

Step 6. Interpolate these wavelet coefficients produced in step 5 with B-Spline function.
Step 7. Perform inverse WT with these interpolated coefficients obtained in step 6.

The difference between BSWSI and three other proposed algorithms, BSWI, LWI and HWI, are listed as below

1. BSWI: The process neglects steps 3 and step 4. In step 5, WT is applied to the entire boundary curves.
2. LWI: Same as BSWI, except the interpolation is linear in step 6. That is, using Eq. (15), we calculate the wavelet coefficients $W(C_i)$ required for the ith interpolated contour between the contours $\hat{C}_k$ and $\hat{C}_{k+1}$. The formula is given as below.

$$W(C_i) = \frac{i}{N} W(\hat{C}_k) + (1 - \frac{i}{N}) W(\hat{C}_{k+1}), \quad 0 < i < N \tag{18}$$

3. HWI: Same as BSWI, except the interpolation is linear interpolation for details and B-Spline interpolation for approximation in step 6.

As mentioned above, the usual interpolation strategies cannot be applied to objects with branch structure. However, by using our contour-based interpolation algorithm, only minor modification is required. For the convenience of explanation, the simplest case "one-to-two" structure is used to illustrate the modification process required for the interpolation strategy. When this branch problem occurs, we just need to do minor change as the "single tube" process. Dealing with the two curves within single slice, the strategy of "virtual connect" is employed to connect them into one. The main difference with "single tube" interpolation is on the manner of tracing curve data and the post-processing for the interpolation results.

After finding the centroid of each boundary curves, we connect the two centroids with a straight line. The line will intersect the boundary curves at the contacted points on the boundaries. The two segments are then merged into one by clockwise boundary tracing. This is called "virtual connection". A simple criterion to determine which points on the interpolated boundaries should be connected is given as below,

if ((d1+d2)<(s1+s2))
    {
                // remark: Constructing Single Connected Curves
                connect the points p11 *and* p21 *by B-Spline curves.*
                Connect the points p12 *and* p22 *by B-Spline curves.*

    }
    else
    {

// remark: Constructing Two Separated Curves
connect the points p11 *and* p12 *by B-Spline curves.*
Connect the points p21 *and* p22 *by B-Spline curves.*

    }

end if

where p11 and p12 are the discontinuities of left curve, p21 and p22 are the discontinuities of right curve, s1 is the distance between p11 and p12, s2 is the distance between p21 and p22, d1 is the distance of p11 and p21, d2 is the distance of p12 and p22.

      In general, for an object with branch structure, if the number of the contour per slice exceeds two, "virtual connection" is also available. Furthermore, this algorithm can solve the interpolation problem for adjacent slices with multi-tube structure via the virtual connection and boundary decision process.

V. EXPERIMENTAL RESULTS

      The source images used in the experiment consist of 15 CT chest images, 40 CT head images, and 40 MR head images. Due to the branch structure existed in the CT chest images (i.e., the bronchus), we use this set of image as an example to illustrate each step in the interpolation strategy. For example, in the set of CT chest images, the thickness of each slice and the inter-distance between adjacent slices are 1 mm and 5 mm, respectively. The regions of interest are the bronchi with branch structure on each CT chest image. The developed algorithms are implemented on a SUN Ultra II workstation. Once we obtain the CT images, the boundary detection stage is performed to extract the desired object, i.e., the bronchus, by radial search with scanning step=30°. Next, the detected boundary points are connected with B-Spline function to obtain the entirely close boundary.

      To obtain the whole-interpolated curves, it is needed to know the distance between adjacent source images. Here, the CT images are sampled per 50 mm and the distance between the pixels on the general display is more than 0.25 mm. Thus, 20 interpolated slices data are needed to construct the whole 2-D curves for visualization process.

      We next analyze the boundary curves that are detected from the source images by WT, extract the features of the curves by selecting the position of zero-crossings, and align these features of adjacent two slices. Here, feature matching is used to match the corresponding features, such that the boundary segments between adjacent matched features can be employed to interpolate the lost slice data. For feature matching, two assumptions are made: The scale (reference size) of shapes should be the same, and no rotation is allowed. Translation will not affect the matching result because we have adjusted these curves to its centroid.

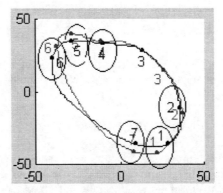

Fig. 4. The result after feature matching.

      According to the distance between two candidate features located on adjacent slices, Fig. 4 illustrates the result after superimposing curve 1 on curve 2. The matching result is listed in Table 1. In Table 1, 'x' means the feature point does not match any other points. In other words, features of curve 1 and curve 2 match at 1st, 2nd, 4th, 5th, 6th and 7th feature points. Other feature points of curve 1 and curve 2 are considered mismatched because their distances are too far. Once the corresponding relationship between curve 1 and curve 2 are obtained, we perform the interpolation for each matched segments by interpolating their wavelet coefficients with B-Spline function as described in previous section to complete 3-D object reconstruction.

To evaluate the performance of the proposed algorithms, various measures based on *area*, *curve length*, and *curve shift* are presented as below, respectively.

Measure based on *Area*

Compute the area of known data (A_0) and interpolated data (A_I)

Area matched:

$A_0 \cap A_I * 100\%$ (19)

Area mismatched:

$A_0 \oplus A_I * 100\%$ (20)

Exclusive-Or Error:

$\xi_E = (A_0 \oplus A_I)/A_0 * 100\%$ (21)

Set-Difference Error:

$\xi_S = (A_0 \backslash A_I)/A_0 * 100\% = (A_0 - A_0 \cap A_I)/A_0 * 100\%$ (22)

Match to Mismatch Area Ratio(MMAR)

$MMAR = A_0 \cap A_I/A_0 \oplus A_I$ (23)

Measure based on *Curve length*

Curve length fittness = $(1-abs(L_0-L_I)/L_0) * 100\%$ (24)

Measure based on *Average Curve Shift*

Euclidean Distance$((x_{co}, y_{co}),(x_{ci}, y_{ci}))$ (25)

Here, the operation $A_0 \cap A_I$ denotes those points that are in both A_0 and A_i. The operation $A_0 \oplus A_I$ denotes those points that are in either A_0 or A_I but not both. The operation $A_0 \backslash A_I$ denotes those points that are in A_0 but not in A_i.

In the experiments, we remove one of these ten slices, and perform interpolation by using the adjacent slice data of the removed slice. Difference of original slice and the interpolated slice is then calculated with ξ_E, ξ_S, *MMAR* and *average curve shift*. It is observed that the maximum difference occurs between 3rd slice and 4th slice. Thus, we remove the 4th original slice data and re-build an interpolated 4th slice data by using the 3rd and the 5th slice data with various interpolation techniques, including linear, B-spline, and four wavelet–based methods. The performance comparison of these methods using different measures is listed in Table 3.

Once we obtain the interpolated data from the above procedures, the visualization process is used to construct a 3-D view of the desired object. In general, to construct a 3-D visualized environment, there are 3 major components to be concerned, i.e., the light source, view port, and reflectivity of object surface. Furthermore, the transparency of object or other consideration can also be added. Here, we employ *Phong specular-reflection model*[32-33] to achieve the shading task. That is, given a light source and the surface data, the luminance (reflection) of the surface can be generated via normal vector calculation.

For a diffuse-reflection coefficient k_d and an ambient-reflection coefficient k_a for each surface, the total diffused reflection equation is written as

$$I_{diff} = k_a I_a + k_d I_l (\mathbf{N} \bullet \mathbf{L})$$ (26)

where I_a is the ambient-light intensity, I_l the light-source intensity, $\mathbf{N}$ the unit surface normal, $\mathbf{L}$ the unit light-source direction vector, and I_{diff} the illumination of single point-source. Once the luminance of each surface point is obtained, the visualized data are displayed with z-buffer method[32-33].

VI. CONCLUSIONS

In medical applications using image processing, doctors need more accurate information about the organs of the interest for diagnosis. The best solution is to construct a full 3-D visualization of the desired objects of human body. With the assistance, doctors do not need to imagine the appearance of the organs by themselves. However, the main difficulty of 3-D reconstruction in medical images is the branch structure of human organ. In this paper, four new approaches based on WT for 3-D reconstruction of serial cross-sectional medical images are presented. From the experimental results, our algorithms can solve both the single tube and branch structured interpolation problems. Generally speaking, the HWI and BSWI schemes perform better. More specifically, although the measures ξ_S and *MMAR* for BSWI scheme are better than those of HWI scheme, the measure *Average Curve Shift* for HWI scheme performs much better than that of BSWI scheme. This means that the localizability of HWI scheme is better than others. The computation cost of BSWI scheme can be reduced with HWI scheme. In summary, single level wavelet decomposition of HWI scheme achieves the best performance among various curve interpolation schemes, and different bases seem to slightly influence the interpolation results. As a general case, the basis "Haar" with single scale wavelet analysis by HWI scheme is a good solution for 3-D reconstruction in our case. The proposed approach in this paper can provide doctors more accurate positions and precise shapes for any specific organs from a series of cross-sectional CT images. The technique with wavelet transform can also be applied to the other image processing procedures.

REFERENCES

1. W. Cheney and D. Kincaid, Numerical Mathematics and Computing, Monterey, CA: Brooks/Cole, 1980.
2. G. T. Herman, S. W. Rowland and M. M. Yau, " A comparative study of the use of linear and modified cubic spline interpolation for image reconstruction," *IEEE Trans. Nucl. Sci.*, vol. NS-26, pp. 2879-2894, 1979.
3. M. R. Stytz and R. W. Parrott, " Using Kriging for 3D medical imaging," *Computerized Med. Imag. Graphics*, vol. 17, no. 6, pp. 421-442, 1993.
4. W. E. Higgins, C. Morice, and E. L. Ritman, "Shape-based interpolation of tree-like structures in three-dimensional images," *IEEE. Trans. Med. Imaging*, vol. 12, no. 3, pp. 439-449, 1993.
5. G. T. Herman, J. Zheng and C. A. Bucholtz, " Shape –based interpolation ," *IEEE. Comput. Gtraphics Appl.*, vol. 12, pp. 69-79, 1992.
6. G. J. Grevera and J. K. Udupa, "Shape-based interpolation of multi-dimensional grey-level images," *IEEE. Trans. Med. Imaging*, vol. 15, no. 3, pp. 881-892, 1996.
7. G. J. Grevera and J. K. Udupa, "An objective comparison of 3D image interpolation methods," *IEEE. Trans. Med. Imaging*, vol. 17, pp. 642-652, 1998.
8. W. C. Lin, C. C. Liang, and C. T. Chen, " Dynamic elastic interpolation for 3-D medical reconstruction from serial cross-sections," *IEEE Trans. Med. Imaging*, vol. 7, pp. 225-232, 1988.
9. E. Maeland, " On the comparison of interpolation methods," *IEEE Trans. Med. Imaging*, vol. 7, pp. 213-217, 1988.
10. W. C. Lin, S. Y. Chen, and C. T. Chen, "A new surface interpolation technique for reconstructing 3-D objects from serial cross-sections," *Comput. Vision, Graphics, Image Processing*, vol. 48, pp. 124-143, 1989.
11. S. Y. Chen, W. C. Lin, C. C. Liang, and C. T. Chen, "Improvement on dynamic elastic interpolation technique for reconstructing 3-D objects from serial cross-sections," in *Proc. Comp. Assisted. Radiology*, Berlin, pp. 702-706, July, 1989.
12. Michael Unser, "A review of wavelets in biomedical applications," *Proceedings of the IEEE*, vol. 84, no. 4, pp. 626-638, 1996.
13. Alejandra Figliola and Eduardo Serrano, "Analysis of physiological time series using wavelet transforms," *IEEE Engineering in Medicine and Biology*, pp. 74-79, 1997.
14. Gilbert Strang, Truong Nguyen, *Wavelets and Filter Banks*. Wellesley-Cambridge Press, 1996.
15. Albert Cohan and Jelena Kovacevic, "Wavelets: the mathematical background," *Proceedings of the IEEE*, vol. 84, no. 4, pp. 514-522, 1996.
16. Jean-Christophe Olivo, "Automatic threshold selection using the wavelet transform," *CVGIP: Graphical Models and Image Processing*, vol. 56, no. 3, pp. 205-218, 1994.
17. Jiann-Der Lee, "A genetic approach to select wavelet features for contour extraction in medical ultrasonic imaging," *Electronics Letters*, vol. 32, no. 23, pp. 1820-1821, 1996.
18. Wenwu Zhu, Yao Wang, Yuqi Yao, and Randall L. Barbour, "A wavelet-based multiresolution regularized least squares reconstruction approach for optical tomography," *IEEE Transactions on Medical Image*, vol. 16, no. 2, pp. 210-217, 1997.
19. Alex P. Pentland, "Interpolation using wavelet basis," *IEEE Trans. Pattern Analysis and Machine Intelligence*, vol. 16, no. 4, pp. 410-414, 1994.
20. Jun Wang and H. K. Huang, "Medical image compression by using three-dimensional wavelet transform," *IEEE Trans. Med. Imaging*, vol. 15, no. 4, pp. 547-554, 1996.
21. Jiann-Shu Lee, Chin-Hsing Chen, Yung-Nien Sun and Guan-Shu Tseng, "Occluded objects recognition using multiscale features and hopfield neural network," *Pattern Recognition*, vol. 30, no. 1, pp. 113-122, 1997.
22. Donald Hearn and M. Pauline Baker, *Computer Graphics*. 2nd Ed., Prentice-Hall, 1986.
23. Rafael C. Gonzalez and Richard E. Woods, *Digital Image Processing*. Addison-Wesley, 1992.
24. J. R. Parker, *Algorithms for Image Processing and Computer Vision*. John Wiley & Sons, 1997.
25. Quang Minh Tieng, "Wavelet-based affine invariant representation: a tool for recognizing planar objects in 3D space," *IEEE Trans. Pattern Analysis and Machine Intelligence*, vol. 19, no. 8, pp. 846-857, 1997.

26. J. A. Garcia and J. Fdez-Valdivia, "Representing planar curves by using a scale vector," *Pattern Recognition Letters*, pp. 937-942, 1994.

27. G. Cortelazzo, G. A. Mian, G. Vezzi, and P. Zamperoni, "Trademark shapes description by string-maching techniques," *Pattern Recognition*, vol. 27, no. 8, pp. 1005-1008, 1994.

28. Jiann-Der Lee, Jau-Yien Lee, and Chin-Hsing Chen, "A new algorithm for two-dimensional object inspection using string matching," *Mathl. Comput. Modeling*, vol. 27, no. 1, pp. 101-106, 1998.

29. Yvette Mallet, Danny Coomans, Jerry Kautsky, and Olivier De Vel, "Classification using adaptive wavelets for feature extraction," *IEEE Trans. Pattern Analysis and Machine Intelligence*, vol. 19, no. 10, pp. 1058-1066, 1997.

30. Kai Xin, Kah Bin Kim, and Geok Soon Hong, "A scale space filtering approach for visual feature extraction," *Pattern Recognition*, vol.28, no. 8, pp. 1145-1158, 1995.

31. Quang Minh Tieng, and W. W. Boles, "Recognition of 2D object contours using the wavelet transform zero-crossing representation," *IEEE Trans. Pattern Analysis and Machine Intelligence*, vol. 19, no. 8, pp. 910-916, 1997.

32. Christian Barillot, "Surface and volume rendering techniques to Display 3-D Data," *IEEE Engineering in Medicine and Biology*, pp. 111-119, 1993.

33. Derek R. Ney, Elliot K. Fishman, and Donna Magid, "Volumetric rendering of computed tomography data: principles and techniques," *IEEE Computer Graphics & Applications*, pp. 24-32, 1990.

A Multi-Scale Application of the N3 Method for Intensity Correction of MR Images

Craig K. Jones and Erick B. Wong

MS/MRI Research Group, 211-2386 East Mall, Vancouver BC, Canada

ABSTRACT

Spatial inhomogeneity due to the radio-frequency coil in MR imaging can confound segmentation results. In 1994, Sled introduced the N3 technique, using histogram deconvolution, for reducing inhomogeneity. We found some scans whose steep inhomogeneity gradient was not fully eliminated by N3. We created a multi-scale application of N3 that further reduces this gradient, and validated it on MNI BrainWeb and actual MRI data. The algorithm was applied to proton density simulated BrainWeb scans (with known inhomogeneity) and 100 standard MRI scans. Intra-slice and inter-slice inhomogeneity measures were created to compare the technique with standard N3. The slope of the estimated bias versus the known bias of BrainWeb data was 1.0 (r=0.9844) for N3 and 1.04 (r=0.9828) for multi-scale N3. The bias field estimated by multi-scale N3 was within 1% root-mean-square of that of standard N3. Over 100 MS patient scans, the average intra-slice measure (0 meaning bias-free) was 0.0694 (uncorrected), 0.0530 (N3) and 0.0402 (multi-scale). The average inter-slice measure (1 meaning bias-free) was 0.9121 (uncorrected), 0.9367 (N3) and 0.9508 (multi-scale). The multi-scale N3 algorithm showed a greater inhomogeneity reduction than N3 in the small percentage of scans bearing a strong gradient, and results similar to N3 in the remaining scans.

Keywords: RF Inhomogeneity Correction, Image Processing, Magnetic Resonance Imaging

1. INTRODUCTION

Magnetic resonance imaging (MRI) is an important tool to diagnose disease and assess treatment. Signal intensties in standard clinical images are a function of both the tissue (water environment), the scanner hardware and the interaction between the hardware and the object scanned. Typically, one is interested in signal intensities as a function of only the tissue and there has been great effort to remove unwanted signal changes due to hardware and the interaction between the hardware and the object. One signal change (artifact) is a shading across the image typically referred to as an intensity non-uniformity or inhomogeneity. The inhomogeneity can arise from imperfect radiofrequency (RF) pulses, inhomogeneities in the RF coil (transmit or receive), a mistuned coil or electrodynamic interaction with the object being scanned. Inhomogeneities such as this are typically not a problem for the radiologist, but can confound automatic computer processing of the data.

Many techniques have been applied to MRI images to correct for the RF inhomogeneity. They can be categorized as: homomorphic methods,[1,2] gradient methods[3] and histogram methods.[4] A survey of six techniques[5] showed that the N3 technique[4] was a robust and accurate method of correcting the RF inhomogeneity. We have also determined the N3 technique to be a reliable method, but a small percentage of scans had a strong linear intensity gradient that the N3 algorithm was not able to fully correct.

We created a multi-scale N3 algorithm to correct MRI volume data with strong inhomogeneity gradients that the standard N3 algorithm was not able to fully correct. The new multi-scale N3 algorithm was applied to simulated data and the estimated bias field was compared to the true bias field as well as the estimated bias field calculated by the standard N3 algorithm. The multi-scale algorithm was applied to 100 randomly-sampled multiple sclerosis (MS) patients' scans and the estimated bias field was compared to that calculated by the standard algorithm.

Further author information: (Correspondence to C.K.J.)

C.K.J.: E-mail: craig@msmri.medicine.ubc.ca, Telephone: 1 604 822 0760

E.B.W.: E-mail: erick@msmri.medicine.ubc.ca

2. METHODS

2.1. Data

Three simulated proton-density (TE $\approx$ 35 ms and TR $\approx$ 3000 ms) MRI volumes based on normal brains were downloaded from BrainWeb.[6-10] The first was a volume with no RF inhomogeneity and no noise. The second was a volume with 40% RF inhomogeneity and no noise. The third was a volume with 40% RF inhomogeneity and 3% Rician noise (quadrature, Gaussian random noise). The true bias field was calculated as the ratio of the second volume to first volume. Each data file was downloaded in MINC format with dimensions $181 \times 217 \times 36$ and a slice thickness of 5mm.

The MS patient MRI data analyzed was proton density weighted volumes of 24 slices with 5mm thickness, acquired using a multi-echo spin-echo pulse sequence with TE $\approx$ 20/80 ms and TR $\approx$ 2600 ms (FOV $\approx$ 23cm, 192×256 acquisition). The data was from a study[11] of relapsing-remitting MS patients.

2.2. Processing

For both the simulated and patient MRI data three algorithms were applied to each data volume: 1) the standard N3 algorithm (version 1.0, denoted N3), 2) the standard algorithm applied five times consecutively (denoted as N3^5) and 3) the multi-scale N3 algorithm (five applications of N3 with different command line parameters for each application as shown in Table 1, denoted N3^{ms}). The application of N3^5 was used to verify that the estimated bias field as calculated by N3^{ms} was different from that calculated by N3^5.

Table 1: Command line parameters (for `nu_correct`) used for each application of the N3^{ms} algorithm.

Application	FWHM	Stop	Distance
1	0.50	0.002	150
2	0.30	0.001	150
3	0.20	0.001	200
4	0.10	0.0005	200
5	0.05	0.0005	200

2.3. Analysis

To validate N3^{ms} on simulated data, N3^{ms} was used to estimate the bias field which was then compared graphically to the true bias field. A straight line fit was calculated for the estimated bias field from N3 to true bias field and for the estimated bias field from N3^{ms} to true bias field. The perecent relative difference in the estimated bias field from N3 and N3^{ms} was calculated as $D = \frac{b^{N3^{ms}} - b^{N3}}{b^{N3}} \times 100$ where b^X was the bias field calculated by algorithm X. The root-mean-square (RMS) of the percent relative difference was calculated over the volume of data.

The N3, N3^5 and N3^{ms} algorithms were compared, based on MRI volumes of MS patients, both qualitatively and quantitatively. We implemented two simple methods to quantify the RF inhomogeneity. One method measured *inter-slice* inhomogeneity, the variation in brightness between slices, and the other measured *intra-slice* inhomogeneity, the variations in intensity from one end of a slice to another. (This distinction was only relevant due to the non-cubic aspect ratio of the voxels.)

The inter-slice method calculated the histogram of the signal intensities to determine the peak intensity on each slice. Within the relevant portion of the head, this value should be relatively constant from slice to slice, so the ratio of the darkest peak to the brightest peak was used as an estimate of the inter-slice RF inhomogeneity.

The intra-slice method subdivided each slice into four quadrants and measured the peak intensity of each quadrant, which should be approximately equal. These four values are sorted, and the brightest (resp. darkest) intensity was compared to the second-darkest (resp. second-brightest) intensity. This was found to be more robust than simply comparing the brightest to the darkest, but still sufficiently sensitive to detect strong gradients.

All processing was done using N3 and Matlab (Natick, Mass).

3. RESULTS AND DISCUSSION

The new technique was applied to simulated data (BrainWeb) to verify that the estimated bias field was similar to the applied bias field and similar to the estimated bias field as calculated by N3. The new technique was then applied to MS patients' proton density weighted data and the estimated bias field compared to that estimated by N3.

The coarse-grained parameters in the first stage of the multi-scale method serve to correct the steepest gradient effects. These have a widely diffusive (blurring) effect on the histogram, and in the unavoidable presence of noise, the range of this effect may not be adequately detected by smaller-width deconvolution kernels. Each stage was therefore intended to sufficiently reduce relatively strong inhomogeneity artifacts so that the finer parameters of the next stage were more effective. By the third stage, the parameters are comparable to those of the standard algorithm, but the histogram was sharpened with typically fewer applications of the wider deconvolution kernels in the prior stages.

3.1. Simulated Data

The plots of the actual applied bias versus the bias estimated by each of the three algorithms are shown in Figure 1. The axes have been plotted in logarithmic space, so 0 represents no bias, positive values represent brightening, and negative values represent darkening. A square root function has been applied to the grayscale intensities in order to show greater detail at the low end.

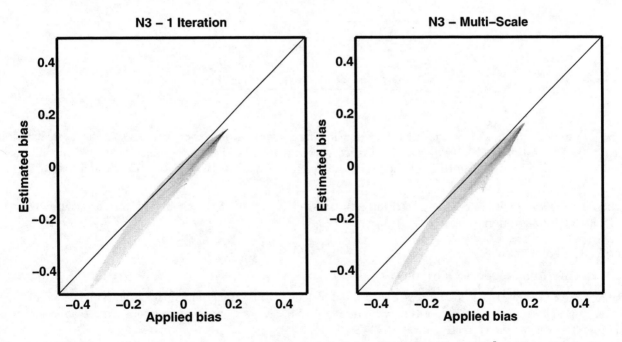

Figure 1. Histogram of the estimated vs. applied bias for N3 (left), and N3^{ms}(right). (N3^5 results were similar to N3^{ms}). A logarithmic scaling was used for the axes and the line shown is unity slope.

The slope, intercept and correlation coefficient were calculated from the scatter plots (as in Figure 1) of the estimated bias field of each algorithm to the true bias field. The slope of the scatter plots was 1.0 for 1.0 for each of the algorithms and very little bias was present (see Table 2). The correlation coefficients were 0.98 for each algorithm.

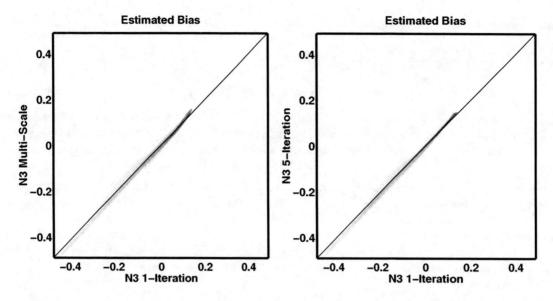

Figure 2: Histograms of the estimated bias calculated by N3 compared to $N3^{ms}$ and $N3^5$.

Table 2. The slope, intercept and coerrelation coefficient calculated from the scatter plot of the estimated bias from each algorithm relative to the true bias.

Algorithm	Slope	Intercept	r
N3	1.00	-0.03	0.9844
$N3^5$	1.04	-0.04	0.9814
$N3^{ms}$	1.04	-0.04	0.9828

Histograms (Figure 2) showed that there was excellent agreement between the estimated bias field calculated by $N3^{ms}$ and the estimated bias field from N3. As well, there was an excellent agreement for the estimated bias calculated by N3 and $N3^5$. The RMS of this relative difference (from N3) for $N3^5$ was 0.82%, and for $N3^{ms}$ it was 1.00%.

Based on these results, the $N3^{ms}$ algorithm estimates the bias field of the simulated data as accurately as the standard N3 algorithm.

3.2. MRI Data

3.2.1. Strong Inhomogeneity Gradient

A small percentage of MRI scans that we have looked at have had a strong inhomogeneity gradient present in the image that the standard N3 algorithm was not able to fully correct. One example of such a scan is shown in Figure 3 as well as the corrected images (N3, $N3^5$ and $N3^{ms}$).

All MS patient inhomogeneity estimates were restricted to slices 10 to 22 to improve the reliability of the intra-slice measure, which can be affected by the lower slices (e.g. jaw) and the top two slices, which were often too small from which to take good measurements. Although both RF estimates were relatively unsophisticated in nature, we found that they correlated well with the qualitatively observed artifacts present in the scans with strong intensity gradients. Thus they enabled an independent, quantitative means of comparing how effectively the different correction methods removed those artifacts.

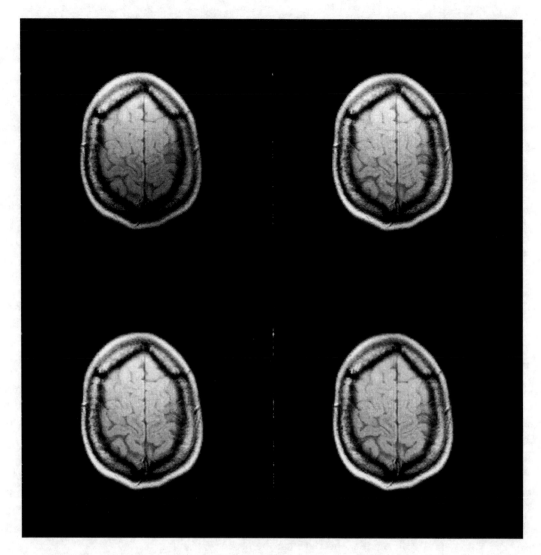

Figure 3. Example slice of an MRI image with a strong inhomogeneity gradient (primarly top to bottom). Shown are the original image (top left), N3 (top right), $N3^5$ (bottom left) and $N3^{ms}$ (bottom right).

Table 3: Intra-slice correction measure (0 represents no inhomogeneity).

Algorithm	Mean	Standard Deviation
Original	0.0694	0.0518
1 Iteration	0.0530	0.0406
5 Iterations	0.0435	0.0347
Multi-Scale	0.0402	0.0291

3.2.2. Random Sample Study

To verify that the multi-scale technique was not incorrectly estimating the bias field on scans with "simpler" RF inhomogeneity, a random sample of 100 proton density weighted scans was selected. Each of the 3 RF inhomogeneity algorithms was applied to a scan and the inter- and intra-slice RF measures were compared (based on the measures in Section 2.3).

Table 4: Inter-slice correction measure (1 represents no inhomogeneity).

Algorithm	Mean	Standard Deviation
Original	0.9121	0.0465
1 Iteration	0.9367	0.0383
5 Iterations	0.9483	0.0348
Multi-Scale	0.9508	0.0349

Table 3 shows the mean and standard deviation of the intra-slice correction measure (0 refers to no inhomogeneity) over the 100 randomly selected scans. There were 33/100 scans where the 1-iteration method had a lower measure than the multi-scale measure. A two-tailed t-test was done on the difference between the intra-slice measure from 1-iteration and the intra-slice measure from the multi-scale and they were found to be different ($p < 0.0001$).

Table 4 shows the mean and standard deviation of the inter-slice correction measure (1 represents no inhomogeneity) over the 100 randomly selected scans. There were 6/100 scans where the 1-iteration method had a higher measure than the multi-scale measure. A two-tailed t-test was done on the difference between the inter-slice measure from 1-iteration and the inter-slice measure from the multi-scale and they were found to be different ($p < 0.0001$).

Timing

A single application of N3 actually takes place over a number of iterative steps, each successively refining the estimated inhomogeneity field until stopping criteria are met. For a given volume size, the time required for each step is essentially constant, provided certain N3 parameters such as *shrink* are not altered. Thus, the total number of iterative steps (over all stages of the multi-scale and 5-iteration methods) constitutes a measure of processing time that is independent of processor type and system load.

The total number of iterative steps over the 100 scans was: 1666 (1-iteration), 3915 (5-iterations), 3447 (multi-scale). There were 56 scans for which the number of steps used by the multi-scale method was less than the number of steps used by the 5-iteration method. There are 5 scans where the multi-scale method used fewer iterative steps than the 1-iteration method.

The number of iterative steps of the N3 algorithm doubled for N3^{ms} compared to N3, but because all the algorithms based on N3 were fully automatic, the data can be processed offline.

4. CONCLUSIONS

We have developed a fully automatic multi-scale extension to the original N3 RF inhomogeneity correction technique. For simulated data, the estimated bias field from N3^{ms} was within 1% (rms) of the estimated bias field from N3. On a random sample of 100 MRI volumes the N3^{ms} algorithm tended to result in a smaller inter-slice and intra-slice inhomogeneity compared to N3. On the small number of MRI volumes that had a strong inhomogeneity gradient, N3^{ms} was more successful in removing the inhomogeneity. The N3^{ms} algorithm was shown to be at least as good as N3 on MRI data with expected inhomogeneity and better when a strong inhomogeneity gradient is present.

ACKNOWLEDGMENTS

We wish to thank Serono for supporting the MS study from which the sample data was obtained, and also John Sled at MNI for publishing the implementation of his N3 algorithm as well as helpful correspondence.

REFERENCES

1. B. Brinkmann, A. Manduca, and R. Robb, "Optimized homomorphic unsharp masking for MR grayscale inhomogeneity correction," *IEEE Trans Med Imaging* **17**, pp. 161–71, Apr. 1998.

2. M. Cohen, R. DuBois, and M. Zeineh, "Rapid and effective correction of RF inhomogeneity for high field magnetic resonance imaging," *Hum Brain Mapp* **10**, pp. 204–11, Aug. 2000.

3. E. Vokurka, N. Thacker, and A. Jackson, "A fast model independent method for automatic correction of intensity nonuniformity in MRI data," *J Magn Reson Imaging* **10**, pp. 550–62, Oct. 1999.

4. J. Sled, A. Zijdenbos, and A. Evans, "A nonparametric method for automatic correction of intensity nonuniformity in MRI data," *IEEE Trans Med Imaging* **17**, pp. 87–97, Feb. 1998.

5. J. Arnold, J. Liow, K. Schaper, J. Stern, J. Sled, D. Shattuck, A. Worth, M. Cohen, R. Leahy, J. Mazziotta, and D. Rottenberg, "Qualitative and quantitative evaluation of six algorithms for correcting intensity nonuniformity effects," *Neuroimage* **13**, pp. 931–43, May 2001.

6. D. Collins, A. Zijdenbos, V. Kollokian, J. Sled, N. Kabani, C. Holmes, and A. Evans, "Design and construction of a realistic digital brain phantom," *IEEE Transactions on Medical Imaging* **17**(3), pp. 463–468, 1998.

7. R.-S. Kwan, A. Evans, and G. Pike, "An extensible MRI simulator for post-processing evaluation," *Visualization in Biomedical Computing (VBC'96). Lecture Notes in Computer Science* **1131**, pp. 135–140, 1996.

8. R.-S. Kwan, A. Evans, and G. Pike, "MRI simulation-based evaluation of image-processing and classification methods," *IEEE Transactions on Medical Imaging* **18**(11), pp. 1085–1097, 1999.

9. C. Cocosco, V. Kollokian, R.-S. Kwan, and A. Evans, "Brainweb: Online interface to a 3D MRI simulated brain database," *NeuroImage* **5**(4), p. S425, 1997.

10. "http://www.bic.mni.mcgill.ca/brainweb/."

11. M. S. Freedman, "Dose-dependent clinical and magnetic resonance imaging efficacy of interferon β-1a in multiple sclerosis," *Ann. Neurology* **44**, December 1998.

Multiwavelet grading of prostate pathological images

Hamid Soltanian-Zadeh [*a,b], Kourosh Jafari-Khouzani [**c]

[a]Radiology Image Analysis Lab, Henry Ford Health System, Detroit
[b]Dept. of Electrical and Computer Engineering, University of Tehran, Tehran, Iran
[c]Dept. of Computer Science, Wayne State Univ., Detroit

ABSTRACT

We have developed image analysis methods to automatically grade pathological images of prostate. The proposed method generates Gleason grades to images, where each image is assigned a grade between 1 and 5. This is done using features extracted from multiwavelet transformations. We extract energy and entropy features from submatrices obtained in the decomposition. Next, we apply a k-NN classifier to grade the image. To find optimal multiwavelet basis, preprocessing, and classifier, we use features extracted by different multiwavelets with either critically sampled preprocessing or repeated row preprocessing and different k-NN classifiers and compare their performances, evaluated by total misclassification rate (TMR). To evaluate sensitivity to noise, we add white Gaussian noise to images and compare the results (TMR's). We applied proposed methods to 100 images. We evaluated the first and second levels of decomposition using Geronimo, Hardin, and Massopust (GHM), Chui and Lian (CL), and Shen (SA4) multiwavelets. We also evaluated k-NN classifier for $k=1,2,3,4,5$. Experimental results illustrate that first level of decomposition is quite noisy. They also show that critically sampled preprocessing outperforms repeated row preprocessing and has less sensitivity to noise. Finally, comparison studies indicate that SA4 multiwavelet and k-NN classifier ($k=1$) generates optimal results (with smallest TMR of 3%).

Keywords: Gleason grading system, multiwavelet transform, k-NN classifier, simulated annealing, image analysis, classification

1. INTRODUCTION

1.1 Background and motivation

Cancer is the second killer of American people, and only cardiovascular diseases take a higher toll.[1] Histological grading is a very important task in the framework of prostate cancer prognosis, since it is used for treatment planning. If infection of cancer disease was not rejected by non-invasive diagnostic techniques like MRI, CT scan, and ultrasound, then a biopsy specimen of the tissue is tested. For prostate, the tissue is usually stained by H&E (Hematoxyline and Eosine) technique. Then the histological grading is done by viewing the microscopic image of the tissue. This task is done by pathologists. Manual grading is very subjective due to inter- and intra-observer variations. So an automatic and repeatable technique is needed for grading. Gleason grading system is the most common method for histological grading of prostate.[2] The goal of this paper is to automate the Gleason grading.

For data classification, the decision is made based on a set of features. Since most pattern recognition tasks are first done by humans and are automated later, the most appropriate source of features has been those used by the experts to classify the objects. Automating the classification of objects using the same features as those used by experts can be a difficult task, but fortunately the features used by machines need not be precisely those used by humans. Sometimes features that would be impossible or difficult for humans to estimate are useful in automated systems.[3] In this research, we used energy and entropy features calculated from multiwavelet coefficients of the image. Then a k-NN classifier was used to classify each image to appropriate grade. The leaving-one-out technique was used for error rate estimation.

---

* hamids@rad.hfh.edu; phone 1 313 874-4482; fax 1 313 874-4494; http://Radiologyresearch.com; Radiology Image Analysis Lab, One Ford Place, 2F, Detroit, Henry Ford Health System, Detroit, MI48202, USA; ** kjafari1@yahoo.com; phone 1 313 577-5070; fax 1 313 577-6868; www.cs.wayne.edu; Dept. of Computer Science, 431 State Hall, Wayne State Univ., Detroit, MI48202, USA

1.2 Gleason grading system

There is a great need for methods to quantify the probable clinical aggressiveness of a given neoplasm, and further to express its apparent extent and spread in patients.[1] Histological grading is one of these methods. The grading of a cancer attempts to establish some estimate of its aggressiveness or level of malignancy. In Gleason grading system, the prostate cancer may be classified as grade 1, 2, 3, 4 or 5 with increasing or lack of glands differentiation as explained below.

Gleason has provided a conceptual diagram in Fig. 1 to show the continuum of deteriorating cancer cell architecture, and the four dividing lines along this continuum that he discovered are able to identify patients with significantly different prognosis. The Gleason system is based exclusively on the architectural pattern of the glands of the prostate tumor. It evaluates how effectively the cells of any particular cancer are able to structure themselves into glands resembling those of the normal prostate.[2] The ability of a tumor to mimic normal gland architecture is called its *differentiation*, and experience has shown that a tumor whose structure is nearly normal (well differentiated) will probably have a biological behavior relatively close to normal (that is not very aggressively malignant). Gleason grading from very well differentiated (grade 1) to very poorly differentiated (grade 5) is usually done by viewing the low magnification microscopic image of the prostate tissue.

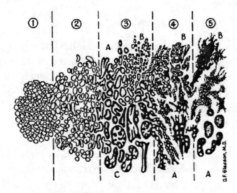

Figure 1. Gleason grading diagram.

If there exits two patterns in the specimen, a combined score is calculated which is the sum of two grades. So combined score varies from 2 to 10. Fig. 2 shows two tissue samples of grades 2 and 5. For grade 2, the glands are well-differentiated with respect to grade 5. Fig. 2(b) shows only a sea of black nuclei with no pattern.

The grade of a prostate cancer specimen is very valuable to doctors in understanding how a particular case of prostate cancer can be treated. An accurate Gleason score can help one decide which treatment may be most beneficial. In general, the time for which a patient is likely to survive following diagnosis of prostate cancer is related to the Gleason score. The lower the Gleason score, the better the patient is likely to do. Patients with score of 2 to 4 almost never develop aggressive disease, whereas most patients with a score of 8 to 10 die of prostatic carcinoma.[2]

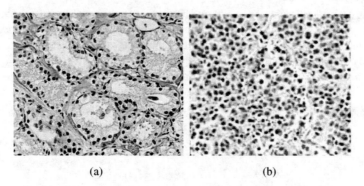

(a)   (b)

Figure 2. Two samples of prostate tissue. (a) Grade 2. (b) Grade 5.

1.3 Previous work

Analysis of pathological images has been an area of interest during the last few years.[4-13] The aim of these researches has been distinguishing the normal and abnormal tissues. Stotzka *et al.*[4] proposed a method to distinguish the moderately and poorly differentiated lesions of prostate tissues. The decision is based on a number of features based on shape and texture of the image. In reference[5] a technique using pyramid node linking to segment and classify the given cell images is described. The proposed method was used for microscope slides of cultured rat liver cells, to classify these cells into one of three possible classes. The decision is based on previous knowledge of gray levels in these groups. A method for automatic grading of breast cancer based on Bloom and Rechardson grading system has been proposed in reference[6]. Features based on fuzzy co-occurrence matrix are calculated and then the decision is made using an artificial neural network. A nonlinear technique is proposed in reference[7] to segment and extract features from the area of each individual cell in biopsy images of breast. Then a fuzzy classifier is used which determine the probability of the biopsy to belong to a high or low cancer level.

Schnorrenberg *et al.*[8] developed a method to detect tissue cell nuclei in histological sections of breast with immuno-cytochemistry staining. The detection system uses a receptive field filter to enhance negatively and positively stained cell nuclei and a squashing function to label each pixel value as belonging to the background or a nucleus. Some statistical features of color values of cell pixels are calculated, and then a neural network is used to classify each cell to one of five classes.

An automatic system was presented in reference[9] to analyze a cell nucleus in a given biopsy of mammary tissue, which is cancerous. Images are enhanced and segmented using morphological transformations. An ultimate erosion is used in two steps to separate cell nuclei in contact. It is based on a combination of symmetrical ultimate erosion with directional ultimate erosion. Wouwer[10] has proposed a method for classification of pathological images of breast. Features based on wavelet transform are extracted from each segmented cell and the cell is classified to one of four grades. The grading is based on distribution of chromatin in the cell.

Hallinan proposed a method for detection of malignancy in cervical cells[11]. The cytological image is first segmented to cells. A number of features are defined for each cell. Then an artificial neural network is used for classification. A similar study was done in reference[12] to determine malignant mesothelioma. A number of shape features are calculated for each nucleus and a k-NN classifier is used for classification. An automatic algorithm for the categorization of normal and cancerous colon mucosa was reported in reference[13] where a number of features were derived using the co-occurrence matrix and a parametric linear-discriminate function was used to determine the classification rule.

A major difference between our work and most previous techniques is that they use the shape information of individual cells or glands and/or its texture information, but we use features of the entire image. Another difference is that we use multiwavelets which have not been used in previous work.

2. FEATURE EXTRACTION

2.1 Multiwavelet transform

While in scalar wavelet transform there is only one scaling function, in multiwavelet transform we can have more than one scaling function. Multiwavelets have some advantages compared to scalar ones. For example, features such as short support, orthogonality, symmetry and vanishing moments are known to be important in signal and image processing. A scalar wavelet cannot possess all of these properties at the same time. On the other hand, a multiwavelet system can simultaneously provide perfect reconstruction while preserving length (orthogonality), good performance at the boundaries (via linear-phase symmetry), and a high order of approximation (via vanishing moments). This suggests that multiwavelets may perform better in various applications.[14]

In multiwavelet analysis, the multiscaling function $\boldsymbol{\Phi}(t) = [\phi_1(t), ..., \phi_r(t)]^T$ satisfies a two-scale equation:

$$\boldsymbol{\Phi}(t) = \sqrt{2} \sum_k H_k \boldsymbol{\Phi}(2t - k) \tag{1}$$

where H_k is an $r \times r$ matrix of lowpass filter coefficients and r is called multiplicity. Like scalar wavelet function, multiwavelet function $\boldsymbol{\Psi}(t) = [\psi_1(t), \ldots, \psi_r(t)]^T$ must satisfy the two-scale wavelet equation:

$$\boldsymbol{\Psi}(t) = \sqrt{2} \sum_k G_k \boldsymbol{\Phi}(2t - k) \tag{2}$$

where G_k is an $r \times r$ matrix of highpass filter coefficients.

Corresponding to each multiwavelet system is a matrix-valued multirate filterbank, or multifilter shown in Fig. 3. The lowpass filter and highpass filter consist of coefficients corresponding to the dilation equation (1) and wavelet equation (2) and these coefficients are matrices, so during the convolution step they must multiply vectors (instead of scalars). This means that multifilter banks need input rows. Thus, some methods for vectorization of scalar input should be used. These are called preprocessing methods and different approaches to preprocessing have been developed.[15-17] In this research, we use repeated row and critically sampled approaches.

In repeated row approach the input signal is repeated to get an input vector.[14] So it introduces oversampling of the data by a factor of two. There is an alternative version of repeated row preprocessing in which the first row of input vector is the signal and the second row is the signal with a factor of α. This factor is chosen so that if the input signal is constant, then the output from the high-pass multifilter is zero.[18] We use this kind of repeated row preprocessing.

In critically sampled approach the input signal is preprocessed such that a critically sampled representation is maintained: If the data enters at rate R/2, preprocessing yields two streams at rate R/2 for input to the multifilter.[14] The symmetric extension of signal also is also used as described in reference[14] to preserve critically sampling nature of system in filtering the signals at their boundaries. This approach can be used for symmetric or antisymmetric filter banks. All the multiwavelets that we used in this research have symmetric or antisymmetric filter banks except cardinal balanced multiwavelets which do not need preprocessing.

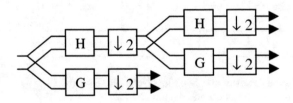

Figure 3. Multiwavelet filterbank, showing 2 levels of decomposition.

2.2 Multiwavelet transform of images

For calculating multiwavelet transform images, we can use tensor product method, i.e., performing the 1-D algorithm in each dimension separately.[14,17] Fig. 4 shows the submatrices resulted from 2-D multiwavelet decomposition. The result after first decomposition can be realized as the following matrix:

$$
\begin{array}{cccc}
L_1L_1 & L_2L_1 & H_1L_1 & H_2L_1 \\
L_1L_2 & L_2L_2 & H_1L_2 & H_2L_2 \\
L_1H_1 & L_2H_1 & H_1H_1 & H_2H_1 \\
L_1H_2 & L_2H_2 & H_1H_2 & H_2H_2
\end{array}
$$

in which each entry represents a subband, which corresponds to lowpass and/or highpass filters used in vertical and horizontal directions. For example, the subband labeled L_1H_2 corresponds to data obtained by applying the highpass filter on the horizontal direction and taking its 2nd channel, then applying lowpass filter on the vertical direction and taking its first channel (Fig. 3). The next level of decomposition will decompose the following "low-low pass" submatrix, in a similar manner:

$$L_1L_1 \quad L_2L_1$$
$$L_1L_2 \quad L_2L_2$$

This is shown in Fig. 4(b). The number of submatrices will be equal to $4+12l$ where l is the number of levels of decomposition. The energy and entropy of the multiwavelet coefficients are calculated as features for image classification. As indicated in Fig. 4, the result of decomposition is a number of submatrices. From each submatrix $[x_{ij}]$, the following features are calculated:

$$Energy = \frac{\sum_i \sum_j x_{ij}^2}{N \times N} \tag{3}$$

$$Entropy = \frac{-1}{\log N^2} \sum_i \sum_j \left[\frac{x_{ij}^2}{norm^2} \right] \log \left[\frac{x_{ij}^2}{norm^2} \right] \tag{4}$$

where $norm^2 = \sum_i \sum_j x_{ij}^2$ and N is the dimension of each submatrix and its use in the above equation permit features be independent of submatrix dimensions.

In this work we use 10 different multiwavelets: GHM, CL, SA4, BiGHM2, BiH52s, BiH32s, BiH54n, CardBal2, CardBal3 and CardBal4. A brief description of each multiwavelet is given in Appendix.

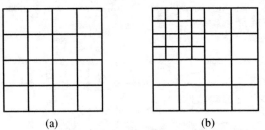

(a)   (b)

Figure 4. Result of 2-D multiwavelet decomposition.
(a) One level of decomposition. (b) Two levels of decompostion.

3. CLASSIFICATION

3.1 k-NN classifier

Having generated a feature vector for each image, we use a k-nearest neighbors (k-NN) classifier using Euclidean distance to classify it to appropriate grade. Because limited number of images for each grade was available, we use the leaving-one-out technique to evaluate accuracy of classification. Before classification, we normalize features. Recall that if one of the features has a very wide range of possible values compared to the other features, it will have a huge effect on the dissimilarity (distance), and the decisions will be based primarily upon this single feature. To overcome this, it is necessary to apply scale factors to the features before computing the distances.[3] In this research, we normalized each feature to have mean of zero and standard deviation of one for the entire data set. Furthermore, because some features may be more important than others, we used weight for each normalized feature. To calculate the best weight vector for the feature vector, we minimized the error rate estimated by the leaving-one-out technique. This minimization was done using Simulated Annealing algorithm.[18] The k-NN algorithm classifies each image by assigning it the label most frequently represented among the k nearest samples; in other words a decision is made by examining the labels on the k nearest neighbors and taking a vote. If the label coincides with the Gleason grade of the sample, this is considered a correct classification

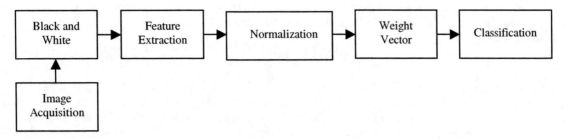

Figure 5. Stages of prostate image analysis: Image acquisition, generating black and white images, feature extraction, normalization, exerting weight vector, and classification.

3.2 Noise effect

To evaluate the noise effect we added Gaussian noise with signal to noise ratio SNR=5 to each image before classification in leaving-one-out technique. SNR is defined by the ratio of signal expectation to the noise standard deviation.

4. RESULTS

In our experiments, 100 prostate tissue sample images were processed by the proposed approach. These color images were of grades 2 to 5 and of magnification ×100 with different sizes.The specimens were stained using Hematoxyline and Eosine technique. Grade 1 was excluded because it is a very rare pattern and should be avoided. All of the images were captured in equal conditions of light. Our image set consisted of 21, 20, 32, 27 images of grades 2, 3, 4, 5, respectively. Because different portions of a specimen may have more than one grade, we captured our images in a manner so that each image has a single grade. The grading of these images was done by pathologists.

We first made each image black and white to simplify the calculations, since the color does not have important information. For multiwavelet features, each image was decomposed to submatrices as explained in Section 2.2. A set of features using relations (3) and (4) was calculated using submatrices, and then normalized as described in Section 3.1. Submatrices of the first and second levels of decomposition were tested separately using GHM, CL and SA4 multiwavelets. For each set of features, the k-NN classifier was tested for k=1, 3, 5 and 7, and the error was calculated using leaving-one-out technique. Tables 1-3 show the error rates before and after using weight vectors. In these tables, r.r. and c.s. show repeated row and critically sampled preprocessing, respectively.

Likewise because of similar results, we evaluated the effect of noise for only these three multiwavelets. The results of noise effect are given in Tables 1-3. These results are the average of error for 10 realization of Guassian noise. The results are rounded. We can see that the first level of decomposition is very sensitive to noise and should be avoided for feature extraction. This also helps for noise reduction. Furthermore for the first level of decomposition, critically sampled preprocessing leads to more errors compared to repeated row technique. This is because critically sampled preprocessing creates a compact form, so the coefficients resulted from signal in first level of decomposition are small compared to noise. As a result the SNR in this level is low, leading to a higher noise sensitivity.

As we see, for the second level of decomposition, critically sampled preprocessing has lower sensitivity to noise compared to repeated row preprocessing. This is also due to compact form that critically sampled technique can produce. This leads to higher energy and higher SNR at low resolutions and resulting in sensitivity to noise.

To compare different multiwavelets, we calculated the errors for the second level of decomposition using 10 different of multiwavelets with critically sampled preprocessing[1] and leaving-one-out technique to calculate the error rate. The results are graphed in Fig. 6. The results show that the multiwavelet basis determines the classification accuracy. As shown in Fig. 6, SA4 multiwavelet shows better results compared to other multiwavelets. Note that for high k's the error

---

[1] As described in Appendix, cardinal multiwavelets (CardBal2, CardBal3, CardBal4) do not need preprocessing step.

grows rapidly. This is because of the number of data points is small compared to the number of classes. This causes that in the feature space there are not enough neighbors for an image with the same class.

5. CONCLUSIONS

We proposed a method for grading the pathological images of prostate. The color image is converted to black and white and then decomposed to multiwavelet submatrices. For each submatrix, the energy and entropy features are calculated and then normalized. Weight vectors are exerted and classification is done using k-NN classifier. The weight vectors are found using Simulated Annealing algorithm. This study demonstrates that energy and entropy features drived from multiwavelet transform can result in accurate classification and discrimination of various cancer grades in pathological images of prostate. It was shown that the multiwavelet basis affects the classification. The second level of decomposition has less sensitivity to noise. Because in this level the SNR is more than the first level. Furthermore for second level of decomposition, critically sampled preprocessing leads to less sensitivity compared to repeated row preprocessing. This is because critically sampled preprocessing creates better compactness.

One of the drawbacks of multiwavelets in feature extraction is the large number of produced features. Coarser resolutions may have important information, but with higher decomposition levels, the number of submatrices grows rapidly. In future studies, we are planning to reduce the dimention of the feature space.

Table 1. Error rates for first and second levels of decomposition using GHM multiwavelet.

		1st level				2nd level			
	k	1	3	5	7	1	3	5	7
r.r.	Without Weight	20	28	31	40	16	22	28	25
	With Weight	13	16	22	28	14	17	20	20
	With Noise	26	28	27	36	33	31	30	36
c.s.	Without Weight	12	12	17	22	11	12	18	26
	With Weight	8	9	13	18	6	9	14	20
	With Noise	43	51	34	34	11	14	16	21

Table 2. Error rates for first and second levels of decomposition using CL multiwavelet.

		1st level				2nd level			
	k	1	3	5	7	1	3	5	7
r.r.	Without Weight	17	27	32	35	10	18	17	24
	With Weight	13	18	20	27	8	11	13	16
	With Noise	30	29	30	37	20	18	18	26
c.s.	Without Weight	11	11	15	19	11	12	14	26
	With Weight	7	9	13	15	6	10	12	19
	With Noise	36	43	34	41	11	12	15	25

Table 3. Error rates for first and second levels of decomposition using SA4 multiwavelet.

		1st level				2nd level			
	k	1	3	5	7	1	3	5	7
r.r.	Without Weight	17	23	26	27	16	22	29	29
	With Weight	11	15	19	18	15	17	19	24
	With Noise	25	34	36	34	53	44	55	57
c.s.	Without Weight	10	10	16	18	9	11	15	25
	With Weight	5	6	11	14	3	7	10	17
	With Noise	77	73	73	84	5	11	11	21

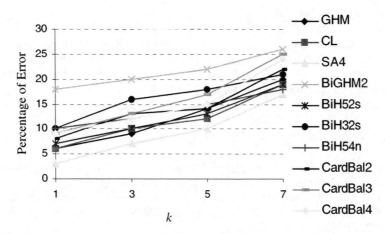

Figure 6. Comparison of error results, using different multiwavelet transforms. The features were extracted using second level of decomposition and critically sampled preprocessing.

6. APPENDIX

1) GHM: This multiwavelet was introduced by Geronimo, Hardin and Massopust. Both scaling functions are symmetric and multiwavelet functions are symmetric-antisymmetric.[19] It has approximation order of 2.
2) CL: This multiwavelet was introduced by Chui and Lian[20] and has approximation order of 2.
3) SA4: Shen *et al.*, showed how to create symmetric-antisymmetric orthonormal multiwavelets from orthonormal scalar wavelets.[21] Then they obtained the SA4 multiwavelet with length 2 from Daubechies scalar wavelets with length 4.
4) BiGHM2: This is a biorthogonal multiwavelet with length 2. Strela suggested a method to design biorthogonal multiwavelets with desired approximation order from ordinary multiwavelets.[22] BiGHM2 multiwavelet was made from GHM multiwavelet using this method.
5) BiH52s: This is a symmetric-antisymmetric biorthogonal multiwavelet with length 5 and approximation order of 2. It was proposed by Turcajova using Hermite splines.[23]
6) BiH32s: This multiwavelet is the dual of BiH52s.[23]
7) BiH54n: This is a biorthogonal multiwavelet with length of 5 and approximation order of 4. It can be obtained with the same proposed method in reference[22] but starting with Hermite multiwavelet.[23]
8) CardBal2: Cardinal multiwavelets were introduced to avoid the prefiltering step in multiwavelet computations.[24] Multiwavelet bases, for which the zero moment properties carry over to the discrete-time filter bank, are called balanced.[25] CardBal2 is a cardinal balanced multiwavelet introduced in reference[26] with length of 6 and approximation order of 2.
9) CardBal3: Cardinal balanced multiwavelet with length 8 and approximation order of 3 introduced in reference.[26]
10) CardBal4: Cardinal balanced multiwavelet with length 12 and approximation order of 4 introduced in reference.[26]

REFERENCES

1. Kumar, Cotran, Robbins, *Basic Pathology*, W.B. saunders company, 1997.
2. J. Rosai, L.V. Ackerman, *Ackerman's Surgical Pathology*, Mosby Inc., 1996.
3. E. Gose, R. Johnsonbaugh, and S. Jost, *Pattern Recognition and Image Analysis*, Prentice Hall, 1996.
4. Stotzka R., Männer R., Bartels P.H., and Thompson D. "A hybrid neural and statistical classifier system for histo-pathologic grading of prostate lesions," in *Analytical and Quantitative Cytology and Histology*, **17(3)**, pp. 204-218, 1995.
5. F. Arman, and J.A. Pearce, "Unsupervised classification of cell images using pyramid node linking," *IEEE Trans. Biomed. Eng.*, **37(6)**, pp. 647-650, June 1990.

6. H. D. Cheng, C. H. Chen, and R. I. Freimanis, "A neural network for breast cancer detection using fuzzy entropy approach," in *Proc. Int. Conf. Image Processing*, **3**, pp. 141-144, 1995.

7. S. M. Marroquin, C. Vos, E. Santamaria, X. Jove, and J.C. Socoro, "Non linear image analysis for fuzzy classification of breast cancer," in *Proc. Int. Conf. Image Processing*, **2**, pp. 943-946, 1996.

8. F. Schnorrenberg, C. S. Pattichis, K. C. Kyriakou, and C. N. Schizas, "Computer-aided detection of breast cancer nuclei," *IEEE Trans. Infor. Tech. in Biomed.*, **1(2)**, pp. 128-140, June 1997.

9. E. M. Marroquin, E. Santamaria, X. Jove, and J. C. Socoro, "Morphological analysis of mammary biopsy images," in *Electrotechnical Conf., 1996. MELECON '96., 8th Meditarranean*, **2**, pp. 1067-1070.

10. G. Van de Wouwer, "Wavelet for Multiscale Texture Analysis," *Ph.D. Thesis*, University of Antwerpen, Dept. Natuurkunde, 1998.

11. J. S. Hallinan, "Detection of malignancy associated changes in cervical cells using statistical and evolutionary computation techniques," *Ph.D. thesis, The University of Queensland, Australia*, 1999.

12. B. Weyn, G. V. Wouwer, Samir Knmar-Singh, A. Van Daele, Paul Scheunders, Eric Van Marck, and Willem Jacob, "Computer-assisted differential diagnosis of malignant mesothelioma based on syntactic structure analysis", Cytometry, **35**, pp. 23-29, 1999.

13. A. N. Esgiar, R. N. G. Naguib, B. S. Sharif, M. K. Bennett, and A. Murray, "Microscopic image analysis for quantitative measurement and feature identification of normal and cancerous colonic mucosa", *IEEE Trans. on Information Technology in Biomedicine*, **2(3)**, pp. 197-203, 1998.

14. V. Strela, P. Heller, G. Strang, P. Topiwala, and C. Heil, "The application of multiwavelet filter banks to signal and image processing," *IEEE Trans. Image Processing*, **8(4)**, pp. 548-563, 1999.

15. X.G. Xia, J.S. Geronimo, D.P. Hardin, and B.W. Suter, "Design of prefilters for discrete multiwavelet transforms," *IEEE Trans. Signal Processing*, **44**, pp. 25-35, 1996.

16. D.P. Hardin and D.W. Roach, "Multiwavelet prefilters I: Orthogonal prefilters preserving approximation order p<=2," *IEEE Trans. Circuits and Systems*, **45(8)**, pp. 1106-1112, Aug. 1998.

17. V. Strela and A. T. Walden, "Signal and image denoising via wavelet thresholding: Orthogonal and biorthogonal, scalar and multiple wavelet transforms," *Imperial College, Statistics Section, Technical Report* TR-98-01, 1998

18. P.J.M. van Laarhoven and E.H.L. Aarts, *Simulated Annealing: Theory and Applications*, Kluwer Academic Publishers, 1987.

19. J.S. Geronimo, D.P. Hardin, and P.R. Massopust, "Fractal functions and wavelet expansions based on several functions," *J. Approx. Theory*, **78(3)**, pp. 373-401, 1994.

20. C.K. Chui and J.A. Lian, "A study of orthonormal multiwavelets," *Appl. Numer. Math.*, vol. 20, pp. 273-298, 1995.

21. L.-X. Shen, H.H. Tan, and J.Y. Tham, "Symmetric-antisymmetric orthonormal multiwavelets and related scalar wavelets," *Applied and Computational Harmonic Analysis (ACHA)*, **8(3)**, pp. 258-279, May 2000.

22. V. Strela, "A note on construction of biorthogonal multi-scaling functions," in *Contemporary Mathematics*, A. Aldroubi and E. B. Lin (eds.), pp.149-157, AMS, 1998.

23. R. Turcajova, "Hermite spline multiwavelets for image modeling," Wavelet applications V, Orlando, FL, *SPIE Proc.*, **3391**, pp. 46-56, April 1998.

24. I.W. Selesnick, "Interpolating multiwavelet bases and the sampling theorem," *IEEE Trans. Signal Processing*, **47(6)**, pp. 1615-1621, June 1999.

25. I.W. Selesnick, "Cardinal multiwavelets and the sampling theorem," In *Proc. of IEEE Int. Conf. Acoustics, Speech, and Signal Processing*, **3**, pp. 1209 -1212, 1999.

26. J. Lebrun, M. Vetterli, "Balanced multiwavelets Theory and design," *IEEE Trans. Signal Processing*, **46(4)**, pp.1119-1124, April 1998.

Soft Parametric Curve Matching in Scale-Space

Brian Avants[1] and James Gee[1,2]

Departments of Bioengineering[1] and Radiology[2]

University of Pennsylvania

Philadelphia, PA 19104-6389

ABSTRACT

We develop a softassign method for application to curve matching. Softassign uses deterministic annealing to iteratively optimize the parameters of an energy function. It also incorporates outlier rejection by converting the energy into a stochastic matrix with entries for rejection probability. Previous applications of the method focused on finding transformations between unordered point sets. Thus, no topological constraints were required. In our application, we must consider the topology of the matching between the reference and the target curve. Our energy function also depends upon the rotation and scaling between the curves. Thus, we develop a topologically correct algorithm to update the arc length correspondence, which is then used to update the similarity transformation. We further enhance robustness by using a scale-space description of the curves. This results in a curve-matching tool that, given an approximate initialization, is invariant to similarity transformations. We demonstrate the reliability of the technique by applying it to open and closed curves extracted from real patient images (cortical sulci in three dimensions and corpora callosa in two dimensions). The set of transformations is then used to compute anatomical atlases.

Keywords: curve matching, non-linear deformations, anatomical atlases, deterministic annealing, softassign, dynamic programming

1. INTRODUCTION

Curve matching[1] has important applications in the medical domain. In particular, non-rigid correspondences are needed to compensate for the dynamics of development, disease and motion in the human body. Such results may be used to perform statistical shape analysis,[2] to gain insights into time series data,[3] in clinical tracking of patient motion[4] and as initialization for algorithms which register surfaces or volumes.[5] Curve matching is also useful in computer aided surgery and for registration between imaging modalities where only structural borders may contain shared information. The increasing availability of images in large databases further motivates these methods as non-lexical search strategies.

Matching is particularly useful in generating anatomical atlases from datasets that are too large or complex to handle manually.[6,7] A good atlas may be used to guide the analysis of new data, to study the statistics of shape over populations, for medical instruction and possibly to assist in quantitative diagnosis.[8] Thus, it is important for biological matching algorithms to be both highly reliable and amenable to atlas computation. The authors in Ref 2 point out that a hallmark of good matching is that it allows a sparse "minimum description length" representation of the training set. They use principal components analysis to define this representation.

Previous work has approached the problem with image registration, pattern matching, as well as purely geometric methods. We are concerned with the latter, which use properties intrinsic to the curve geometry to guide the matching. We believe this is particularly important in the medical domain where the shape descriptions themselves may benefit diagnosis and where intensity methods often fail to align important anatomical features. Geometric techniques work, typically, either through feature matching or dense parametric matching. Feature methods focus on some organization of curve attributes, while parametric methods attempt to minimize a variational energy function. Matching based on curve parameterizations lends itself naturally to atlas generation as pairings of arc lengths can be used directly and unambiguously to generate anatomical atlases.[6,9]

Feature matching is used successfully on articulated shapes,[10] in dealing with occlusion[11] as well as on biological data.[12] These methods, though very different in detail, rely on a small set of features through which

---

For correspondence, e-mail: {avants,gee}@grasp.cis.upenn.edu

shapes are compared. Developing a full curve atlas from sparsely distributed points is not straightforward, perhaps requiring optimization of landmark positions or another interpolation step.

Pure parametric matching eliminates these issues by optimizing the match over the full domain of the data. Many methods have used functionals based on bending and stretching energy which can be optimized in a small window of comparison along arcs.[7, 13] In this case, however, no global information about curve similarities is used. In addition, as noted in Ref 8, matching patterns of curvature, rather than specific values, is more biologically meaningful. Other methods impose smoothness of the transformation between reference and target without taking any account of noise. The finite-element technique provided in Ref 4 relies on a smooth deformation field to find a match, thus penalizing sudden deletion of segments, which may be necessary when dealing with noisy data or matching normal and atrophied anatomy. The approach used by Ref 2 define parametric matchings but their methods are somewhat heuristic and it is not clear what kind of energy minimizing properties they have. We will address these issues by using energy function smoothing and by allowing outlier rejection.

Formulation of the parametric matching problem can be quite elegant. The basic requirements for good match functionals and a theoretical framework are well-defined in Refs 14, 15. However, the theory does not always translate algorithmically, requiring approximations to be made. An iterative hierarchical approach is used in Ref 14 to make some difficult problems tractable. However, no extension to higher than two dimensions has been given, nor is it clear how noise might effect the procedure.

Softassign matching[16] provides a flexible framework with outlier rejection for robustness to noise. The method was initially designed for rigid matchings of unordered point sets. Recently, it was extended to provide thin-plate spline matchings[17] and shown to out-perform iterative closest point (ICP) in the examples given. Issues of topology (e.g. self-intersection) are not dealt with though, and may be induced by the thin-plate spline. The method performs a coarse to fine scale match, but it does so implicitly without clearly defining the nature of the smoothing, which is likely non-linear and apt to create artificial features. Nor is it stated how to extract a match explicit from the possibly real valued match matrix.

It follows from the discussion above that parametric methods may need to delete or truncate curve segments to work robustly with noisy data or data from diseased patients. The method should also incorporate some global notion of the curves and insure topological correctness. If this is not accounted for, possibly large segments of reference curve will be mismatched whenever occlusion, noise or anatomic deterioration is present in the target. We will address some of these issues with respect to curve matching, focusing especially on the correctness of the match function, natural smoothing and also robustness.

2. SOFT PARAMETRIC CURVE MATCHING

Our model of the matching problem builds on the above mentioned work and naturally fuses a hierarchical curve description and parametric matching, while allowing controlled rejection of noisy data. The method is an iterative process which is invariant to similarity transformation. We alternate optimization of the parametric matching and the rigid transformation between target and reference curves. The framework given will be probabilistic, which will lead to some unexpected side benefits in the analysis. This amounts to a novel method for regularizing the linear and non-linear transformations on which parametric curve matching is based.

2.1. Curves and Reparameterization

We assume the data is given to us in the form of an ordered point set. We desire a continuous curve model for the discrete data so that we have $C: s \in \tau \to \mathbb{R}^d$ where τ is the closed interval $[0, 1]$ and s denotes the (arc-length) parameter. In practice, we use a spline to obtain this parameterization as well as derivative information.[18] In matrix form, we have

$$C(s) = BX, \tag{1}$$

where B is the $1 \times p$ vector of basis functions and X is the $p \times d$ matrix of control vectors with $p - 1$ the degree of the spline. This allows us to reparametrize the curves at any time and choose either B-spline (for approximation) or Hermite basis functions (for interpolation.) If the points are unordered, methods exist for obtaining error minimizing ordered (sub)sets of the original points for use as control vectors.[19]

Given a pair of such curves, (C_1, C_2), we want to find a reparameterization such that the pair is better aligned with respect to some cost. We define the reparameterization curve $g: \xi \in [0, 1] \to \tau \times \tau$ with L the length of g. We then have $g(\xi) = (s_1(\xi), s_2(\xi))$ which is a pairing of curve parameters for (C_1, C_2). We will suppress the dependence of s on ξ from here except where necessary. We require that topology should also be preserved by reparameterization. That is, if a curve does not self intersect, no self intersections should be created (for example, by a reordering of the points.) For this reason, the space of permissible reparameterizations requires that g is monotonic; its first derivative does not change sign. The identity reparameterization simply pairs every value with itself so $g_I(\xi_I) = (s, s)$ with subscript I denoting the identity. This is also the shortest possible curve linking the points $(0, 0)$ and $(1, 1)$ in $\tau \times \tau$.

The derivative of g will give us the rate of reparameterization. We will use this later as a penalty term in our energy function. We have

$$\frac{dg}{d\xi} = \left(\frac{ds_1}{d\xi}, \frac{ds_2}{d\xi}\right). \tag{2}$$

We can write the length of g using its first derivative,[23] to find

$$L = \int_0^1 \sqrt{(s_1')^2 + (s_2')^2} d\xi. \tag{3}$$

We recall that the identity provides the shortest path in the reparameterization space. Any deviation from this will result in $L > L_I$ where L_I is the length of the identity curve. Thus, we can penalize non-identity parameterizations by penalizing the incremental length of g. This can also be used as a measure of "stretching", that is, the extent to which the reparameterization is compressing one arc length relative to the other. The length of g is also a metric of the parameterization deformation needed to align curves. This may prove a useful index for ranking curve similarities.

The approach given here addresses the issue of reparameterization curve symmetry dealt with previously by other authors.[7, 20] We prefer our formulation over those that use a diffeomorphism[21] because of its simplicity and direct geometric nature. Additionally, it is unbiased to the choice of reference and target when used in matching. This is in contrast to the asymmetry that arises when g is defined as $g: s_1 \to s_2$ (as the derivative is undefined when $ds_1 = 0$). With our approach, asymmetry is not an issue due to the arbitrariness for ordering s_1 and s_2. We also apply g to the curve pair in an unbiased way to creating the reparametrized curve pair,

$$g: (\, C_1(s_1), C_2(s_2) \,) \to (\, C_1 \circ (g(\xi) \cdot (1, 0)), C_2 \circ (g(\xi) \cdot (0, 1)) \,). \tag{4}$$

We will denote the reparameterization as $C(g)$ or $C \circ g$ for either curve. New reparameterizations can be found by composing sets of g_i so

$$g_n = g_0 \circ g_1 \circ \cdots \circ g_{n-1}. \tag{5}$$

This operation can be thought of, in discrete form, as a matrix-vector multiplication. An example of a reparameterization based matching and a symmetric match function is found in Figure 1.

2.2. Reparameterization Energy Function

We view the curve matching problem in terms of finding g that minimizes an energy or cost function, E, by optimally aligning a pair of curves,

$$g = argmin\ E(C_1, C_2, g). \tag{6}$$

If C_2 is geometrically equivalent to C_1, then g captures the translational difference in parameterizations. If the curves are not geometrically equivalent, but are similar, then g will be a reparameterization that brings the features measured by the energy function into minimum energy correspondence. There are a number of well known energy functions for curve matching.[4, 7–9, 14, 22] We choose one that combines aspects of functionals in previous work and that will illustrate the benefits of our approach,

$$E(g) = \int \left(w_1 \|g'\|^2 + w_2 \|R(C_1 \circ g(\xi))' - (C_2 \circ g(\xi))'\|^2 + w_3(\kappa_1 \circ g(\xi) - \kappa_2 \circ g(\xi))^2\right) d\xi. \tag{7}$$

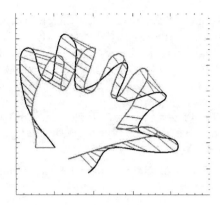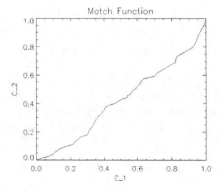

Figure 1. The simulated hand correspondence is reasonable despite a bad initialization. The associated symmetric match function is on the right.

The first term penalizes stretching of the parameterizations, the second term penalizes differences in the tangents (after rotation R) and the third term penalizes differences in curvature. Recall that curvature is invariant to rotation and translation and the tangents are invariant to translation and scale.[23] Thus, the term R should provide an estimate to the optimal rotation and scaling. The w_i are weights.

In $\mathbb{R}^d$, this matching implies a physical transformation that can be decomposed into,

$$T(X) = R(X) + V(X),\tag{8}$$

where R is a linear transformation and $V(X)$ is non-linear. Either might be the identity element. We will use R as a similarity or rigid transformation and V as a non-linear vector field acting on $R(X)$.

2.3. Scale-space

We intend to alternate calculations of V and R in a coarse to fine fashion. Thus, we need to process our data at multiple scales. The scale-space method, based on Gaussian filtering, provides the most natural way to do this.[24, 25] Properties of Gaussian filtering are well documented,[26] and often used for evolving digital signals through scale. The main advantage of the Gaussian kernel is that no new inflection points are created as the curve is filtered. In addition, features of different sizes will eventually be smoothed away. The scale at which a feature disappears is known as its characteristic scale and is linked to the size or visual importance of the feature. Thus, scale-space combined with an iterative process allows us to focus on matching the most salient features first, worrying about matching finer details later. We denote C at scale σ,

$$C(\sigma) = C \star G_\sigma,\tag{9}$$

where $\star$ denotes convolution and σ is the square root of the continuous scale parameter (or standard deviation). The traditional Gaussian kernel is represented by G. Our goal is to incorporate this scale-space evolution of curves with softassign.

2.4. Deterministic Annealing

The idea in deterministic annealing,[27] and softassign,[16] is to map a non-convex energy function into a smoother probability-based energy space using the principles of statistical physics. Using the physical analogy with annealing (heating and cooling a material to increase its stability) as justification, we formulate an energy of the following form,

$$E_{DA}(g) = \int \Pr(g(\xi))\big(E(C_1, C_2, g) + T \ln \Pr(g(\xi))\big)d\xi,\tag{10}$$

where T is a temperature parameter controlling the free energy. The term $E(\cdot)$ is the cost function we want to anneal. The probability term, $\Pr(g)\ln\Pr(g)$, is the entropy of the distribution, which is as yet unknown. The integral is over a path through the $s_1 \times s_2$ space of arc length pairings. This is also the space over which the probability functions lie. Thus, we hope to maximize the probability of this path in order to smoothly minimize the energy E. This will be accomplished by beginning with a high temperature, estimating the parameters of the energy function and reducing the temperature (and free energy) deterministically. We repeat this until $\mathcal{T} \to 0$ which gives the full resolution of the energy function.

We want to find the minimum of this function first with respect to Pr,

$$\frac{\partial E_{DA}}{\partial \text{Pr}} = E(C_1, C_2, g) + \mathcal{T} \ln \text{Pr}(g) + \mathcal{T}, \tag{11}$$

Setting this equal to zero and solving for Pr (dropping the constant) we find,

$$\text{Pr}(g(\xi)) = exp\left(-\frac{E(C_1, C_2, g)}{\mathcal{T}}\right). \tag{12}$$

Recall that $g(\xi) = (s_1, s_2)$ and so $\text{Pr}(g(\xi)) = \text{Pr}((s_1, s_2))$. We want to enforce that each $\text{Pr}((s_1, s_2))$ is a member of the family of Gibbs distributions, as these are maximally robust with respect to noise.[27] It is possible to impose the Gibbs distribution on this probability by normalizing it. That is, we want to impose that the probability of all s_2 in the pair $\text{Pr}(s_1, s_2)$ is such that,

$$\text{Pr}((s_1, s_2)) = \frac{exp\left(-\frac{E(C_1,C_2,g)}{\mathcal{T}}\right)}{\int exp\left(-\frac{E(C_1,C_2,g)}{\mathcal{T}}\right) ds_2} \tag{13}$$

and likewise for s_1. Sinkhorn's method (discussed below) accomplishes this in the discrete case when the probability matrix is square. This is equivalent to using Lagrange multipliers[16] with a penalty term in the energy function E_{DA}.

This method of normalization enforces probability constraints written, without outliers,

$$\int \text{Pr}((s_2, s_1)) \left(\int \text{Pr}((s_1, s_2)) ds_1\right) ds_2 = 1. \tag{14}$$

If we want to incorporate outlier probability, we have

$$\int_0^{1+\epsilon} \text{Pr}((s_1, s_2)) ds_1 = 1. \tag{15}$$

The same is done for s_2. The constant ϵ can be thought of as the tail of the probability function corresponding to outlier likelihood. If $\text{Pr}((s_1, s_2))$ is maximal with respect to s_1 when $s_1 > 1$, then the specific arc length value s_1 is considered to have no likely match. It is rejected as an outlier.

We now see that g defines a path through a series of Gibbs distributions, each of which is derived from the cost of pairing a fixed s_1 to all possible partners, s_2. Thus, if $g(0)$ is $(0,0)$ and $g(L)$ corresponds to the arc length pair $(1, 1)$, we have a path in both spaces $E: \tau \times \tau \to \mathbb{R}^+$ and $\text{Pr}: \tau \times \tau \to [0,1]$. We intend this path to be of maximal probability for a given temperature. It therefore gives us a solution to a smoothed version of E. Note, however, that the map between $E \in \mathbb{R}^+$ and $\text{Pr} \in [0,1]$ is surjective but not injective. To see this, consider the case where for some s_1^1 and some other s_1^2, $E(C_1, C_2, (s_1^1, s_2)) = \gamma E(C_1, C_2, (s_1^1, s_2))$ for all $s_2 \in [0,1]$, where γ is a constant. Then the probability map results in $\text{Pr}(s_1^1, s_2) = \text{Pr}(s_1^2, s_2)$ and we cannot recover E.

In the discrete domain, Pr is represented as a probability matrix M, so that $\text{Pr}(s_1, s_2) = M(i, j) = M_{ij}$. Given that we have computed the exponential of the energy, the constraints on this match matrix must now be enforced. We use Sinkhorn's algorithm, which we iterate until convergence. Outlier columns are not normalized themselves, though their values are included in the normalization of other rows. That is, for each row $i \in \{1, \cdots, m\}$, and column $j \in \{1, \cdots, n\}$,

$$\hat{M}_{ij}^{t+1} = \frac{M_{ij}^t}{\sum_{j=1}^{n+1} M_{ij}^t}, \quad \hat{M}_{ij}^{t+2} = \frac{M_{ij}^{t+1}}{\sum_{i=1}^{m+1} M_{ij}^{t+1}}. \tag{16}$$

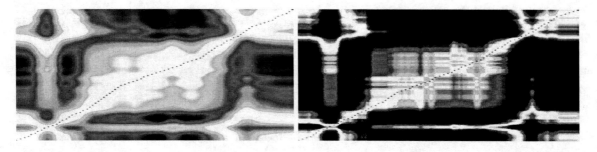

Figure 2: The path through the probability matrix, M, at consecutive temperatures. The path is the dotted line.

The normalized rows are denoted $\hat{M}^{t+1}$ and the normalized columns are $\hat{M}^{t+2}$ where t is the step of the iteration. If $n = m$, this procedure converges to a doubly stochastic match matrix (each row and each column sums to one.) If $n \neq m$, this is not possible. Let r_i denote the sum of row i, c_j the sum of column j and μ the sum of all matrix entries M_{ij}. If $\sum_i r_i = \mu$ and all $r_i = 1$ then $\mu = m$. If also $\sum_j c_j = \mu$ and all $c_j = 1$ then $\mu = n$. This is a contradiction unless $n = m$. Thus, if the matrix is rectangular, either the sum of all $r_i = m$, $\mu = m$ and the c_j are not normalized or the sum of all $c_j = n$, $\mu = n$ and the r_i are not normalized.

It is not possible to enforce probability constraints on a rectangular matrix. We can remedy this situation, if necessary, by sampling the curves such that the number of points is always equal. A single application of the reparameterization curve, g, will accomplish this. However, this is not always necessary. One may also normalize with respect to the rows or columns that correspond to the reference curve. This ensures that $P((s_1, s_2))$ is always a true probability. Another option is to use a constant arc length parameterization with a fixed sampling of τ. Fast approximations to this can be found.[18]

We can now extract an optimal correspondence from the matrix M, enabling the analytical computation of the transformation, T. One way to estimate the matched curve pair is to simply perform the matrix multiplication.[17] This gives us the suboptimal pair $(C_1, M \cdot C_2)$. This is suboptimal because any match fuzziness will result in an averaging of the points on C_2. This effect may be unimportant or even appear desirable in some cases, but it is not clear what kind of scaling is being done. It is possible that spurious features may be generated and that the topology of the curve not respected. This issue is not a problem, in our experience, when computing rigid transformations of unordered point sets as in Ref 16, but degrades performance of curve matching. Therefore, we give an optimal and topologically correct method for extracting the correspondence g at each step of the algorithm. The energy smoothness caused by the annealing process is shown in Figure 4.

2.5. Curve Matching Energy and Dynamic Programming

We assume that we have rejected outliers by thresholding.[16] We are now prepared to find an optimal reparameterization curve. We incorporate scale-space with (7) to give the energy we minimize,

$$E(g) = \int \left(w_1 \|g'\|^2 + w_2 \|R(C_1(\sigma_1) \circ g(\xi))' - (C_2(\sigma_2) \circ g(\xi))'\|^2 + w_3(\kappa_1(\sigma_1) \circ g(\xi) - \kappa_2(\sigma_2) \circ g(\xi))^2 \right) d\xi. \quad (17)$$

The associated probability is then given by (12) and (14). We will locate from within the match matrix, a monotonic path maximizing the Gibbs probabilities derived from this energy,

$$g = argmax \, \Pr((s_1^f, s_2^f)). \quad (18)$$

The pair (s_1^f, s_2^f) denotes the final state of g, i.e. its endpoint. We assume the start state is given, then g is the path that connects them.

Dynamic programming is a useful tool for solving problems of path optimization.[28] Dynamic programming relies on a problem's 'optimal substructure,' the property that, at each step, the optimal solution can be found.

For example, optimal substructure exists for the discrete shortest path problem. This is because the triangle inequality holds for Euclidean distance,

$$d(x, z) \leq d(x, y) + d(y, z). \tag{19}$$

The recursive solution for this problem is then given by,

$$\mathcal{C}(i) = \min_j \{c(i, j) + \mathcal{C}(j)\}, \tag{20}$$

where $\mathcal{C}$ is a cumulative optimal cost and c are the known distances between neighbors. Here, $\mathcal{C}(j)$ has already been computed and we are finding $\mathcal{C}(i)$. For example, given a graph with nodes N, we compute at each step,

$$\mathcal{C}(N_n) = \min\{c(N_n, N_{n-1}) + \mathcal{C}(N_{n-1}), \cdots, c(N_n, N_1) + \mathcal{C}(N_1)\}, \tag{21}$$

where each N_i is a node with $c(\cdot, \cdot) = \infty$ if N_n is not reachable and finite otherwise.

The problem of (18) can be formulated in terms of transition probabilities to yield the Viterbi algorithm,[29]

$$P(i) = \max_j \{p(i, j) P(j)\}, \tag{22}$$

where p denotes a transition probability and P denotes a cumulative (path) probability. Noting that maximizing the product of probabilities is equivalent to minimizing the sum of minus log-likelihoods, we have

$$-\ln P(i) = \min_j \{-\ln p(i, j) - \ln P(j)\}. \tag{23}$$

If we identify $\ln P = -\mathcal{C}$ and $\ln p = -c$, this is identical to the shortest path problem for which efficient $N log(N)$ algorithms are known, e.g., Dijkstra's algorithm implemented with a priority queue.

We can now solve (18) in terms of dynamic programming.

$$-\ln \Pr(g(L)) = \min_j \{-\ln pr((s_1^f, s_2^f), (s_1^j, s_2^j)) - \ln \Pr((s_1^j, s_2^j))\}, \tag{24}$$

where $g(L) = (s_1^f, s_2^f)$, recalling L denotes the total length of g. Here, pr denotes the transition probability and $\Pr$ the total probability at (s_1^j, s_2^j). The set of allowable transitions is selected such that only permissible reparameterization curves are allowed.[7] These methods can be shown to return globally optimal, though not necessarily unique solutions (different paths may have the same cost).[28] The path, g, is recovered by backtracking along the locally optimal choices. Figure 2 shows a path through the probability matrix.

2.6. Algorithm

The full algorithm is summarized in Algorithm 1. The states of the algorithm in the case of two closed planar curves are shown in Figure 3.

The initialization sets all the parameters of the algorithm. In general, it is enough to choose the initial scale, σ_0, with respect to the arc length parameter. Depending on the expected noise of the curve, we choose values between 0.25 and 1.0. We also use the scale-space parameter to set the value of the temperature, such that $\mathcal{T} = c \sigma$ where c is a constant. Then the annealing rate and the (usually dyadic) scale-space rate are the same. We choose c in accord with the amount of regularization we need for the problem; often it is one. Conveniently, this leads to a desireable trajectory through the energy space as shown in Figure 4. The only other initialization step is to find the minimum energy translation. This amounts to shifting the parameterization linearly until the energy of (7) is minimal. In addition, one must also choose a starting point for the matching. If the curves are closed, we choose the point with minimum energy under translation. This point becomes both the start and end of the match function at that iteration. If the curves are open, then we simply match the beginnings and the ends of the curves.

Algorithm 1 *Scale-space soft parametric curve matching*

Initialize M with outlier values ϵ, linear transformation R as identity, σ as the starting scale, σ_f as the final scale, $\mathcal{T}$ as the start temperature, and $\Delta\mathcal{T}$, $\Delta\sigma$ as the annealing and scale-space rates. Also initialize g with minimum energy arc-length translation, t,

$$g_{init} = g_I + \min_t E(C_1, C_2, g_I + t). \qquad (25)$$

We find the minimal energy t by parametric search.

> **while** $\sigma \geq \sigma_f$ **do**
> 0. $C_1^k \Leftarrow R(C_1) \star \sigma$ apply R and scale-space to C_1
> 1. $C_2^k \Leftarrow C_2 \star \sigma$ apply scale-space to C_2
> 2. Compute E given g Equation 17
> 3. $M \Leftarrow exp(-E/\mathcal{T})$ Equation 12
> 4. $Sinkhorn(M)$ Equation 16
> 5. $g_i = ExtractMatch(M)$ Equation 24
> 6. $g \Leftarrow g \circ g_i$ Equation 5
> 7. Update R gradient descent
> 8. $\sigma \Leftarrow \sigma * \Delta\sigma$ change scale space parameter
> 9. $\mathcal{T} \Leftarrow \mathcal{T} * \Delta\mathcal{T}$ anneal
> 10. find minimum translation, t.   Equation 25
> 11. reparametrize C_2 by g; set $g = g_I$ (optional).
> **end while**

The procedure *ExtractMatch* is the dynamic programming step and assumes outliers have been rejected (that is, removed from the point set.) Because *ExtractMatch* gives an optimal solution for each temperature, we do not have to force the correspondence matrix to be binary. We can choose to find, use and compare solutions at any temperature.

The steps zero to nine are exactly the equations referenced in the comments. Step ten points out that it is sometimes advantageous to estimate a new optimal translation (and starting point) for the matching at each iteration. Similarly, step 11 provides another option for the matching, which we have used. We will now discuss step seven in more detail.

Subsequent to estimating the correspondence, we update the transformation, R. We then return to the energy computation step. In our example of the similarity transformation, R, we initialize using the method given in Ref 30. A least squares estimate with the singular-value decomposition is used to compute the optimal rotation. The scaling is then found from the points' covariance matrix. In addition, reflections are preventable. Another method, based on Fourier transformations, is given in Ref 31. After a few iterations of the least squares method, we then update R at each step with a conjugate gradient method.

One advantage of using this probabilistic formulation is that at each point $g(\xi)$ on the reparameterization curve, we have an estimate of the uncertainty of the match with respect to s_1 and also s_2 if the matrix is square. We can characterize the uncertainty by fitting a Gaussian to the local distribution. Then the full width at half maximum provides a measure of the match resolution. However, this uncertainty is dependent upon the free energy of the final solution and only has relative meaning. That is, it reveals the certainty of correspondences along g relative to each other. This is a subject of further investigation. We have mainly used, to this point, the log of the path probability, given by $\ln(\Pr(g(\xi)))$, to evaluate the certainty of correspondences along the matched curve pair. Aspects of these path probabilities are shown in Figures 2, 4 and 5.

2.7. Atlas Computation

We must now distinguish the reference and target curves. Assume C_1 is the reference and that it is optimally aligned by the linear transformation R. Given the reparameterization, g, we would like to compute a non-rigid

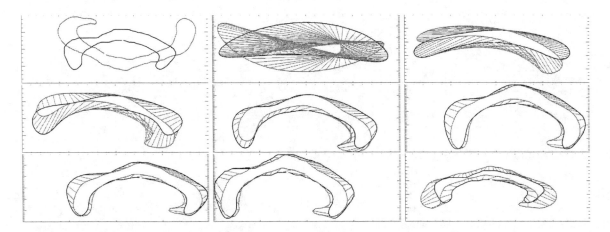

Figure 3. The states of our matching algorithm for a pair of callosa. From left to right, top to bottom, the first panel is initialization which is followed by the alignment at intermediate dyadic scales. The last panel holds the final solution at the original scale.

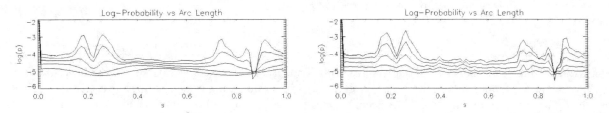

Figure 4. The trajectory of the path log-probabilities as the temperature decreases with temperature annealing and scale-space (left) and only temperature annealing (right).

vector field, $V: C_1 \rightarrow C_2$. Thus, we apply the match function g to find the matched pair (C_1, C_2). From this transformed curve we get the vector field directly, using (4),

$$V(s_1) = C_2 \circ g - C_1 \circ g. \tag{26}$$

This gives us a direct way to compute atlases. Given a set of K vector fields, V_k, taking C_1 to C_k, we can compute the average and standard deviation of these fields for every point on C_1. For example,

$$V_{avg}(s_1) = \frac{1}{K} \sum_{k=1}^{K} V_k(s_1), \tag{27}$$

noting we can assume if $C_1(s_1)$ matches $C_2(s_2)$ and $C_3(s_3)$ then $C_2(s_2)$ matches $C_3(s_3)$ because this is simply a composition of match functions as in (5). Recall, we have computed this vector field from a bending and stretching energy and after the linear transformation was applied, so we expect the curves to be exactly aligned. In addition, the transformation is decomposed into two parts, the rigid part and the non-linear part, which can be analyzed separately.

3. RESULTS

We compare the performance of the algorithm when parameters are varied and supply results from patient images.

3.1. Performance

We tested a few variations of the algorithm. We first investigated using temperature annealing without scale-space. We found that in two dimensions the results were similar to using annealing with both temperature and

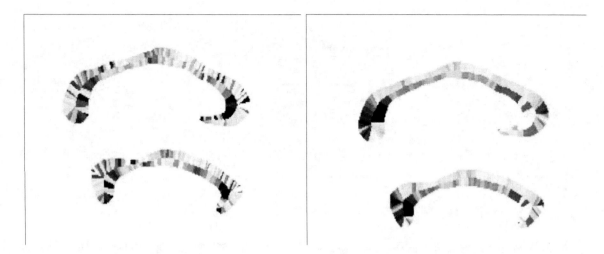

Figure 5. The path probabilities mapped to the associated area intervals. Darker colors represent higher confidence correspondences. The curve pair is the same as in Figure 3. The image on the left is a result from using curvature. The image on the right resulted from using only the first derivatives.

scale, however, the energy of the solution was generally somewhat lower. This can be expected to some extent because, when using scale-space, we actually solve a different problem at each iteration. On the other hand, in three dimensions, we found some degradation of the results when not using scale-space; that is, the energy was lower with scale-space than without. This occurred mainly because the three dimensional curves were much noisier than the planar curves. The performance of the similarity transformation suffered accordingly. This, in turn, affects the computation of the match, especially when using the first derivative term. We also tried using scale-space only, with a constant temperature. The results were significantly degraded in both two and three dimensions. This was due mainly to the noise in the unsmoothed probability matrix, which resulted in lower quality match functions. Overall, the best performance was found when using both scale-space and annealing. This was especially apparent in three dimensions. The log probability along the path resulting from the $\sigma = \mathcal{T}$ annealing schedule is shown in Figure 4. The outliers appear as probability sinks. The case of scale-space with annealing and annealing only are shown. The path probability (at higher temperature) is smoother when both are used.

We also give a result in Figure 5 illustrating performance of two different energy functions in terms of the path probabilities. We have mapped the probability along the boundary to the interior using the computed correspondence and a distance transform. Thus, each matched region is colored according to the relative confidence of the correspondence. The energy functions provided similar practical results, but the uncertainties are very different. In the case of the curvature energy, one can see that regions that have similar curvature correspond most strongly (that is, are darker in the image). The first derivative energy gives stronger correspondence in regions where curve tangents are similar and weaker similarity (and the image pair is brightly colored) where the tangents are different. Bright areas also appear when neighboring regions of the curve have similar tangents and thus "share" probability. That is, if all the neighbors have similar values, then the match is less unique. The two examples were annealed to the same temperature. To test the first derivative energy, we used the values $w_1 = 0.0$, $w_2 = 1.0$, $w_3 = 0.0$. To test the curvature energy, we chose $w_1 = 0.0$, $w_2 = 0.0$, $w_3 = 1.0$. We often use the following operating point, $w_1 = 1.0$, $w_2 = 0.1$, $w_3 = 0.9$, as we find it provides a good balance between the terms.

3.2. Patient Data

We give results of soft parametric matching on instances of real patient data as well as on a large dataset. The mid-sagittal direction of the corpus callosum was automatically segmented from MRI for each of 87 human controls matched roughly for age and handedness. Because of noise in the segmentation, we applied a small

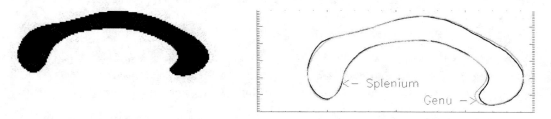

Figure 6. The average callosum computed from 87 segmented callosa is on the left. The average male and female callosa are superimposed on the right. The male has the larger genu.

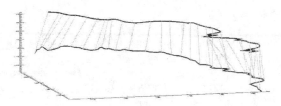

Figure 7: Match between the sylvian fissures of two different subjects.

Gaussian smoothing with constant width to all boundaries before extracting them from the binary images. No adjustments for scale were made before the algorithm was run. Curvature information was gained from a natural cubic spline fit.

Figure 6 shows the average callosa computed from this dataset with respect to an arbitrarily chosen reference. The average is of 55 female and 32 male callosa. Figure 6 also shows the average male and female callosa. One can see the splenium of the average female appears slightly larger than the average male. Figure 7 displays a sulcal curve result. The curves are drawn with a GUI on noisily segmented volumetric MRI images.

4. SUMMARY AND CONCLUSIONS

We have shown a solution to the curve correspondence problem that incorporates scale space with the softassign algorithm. We also develop a moderately unique formulation of the reparameterization problem. In addition, we have given a procedure for reliably extracting the match function from the correspondence matrix generated by softassign. This function satisfies monotonicity and symmetry. We also use the probabilistic match to show some of the properties of the algorithm and its performance. The statement of the solution is flexible and general enough that it may be adapted to find minima of a large range of energy functions. Preliminary experiments have also shown its reliability for plane and space curves, as indicated by our generation of atlas results for corpora callosa and matching of cortical sulci. In the future, we hope to perform a more thorough analysis of the energy minimizing properties of the algorithm and to approximate parametric matching on unordered point sets. We will also further investigate the usefulness of this algorithm for occlusion.

ACKNOWLEDGMENTS

This work was funded in part by the USPHS under grants NS33662, LM03504, MH62100, AG15116 and AG17586.

REFERENCES

1. Guziec A., Ayache N., "Smoothing and matching of 3D space curves," Springer-Verlag, European Conference on Computer Vision (ECCV), Santa Margherita (Italy), May 1992.

2. Davies R., Cootes T., Waterton J., Taylor C.J., "An Efficient Method for Constructing Optimal Statistical Shape Models." Medical Image Computing and Computer Assisted Intervention, 57-65, 2001.

3. Amini A., Duncan J., Pointwise tracking of left ventricular motion. Proceedings of the IEEE Workshop on Visual Motion, Princeton, NJ., 1991.

4. Cohen I., Ayache N., Sulger P., "Tracking points on deformable objects using curvature information," ECCV, 458-466, 1992.

5. Luo S., Evans A. C., "A Method to Match Human Sulci in 3D-Space." IEEE Engineering in Medicine and Biology 17th Annual Conference and 21st Canadian Medical and Biological Engineering Conference, 1995.

6. Subsol G., Thirion J., Ayache N., "First Steps Towards Automatic Building of Anatomical Atlases," INRIA, Technical Report No. 2216, 1994.

7. Sebastian T., Klein PN., Kimia BB., Crisco J., "Constructing 2D Curve Atlases," MMBIA, 70-77, 2000.

8. Davatzikos C., "Measuring biological shape using geometry-based shape transformations," Image and Vision Computing, 19, 63-74, 2001.

9. Grenander U. and Miller M., "Computational Anatomy: An Emerging Discipline," Quarterly of Applied Mathematics, LVI, 4, 617-694, December, 1998.

10. Liu T., Geiger D., "Approximate Tree Matching and Shape Similarity," ICCV. 456-462, 1999.

11. Ansari N., Delp E., "Partial shape recognition: a landmark based approach," IEEE Transactions on Pattern Analysis and Machine Intelligence (PAMI), 12, 470-489, 1990.

12. Bookstein F., Morphometric Tools for Landmark Data: Geometry and Biology. Cambridge University Press, 1991.

13. Bakircioglu M., Grenander U., Khaneja N., Miller MI., "Curve Matching on Brain Surfaces Using Induced Frenet" Distance Metrics. Human Brain Mapping. 6(5), 329-331, 1998.

14. Younes L., "Computable Elastic Distance Between Shapes," SIAM J. Appl. Math, 58, 565-586, 1998.

15. Trouve A., Younes L., "On a Class of Diffeomorphic Matching Problems in One Dimension," SIAM Journal on Control and Optimization, 39(4), 1112-1135, 2000.

16. Rangarajan A., Chui H., Mjolsness E., Pappu S., Davachi L., Goldman-Rakic P., Duncan J., "A robust point matching algorithm for autoradiograph alignment," Medical Image Analysis, 4(1), 379-398, 1997

17. Chui H., Rangarajan A., "A New Algorithm for Non-Rigid Point Matching," Computer Vision and Pattern Recognition (CVPR), 2, 44-51, 2000.

18. Piegl L., Tiller W., The NURBS Book, Springer-Verlag, 1995

19. Lee I., "Curve reconstruction from unorganized points," Computer Aided Design, 17, 161-177, 2000

20. Tagare H. D. , O'Shea D. and Rangarajan A., "A geometric criterion for shape based non-rigid correspondence," Fifth Intl. Conf. on Computer Vision (ICCV), 434-439, 1995.

21. Trouve A., Younes L., Diffeomorphic matching in 1d: designing and minimizing matching functionals, ECCV, 2000.

22. Geiger D., Gupta A., Costa L., Vlontzos J., "Dynamic programming for detecting, tracking and matching deformable contours," PAMI 17, 294-302, 1995.

23. DoCarmo M., Differential Geometry of Curves and Surfaces. Prentice-Hall. Englewood Cliffs, NJ, 1976.

24. Babaud J., Witkin A., Baudin M., Duda R., "Uniqueness of the Gaussian kernel for scale space filtering," PAMI, 8, Jan 1986.

25. Lindeberg T., "Scale-space for discrete signals," PAMI, 12, March 1990.

26. Mokhtarian F., Mackworth A., "Scale-based description and recognition of planar curves and two-dimensional shapes," PAMI 8, 34-44, 1986.

27. Hofmann T., Buhmann J., "Pairwise data clustering by deterministic annealing," PAMI, 19(1), 1997.

28. Amini A., Weymouth T., Jain R., "Using dynamic programming for solving variational problems in vision." PAMI, 12(9), 855-867, 1990.

29. Viterbi A.,"Error bounds for convolutional codes and an asymptotically optimum decoding algorithm," IEEE Transactions on Information Theory, 260-269, 1967.

30. Umeyama S., "Parameterized point pattern matching and its application to recognition of object families", PAMI 15, 136-144, 1993.

31. Marques J., Abrantes A., "Shape alignment - optimal initial point and pose estimation," Pattern Recognition Letters, 18, 49-53, 1997.

Wavelet Median Denoising of Ultrasound Images

Katherine E. Macey[a] and Wyatt H. Page[b]

[a]University of California at Los Angeles, Los Angeles, CA, USA
[b]Open Networks Ltd, Wellington, New Zealand

ABSTRACT

Ultrasound images are contaminated with both additive and multiplicative noise, which is modeled by Gaussian and speckle noise respectively. Distinguishing small features such as fallopian tubes in the female genital tract in the noisy environment is problematic. A new method for noise reduction, Wavelet Median Denoising, is presented. Wavelet Median Denoising consists of performing a standard noise reduction technique, median filtering, in the wavelet domain. The new method is tested on 126 images, comprised of 9 original images each with 14 levels of Gaussian or speckle noise. Results for both separable and non-separable wavelets are evaluated, relative to soft-thresholding in the wavelet domain, using the signal-to-noise ratio and subjective assessment. The performance of Wavelet Median Denoising is comparable to that of soft-thresholding. Both methods are more successful in removing Gaussian noise than speckle noise. Wavelet Median Denoising outperforms soft-thresholding for a larger number of cases of speckle noise reduction than of Gaussian noise reduction. Noise reduction is more successful using non-separable wavelets than separable wavelets. When both methods are applied to ultrasound images obtained from a phantom of the female genital tract a small improvement is seen; however, a substantial improvement is required prior to clinical use.

Keywords: Noise reduction, denoising, separable, non-separable, wavelets, soft-thresholding, median filter, Gaussian, speckle, ultrasound

1. INTRODUCTION

Ultrasound images of the uterine cavity are contaminated by noise, making it difficult to distinguish fine details such as fallopian tubes. Noise in the images is both additive and multiplicative and can be modelled by Gaussian and speckle noise. Noise reduction aims to enhance an image, facilitating observation of anatomical details of interest.

There are a wide variety of noise reduction techniques currently available. One of the most common filtering techniques used for noise reduction is the median filter.[1] The median filter assumes that, in general, signals will not vary greatly within a small region and generally preserves edge information moderately well. In the 2-D case, a small window is centered over each pixel in an image. At each pixel, the surrounding pixel values within the window are sorted according to intensity (assuming a greyscale image) and the median value replaces the original pixel value.

Wavelet based denoising techniques employ band pass filtering to reduce the bandwidth at which noise reduction is applied. A signal is transformed, or filtered, into the wavelet domain giving wavelet coefficients in different decomposition levels; each level represents a spectral band, with the first bands representing higher frequencies. The denoising technique of choice is applied to the wavelet coefficients and the altered coefficients are reconstructed back into the image domain. An early approach to denoising in the wavelet domain was to omit bands that contained noise from the reconstruction.[2] If noise is limited to a single spectral band and that band does not contain any components of the signal, then this approach works well. However, frequently the signal and noise are not spectrally separated as edge information tends to be in the same spectral bands as

---

Further author information: (Send correspondence to K.E.M.)

K.E.M.: E-mail: kmacey@mednet.ucla.edu, Telephone: +1 310 206 1679, Fax: +1 310 825 2224, Address: Department of Neurobiology, University of California at Los Angeles, 10833 Le Conte Ave, Los Angeles, CA 90095-1763, USA

W.H.P.: E-mail: Wyatt.Page@opennw.com, Telephone: +64 4 382 4824, Fax: +64 4 384 8025, Address: Open Networks Ltd., 32-42 Manners Street, Wellington, New Zealand

noise in the signal, resulting in blurred reconstructed images if the spectral bands containing noise are simply omitted from the reconstruction. The next development was to employ hard thresholding in bands that were likely to contain noise - typically the first and second decompositions in the wavelet domain containing the high frequency information. Hard thresholding reduces to zero any coefficients below a threshold,[2] leaving the remaining coefficients unchanged. In soft-thresholding[3] coefficients below a threshold are reduced to zero as in hard thresholding, but the coefficients above the threshold are reduced towards zero by the threshold amount.

Both hard and soft thresholding assume that the individual coefficients are independent from their neighbors. The underlying assumption is that noise causes isolated wavelet coefficients to have high (or low) valued components compared to their neighbours. Conversely, a wavelet coefficient is likely to have adjacent coefficients of a similar magnitude. This effect is known as *clustering*.[4] For example, wavelet coefficients due to edges will tend to be grouped spatially with several coefficients in the vicinity having a high intensity. A new method, *Wavelet Median Denoising*, is proposed to take advantage of clustering. The method uses a classical image enhancement technique, median filtering, but applied in the wavelet domain to reduce noise.

2. METHODS

Selected images are transformed into the wavelet domain and denoising is performed, followed by reconstruction to the image domain. Unlike the Fourier Transform, the wavelet transform has a myriad of possible transforms. We investigate differences between separable and non-separable wavelet transforms in relation to the denoising problem. Wavelet Median Denoising is applied and compared with denoising using soft thresholding.

2.1. Separable and non-separable wavelets

In general, two-dimensional wavelets are classified as separable or non-separable. Separable wavelet transforms may be performed separately in each dimension, whereas non-separable wavelet transforms are performed simultaneously in all dimensions. Separable wavelets have the advantage of having lower computational complexity, but non-separable wavelets have more degrees of freedom in their design, potentially leading to wavelets more suited to the application.[5] Non-separable wavelets give greater freedom for designing sub-sampling schemes.[5] One such scheme is quincunx sub-sampling, which leads to smaller bandwidths in the frequency domain for each level, giving greater control in denoising schemes. It is also possible to design non-separable filters that are non-directional. Using non-directional wavelet transforms may be appropriate for images of natural objects, such as medical images, as these images often do not have inherent directional biases.[6]

The two-dimensional separable wavelet transform can be described by the sub-band filtering approach. Considering an image as an array, sampled on a rectangular grid, $x[n]$, then the filtering functions are applied separately to the rows and columns of the array,[7] as illustrated in Figure 1. The filtering functions, $h_1[n]$ and $h_0[n]$, are high and low filters, respectively. After filtering, the coefficients are downsampled by 2 (every second sample is removed.) After filtering in both directions, four images in the wavelet domain are obtained; three detail images, $d_{1,1}$, the image obtained by the high pass filter of $x[n]$ in both rows and columns, $d_{1,0}$, the image obtained by the high pass filter of the rows and low pass filter of the columns, $d_{0,1}$, the image obtained by the low pass filter of the rows and high pass filter of the columns, and an approximation image, $a_{0,0}$, the image obtained by the low pass filter of both the rows and columns. These images taken together give the first level of decomposition. 2-D filters may be constructed using tensor products of the low and high pass filters. Reconstruction, or synthesis, is performed in a similar manner, but upsampling (inserting zeros between every sample) prior to filtering. The reconstructed image is $\hat{x}[n]$. The decomposition and reconstruction filters are designed so that perfect reconstruction occurs, that is $x[n] = \hat{x}[n]$. Iteration of the transform is achieved by taking the approximation, $a_{0,0}$, as the input to the next level of filter banks, just as in the one-dimensional case.

When performing wavelet transforms, the signal is filtered and then downsampled. Downsampling can be described using a sub-lattice of the initial lattice.[8] The sub-lattice resulting from separable two-dimensional sub-sampling is represented by solid dots in Figure 2(a). There is an overall downsampling rate of 4, i.e., only one in every four samples is kept. If, as in the one-dimensional case, a downsampling rate of 2 is desired, then a different sub-lattice is required. One solution is the quincunx sub-lattice[8,9] illustrated in Figure 2(b). The

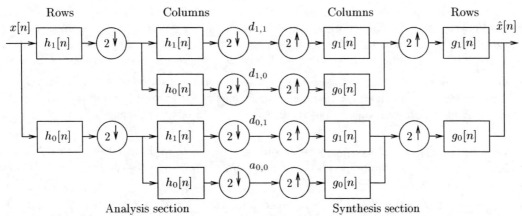

Figure 1: A two-dimensional separable analysis and synthesis filter bank.

quincunx sub-lattice gives an overall sub-sampling rate of 2 whilst still reducing the number of samples in both the horizontal and vertical directions. It is a non-separable sub-lattice.[5, 8]

Sub-lattices can be represented by a dilation matrix $\mathbf{D}$.[5, 8] The index points of the sub-lattice are given by weighted integer combinations of the columns of $\mathbf{D}$. A separable lattice is a lattice that can be represented by a diagonal matrix. For example, the separable sub-lattice in Figure 2(a) may be represented by $\mathbf{D}_0 = \left(\begin{smallmatrix} 2 & 0 \\ 0 & 2 \end{smallmatrix}\right)$. The sampling rate, N, is given by $N = |Det(\mathbf{D}_i)|$. Notice that $N_0 = |Det(\mathbf{D}_0)| = 4$.

The matrix $\mathbf{D}$ is not unique for any given lattice. Some examples of dilation matrices for the non-separable quincunx lattice are:

$$\mathbf{D}_1 = \begin{pmatrix} 1 & 1 \\ 1 & -1 \end{pmatrix}, \quad \mathbf{D}_2 = \begin{pmatrix} 1 & -1 \\ 1 & 1 \end{pmatrix}, \quad \mathbf{D}_3 = \begin{pmatrix} 2 & 1 \\ 0 & 1 \end{pmatrix}. \tag{1}$$

A dilation matrix in two-dimensional downsampling takes the place of the dilation function in the one-dimensional two-scale difference equation for wavelets, leading to the two-dimensional two-scale difference equation:

$$\Psi_i(\mathbf{t}) = \sqrt{N} \sum_{k=\mathcal{Z}^n} h_i[k]\phi(\mathbf{D}\mathbf{t} - \mathbf{k}). \tag{2}$$

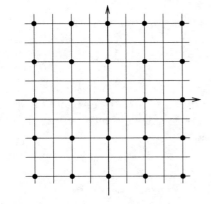

(a) Original sampling lattice represented by crossing of horizontal and vertical lines. A separable sub-lattice is represented by solid dots.

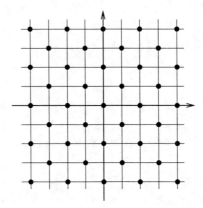

(b) Original sampling lattice represented by crossing of horizontal and vertical lines. A non-separable quincunx sub-lattice is represented by solid dots.

Figure 2: Initial sampling and sub-sampling lattices; (a) separable sub-sampling, and (b) quincunx sub-sampling.

When iterating the filter bank, sub-sampling by $\mathbf{D}$ is also iterated. Therefore, different dilation matrices can produce very different results.[8] For instance, iterating $\mathbf{D}_1$ twice results in a diagonal matrix equivalent to iterating $\mathbf{D}_0$ once and, therefore, results in separable sub-sampling every second iteration. Iterating $\mathbf{D}_3$, however, will never result in a diagonal matrix and, therefore, will never result in separable sub-sampling.

Another consideration in choosing the matrix $\mathbf{D}$ is whether it represents a dilation in all directions. If it does, the associated wavelet will also increase its size in all dimensions over successive iterations. Dilation in all dimensions is equivalent to requiring that all eigenvalues of $\mathbf{D}$ should have a magnitude strictly greater than one.[8]

Here, the dilation matrix $\mathbf{D}_1$ is used as it gives equal sub-sampling in both dimensions, and every second iteration is equivalent to separable sub-sampling, allowing comparison between the two classes of two-dimensional wavelets.

We compare examples of orthogonal wavelets and linear phase wavelets that are separable with those that are non-separable. We use the non-separable wavelets developed by Kovačević and Vetterli[8] and chose separable wavelets that were similar in construction and size. Therefore tensor products of the Daubechies order 2 and the biorthogonal 3.1 wavelets were used to create 2-D separable orthogonal and linear phase wavelets, respectively.

2.2. Denoising

Two denoising schemes are considered. The first, *soft-thresholding*, was introduced to compensate for the noise in images around edges remaining after hard thresholding.[3] Soft-thresholding reduces to zero any signal component that is less than a threshold and reduces all other components towards zero. For a signal, $x(t)$, the soft-threshold function is given by:

$$x'(t) = sign(x(t))max(0, |x(t)| - \lambda), \tag{3}$$

where $sign(x(t)) = \pm 1$ according to the sign of $x(t)$, and λ is the threshold value. The threshold value, λ_n, is given by[3]:

$$\lambda_n = s_m \sqrt{2 \log(n)}, \tag{4}$$

where n is the number of coefficients and s_m is given by the variance of the wavelet coefficients $Var(d_{j_i}) \leq s_m^2, i = 0, \ldots n$ and for each scale, j. This approach has been used by others successfully.[10]

Another estimate for the threshold is based on the sample variance, s_s of the first decomposition level of the wavelet transform coefficients.[11] The sample variance s_s is given by:

$$s_s^2 = \frac{\sum (d[n_1, n_2] - \bar{d})}{N},$$

where

$$\bar{d} = \frac{\sum d[n_1, n_2]}{N} \tag{5}$$

and N is the number of samples. The sample variance is used because it is a reasonable estimate of the noise power of the image.[11] The estimate of the noise power at other levels can be calculated using the known decomposition filters. The following has been used for uniform thresholding[11] :

$$\lambda = 1.8 s_s. \tag{6}$$

where the constant 1.8 was determined empirically.

Soft thresholding considers each wavelet coefficient to be independant of its neighbors. The second denoising scheme, *Wavelet Median Denoising* (WMD) attempts to exploit spatial clustering between adjacent scales in the wavelet domain. Median filtering in the spatial domain is a statistical approach in which the pixels in a neighbourhood are ranked according to brightness and the central pixel is replaced by the median value of the ranked pixels.[1] For WMD, the filtering is performed in the wavelet domain. A cluster of high intensity

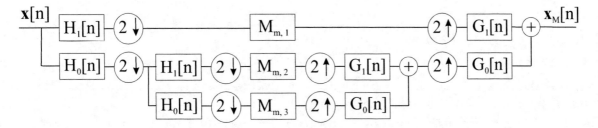

Figure 3. Schematic of Wavelet Median Denoising. The image $\mathbf{x}[n]$ is decomposed. The median filter, $M_{m,j}$, of width m is applied in the wavelet domain at scales j and the modified wavelet coefficients are reconstructed to form the denoised image, $\mathbf{x}_M[n]$. $M_{m,j}$ may be different for each scale.

wavelet coefficients due to an edge will tend to have a higher median value, compared with the median value of a wavelet coefficients due to a uniform surface contaminated with noise. This approach should change the wavelet coefficients due to noise to the same as the local neighbourhood, but should retain the wavelet coefficients due to edges. Therefore, noise in the image will be reduced, whilst the edges of objects will be retained. A schematic of the process is shown in Figure 2.2. An image $\mathbf{x}[n]$ is decomposed. The median filter, $M_{m,j}$, of width m is applied in the wavelet domain at scales j and the modified wavelet coefficients are reconstructed to form the denoised image, $\mathbf{x}_M[n]$.

The median filter has two parameters that may be varied: the width of the median filter window and the range of scales over which it is applied. A range of values for these parameters was tested.

2.3. Image processing

The denoising methods were applied to a test image from our own library, rose window, as well as an additional eight images obtained from the Matlab library, amfsurf, alumgrns, cameraman, checker, ngc4024m (an image of a galaxy), moon, saturn, and tire. The images had a variety of characteristics; some with prominent straight lines at various angles, some with circular images, some with large objects, some with small objects.

Gaussian noise or speckle noise was applied to the images for various levels of noise. The levels tested for Gaussian noise are given in Table 1. The levels for Gaussian noise were altered by mean and variance. The levels tested for speckle noise are given in Table 2 and had different variances.

2.4. Evaluation

Success of the denoising techniques was measured subjectively and using a Figure of Merit (FOM),[12] being the ratio of the signal to noise ratios for the denoised and original images:

Table 1: Noise levels applied for Gaussian noise.

Gaussian noise level	1	2	3	4	5	6	7	8	9	10
Mean of noise	0	0	-0.1	-0.05	0	0.01	0.05	0	0	0
Variance of noise	0.001	0.005	0.01	0.01	0.01	0.01	0.01	0.05	0.1	0.5

Table 2: Noise levels applied for speckle noise.

Speckle noise level	1	2	3	4
Variance of noise	0.01	0.05	0.1	0.5

$$FOM = \frac{SNR_d}{SNR_o} = \frac{log_{10}\left(\frac{\sum X_i'^2}{\sum(X_i - N_i)^2}\right)}{log_{10}\left(\frac{\sum X_i^2}{\sum(X_i - N_i)^2}\right)} \tag{7}$$

The FOM is greater than one if the denoised image has a better signal to noise ratio than the original. The tests were repeated three times to test the robustness of the results.

Ultrasound images of a phantom of a female genital tract were denoised. Each of the four wavelets were used for decomposition into the wavelet domain. Both denoising methods were applied in the wavelet domain and each set of coefficients was reconstructed. The resulting denoised images were assessed subjectively.

3. RESULTS

Both methods showed improvements in the Figure of Merit (FOM) for all the images. Figure 4 shows the FOM results obtained for the rose window test image for Gaussian noise (mean = 0, variance = 0.1) for Wavelet Median Denoising in 4(a) and for soft thresholding in 4(b). The results for the different wavelets are shown in individual graphs with all the results from different denoising parameters grouped in each graph. In this example, the non-separable orthogonal wavelet using soft thresholding produced the best results. The best result was a FOM of 2.02 for 4 levels of denoising with a soft threshold of 2. The best result for the WMD for this image and level of noise was for the non-separable wavelet, denoised to 3 levels using a window width of 7, giving a FOM of 1.91. These results are indicative with the non-separable wavelets generally achieving a higher FOM than the separable wavelets. The inverted U-shaped curve for the FOM over various denoising levels is also typical. The peak of the curve does not occur at the same denoising level for the different images and noise parameters. The larger window width of 7 pixels seemed to perform best for WMD from a FOM standpoint. Soft threshold denoising seemed to perform best with a threshold constant of 2.

Rose window test images are illustrated in Figure 5, denoised using the parameters that gave the best results for WMD and soft thresholding from Figure 4. The original image is shown in Figure 5(a), with the noisy image in Figure 5(b). The image denoised using WMD (3 denoising levels and a median filter of width 7) is shown in (Figure 5(c)), and the image denoised using soft thresholding (4 denoising levels and a threshold constant of 2) is shown in Figure 5(d). Both methods tend to blur the image as denoising is performed in decomposition levels representing lower frequency spectral bands.

In general, Wavelet Median Denoising performed comparably to soft thresholding. While only 1% of the images with Gaussian noise were denoised more successfully using the WMD than soft thresholding, 67% were within 5% of the result for soft thresholding. Similarly, for speckle noise 72% of the results were within 5% of the results for soft thresholding (see Figure 6(a).) However, WMD performed better against soft thresholding for speckle noise than for Gaussian noise; 12% of WMD performed better than soft thresholding for speckle noise. A comparison is shown in Figure 6(a). Results were stable for all three of the test runs.

The best wavelet for noise reduction of either Gaussian or speckle noise, disregarding the method of denoising, was the non-separable orthogonal wavelet. The wavelet with the best FOM for a given class of noise was evaluated for all the images and noise levels. The number of times each wavelet scored the best FOM was expressed as a percentage of total number of trials over all images and noise levels and is given in Figure 7(a). Similarly, the wavelet with the best FOM for a either WMD or soft thresholding was the non-separable orthogonal wavelet. The results for a given denoising method are shown in Figure 7(b), again with the number of times each wavelet scored the highest FOM expressed as a percentage of the total number of trials.

One image from the volume of ultrasound images that was tested is shown in Figure 8. The original image is shown in Figure 8(a) with an orientation image shown beside it in Figure 8(b). The result of denoising using the Wavelet Median Denoising with the non-separable orthogonal wavelet to one decomposition level with a median filter of width 7 is shown in Figure 8(c). The result for the same wavelet and decomposition level, but for soft thresholding with a threshold constant of 2 is shown in Figure 8(d).

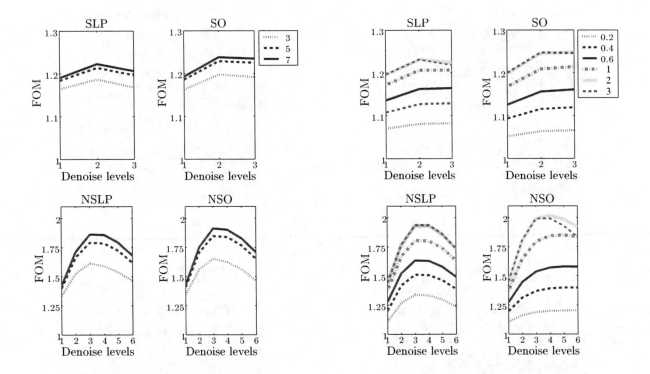

(a) Figure of Merit (FOM) for Wavelet Median Denoising (WMD) for various window widths (dotted: 3; dashed: 5; solid 7.)

(b) Figure of Merit (FOM) for soft thresholding for various threshold constants (thin dotted: 0.2; thin, dark dashed: 0.4; thin, dark solid: 0.6; thick dash dotted: 1; thick, light solid: 2; thick, light dashed: 3.)

Figure 4. Figure of Merit (FOM) for (a) Wavelet Median Denoising (WMD) and (b) soft thresholding (ST) for the rose window test image with added Gaussian noise with mean = 0 and variance = 0.1.

4. DISCUSSION

Using the Figure of Merit (FOM) measure of image quality, Wavelet Median Denoising (WMD) performs similarly to soft thresholding reducing Gaussian noise from test images. WMD performs better than soft thresholding reducing speckle noise more often than when reducing Gaussian noise.

These results were verified subjectively. However, quality of images is difficult to assess. Traditional methods using signal-to-noise ratio or mean squared error do not fully take into account undesirable features such as blurring of the image. Enhancing contrast in images can improve quality, but this also is difficult to assess.

Neighboring pixels in the wavelet domain may exhibit clustering where groups of wavelet coefficients are of a similar intensity due to some underlying feature in the image, such as an edge. Where clustering occurs, neighboring pixels are not truely independent. Soft thresholding treats the coefficients as if they were independent, whereas Wavelet Median Denoising assumes dependency between neighbors. Other, more complex denoising techniques, such as applying the Hidden Markov Model (HMM) in the wavelet domain take into account not only clustering, but also *persistence*.[4] Persistence is related to the likelihood of a group of pixels in one decomposition level having a geographically related group of pixels in the next decomposition level showing the same characteristics. However, persistence in ultrasound images for the objects of interest such as Fallopian tubes is likely to be low, so including these methods is unlikely to significantly improve the results. Additionally, including clustering and persistence in a denoising solution such as the HMM substantially increase the complexity of

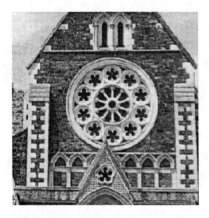

(a) Original image

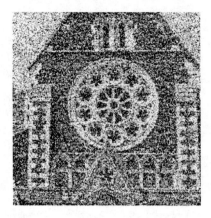

(b) Image contaminated with Gaussian noise

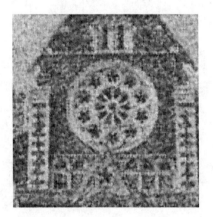

(c) Denoised using Wavelet Median Denoising.

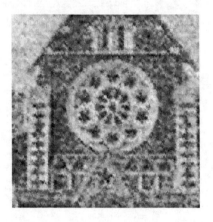

(d) Denoised using soft thresholding.

Figure 5: Comparison of denoising methods for ultrasound image.

the denoising solution. Complexity in a method increases the computational time taken to perform the method. This is a consideration for ultrasound images as a radiologist typically views ultrasound images in real time.

Non-separable wavelets performed better than the separable wavelets, with the non-separable orthogonal wavelet performing the best overall. This was somewhat surprising as, in general, linear phase wavelets produce less distortion than orthogonal wavelets. The results may be related to the concentration of power in the wavelet domain as the non-separable linear phase wavelet tends to concentrate the power of the wavelet coeffients in the first decomposition level. The other wavelets are all able to spread out the power concentration, indicating perhaps that the non-separable linear phase wavelet was not well matched to the data.

5. CONCLUSIONS

Wavelet Median Denoising performs similarly to soft thresholding for Gaussian and speckle noise. The non-separable orthogonal wavelet performed the best of the wavelets tested. Non-separable wavelets provide greater flexibility for the design of the wavelet and allow finer downsampling leading to finer spectral band decomposition and better denoising. They are, however, computationally more expensive. The WMD performed better for speckle noise, relative to soft thresholding, suggesting that an approach to denoising in the wavelet domain that assumes dependence between neighboring coefficients may be better at denoising multiplicative noise.

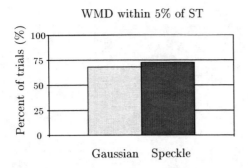

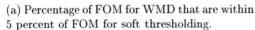

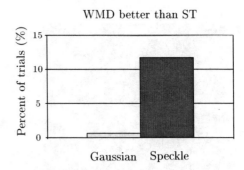

(a) Percentage of FOM for WMD that are within 5 percent of FOM for soft thresholding.

(b) Percentage of FOM for WMD that scored better than soft thresholding.

Figure 6. Relative measures of Figure of Merit (FOM) for Wavelet Median Denoising (WMD) and soft thresholding (ST).

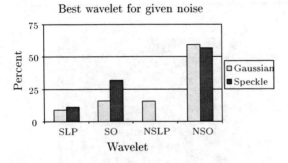

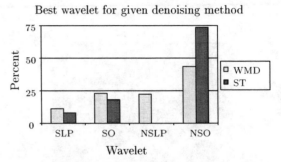

(a) Number of times each wavelet scored the best FOM for a given class of noise expressed as a percentage of total number of trials over all images and noise levels.

(b) Number of times each wavelet scored the best FOM for a given method of noise reduction expressed as a percentage of total number of trials over all images and noise levels. (WMD: Wavelet median denoising; ST: soft thresholding)

Figure 7. Number of each wavelet scoring the best Figure of Merit (FOM) for (a) given noise and for (b) given denoising method. (SLP: Separable linear phase; SO: Separable orthogonal; NSLP: Non-separable linear phase; NSO: Non-separable orthogonal)

ACKNOWLEDGMENTS

We acknowledge Mr. Nigel Anderson and Dr. Richard Fright for access to the ultrasound phantom images from Christchurch Hospital, New Zealand. Support for KM was provided by Dr. Ronald Harper and HD22695.

REFERENCES

1. J. C. Russ, *The Image Processing Handbook*, CRC Press in cooperation with IEEE Press, Forida, USA, 3rd ed., 1998.

2. A. Laine, J. Fan, and W. Yang, "Wavelets for contrast enhancement of digital mammography," *IEEE Engineering in Medicine and Biology* **14**, pp. 536–550, September/October 1995.

3. D. L. Donoho, "De-noising by soft-thresholding," *IEEE Transactions on Information Theory* **41**, pp. 613–627, May 1995.

4. M. S. Crouse, R. D. Nowak, and R. Baranuik, "Wavelet-based statistical signal processing using hidden markov models," *IEEE Transactions on Signal Processing* **46**, pp. 886–902, April 1998.

5. J. Kovačević and M. Vetterli, "Nonseparable two- and three-dimensional wavelets," *IEEE Transactions on Signal Processing* **43**, pp. 1269–1273, May 1995.

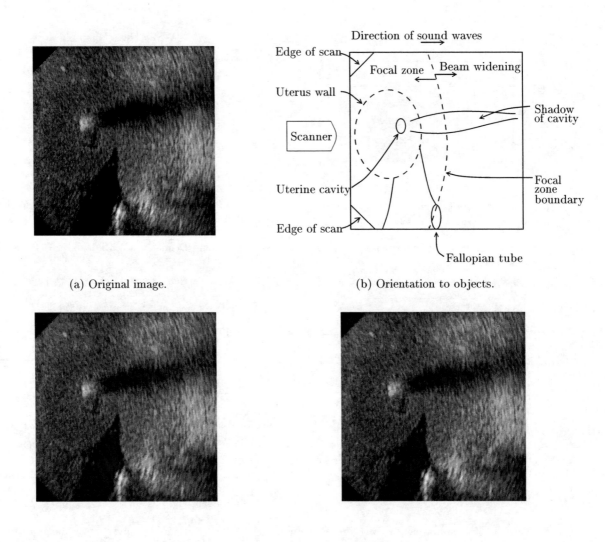

(a) Original image.

(b) Orientation to objects.

(c) Denoised using Wavelet Median Denoising.

(d) Denoised using soft thresholding.

Figure 8: Comparison of denoising methods for ultrasound image.

6. S. Mallat, "A theory for multiresolution signal decomposition: The wavelet representation," *IEEE Transactions on Pattern Analysis and Machine Intelligence* **11**, pp. 674–693, July 1989.

7. I. Daubechies, *Ten Lectures on Wavelets*, Society for Industrial and Applied Mathematics, Philadelphia, Pennsylvania, 1992.

8. J. Kovačević and M. Vetterli, "Nonseparable multidimensional perfect reconstruction filter banks and wavelet bases for $\mathcal{R}^n$," *IEEE Transactions on Information Theory* **38**, pp. 533–555, March 1992.

9. O. Rioul and M. Vetterli, "Wavelets and signal processing," *IEEE Signal Processing Magazine* **8**, pp. 14–38, October 1991.

10. R. Herrera, R. Sclabassi, S. Mingui, and R. Dahl, "Single trial visual event–related potential EEG analysis using the wavelet transform," in *Proceedings of the First Joint BMES/EMBS Conference*, **2**, p. 947, IEEE, (Piscataway, NJ, USA), 1999.

11. S. G. Chang and M. Vetterli, "Spatial adaptive wavelet thresholding for image denoising," in *Proceedings of the IEEE International Conference on Image Processing*, pp. 374–377, 1997.

12. S. Haykin, *Communication Systems*, John Wiley & Sons, New York, NY, USA, 1983.

APPLICATION OF AN ADAPTIVE CONTROL GRID INTERPOLATION TECHNIQUE TO MR DATA SET AUGMENTATION AIMED AT MORPHOLOGICAL VASCULAR RECONSTRUCTION

Frakes, David H.[1], Sinotte, Christopher M.[1], Conrad, Christopher P.[1], Healy, Timothy M.[1], Sharma, Shiva[2], Fogel, Mark[4], Monaco, Joseph W.[3], Smith, Mark J.T.[3], Yoganathan, Ajit P.[1]

[1]School of Biomedical Engineering, Georgia Institute of Technology, Atlanta, Georgia, USA
[2]Egleston Children's Hospital, Atlanta, Georgia, USA
[3]School of Electrical and Computer Engineering, Georgia Institute of Technology, Atlanta, Georgia, USA
[4]Children's Hospital of Philadelphia (CHOP), Philadelphia, Pennsylvania, USA

ABSTRACT

The total cavopulmonary connection (TCPC) is a palliative surgical repair performed on children with a single ventricle (SV) physiology. Much of the power produced by the resultant single ventricle pump is consumed in the systemic circulation. Consequently the minimization of power loss in the TCPC is imperative for optimal surgical outcome. Toward this end we have developed a method of vascular morphology reconstruction based on adaptive control grid interpolation (ACGI) to function as a precursor to computational fluid dynamics (CFD) analysis aimed at quantifying power loss. Our technique combines positive aspects of optical flow-based and block-based motion estimation algorithms to accurately augment insufficiently dense Magnetic Resonance (MR) data sets with a minimal degree of computational complexity. The resulting enhanced data sets are used to reconstruct vascular geometries, and the subsequent reconstructions can then be used in conjunction with CFD simulations to offer the pressure and velocity information necessary to quantify power loss in the TCPC. Collectively these steps form a tool that transforms conventional MR data into more powerful information allowing surgical planning aimed at producing optimal TCPC configurations for successful surgical outcomes.

I. INTRODUCTION

The total cavopulmonary connection (TCPC) is a palliative surgical repair performed on children born with single ventricle (SV) physiology. Children with such physiology have a mixing of oxygenated and deoxygenated blood, which when left untreated leads to inadequate tissue oxygenation and cyanosis [4]. The anatomy of a normal heart is displayed in Fig. 1 and the overlap of pulmonary and systemic circuits leading to oxygenated and deoxygenated blood mixing is displayed in Fig. 2. In order to prevent systemic and pulmonary blood from mixing, the surgeon will disconnect the pulmonary artery from its ventricular origin, anastomose the superior vena cava to the unbranched right

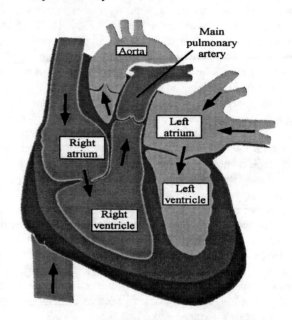

Fig. 1. Anatomy of normal heart.

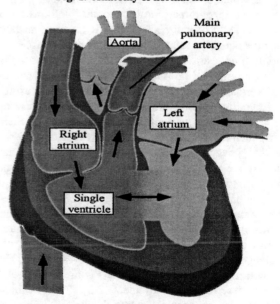

Fig. 2. Anatomy of single ventricle heart defect.

pulmonary artery (RPA), and construct a lateral tunnel through the right atrium connecting the inferior vena cava with the RPA. The procedure results in a complete bypass of the right heart with the single ventricle driving blood through the entire circulatory system.

Much of the power produced by the single ventricle pump is consumed in the systemic circulation. For this reason minimizing power loss in the modified district is critical for optimal surgical outcomes. Presently, the surgeon's experience dictates the implemented intervention with little attention paid to achieving minimal power loss. To refocus connection choice on fluid dynamics, our group is developing surgical planning techniques for the TCPC. Such techniques will aid the surgeon in selecting the optimal TCPC among possible alternatives for specific patients. The proposed methodology employs combined use of magnetic resonance (MR) imaging and computational fluid dynamics (CFD) to study flow conditions among alternative post-operative morphologies prior to performing the surgical procedure. First MR images containing anatomical information will be acquired and used to reconstruct morphological models of pre-operative anatomy. Next, the surgeon and engineers collaboratively construct computer models of possible connections within the framework of the pre-operative reconstructions. Finally computer simulations are performed for each connection alternative to provide pressure and velocity information thereby allowing the surgeon to select the best potential alternative in terms of power loss. In addition the detailed velocity information generated by CFD can also be utilized to predict the occurrence of longer-term problems such as thromboembolic episodes and flow induced vascular damage.

In order to execute CFD simulations at any stage, comprehensive three-dimensional anatomical information is required. Volumetric morphological MR imaging methods extract high quality information, but demand excessive acquisition time even for relatively small volumes. Our reconstruction method is an alternative that provides the desired information without exorbitant scan time. By using a series of two-dimensional morphological MR images we are able to reconstruct an accurate three-dimensional geometry which can then be analyzed using CFD. Reconstruction from a series of images necessitates the approximation of data contained in the original three-dimensional structure, but not captured with two-dimensional imaging. Numerous methods of interpolation have been proposed to accomplish this task [1]. Reconstruction methods customarily require a method for establishing a correlation between points in related images as a precursor to interpolation [5-8]. We have developed a new technique to accomplish this task, whereby a modified form of control grid interpolation (CGI) is used to calculate vectors that describe pixel movement [2-3]. This technique provides us with an accurate morphological reconstruction suitable for importation into CFD software.

II. METHODOLOGY

The starting point for our reconstruction process is a series of transverse black blood MR images taken at uniformly spaced depths through a patient's chest. The parameters associated with image acquisition are displayed in Table 1.

MR System Type	General Electric
Pulse Sequence Type	Spin Echo
Image Acquisition Plane	Transverse
Images Acquired	~30
Slice Thickness	5mm
Field of View	200mx200mm
Flip Angle	50 degrees
Repetition Time	350-1000ms
Echo Time	15ms
Number of Signals Averaged	3
Matrix size	256x256

Table 1. MR data acquisition parameters associated with the acquisition of original images.

Fields of motion vectors are then calculated describing the displacement of pixels from one image to another. In the CGI representation, the motion field is obtained by segmenting the image into contiguous rectangular regions. The corners of these regions form control points that are used as the anchors from which the motion vectors in between are derived via bilinear interpolation. There is a trade off between the expense in terms of calculation time and the error associated with the resultant motion field when the block size bounded by control points is varied. Smaller block sizes lead to a more accurate motion field, but require more intense computation. This fact is displayed in Fig. 3A and Fig. 3B where total squared error and computation time for a sample image set are plotted as a function of pixel block size.

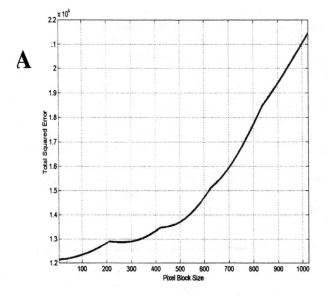

A

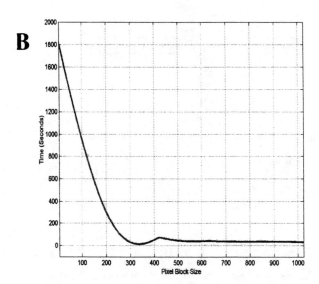

B

Fig. 3. Total squared error (A) and computation time (B) plotted versus pixel block size.

of the field of motion vectors at a minimal cost in terms of computational complexity.

The first pass of this motion vector calculation algorithm yields the best approximation of a control point pixel's destination on the dense grid of dimension determined by the MR scan. Following this portion of the technique a recursive interpolation scheme is employed to further increase the accuracy of each motion vector to a specified degree. Assuming that the actual destination of a given pixel lies somewhere between the best approximation on the dense grid and one of it's surrounding neighbors, the search region is pinpointed. Interpolants are then interleaved between the members of this nine pixel neighborhood until a motion solution decreasing error below the specified threshold is located. In doing so an arbitrary degree of sub-pixel accuracy is incorporated into the routine. With each iteration of this procedure the marginal benefit in terms of error reduction decreases. For this reason only a few iterations are usually required to realize the benefits of the algorithm. This can be done without incurring any significant increase in computation time. The total squared error is plotted against the number of iterations in Fig. 4.

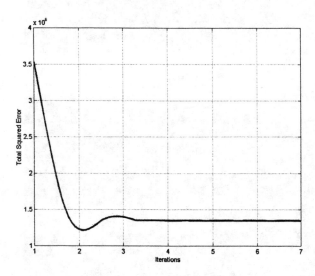

Fig. 4. Total squared error versus iterations of sub-pixel accuracy phase.

In contrast to traditional block matching approaches, which are commonly used for motion vector estimation, CGI is attractive for this application because it allows for the representation of complex non-translational motion. In this work we employ an adaptive CGI algorithm to partition the image into sub-blocks of size sufficient to capture characteristics of complex anatomical transition. In addition, we employ optical flow equations to calculate the motion of the CGI control points instead of an iterative search-based method. These characteristics of the algorithm are important, since we wish to obtain an accurate and dense representation

As a result of the recursive interpolation scheme for each control point, and the aforementioned bilinear interpolation, a dense field of motion vectors is obtained. By following one of these vectors a portion of the way from one image to the next, a linear approximation of where a given pixel would be found in an intermediate image can be made. Repeating this process for an entire image yields an interpolated intermediate image between two known images. Pairs of these images are then combined in a spatially weighted sum to form a single interpolated frame. This process is then repeated and several interpolated images are stacked between the known images in anatomical proportion to produce a three-dimensional augmented data set. A coronal view of an augmented data set is displayed in Fig. 5 along with the original. Each frame is then segmented with a semi-automated segmentation routine prior to reconstruction. Our segmentation protocol employs thresholding, region growing, and contour-based segmentation strategies, but allows user intervention when these techniques break down. This and the actual reconstruction phase are executed within Mimics software [9].

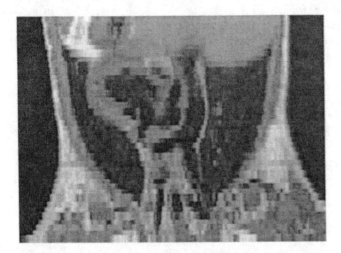

Original

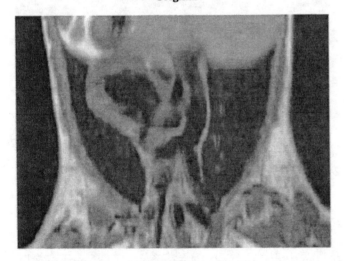

Augmented

Fig. 5. Coronal view of original and augmented MR data.

Taking into consideration the smooth variance of the TCPC vasculature, one might propose that interpolation along any vector would be sufficient to reconstruct an accurate morphology. The appeal of using the adaptive CGI technique to arrive at vectors to interpolate upon is that because of its sensitivity to both intensity and gradient information and its

ability to detect complex non-translational motion, this method is especially adept at creating interpolation vectors that reconstruct accurate data near vessel boundaries. This point is extremely important for reconstructions to be used as CFD models for quantitative analysis of flow characteristics.

III. RESULTS AND DISCUSSION

In order to validate the reconstruction portion of our technique, numerical models of TCPC phantoms were examined. Planes from these phantoms were extracted, blurred in a Gaussian fashion, and then distorted with noise to simulate MR images. The extracted slices from the original model and a sample simulated MR image are shown in Fig. 6A and Fig. 6B respectively.

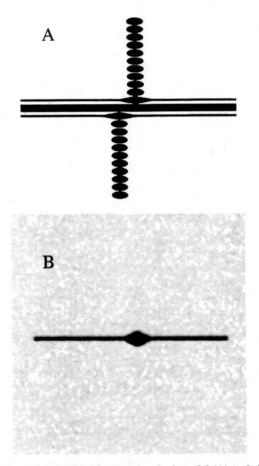

Fig. 6. Slices extracted from numerical model (A) and single simulated MR image (B).

These simulated images were then reconstructed using three different interpolation techniques: linear, spline, and ACGI. Qualitatively these reconstructions affirmed that the ACGI technique did in fact reconstruct with a greater degree of accuracy than the alternatives as shown in Fig. 7 and Fig. 8.

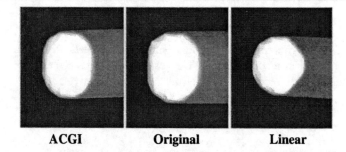

| ACGI | Original | Linear |

Fig. 8. TCPC model reconstruction LPA cross-sections. Deformation is observable in the linear reconstruction.

Two characteristics of the reconstructions, pulmonary artery cross-sectional diameter and connection geometry radius of curvature, were used as a basis for a quantitative comparison. Both of these quantities were obtained using the measurement tool within Mimics software [9]. For the cross-sectional diameter distances, measurements were taken both parallel and perpendicular to the plane of symmetry for each pulmonary artery. These four numbers were then averaged. The radius of curvature was calculated using strait line measurements spanning the distance of the the vena cava to pulmonary artery transitions. The actual radius of curvature was then determined geometrically. Four distances, one for each transition region, were measured and then averaged for each model. The results of the quantitative analysis are diplayed in Table 2.

	Original	ACGI	Spline	Linear
PA Diameter (mm)	13.59	13.72	13.69	12.36
% Error	N/A	0.96%	0.74%	9.05%
Radius of Curvature (mm)	7.92	8.06	9.03	7.46
% Error	N/A	1.77%	14.02%	5.81%

Table 2. Quantitative validation results.

Simple in vitro phantom models were also constructed to aid in validating the reconstruction algorithm. These glass pipe intersection models were scanned and the reconstruction process was then applied to the acquired data sets. The morphological reconstructions displayed dimensions that differed from the original in vitro model by less than six percent by volume and less than four percent by diameter at any cross-section of the pipe. These results collectively affirm that our technique can use non-invasively obtained data to accurately reconstruct complex morphologies from relatively sparse MR data sets. Following this validation,

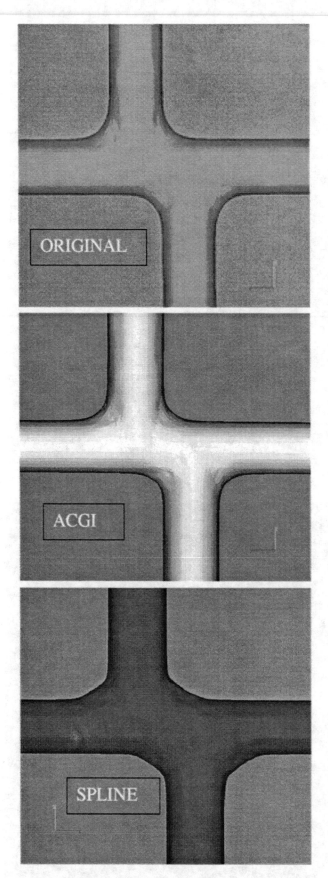

Fig. 7. Views of reconstruction connection geometries. Deformation is observable in the spline reconstruction.

data sets from patients having a surgically created TCPC were used in reconstruction. The results of two such three-dimensional reconstructions from different patients are displayed in Fig. 9 and Fig 10. A multi zone tetrahedral CFD mesh from the reconstruction displayed in Fig. 10 is shown in Fig. 11.

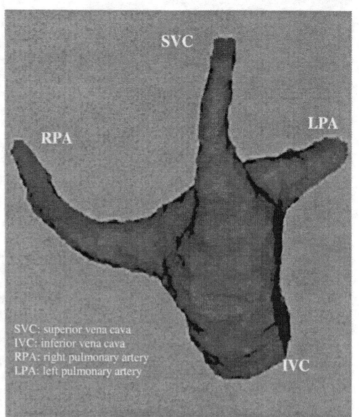

Fig. 10. Reconstruction of patient TCPC vasculature.

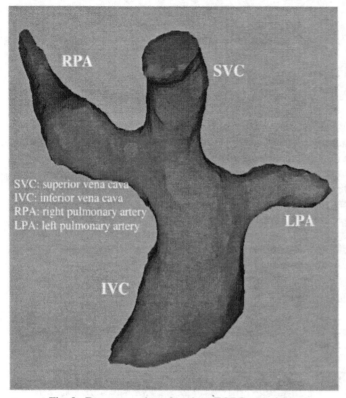

Fig. 9. Reconstruction of patient TCPC vasculature.

IV. CONCLUSIONS

Effective analysis of TCPC performance requires comprehensive three-dimensional pressure and/or velocity information. Due to the difficulty associated with extracting such data in vivo, and the surgical planning context within which that data are ultimately to be used, CFD has been selected as an attractive alternative data acquisition method. However, conventional MR yields data sets insufficiently dense to accurately reconstruct for CFD analysis. Our technique employs ACGI to augment MR data sets to be reconstructed as a necessary precursor to CFD analysis. By combining advantages of block-based and optical flow-based motion models, correlations are established between related images leading to anatomically realistic interpolated data. Results have shown that this reconstruction technique can be carried out using data acquired in a fraction of the time required by volumetric data acquisition methods, while providing accurate three-dimensional information for CFD. CFD simulations then yield data needed to carry out power loss calculations and determinine optimal TCPC configurations for successful patient outcomes.

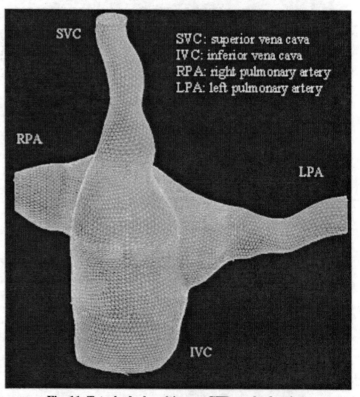

Fig. 11. Tetrahedral multi-zone CFD mesh of patient reconstruction shown in Fig. 10.

V. REFERENCES

[1] A. Docef, M.J.T. Smith, *Digital Image Processing,* 2nd ed., Riverdale: Scientific Publishers, pp.418-426, 1999.

[2] J.W. Monaco, "Motion Models for Video Applications," Ph.D. Thesis, Georgia Institute of Technology, Nov 1997.

[3] J.W. Monaco, M.J.T. Smith, "Video Coding Using Image Warping Within Variable Size Blocks," in ISCAS' 96, Vol II, pp 794-797, May 1996.

[4] M. D. Reller, R. W. McDonald, L. M. Gerlis, K. L. Thornburg, "Cardiac Embryology: Basic Review and Clinical Correlations," *Journal of the American Society of Echocardiography*, vol. 4, pp. 519-532, Jan. 1991.

[5] C. A. Taylor, T. J. Hughes, C. K. Zarins, "Finite Element Modeling of Three-Dimensional Pulsatile Flow in the Abdominal Aorta: Relevance to Atherosclerosis," *Annals of Biomedical Engineering*, vol. 6, pp. 975-987, Nov.-Dec. 1998.

[6] G. Dubini, M. R. de Leval, R. Pietrabissa, F. M. Montevecchi, R. Fumero, "A Numerical Fluid Mechanical Study of Repaired Congenital Heart Defects. Application to the Total Cavopulmonary Connection," *Journal of Biomechnics*, vol. 29, pp. 111-121, Jan. 1996.

[7] F. Migliavacca, M. R. de Leval, G. Dubini, R. Pietrabissa, "A Computational Pulsatile Model of the Bidirectional Cavopulmonary Anastomosis: The Influence of Pulmonary Forward Flow," *Journal of Biomechanical Engineering*, vol. 118, pp. 520-528, Nov. 1996.

[8] F. Migliavacca, G. Dubini, G. Pennati, R. Pietrabissa, R. Fumero, T. Hsia, M. R. de Leval, "Computational Model of the Fluid Dynamics in Systemic-to-Pulmonary Shunts," *Journal of Biomechnics*, vol. 33, pp. 549-557, Dec. 2000.

[9] MATERIALISE, MI. Mimics. [Online]. Available: http://www.materialise.com/mt.asp?mp=mm_main

VI. ACKNOWLEDGEMENTS

This work was partially supported by a grant from the National Institutes of Health. The Children's Hospital of Philadelphia, Egleston Children's Hospital, Emory University, and the University of North Carolina Chapel Hill have also contributed to this research at the Georgia Institute of Technology.

Analysis of myocardial motion in tagged MR images using nonrigid image registration

Raghavendra Chandrashekara[a], Raad H. Mohiaddin[b], Daniel Rueckert[a]

[a]Visual Information Processing Group, Department of Computing,
Imperial College of Science, Technology, and Medicine,
180 Queen's Gate, London SW7 2BZ, United Kingdom
[b]Royal Brompton and Harefield NHS Trust, Sydney Street, London, United Kingdom

ABSTRACT

Tagged magnetic resonance imaging (MRI) is unique in its ability to non-invasively image the motion and deformation of the heart *in-vivo*, but one of the fundamental reasons limiting its use in the clinical environment is the absence of automated tools to derive clinically useful information from tagged MR images. In this paper we present a novel and fully automated technique based on nonrigid image registration using multi-level free-form deformations (MFFDs) for the analysis of myocardial motion using tagged MRI. The novel aspect of our technique is its integrated nature for tag localization and deformation field reconstruction. To extract the motion field within the myocardium during systole we register a sequence of images taken during systole to a set of reference images taken at end-diastole, maximizing the mutual information between images. We use both short-axis and long-axis images of the heart to estimate the full four-dimensional motion field within the myocardium. We have validated our method using a cardiac motion simulator and we also present quantitative comparisons of cardiac motion from nine volunteers.

Keywords: Cardiac Motion Analysis, Image Registration, Tagged MRI, Mutual Information

1. INTRODUCTION

With the development of new imaging and surgical techniques, the care and treatment of patients with cardiovascular diseases (CVDs) has steadily improved over the last 50 years, but they are still the leading cause of death in the western world.[1, 2] The most common form of CVD is coronary heart disease (CHD) which accounts for almost half of all these deaths. A lack of oxygen being supplied to the muscles of the heart due to the atherosclerosis of the coronary arteries can cause the muscles to become ischemic, leading to a reduced contractility and a loss of function. Patients with impaired left ventricular function have a poor prognosis. Those with three-vessel coronary artery disease who successfully undergo revascularization have a better outlook but the decision to revascularize must be tempered with consideration of the appreciable peri-operative mortality in these patients. Viable, under-perfused myocardium improves function following revascularization and the pre-operative identification of this "hibernating myocardium" helps select those patients most likely to benefit from surgery. One way of assessing myocardial viability is with the use of magnetic resonance imaging and wall motion analysis performed at rest, with low dose dobutamine (beta agonists) for detection of viable myocardium and high dose dobutamine for the detection of ischemia. Cine CMR sequences allow qualitative assessment of regional function in a manner similar to echocardiography but without the limitations of acoustic windows, while myocardial tagging offers a method for quantification of regional wall motion and myocardial strain.

Tagged MRI[3–5] is a well known technique which can be used to obtain regional information about the deformation of the left ventricle (LV), and thus potentially help to diagnose CHD. The technique relies on the perturbation of magnetization in the myocardium in a specified spatial pattern at end-diastole. These appear as dark stripes or grids when imaged

---

Further author information: (Send correspondence to R.C.)

R.C.: E-mail: rc3@doc.ic.ac.uk, Telephone: +44 (0)20 7594 8370

R.H.M.: E-mail: r.mohiaddin@rbh.nthames.nhs.uk, Telephone: +44 (0)20 7351 8813, Address: Cardiovascular Magnetic Resonance Unit, Royal Brompton and Harefield NHS Trust, Sydney Street, London SW3 6NP, United Kingdom

D.R.: E-mail: dr@doc.ic.ac.uk, Telephone: +44 (0)20 7594 8333

immediately after the application of the tag pattern, and because the myocardium retains knowledge of this perturbation, the dark stripes or grids deform with the heart as it contracts, allowing local deformation parameters to be estimated. A recent review of MR tagging is given in Reichek.[6]

One of the fundamental reasons limiting the widespread use of tagged MRI in the clinical environment is the lack of automated tools to aid in the extraction and analysis of the motion fields within the myocardium. A number of methods have been proposed in recent years to help with this task, but many need substantial manual intervention and user interaction. The main difficulties arise because of a loss of contrast between tag stripes, due to T1 relaxation, as the heart contracts during its cycle.

2. BACKGROUND

A general trend seen in the literature relating to tagged MR image analysis is the separation of the task of tag localization or tag displacement measurement with that of deformation field reconstruction: Usually the tags are localized in an initial step and then a transformation or deformation model is fitted to the measured displacements.

2.1. Active contour models

The most popular method for the tracking tag stripes in spatial modulation of magnetization [4,5] (SPAMM) MR images is through the use of active contour models or snakes.[7] Amini et al.[8,9] used B-snakes and coupled B-snake grids to track the motion of the myocardium in radial and SPAMM tagged MR images. The B-snake grids were optimized by finding the minimum intensity locations in the tagged MR images. A dense displacement field was then interpolated by calculating a smooth warp based on continuity and intersection constraints. As the authors have noted, their method is limited to 2D analyses of the motion field within the myocardium as cardiac through plane motion is neglected. A specific imaging protocol consisting of a series of short-axis SPAMM tagged MR images lying along the corresponding tag planes in a set of parallel-tagged long-axis images has also been suggested for the analysis of cardiac motion.[10] The intersections of the tag planes, which were modelled as a series of B-spline surfaces, defined a set of points called myocardial beads which could then be visualized as the heart contracted during its cycle.

Active contour models were also used by Young et al.[11] where a weighted combination of energy potentials related to the internal energy of the deforming grid, the energy of the tagged image itself and the energy of user interactions was minimized using a modified gradient descent technique. The displacements obtained were then fitted to a finite element model to calculate deformation indices.

Park et al.[12,13] defined a new class of deformable models parameterized by functions which captured the local shape variation of the LV such as the contraction and axial twist. Again the SPAMM tag pattern was tracked using active contour models and the displacement data obtained was fitted with the deformable models. The main advantage of this method was that the parameter functions were few in number, intuitive, and allowed quantitative analyses to be made easily.

Specific packages have also been designed for the measurement of tag displacements. Kumar and Goldgof [14] used energy minimizing active contour models to track a SPAMM grid in tagged MR images, while Guttman et al. [15] have designed a package called "findtags" which uses a series of image processing steps to find the myocardial contours and tags in parallel and radial tagged MR images. The contours are found by using a morphological closing operator to remove tags in the myocardium followed by the minimization of a nonlinear combination of local cost functions. The tags were then detected using template matching based on expected tag profiles from a tagged spin-echo imaging equation. The package also uses a graphical user interface (GUI) to help users to adjust incorrectly detected contours and tags.

These packages have been used by various researchers to both validate and fit specific models of the LV that reflect its geometry. O'Dell et al.[16] used a truncated series expansion in prolate spheroidal coordinates to fit tag displacement measurements and reconstruct the motion field within the myocardium from a set of orthogonal parallel planar tagged MR images. Declerck et al.[17] also used orthogonal parallel planar tagged MR images, but the motion of the myocardium was modelled using a four-dimensional (4D) planispheric transformation. Again, in an initial step, "findtags" was used to make measurements of tag displacements. The advantage of using a 4D planispheric transformation is that it is continuous both in space and time. Denney and Prince [18] used an estimation theoretic approach modelling the measurement noise in tracking tags with a white random process. Using smoothness and incompressibility constraints, they were able to estimate the motion field within the myocardium using a Fisher estimation framework. A number of the methods discussed in the above paragraphs have been compared in Declerck et al. [19]

2.2. Optical flow methods

Optical flow methods have been proposed which implicitly track the motion of tags. Conventional optical flow methods are insufficient for tagged MR images since the contrast between the tags changes, due to T1 relaxation, during the cardiac cycle. A number of methods have been proposed to model this variation in contrast. The variable brightness optical flow (VBOF) method of Prince and McVeigh [20] used a model of the imaging process to estimate the variation in the brightness of material points in the myocardium as it undergoes deformation. The key difficulty with this method is that it requires prior knowledge of the longitudinal and transverse relaxation parameters, the proton density, and the tagging pattern itself over the entire field of view at end-diastole. Gupta and Prince [21] used a local linear transformation model to take account of the brightness variation in the tagged MR images. The linear transformation was approximated using the spin-echo tagging equation from MR physics. Although the method requires less knowledge of the MR imaging parameters it is still dependent on an appropriate approximation of the longitudinal relaxation parameter of the imaged tissue. Dougherty et al. [22] circumvented the problem of the modelling the brightness variation of tagged MR images by preprocessing the images with a series of Laplacian filters to estimate the motion between two consecutive images. Although these optical flow methods can be extended to three dimensions, the authors have limited their analyses and validations to only two dimensions. A summary of the work done on tagged MR image analysis is given in table 1.

2.3. Overview

In this paper we propose a new method for the extraction and analysis of the deformation field within the myocardium based on nonrigid image registration. The registration algorithm we use is based on the one developed by Rueckert et al., [23] which was originally developed for the registration of contrast enhanced MR breast images for the detection of cancerous lesions. We have modified this algorithm in a way so that it may be used for extraction and analysis of the full four-dimensional deformation field within the myocardium of the LV. To do this we make use of both short-axis and long-axis images of the LV. The advantage of using our approach is that tag localization and deformation field reconstruction are done simultaneously.

The paper is organized as follows. In section 3 we discuss the nonrigid registration algorithm and how we have used it recover the deformation field within the myocardium. In section 4 we present validation results using a cardiac motion simulator and experiments conducted on volunteer data. Finally, in section 5, we summarize and conclude our work and make suggestions for future directions of our research.

3. METHOD

In a normal healthy adult the left ventricle undergoes a number of different types of deformation as it pumps blood out to the body. [24] Not only does the myocardium thicken as the LV contracts but it also undergoes a twisting motion. It is also known that the base of the LV moves approximately 10 mm from base to apex during systole. [16] Since the imaging planes defined in an MR scanning session are stationary with respect to the coordinate system of the scanner, this results in a problem for the tracking of material points within the myocardium—not all points will stay within a single plane during the cardiac cycle. Thus, to fully reconstruct the deformation field within the myocardium, we need to acquire multiple-slice short-axis (SA) and long-axis (LA) images of the LV.

In figure 1 we see a typical configuration of imaging planes which could be used to reconstruct the deformation field within the myocardium. The figure shows a series of short-axis planes $(SA_1, SA_2, \ldots, SA_{10})$ and a series of long-axis planes $(LA_1, LA_2, \ldots, LA_5)$ which define an imaging volume enclosing the LV. A set of SA and LA images are also shown, to the right in the figure, corresponding to one of the SA imaging planes and one of the LA imaging planes. The LA planes are shown to be perpendicular to the SA planes, and also in a contiguous block, but the algorithm used in this paper need not be limited to these restrictions as will be explained in the following.

Consider a material point P in the myocardium at a position $\mathbf{u} = (x, y, z)$ at time $t = 0$ (corresponding to end-diastole)

Authors	Tagging Method	2D/3D	Tag Local-ization	Motion Reconstruction	Validation
Amini et al.[8,9]	radial & SPAMM	2D	ACM	thin-plate splines	motion simulator
Amini et al.[10]	SPAMM	3D	ACM	B-spline surfaces	motion simulator
Young et al.[11]	SPAMM	3D	ACM	finite-element model	gel phantom
Park et al.[12,13]	SPAMM	3D	ACM	deformable models	none
Kumar & Goldgof[14]	SPAMM	2D	ACM	thin-plate splines	manual tracking
Guttman et al.[15]	radial & parallel	2D	ACM/TM	none	none
O'Dell et al.[16]	parallel	3D	ACM/TM	series expansion	motion simulator
Declerck et al.[17]	parallel	3D	ACM/TM	planispheric transformation	none
Denney & Prince[18]	parallel	3D	ACM/TM	Fisher estimation framework	motion simulator
Prince & McVeigh[20]	SPAMM	2D	OF	velocity fields	motion simulator and phantom
Gupta & Prince[21]	SPAMM	2D	OF	velocity fields	motion simulator
Dougherty et al.[22]	SPAMM	2D	OF	velocity fields	gel phantom

Table 1. This table summarizes the work which has been done in tagged MR image analysis. The abbreviations used in the table are: spatial modulation of magnetization (SPAMM), 2-dimensional/3-dimensional (2D/3D), active contour models (ACM), template matching (TM), optical flow (OF).

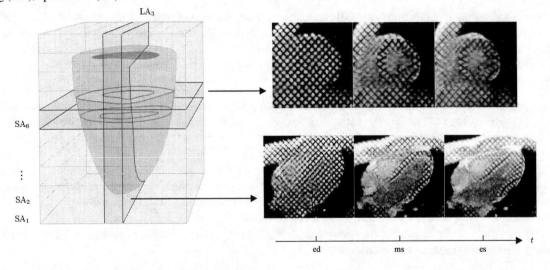

Figure 1. A typical configuration of imaging planes required to fully reconstruct the deformation field consists of both short-axis (SA) planes as well as long-axis (LA) planes. The images on the right show a set of SPAMM images for the corresponding SA and LA imaging planes at three time points, end-diastole (ed), mid-systole (ms), and end-systole (es).

that moves to another position $\mathbf{u}'$ at time t = i (figure 2). The problem, simply stated, is to find the transformation $\mathbf{T}$ for all times t such that:

$$\mathbf{T}(\mathbf{u}, t) = \mathbf{u}' \qquad (1)$$

We derive $\mathbf{T}$ using a series of free-form deformations[25] as described in the next subsection.

3.1. Combined nonrigid registration of SA and LA images

The algorithm used to calculate the transformation $\mathbf{T}(\mathbf{u}, t)$ is based on the nonrigid registration algorithm of Rueckert et al.[23] In their paper, registration was achieved by optimizing a cost function measuring the similarity between two images as well as the smoothness of the deformation needed to align the images. The similarity measure used was

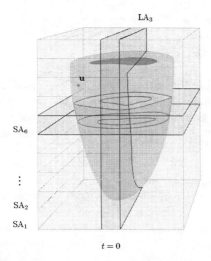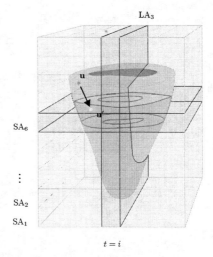

Figure 2. To reconstruct the deformation field within the myocardium we must relate points in the myocardium from images taken at time $t = 0$ (end-diastole) to their corresponding positions in images taken at a later time $t = i$. This figure also shows that the myocardium moves through the short axis imaging planes as the LV contracts.

based on normalized mutual information (NMI) and is particularly suited for application to tagged MR images since it is not dependent on changes in intensity in the images, as is the case in our application. Although the transformation model is a hierarchical one consisting of a global affine transformation and a local transformation (defined by a free-form deformation (FFD)), the motion of the heart is predominantly nonrigid, so we focus on the local transformation. We also set the regularization term in the cost function to be zero.

For the purposes of explanation we will assume that we have acquired a series of multiple-slice SA and LA images enclosing the whole of the LV and for the entire cardiac cycle as shown in figure 1. A volumetric free-form deformation (FFD) is defined on a domain Ω by a mesh of $n_x \times n_y \times n_z$ control points Φ. The domain Ω corresponds to the volume of interest V_i and includes both the short-axis image slices SA_j as well as long-axis image slices LA_j. The domain Ω defines a single coordinate system in which to perform the tracking of the LV throughout the cardiac cycle. We have chosen a coordinate system which is aligned with the short-axis image slices. To calculate the positions of the long-axis slices in this coordinate system, we use a transformation between the relative positions of short-axis and long-axis imaging planes in the coordinate system of the MR scanner that is recorded in the DICOM file format. The spacings between the control points $\phi_{i,j,k}$ in the x- and y-directions are chosen to be approximately equal to the tag spacing, while the spacing in the z-direction is chosen to be equal to the distance between the SA slices.

Since we are concerned only with recovering the deformation field within the myocardium, control points which cannot affect this field are marked as passive and not optimized. To do this we need a segmentation of the myocardium at end-diastole. This we obtain by noting that although the SPAMM tag pattern is retained by the myocardium as the LV contracts, the tag pattern in the center of the LV is completely spoiled by the blood flowing within it. At the end of the cardiac cycle the configuration of the tag pattern has returned to the state it was in at end-diastole except for its absence within the blood pool. This fact allows us to segment the myocardium in the images taken at end-diastole by segmenting the image taken at the end of the cardiac cycle. The segmentation obtained is then registered to the images taken at end-diastole to define the myocardium at that time point. Thus the blood pool, the right ventricle and other parts of the body are not considered during the registration process. This allows us to not only obtain more accurate results, but also to perform the registration more quickly.

We use a multi-level FFD as suggested by Schnabel *et al.* [26] where the transformation $\mathbf{T}(\mathbf{u}, t)$ is represented as the sum of a series of local FFDs:

$$\mathbf{T}(\mathbf{u}, t) = \sum_{h=1}^{t} \mathbf{T}_{\text{local}}^{h}(\mathbf{u}) \tag{2}$$

Parameter	Type of Motion
k_1	Radially dependent compression
k_2	Left ventricular torsion
k_3, k_4	Ellipticallization in LA and SA planes respectively
k_5, k_6, k_7	Shear in x, y, and z directions respectively
k_8, k_9, k_{10}	Rotation about x, y, and z axes respectively
k_{11}, k_{12}, k_{13}	Translation in x, y, and z directions respectively

Table 2: The 13 k-parameters controlling the cardiac motion simulator.

where

$$\mathbf{T}^h_{\text{local}}(\mathbf{u}) = \sum_{l=0}^{3} \sum_{m=0}^{3} \sum_{n=0}^{3} B_l(u) B_m(v) B_n(w) \phi_{i+l, j+m, k+n} \qquad (3)$$

and where the ϕ's represent the nearest 64 control point locations (because we are using cubic B-splines) that are used to calculate the deformation at $\mathbf{u}$. Here u, v, w are the relative positions of $\mathbf{u}$ with respect to the nearest 64 control points, and the B_i are the cubic B-spline functions.[23]

The estimation of the deformation field $\mathbf{T}(\mathbf{u}, t)$ proceeds in a sequence of registration steps as shown in figure 3. In this figure the series of volumes $V_1, V_2, \ldots, V_e$, where the subscript e denotes the volume at end-systole, are registered to V_0, with the registration of the SA images and the LA images being performed simultaneously. This is done by optimizing a cost function which is now dependent on the degree of similarity between both the SA images and the LA images:

$$\mathcal{C}(\Phi) \quad = \quad -\mathcal{C}_{\text{similarity}}(V_0, \mathbf{T}(V_t)) \qquad (4)$$

$$= \quad \frac{H(V_0) + H(\mathbf{T}(V_t))}{H(V_0, \mathbf{T}(V_t))} \qquad (5)$$

where the Φ are the parameters defining the local transformation $\mathbf{T}$, $\mathbf{T}(V_t)$ is the volume V_t transformed so that it is registered with V_0, $H(V_0)$ is the marginal entropy of image intensities in the volume V_0, $H(\mathbf{T}(V_t))$ is the marginal entropy of image intensities of the transformed volume $\mathbf{T}(V_t)$, and $H(V_0, \mathbf{T}(V_t))$ is the joint entropy of image intensities of these two volumes. The transformations $\mathbf{T}$ and the similarity measure are only evaluated within the myocardium.

After registering the volume V_1 to V_0 we obtain a multi-level FFD (MFFD) consisting of a single FFD representing the motion of the myocardium at time $t = 1$. To register volume V_2 to V_0 a second level is added to the sequence of FFDs and then optimized to yield the transformation at time $t = 2$. This process continues until all the volumes in the sequence are registered, as shown in figure 3, allowing us to relate any point in the myocardium at time $t = 0$ to its corresponding point throughout the sequence.

4. RESULTS

4.1. Cardiac motion simulator data

For the purposes of validation, a cardiac motion simulator as described in Waks et al.[27] was implemented. The motion simulator is based on a 13-parameter model of left-ventricular motion developed by Arts et al.[24] and is applied to a volume representing the LV that is modelled as a region between two confocal prolate spheres while the imaging process is simulated by a tagged spin-echo imaging equation.[20] The 13 parameters and the types of motion to which they correspond are shown in table 2. To compare how well the registration algorithm performed in reconstructing the deformation field, when the deformation field is known, nine sets of images were generated from the simulator showing three different types of nonrigid motion. Three sets of images, A_1, A_2, A_3, were generated by varying k_1 as shown below:

$$k_1 = -0.01t \text{ where } t = 0, 1, \ldots, 9 \qquad (6)$$

Gaussian noise with a mean of 0 and standard deviations, σ, of 8 and 16 were added to image sets A_2 and A_3 respectively. No noise was added to image set A_1. Another three sets of images, B_1, B_2, B_3, were generated by varying k_2 in addition

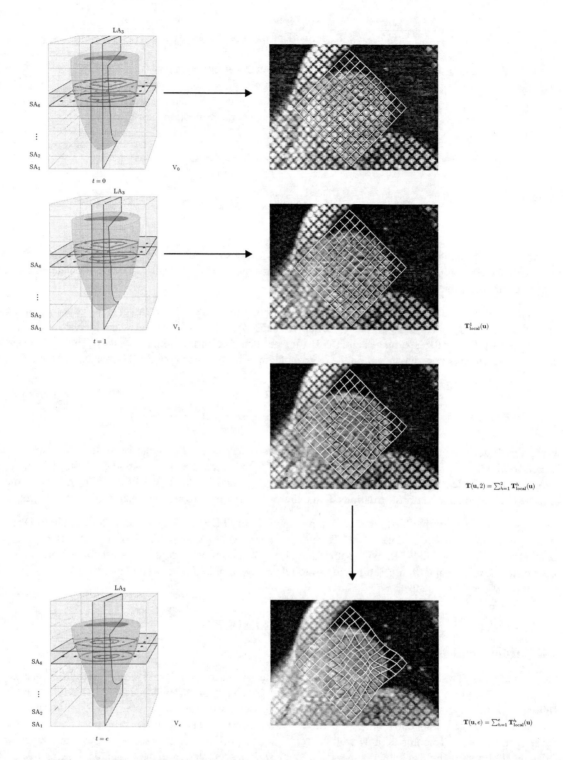

Figure 3. The short-axis SA_i and the long-axis images LA_i taken at time t are registered to their corresponding images taken at time $t = 0$ to to recover the deformation within the myocardium. The SA images on the right show a virtual tag grid which has been aligned with the tag pattern at time $t = 0$. As time progresses the virtual tag grid is deformed by the MFFD and follows the underlying tag pattern in the images.

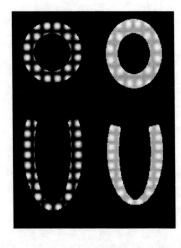

Parameter	Description	Value
λ_i	Inner radius	0.35
λ_o	Outer radius	0.55
δ/cm	Focal radius	4.00
D_0	Spin density	300.0
T_E/s	Echo time	0.03
T_R/s	Pulse repetition time	10.0
T_1/s	Longitudinal relaxation time	0.6
T_2/s	Transverse Relaxation time	0.1
θ	Tip angle of tag pattern	45.0°
$\text{SA}_x \times \text{SA}_y$	SA voxel sizes	0.5×0.5 mm
$\text{LA}_x \times \text{LA}_y$	SA voxel sizes	0.5×0.78125 mm

(a) Simulator images   (b) Simulator parameters

Figure 4. The figure on the left shows a SA image ($z = -5$ mm) and a LA image ($y = 3.2$ mm) for two different times from image set C_1. The images on the left show the LV at time $t = 0$ and the images on the right show the LV at time $t = 9$. The table on the right shows the parameter values used in generating the simulator images.

to k_1:

$$k_1 = -0.01t, \ k_2 = 0.01t \text{ where } t = 0, 1, \ldots, 9 \tag{7}$$

Similarly Gaussian noise with a mean of 0 and standard deviations of 8 and 16 were added to image sets B_2 and B_3 respectively, while no noise was added to image set B_1. The final sets, C_1, C_2, C_3, were generated by varying k_1, k_2, k_3 and k_4 according to:

$$k_1 = -0.01t, \ k_2 = 0.01t, \ k_3 = -0.01t, \ k_4 = -0.01t \text{ where } t = 0, 1, \ldots, 9 \tag{8}$$

Again Gausssian noise with a mean of 0 and standard deviations of 8 and 16 were added to image sets C_2 and C_3 respectively. The images generated consisted of both SA and LA images. The SA slices were located at $z = -45, -35, \ldots, 45$ (in mm) with respect to the origin defined by the LV model.[27] Two sets of LA images were produced which were perpendicular to each other and also to the SA images. The two sets of LA image slices were located at positions $x = -16, -9.6, -3.2, 3.2, 9.6, 16$ (in mm) and $y = -16, -9.6, -3.2, 3.2, 9.6, 16$ (in mm) respectively. Figure 4(a) shows the deformation of the LV in the SA and LA views at two different times frames from image set C_1. The model and imaging parameters used in generating the images are given in table 4(b). The tag spacing in all images was $2\pi/8$ mm.

For each set of images a transformation, $\mathbf{T}$, which gave the deformation of the model LV was calculated using the registration algorithm described in section 3. The root mean square (r.m.s) error in the displacement of points in the LV estimated from the transformation $\mathbf{T}$ was then calculated for each time t as follows:

$$\delta(t) = \sqrt{\frac{1}{N} \sum_{\mathbf{u} \in \text{LV}} |\mathbf{T}(\mathbf{u}, t) - \mathbf{T}_{\text{actual}}(\mathbf{u}, t)|^2} \tag{9}$$

where the summation is over all points in the image at time frame 0 which are within the LV, N is the number of such points, $\mathbf{u}$ is the position of a point, t is the time, and $\mathbf{T}(\mathbf{u}, t)$ and $\mathbf{T}_{\text{actual}}(\mathbf{u}, t)$ are the estimated and actual displacements of the point $\mathbf{u}$ at time t respectively.

Figures 5(a), 5(b), 5(c) show the variation of the r.m.s error in the estimated displacements for the three different types of motion. In each of the figures the r.m.s error is seen to increase with time. In figures 5(a) and 5(b) the r.m.s error increased to only approximately 0.1 mm even when noise had been added. The r.m.s errors in figure 5(c) are larger since the LV performs a more complicated deformation which includes ellipticallization as well as torsional and compressional deformations. But in all the sets of images the r.m.s error was less than the voxel size.

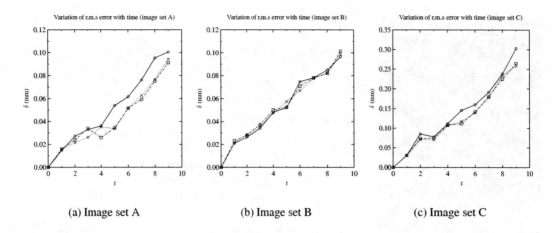

| (a) Image set A | (b) Image set B | (c) Image set C |

Figure 5. This figure shows the variation of the r.m.s error in the estimated displacements for three different types of motion generated from the LV simulator, and for different amounts of Gaussian noise added to the images. Curves drawn with circles correspond to no noise in the images, crosses to Gaussian noise with $\sigma = 8$, and squares with $\sigma = 16$.

4.2. Human data

Tagged MR data from 9 healthy volunteers was acquired with a Siemens Sonata 1.5 T scanner consisting of a series of SA and 0, 2, or 3 LA slices covering the whole of the LV. For two of the volunteers no LA slices were acquired, for one volunteer 2 LA slices were acquired and for the remaining six volunteers 3 LA slices were acquired. A cine breath-hold sequence with a SPAMM tag pattern was used with imaging being done at end expiration. The image voxel sizes were $1.40 \times 1.40 \times 10$ mm, and 10–18 images were acquired during the cardiac cycle, depending on the volunteer. The images taken at end-diastole, mid-systole, and end-systole for one of the volunteers are shown in figure 6. The figure also shows the orientation of the LA images with respect to the SA images. The imaging parameters for this volunteer were a repetition time of 40 ms, an echo time of 4 ms, and a $15°$ flip angle.

The deformation field within the myocardium for each of the volunteers was constructed by using the method described in section 3. To assess how well the registration algorithm performed in tracking the motion of the myocardium for volunteer data, tag-intersection points were detected manually by an observer in a slice midway between the base and the apex for all time frames between end-diastole and end-systole. For the purposes of comparing the registration algorithm with the observer, only SA slices were used to reconstruct the deformation field, since only in-plane displacements were able to be measured by the observer. The r.m.s error between the in-plane displacements estimated from the registration algorithm and the actual in-plane displacements as measured by the observer were then calculated as in section 4.1. The results are shown in figure 7.

The figure shows that for volunteers 2, 4, 6, 8, and 9 the r.m.s error is smaller than the voxel size; for volunteers 3, and 5 the r.m.s error is smaller than the voxel size for most of the cardiac cycle reaching a value just greater than the voxel size at end-systole; and for volunteers 1, and 7 the r.m.s error was below 2.1 mm. These results indicate a very good performance in the motion tracking.

5. CONCLUSIONS

In this paper we have presented a novel method for tracking the motion of the myocardium in the LV using nonrigid image registration. We validated our method using a cardiac motion simulator, where we found that the deformation field could be reconstructed with a r.m.s error which was smaller than a voxel. We also reconstructed the deformation field within the myocardium for nine volunteers and showed that the r.m.s tracking error was below the voxel size for most of the volunteers.

In future work we will extend the registration algorithm to make use of transformations which more closely model the

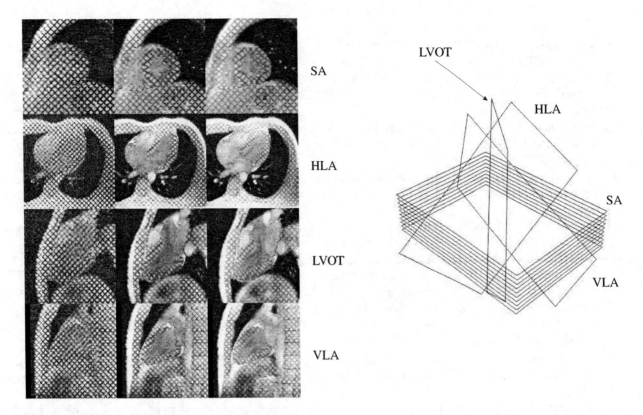

Figure 6. SA and LA images taken from a volunteer at three different times, end-diastole (left column), mid-systole (middle column), end-systole (right column). The top row shows SA images, and the next three rows show horizontal LA (HLA), LV out-flow tract (LVOT), and vertical LA (VLA) images respectively. The orientation of the LA slices with respect to the SA slices is shown on the right.

geometry and motion of the LV. One simple way of doing this would be to use control points which are radially located around the LV. Different modes of motion of the LV, such as torsional and contractional movements, could then be introduced. This extended algorithm should improve the accuracy and speed of the motion field reconstruction.

ACKNOWLEDGMENTS

RC and DR were supported by EPSRC grant no. GR/N24919. We would also like to thank Steve Collins for converting the MR data to DICOM format.

REFERENCES

1. American Heart Association, "2001 heart and stroke statistical update." http://www.americanheart.org/, 2000.
2. M. Rayner and S. Petersen, "European cardiovascular disease statistics." http://www.dphpc.ox.ac.uk/bhfhprg/, 2000.
3. E. A. Zerhouni, D. M. Parish, W. J. Rogers, A. Yang, and E. P. Shapiro, "Human heart: Tagging with MR imaging — a method for noninvasive assessment of myocardial motion," *Radiology* **169**(1), pp. 59–63, 1988.
4. L. Axel and L. Dougherty, "MR imaging of motion with spatial modulation of magnetization," *Radiology* **171**(3), pp. 841–845, 1989.
5. L. Axel and L. Dougherty, "Heart wall motion : Improved method of spatial modulation of magnetization for MR imaging," *Radiology* **172**(2), pp. 349–360, 1989.
6. N. Reichek, "MRI myocardial tagging," *Journal of Magnetic Resonance Imaging* **10**, pp. 609–616, 1999.
7. M. Kass, A. Witkin, and D. Terzopoulos, "Snakes: Active contour models," *International Journal of Computer Vision* **1**(4), pp. 321–331, 1988.

8. A. A. Amini, R. W. Curwen, and J. C. Gore, "Snakes and splines for tracking non-rigid heart motion," in *Proceedings of the Fourth European Conference on Computer Vision*, B. Buxton and R. Cipolla, eds., *Lecture Notes in Computer Science* **1065**, pp. 251–261, Springer, (Cambridge, UK), April 1996.

9. A. A. Amini, Y. Chen, R. W. Curwen, V. Mani, and J. Sun, "Coupled B-snake grids and constrained thin-plate splines for analysis of 2D tissue deformations from tagged MRI," *IEEE Transactions on Medical Imaging* **17**, pp. 344–356, June 1998.

10. A. A. Amini, Y. Chen, M. Elayyadi, and P. Radeva, "Tag surface reconstruction and tracking of myocardial beads from SPAMM-MRI with parametric B-spline surfaces," *IEEE Transactions on Medical Imaging* **20**, pp. 94–103, February 2001.

11. A. A. Young, D. L. Kraitchman, L. Dougherty, and L. Axel, "Tracking and finite element analysis of stripe deformation in magnetic resonance tagging," *IEEE Transactions on Medical Imaging* **14**, pp. 413–421, September 1995.

12. J. Park, D. Metaxas, and L. Axel, "Analysis of left ventricular wall motion based on volumetric deformable models and MRI-SPAMM," *Medical Image Analysis* **1**(1), pp. 53–71, 1996.

13. J. Park, D. Metaxas, A. A. Young, and L. Axel, "Deformable models with parameter functions for cardiac motion analysis from tagged MRI data," *IEEE Transactions on Medical Imaging* **15**, pp. 278–289, June 1996.

14. S. Kumar and D. Goldgof, "Automatic tracking of SPAMM grid and the estimation of deformation parameters from cardiac MR images," *IEEE Transactions on Medical Imaging* **13**, pp. 122–132, March 1994.

15. M. A. Guttman, J. L. Prince, and E. R. McVeigh, "Tag and contour detection in tagged MR images of the left ventricle," *IEEE Transactions on Medical Imaging* **13**, March 1994.

16. W. G. O'Dell, C. C. Moore, W. C. Hunter, E. A. Zerhouni, and E. R. McVeigh, "Three-dimensional myocardial deformations: Calculation with displacement field fitting to tagged MR images," *Radiology* **195**, pp. 829–835, June 1995.

17. J. Declerck, N. Ayache, and E. R. McVeigh, "Use of a 4D planispheric transformation for the tracking and the analysis of LV motion with tagged MR images," in *SPIE Medical Imaging, vol. 3660*, (San Diego, CA, USA), February 1999.

18. T. S. Dennney, Jr. and J. L. Prince, "Reconstruction of 3D left ventricular motion from planar tagged cardiac MR images : An estimation theoretic approach," *IEEE Transactions on Medical Imaging* **14**, pp. 1–11, December 1995.

19. J. Declerck, T. S. Denney, C. Ozturk, W. O'Dell, and E. R. McVeigh, "Left ventricular motion reconstruction from planar tagged MR images: A comparison," *Physics in Medicine and Biology* **45**, pp. 1611–1632, 2000.

20. J. L. Prince and E. R. McVeigh, "Motion estimation from tagged MR images," *IEEE Transactions on Medical Imaging* **11**, pp. 238–249, June 1992.

21. S. N. Gupta and J. L. Prince, "On variable brightness optical flow for tagged MRI," in *Information Processing in Medical Imaging*, pp. 323–334, June 1995.

22. L. Dougherty, J. C. Asmuth, A. S. Blom, L. Axel, and R. Kumar, "Validation of an optical flow method for tag displacement estimation," *IEEE Transactions on Medical Imaging* **18**, pp. 359–363, April 1999.

23. D. Rueckert, L. I. Sonoda, C. Hayes, D. L. G. Hill, M. O. Leach, and D. J. Hawkes, "Nonrigid registration using free-form deformations: Application to breast MR images," *IEEE Transactions on Medical Imaging* **18**, pp. 712–721, August 1999.

24. T. Arts, W. C. Hunter, A. Douglas, A. M. M. Muijtjens, and R. S. Reneman, "Description of the deformation of the left ventricle by a kinematic model," *Biomechanics* **25**(10), pp. 1119–1127, 1992.

25. S. Lee, G. Wolberg, and S. Y. Shin, "Scattered data interpolation with multilevel B-splines," *IEEE Transactions on Visualization and Computer Graphics* **3**, pp. 228–244, July–September 1997.

26. J. A. Schnabel, D. Rueckert, M. Quist, J. M. Blackall, A. D. Castellano-Smith, T. Hartkens, G. P. Penney, W. A. Hall, H. Liu, C. L. Truwit, F. A. Gerritsen, D. L. G. Hill, and D. J. Hawkes, "A generic framework for non-rigid registration based on non-uniform multi-level free-form deformations," in *Proceedings of the Fourth International Conference on Medical Image Computing and Computer Assisted Intervention*, W. J. Niessen and M. A. Viergever, eds., pp. 573–581, Springer, (Utrecht, The Netherlands), October 2001.

27. E. Waks, J. L. Prince, and A. S. Douglas, "Cardiac motion simulator for tagged MRI," in *Proceedings of the IEEE Workshop on Mathematical Methods in Biomedical Image Analysis*, pp. 182–191, June 21–22 1996.

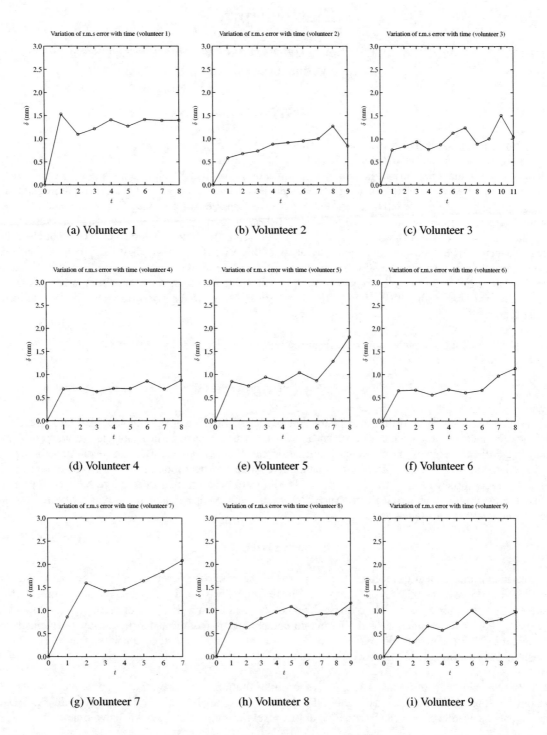

Figure 7. This figure shows the variation of the r.m.s error for displacements estimated from the registration algorithm as compared with the manual tracking of tag intersections in mid-ventricular SA slices for the nine volunteers.

Characterization and Evaluation of Inversion Algorithms for MR Elastography

Armando Manduca, Travis E. Oliphant, David S. Lake, M. Alex Dresner, Richard L. Ehman
Mayo Clinic and Foundation

ABSTRACT

Magnetic resonance elastography (MRE) can visualize and measure acoustic shear waves in tissue-like materials subjected to harmonic mechanical excitation. This allows the calculation of local values of material parameters such as shear modulus and attenuation. Various inversion algorithms to perform such calculations have been proposed. Under certain assumptions (discussed in detail), the problem reduces to local inversion of the Helmholtz equation. Three algorithms are considered to perform this inversion: Direct Inversion, Local Frequency Estimation, and Matched Filter. To study the noise sensitivity, resolution, and accuracy of these techniques, studies were conducted on synthetic and physical phantoms and on in-vivo breast data. All three algorithms accurately reconstruct shear modulus, demarcate differences between tissues, and identify tumors as areas of higher stiffness, but they vary in noise sensitivity and resolution. The Matched Filter, designed for optimal behavior in noise, provides the best combination of sharpness and smoothness. Challenges remain in pulse sequence design, delivering sufficient signal to certain areas of the body, and improvements in processing algorithms, but MRE shows great potential for non-invasive in vivo determination of mechanical properties.

Keywords: MRI, MRE, elastography, stiffness, shear modulus, inversion, reconstruction

1. INTRODUCTION

Magnetic resonance elastography (MRE) is a phase contrast based MRI imaging technique that can directly visualize and quantitatively measure propagating acoustic shear waves in tissue-like materials subjected to harmonic mechanical excitation [1]. Full 3D complex displacement information can be acquired at MR pixel resolution throughout a 3D volume. This data allows the calculation of local quantitative values of shear modulus and the generation of images that depict tissue elasticity or stiffness. Various inversion algorithms to perform such calculations have been proposed. We will discuss the assumptions underlying three such algorithms, and compare their noise sensitivity and resolution on synthetic, phantom and in vivo data sets.

2. THEORY

MRE uses harmonic mechanical displacements as a probe of the material properties of soft tissues, spatially mapping and measuring motions with amplitudes of 1μ or less. The resulting "wave images" reflect the displacement of spins due to acoustic strain wave propagation. Wave images can be obtained at various phase offsets regularly spaced around a motion cycle. This allows extraction of the harmonic component of motion at the frequency of interest, giving the amplitude and the phase (relative to an arbitrary zero point) of the displacement at each point in space [2]. This complex displacement field is the input to all the processing techniques described below.

A single MRE acquisition captures only a single component of motion. However, the experiment can be repeated with three orthogonal sensitization directions. Thus, the data set acquired by MRE can be very rich: full 3D complex harmonic displacement information can be acquired at MR pixel resolution throughout a 3D volume.

Since MRE uses very small displacements (microns), it is a good approximation to model tissue as a linear, viscoelastic solid. In the general case, stress and strain are related by a rank 4 tensor with up to 21 independent quantities [3]. Assuming an isotropic material, this reduces to two independent quantities, the Lame constants λ and μ, related to

Medical Imaging 2002: Image Processing, Milan Sonka, J. Michael Fitzpatrick, Editors, Proceedings of SPIE Vol. 4684 (2002) © 2002 SPIE · 1605-7422/02/$15.00

longitudonal and shear deformation respectively. If local homogeneity is assumed, λ and μ become single unknowns, and the equation for harmonic motion becomes an algebraic matrix equation that can be solved locally [4]:

$$\mu\nabla^2\mathbf{u} + (\lambda + \mu)\nabla(\nabla \cdot \mathbf{u}) = -\rho\omega^2\mathbf{u} \tag{1}$$

with ρ the density, ω the angular frequency of the mechanical oscillation, and $\mathbf{u}$ the displacement vector. The Lame constants can be considered as complex quantities, with the imaginary parts of the constants representing attenuation for a viscoelastic medium. Solving this equation requires the full 3D displacement, since the equations for the individual components are coupled.

In soft tissues, $\lambda \gg \mu$ (typically by 10^4 or more). This makes it difficult to estimate λ and μ simultaneously, but it also effectively decouples the two, allowing partial filtering of longitudonal effects since they occur at very low spatial frequencies. Filtering approaches can also be designed based on the longitudonal wave field being curl-free and the shear wave field divergence-free. In general, the longitudonal wavelength is so long in tissues (tens of meters) that accurate estimation of λ is very challenging.

To formally remove λ from consideration, incompressibility can be assumed, leading to the Helmholtz equation:

$$\mu\nabla^2\mathbf{u} = -\rho\omega^2\mathbf{u} \tag{2}$$

Importantly, the terms involving components in orthogonal directions are now decoupled, and each component satisfies the equation separately. Thus, measurements in only one sensitization direction suffice to determine μ.

3.   INVERSION ALGORITHMS

A variety of techniques have been proposed to perform this inversion, some of which are summarized below. These techniques do not depend on planar shear wave propagation, nor on the presence of only a single wave, but simply on the presence of motion (that satisfies the assumed physical model) in the region of interest. In particular, complex interference patterns from reflection, diffraction, etc. do not pose difficulties, except as these patterns contain areas of low amplitude and hence low SNR.

3.1 Local Frequency Estimation (LFE)

LFE estimates the local spatial frequency of the shear wave propagation pattern, using an algorithm that combines local estimates of instantaneous frequency over several scales. These estimates are derived from filters that are a product of radial and directional components and can be considered to be oriented lognormal quadrature wavelets [5].   The shear stiffness is then $\mu = f_{mech}^2/f_{sp}^2$, with the assumption that $\rho \sim 1.0$ for all soft tissues. It can be shown that this approach is solving the Helmholtz equation obtained under the assumptions of local homogeneity, incompressibility, and no attenuation.   The LFE allows estimation of μ from a single image; i.e., using displacement values for a single sensitization direction and a single phase offset. It is equally applicable to the complex harmonic displacement extracted from multiple phase offsets.

The LFE algorithm has proven to be a robust, useful technique because of the sophisticated multi-scale data averaging in the estimation. It yields accurate and isotropic local frequency estimates and is relatively insensitive to noise [6], and is easily extended to 3D [7]. One disadvantage is the limited resolution; at sharp boundaries the LFE estimate is blurred, and the correct estimate is reached only half a wavelength into a given region. If one considers a stiff object of size equal to (say) an eighth of a spatial wavelength embedded in a less stiff background material, the LFE estimate of $\square$ for the object will never reach the correct value. However, the object is *detectable*; that is, the existence of a stiff object is evident even if quantitative determination of its stiffness is inaccurate.

3.2 Direct Inversion (DI)

The Helmholtz equation can be directly inverted ay every point by simply calculating the required Laplacian within a small spatial window. In practice, this requires data smoothing and the calculation of accurate second derivatives from noisy data. Both of these tasks are performed with Savitsky-Golay filters [8] in this implementation.

3.3 Matched Filter (MF)

The matched filter algorithm uses an adaptive smoothed matched filter and its second derivative to perform the division above. This technique is derived from considerations of attempting to minimize the width of the conditional probability density function of the estimate for μ [9]. Since the filters vary across the image, the need for local calculation of the filters makes this approach computationally more intensive.

3.4 Variational Method (VM)

Romano et al. [10] have suggested using the variational form of (1) above and appropriate test functions to estimate the Lame coefficients. This avoids derivative calculations on noisy data by taking analytic derivatives of smooth test functions and integrating these over local windows in product with the data. In practice, this is similar to our methods of derivative calculations (by filtering with the derivative of a smooth function). Their assumption of constant μ/r also is essentially equivalent to the local homogeneity assumption above. Thus this approach, while providing valuable insights, is very similar to DI, and the results from the two techniques prove to be very similar as well.

4. RESULTS

To study the noise sensitivity, resolution, and accuracy of the processing techniques, we present results on synthetic and physical phantoms of known parameters and on in-vivo breast data.

4.1 Two-Region Phantom

The first phantom is a 2D data set that simulates a perfect plane shear wave propagating through two homogeneous regions separated by a sharp boundary. The regions have no attenuation and their simulated shear moduli are 25.0 and 6.25 kPa. Eight phase offsets were simulated, with Gaussian noise added to simulate a wave image SNR of 5:1. In most MRE experiments, the wave images achieve SNR levels of better than 5:1, so this represents a realistic but fairly noisy situation. These data sets are not simulations of physical wave propagation or the MRE acquisition process, but simply sinusoidal wave patterns with noise added. The images and results were 256x256, but only the central regions of each are shown below.

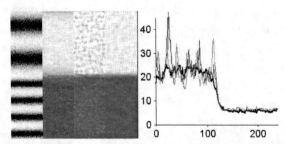

Fig. 1 (left) Sample wave image and results on two-region data set for the LFE, DI and MF algorithms for the central region of the data; (right) profiles through the central columns of the results.

Fig. 1 shows portions of a sample image from the two-region data set, and LFE, DI and MF reconstructions respectively (and vertical profiles of these). The LFE result is smoothest but blurs the boundary more than DI and MF. The DI and MF are more sensitive to noise but depict the boundary more sharply. The MF image is visually smoother and shows less variation in the profiles than the DI. To some extent, the latter two techniques can trade off resolution against noise sensitivity by altering the size of the local window, while LFE can effect a similar tradeoff by altering the analysis filter bank.. All three techniques assume local homogeneity, which breaks down when the boundary between the regions is within the local window, but all simply blur the boundary with no other obvious ill effects.

4.2 Ψ Object

To test the ability of the algorithms to recover complex objects, wave data was simulated for a Ψ–shaped object in a slightly heterogeneous background with and without noise. The plane wave is incoming from the left and undergoes significant refraction and interference after interacting with the object. Significant amplitude nulls and phase discontinuities are evident. From the wave data alone, there is little clue as to the shape of the object.

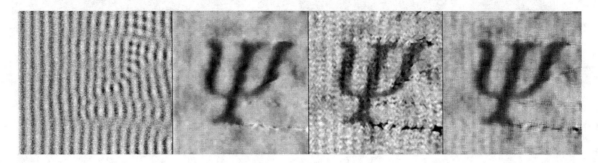

Fig. 2 Sample wave image and LFE, DI and MF results for the simulated psi object.

Fig. 2 shows a sample image and LFE, DI and MF reconstructions for the Ψ data set. All three algorithms do a very good job of visualizing the object, even in the noisy case, although they have some difficulties in the regions of interference. The LFE result is smoother but has poorer boundary definition. The DI result has more artifacts and is more affected by the amplitude nulls. The MF result is slightly sharper and has slightly greater contrast than the LFE and is almost as smooth.

4.3 Prostate Phantom

A 6 cm cylinder of 1.5% agarose gel with a 1.4 cm inclusion of 3% gel was constructed to simulate a palpable tumor nodule in the peripheral zone of the prostate. Separate large (12 cm diameter, 12 cm high) phantoms of pure 1.5% and 3% gels were constructed as references for determining true stiffnesses. The phantoms were excited with shear waves at 400 Hz from a plane wave transducer, and full 7-dimensional data was collected of the propagating waves: volume information (3D spatial) about the vector motion (3D) through time (8 phase offsets).

Fig. 3 shows a sample image and LFE, DI and MF reconstructions for the prostate phantom. Averages over regions of interest in the stiff inclusion and background are given in the Table 1 below. The LFE result is the blurriest and under-estimates the true value significantly (due to the size of the inclusion relative to the wavelength). The DI result has sharper boundaries and is closer to the actual value, but has more artifacts. The MF result gives an accurate and sharp depiction of the inclusion with minimal artifacts. Profiles through the reconstructions are shown in Fig. 4. The DI and MF results have sharper boundaries and are closer to the actual value, but the MF result is smoother, more clearly differentiates inclusion from background, and has fewer artifacts.

Table 1: Average Shear Moduli in Local Regions

	Reference	LFE	DD	MF
Inclusion	56.6 ± 2.1	38.2 ± 1.6	52.9 ± 3.6	47.7 ± 2.0
Backgnd	11.6 ± 0.9	11.0 ± 0.7	13.9 ± 1.0	10.4 ± 0.8

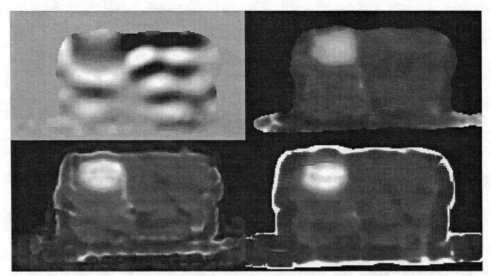

Fig. 3 Sample wave image (top left) and LFE (top right), DI (bottom left) and MF (bottom right) results on prostate phantom.

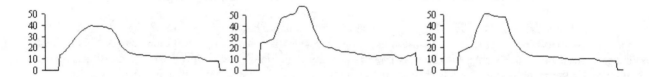

Fig. 4 Profiles through the inclusion for the LFE (left), DI (center) and MF (right) reconstruction of the prostate phantom.

4.4 Breast Data

MRE data was obtained from the breast of a patient with a 4 cm diameter, biopsy-proven breast cancer, using shear waves at 100Hz applied to the skin of the medial and lateral aspects of the breast. The FOV is 12 cm and the slice thickness is 5 mm. Fig. 5 shows a T1-weighted magnitude image of a patient with a biopsy-proven breast cancer and the LFE, DI and MF reconstructions respectively. All three techniques indicate that the shear stiffness of the tumor in the posterior section of the breast is substantially higher than that of normal breast tissues.

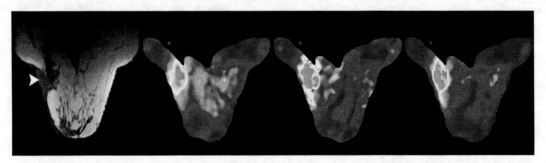

Fig. 5 A T1-weighted breast image of a volunteer with a malignant tumor (arrow), and the LFE, DI and MF reconstructions of MRE data acquired from the volunteer.

5. DISCUSSION

All the inversion algorithms do a reasonable job of reconstructing shear modulus, although with different characteristics. The LFE results are smoother but have more limited resolution. The DI reconstructions are sharper but are more susceptible to noise and artifacts. The MF algorithm, which is explicitly designed for optimal behavior in noise, may provide the best combination of sharpness and smoothness. All three techniques can, to some extent, trade off resolution vs. noise sensitivity by altering the size of the local window or adjusting the filter parameters. More sophisticated techniques that do not assume local homogeneity [11] may yield improved results, but that remains to be proven. It may well be that more important issues are the techniques used for noise smoothing and the estimation of derivatives of noisy data, regardless of the sophistication of the processing algorithm It is also possible to relax the isotropic assumption and solve for anisotropic material properties (and many tissues are anisotropic). Sinkus et al. [12] has proposed such an analysis, although the assumptions they make in terms of material properties are not clear. Finally, attenuation can be solved for with most of the techniques above [4]. However, in our experience, attenuation determinations are very sensitive to noise.

In conclusion, MRE shows great potential for the non-invasive in vivo determination of mechanical properties in a variety of tissues. Reconstruction algorithms have been tested and characterized and, although far from perfect, yield quantitative measures of elasticity that clearly demarcate differences between tissue types and identify tumors as areas of higher stiffness. Challenges remain in pulse sequence design, delivering sufficient signal to certain areas of the body, and improving processing algorithms to generate more accurate, higher resolution elasticity and attenuation maps.all cases where the correction technique was applied, image artifacts were significantly reduced.

ACKNOWLEDGEMENTS

This work was supported in part by NIH grant CA75552.

REFERENCES

1. Muthupillai, R, Lomas, D.J., Rossman, P.J., Greenleaf, J.F., Manduca, A. and Ehman, R.L. (1995) Magnetic resonance elastography by direct visualization of propagating acoustic strain waves. *Science*, 269, 1854-1857.
2. Manduca, A., Smith, J.A., Muthupillai, R., Rossman, P.J., Greenleaf, J.F. and Ehman, R.L. (1997) Image analysis techniques for magnetic resonance elastography. *Proc Int Soc for Magn Reson in Med*, 5, 1905.
3. Auld, B.A. (1990) In *Acoustic Fields and Waves in Solids*, Krieger Publishing Company, Malabar, Florida.
4. Oliphant, T.E., Manduca, A., Ehman, R.L. and Greenleaf, J.F. (2001) Complex-valued stiffness reconstruction for magnetic resonance elastography by algebraic inversion of the differential equation. *Magnetic Resonance in Medicine*, 45, 299-310.
5. Knutsson, H., Westin, C.J. and Granlund, G. (1994) Local multiscale frequency and bandwidth estimation. *Proc of the IEEE Intl Conf on Image Processing*, 1, 36-40.
6. Manduca, A., Muthupillai, R., Rossman, P.J., Greenleaf, J.F. and Ehman, R.L. (1996) Image processing for magnetic resonance elastography. *SPIE Med Imaging* 2710, 616-623.
7. Manduca, A., Muthupillai, R., Rossman, P.J., Greenleaf, J.F. and Ehman, R.L. (1997b) 3-D local wavelength estimation for magnetic resonance elastography. *Radiology* 205(P), 469.
8. Press, W.H., Teukolsky, S.A., Vetterling, W.T. and Flannery, B.P. (1992) In *Numerical Recipes in C*, Cambridge University Press, New York.
9. Oliphant, T.E., Manduca, A., Ehman, R.L. and Greenleaf, J.F. (2001) Adaptive estimation of piecewise constant shear modulus for magnetic resonance elastography. *Proc Int Soc for Magn Reson in Med*, 9, 642.
10. Romano, A.J., Shirron, J.J. and Bucaro, J.A. (1998) On the noninvasive determination of material parameters from a knowledge of elastic displacements. *IEEE Trans Ultra Ferro Freq Cntrl* 45(3), 751-759.
11. Van Houten, E.E.W., Paulsen, K.D., Miga, M.I., Kennedy F.E. and Weaver, J.B. (1999) An overlapping subzone technique for MR-based elastic property reconstruction. *Magnetic Resonance in Medicine*, 42, 779-786.
12. Sinkus, R., Lorenzen, J., Schrader, D., Lorenzen, M., Dargatz, M. and Holz, D. (2000) High-resolution tensor MR elastography for breast tumour detection. *Phys Med & Bio* 45, 1649-1664.

Visualization of Cardiac Wavefronts Using Data Fusion

David B. Kynor[*a], Anthony J. Dietz[a], Eric M. Friets[a], Jon N. Peterson[a], Ursula C. Bergstrom[a],
John K. Triedman[b], Peter E. Hammer[b]

[a]Creare Inc., Hanover, NH, [b]Children's Hospital, Boston, MA

ABSTRACT

Catheter ablation has emerged as a highly effective treatment for arrhythmias that are constrained by known, easily located, anatomic landmarks. However, this treatment has enjoyed limited success for arrhythmias that are characterized by complex activation patterns or are not anatomically constrained. This class of arrhythmias, which includes atrial fibrillation and ventricular tachycardia resulting from ischemic heart disease, demands improved mapping tools. Current technology forces the cardiologist to view cardiac anatomy independently from the functional information contained in the electrical activation patterns. This leads to difficulties in interpreting the large volumes of data provided by high-density recording catheters and in mapping patients with abnormal anatomy (e.g., patients with congenital heart disease). The goal of this is work is development of new data processing and display algorithms that will permit the clinician to view activation sequences superimposed onto existing fluoroscopic images depicting the location of recording catheters within the heart. In cases where biplane fluoroscopic images and x-ray camera position data are available, the position of the catheters can be reconstructed in three-dimensions.

Keywords: x-ray images, cardiac mapping, data fusion, visualization

1. BACKGROUND AND MOTIVATION

Radiofrequency catheter ablation has gained widespread acceptance as a cost-effective cure for many types of arrhythmias.[1,2] The arrhythmias which have been most amenable to catheter ablation have been those types of supraventricular tachycardia (SVT) in which the appropriate site for energy delivery is known and anatomically constant (e.g., AV node reentrant tachycardia)[3], and those in which the accessory fiber mediating the SVT is known to traverse one of the two atrioventricular grooves[4]. For these rhythms, the potentially complicated process of mapping electrical activation patterns in the heart can be reduced to identifying either an anatomic location, or a single point known to be located on the AV groove.

Unfortunately, the largest group of patients, often with severe underlying cardiovascular disease, suffer from other, more intractable atrial or ventricular reentrant arrhythmias, in which the vulnerable sites for ablation are not constrained in any simple manner by known cardiac anatomy. Experimental open-chest procedures in animals and man using endocardial mapping socks containing large numbers of electrodes, have demonstrated that these patients can be treated successfully with catheter ablation, provided the reentrant circuit can be accurately mapped in the presence of numerous, functional barriers.[5] These functional barriers, which often result from wavefront collisions and regions of refractory tissue, are constantly changing and can not be determined before the ablation procedure. Unfortunately, existing technology does not permit mapping of these reentrant circuits with sufficient detail for procedural success. This is reflected in the much lower success rates of catheter ablation when used to treat these arrhythmias.[6,7]

Current clinical mapping techniques are based on analysis of intracardiac electrograms recorded from a small number of electrophysiologic recording catheters. The temporal relationship between the electrogram signals and the relative position of the recording catheters must be jointly analyzed to determine the direction and velocity of the cardiac activation wavefronts. Because of the three-dimensional structure of the endocardium, the tortuous path of the activation wavefronts, and the limited spatial sampling density provided by most catheters, it is usually necessary to make recordings at a number of different catheter positions. Maneuvering the catheters to specific endocardial sites is often a tedious process, complicated by the difficulty of comparing past electrograms with those recorded at the current site and the lack of a quantitative system for measuring catheter position.

---

* Correspondence: David B. Kynor, Creare Inc. PO Box 71, Hanover, NH 03755, dbk@creare.com, 603-643-3800.

Medical Imaging 2002: Image Processing, Milan Sonka, J. Michael Fitzpatrick,
Editors, Proceedings of SPIE Vol. 4684 (2002) © 2002 SPIE · 1605-7422/02/$15.00

This iterative process of catheter placement, catheter localization (based on fluoroscopic imaging), and electrogram analysis is technically difficult, often not reproducible, and time consuming.[8] Solutions to the problem of electrode localization are often *ad hoc*. In some electrophysiology laboratories, it is standard practice to record identifying fluoroscopic features and catheter locations during a complex case by annotating the monitor screen with a wax pencil, which is wiped clean between cases. This problem is compounded by the fact that many cases involve a large volume of intracardiac recordings made by a number of different catheters. As a result, many catheter ablation procedures are very lengthy (one study showed that mean procedure times range from 272 minutes for successful cases to 386 minutes for unsuccessful procedures[9]) and can involve large radiation doses to patient and clinical staff.

Recently, several new technologies have been developed in an effort to provide clinicians with more effective tools for cardiac mapping. One system relies on catheters fitted with electromagnetic position sensors.[10,11] Another system uses a non-contact catheter that is capable of reconstructing a large number of endocardial electrical signals from a central position within the cardiac chamber. However, both of these approaches require dedicated hardware and special-purpose catheters.

2. METHODS

Our work involves development of signal and image processing algorithms that will permit fusion and simultaneous visualization of anatomic and functional data during cardiac electrophysiology procedures (Figure 1). The algorithms are intended to provide three-dimensional visualization of catheter positions, allowing the clinician to link patient-specific anatomical variations with electrophysiological behavior. Three primary classes of processing algorithms are being developed as part of this work. Each class of algorithm is briefly described below.

2.1 Activation event detection

Interventional electrophyiosologic cardiac mapping relies on the use of intravenous recording catheters placed against the endocardial surface. Signals from the catheters are amplified, filtered, and routed to a workstation for display. The signals are examined by the clinician to determine the relative timing of the high-frequency signal events caused by electrical wavefronts passing through the heart muscle in the vicinity of the catheter. Our cardiac mapping system is designed to automatically detect the timing of these cardiac activation events (Figure 2). This is accomplished by detecting all signal complexes exceeding a user-defined signal level, while rejecting lower amplitude complexes caused by distant activation events and measurement noise. The algorithm consists of five different processing steps:

1. Bandpass Filtering—The acquired signal is filtered using a 6th order, zero-phase bandpass filter to reduce low-frequency artifacts and high-frequency measurement noise.

2. Rectification—The filtered signal is rectified to remove any bias in signal polarity associated with the relative orientation between the direction of signal propagation and the recording catheter.

3. Adaptive Thresholding—A signal level threshold is computed based on the shape of the signal. Portions of the signal, whose amplitude falls below this threshold, are set to zero.

4. Amplitude Clipping—A separate amplitude clipping threshold is computed based on previous signal peaks. Signals whose amplitude exceeds the clipping threshold are clipped to the threshold value to minimize the effect of abnormally large signal transients.

5. Peak Detection—The resulting signal is bandpass filtered to yield a peak intensity signal. The peaks of this signal are used to provide the timing of the activation events.

The results of applying this algorithm to endocardial signal recordings are illustrated in Figure 2.

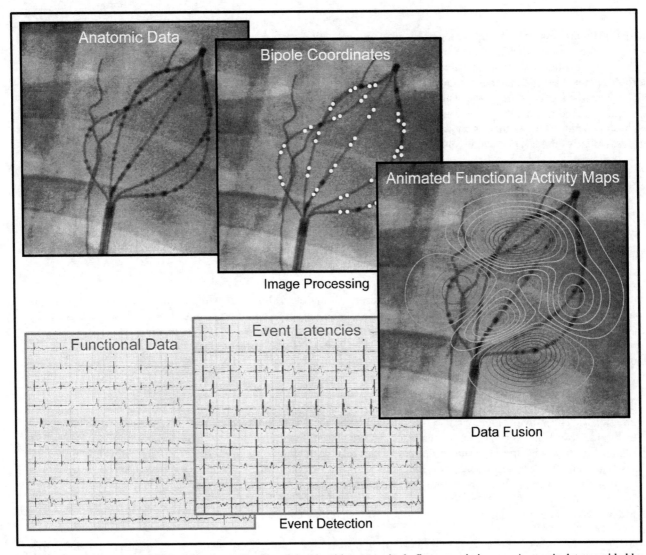

Figure 1. Data flow diagram illustrating the application of the algorithms to a single fluoroscopic image. Anatomic data provided by fluoroscopic images is processed to provide the spatial location of each recording bipole (white dots shown on the catheter). Functional data provided by intracardiac electrogram recordings is processed to provide the timing of endocardial activations. The two sources of data are fused to provide an animated map showing the timing and/or propagation of endocardial wavefronts.

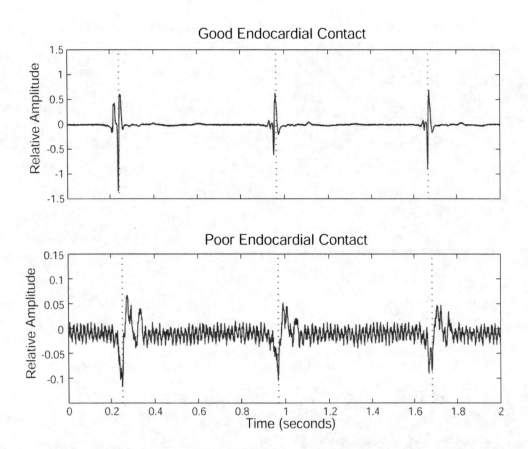

Figure 2. Intracardiac electrical recordings show the results of the activation detection algorithm. Tracings were obtained near the annulus of the tricuspid valve in a patient undergoing catheter ablative treatment for Wolff-Parkinson-White syndrome. The top tracing shows a high-quality tracing indicative of good contact between the recording bipole and the endocardial surface. The bottom tracing shows a poorer quality tracing typically encountered when there is poor contact between the recording bipole and the endocardium. The activation event times as determined by the automated algorithm are shown as vertical dashed lines.

2.2 Catheter bipole detection

Detection of the position of the catheter bipoles in each of the fluoroscopic images is accomplished using an automated algorithm. This algorithm involves three processing steps.

1. Variations in background intensity are normalized by computing the structural opening of the image with a disk-shaped structuring element (upper right panel of the figure). The diameter of the disk is selected to be about twice the diameter of the bipoles (12 pixels).
2. The normalized image is convolved with a kernel designed to enhance the catheter bipoles. The kernel has an outer ring of unit intensity, an inner ring of negative value about the same size as the bipole, and a middle ring of zero intensity. The kernel attenuates (darkens) large structures (e.g., bones) and background noise, while emphasizing objects whose size and shape resemble that of the catheter bipoles. After convolution, pixels with negative values are set to zero and the intensity of each pixel is divided by the average intensity of the neighboring pixels (the size of the neighborhood is ten times the size of an electrode). This process results in the image shown in the lower left panel of Figure 3.
3. The resulting image is converted into binary format using a global threshold. Regions of contiguous pixels above the threshold are then grouped. The shape of each group is then examined and groups whose shape is round are selected as candidate bipole locations.

Raw Image

Background Normalization

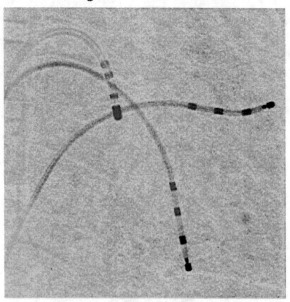

Convolution with Electrode Detection Kernel

Detected Electrodes

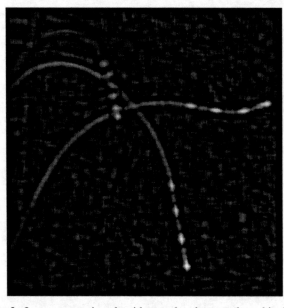
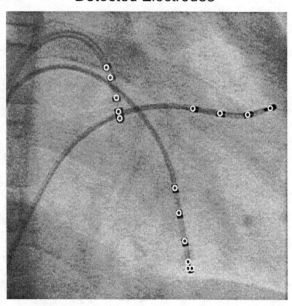

Figure 3. Image processing algorithm used to detect catheter bipoles in fluoroscopic images of the heart. Details of the algorithm are contained in the text.

3. RESULTS

The event detection algorithms were tested by comparing them to a series of 144 electrograms, selected to cover a range of signal quality and activation. One of the authors (J. Triedman) manually marked each electrogram to indicate what he considered to be valid endocardial activations. A total of 1324 events were marked (an average of 9 events in each 2.5 second recording). Mean time between events was 256 $\pm$ 102 ms. The data files were then processed with the automated detection algorithms (the automated algorithms detected 1443 events).

To gauge the accuracy of the detection algorithms, both specificity and sensitivity were calculated. We defined a true positive event as the occurrence of an automatically detected event within ±15 ms of a manually marked event. Under these conditions, the automated algorithms were 91% sensitive and 85% specific. A comparison of the latencies of the automatically detected and manually marked events shows that 50% of the events were within ±3ms and 93% of the events were within ±10 ms (Figure 4).

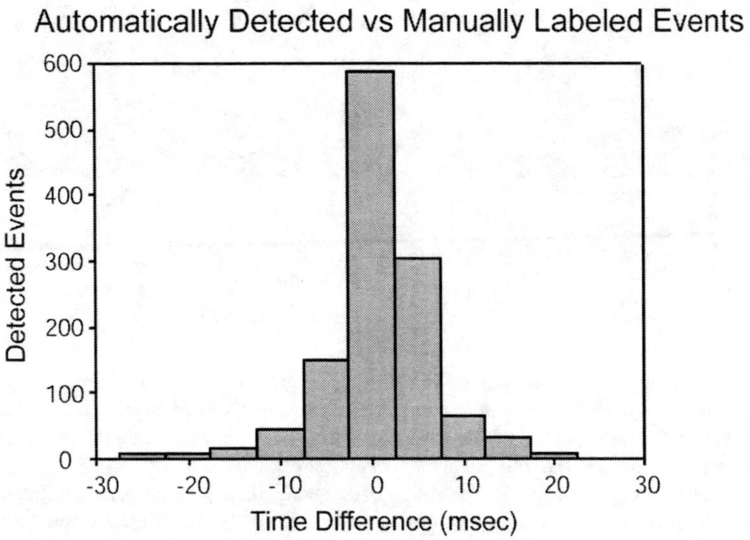

Automatically Detected vs Manually Labeled Events

Figure 4. Timing difference between automatically detected and manually labeled events.

The bipole detection algorithm has not been extensively tested. Preliminary tests on fluoroscopic images obtained during experimental arrhythmia mapping procedures on animals showed that the algorithm correctly identifies 80 to 96% of the 25 bipoles present in each image. The number of false detections in each image ranged from two to six (mean 2.8).

A prototype software system incorporating the algorithms was constructed as a means to demonstrate the use of the system with clinical data. The prototype system was used to process clinical data sets obtained during electrophysiological investigation of patients suffering from a variety of cardiac arrhythmias. For each patient, an animated movie was created by highlighting catheter bipoles during time intervals when electrical activations were detected in the immediate vicinity of the bipole. The animated movies were reviewed by cardiac electrophysiologists and found to be useful in visualizing the propagation of electrical activity within the heart. Three of the clinical data sets are illustrated in the following figures.

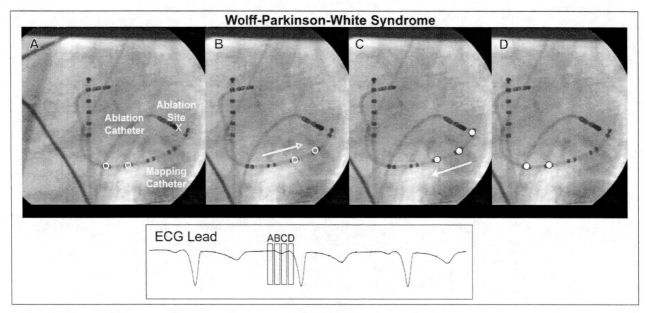

Figure 5. Mapping and Ablation of Wolff-Parkinson-White Syndrome. A typical catheter arrangement for diagnosis and ablation of WPW is shown in this oblique view. A decapolar mapping catheter is placed in the coronary sinus from the superior vena cava. It lies below and defines the lower and lateral border of the mitral annulus. An ablation catheter is located at its tip. Sequential activation of the accessory pathway is shown in the four panels. Panels A and B show late atrial activation (open circles) and panels C and D show early ventricular activation (filled circles). The range of latencies used in each panel is shown on the ECG lead at the bottom of the figure. Note that the earliest ventricular activation occurs at the distal end of the mapping catheter. Catheter ablation applied at this site successfully destroyed the patient's accessory pathway.

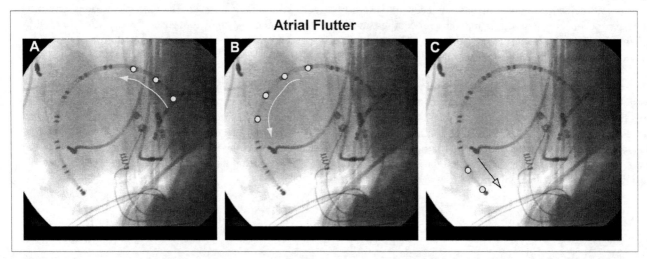

Figure 6. Mapping of Atrial Flutter. This lateral view of a patient with atrial flutter after repair of congenital heart disease shows a halo catheter encircling the tricuspid valve (if the valve were visible we would be looking at it *en face*). The counterclockwise rotation of atrial activation around the tricuspid annulus is clearly depicted in this sequence of images taken at 50 msec intervals.

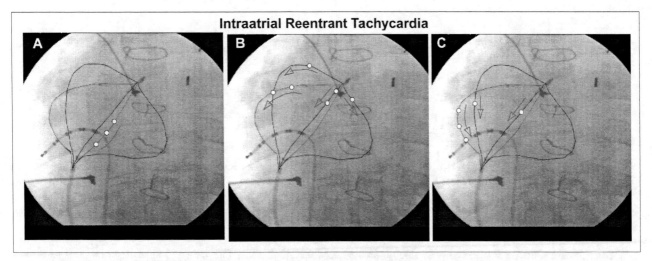

Intraatrial Reentrant Tachycardia

Figure 7. Mapping of Intraatrial Reentrant Tachycardia. This sequence shows a basket catheter placed in the right atrium of a patient with complex cardiac anatomy resulting from surgical repair of congenital heart disease. The splines of the basket catheter have been outlined to enhance visibility and arrows have been added to assist in visualizing the direction of electrical propagation in this set of static images. As the arrhythmia proceeds, activation can be seen moving up the most posterior spline and then spreading down the other splines which are located on the anterior of the atrium.

4. DISCUSSION

We have evaluated the feasibility of using automated algorithms for detection of electrical activation events in intracardiac electrogram data and for detection of bipole locations in fluoroscopic images of catheters in the heart. The resulting data can be combined to produce animated movies of cardiac electrical propagation in the heart. Evaluation of the system by clinicians indicates that this type of display facilitates visualization of movement of electrical wavefronts through the heart muscle and provides a useful adjunct to current technology used in cardiac mapping procedures. The ability to replay the animations more slowly than real-time is particularly useful for evaluating complex activation patterns. However, the present implementation of the system is subject to a number of limitations in the areas of bipole detection, catheter identification, and three-dimensional visualization.

Automated detection of catheter bipoles in fluoroscopic images is complicated by the fact that the images often have large variations in background intensity (portions of the background may be darker than the catheter bipoles) and poor signal-to-noise ratio. In addition, the relative angle between the catheter bipoles and the x-ray camera can have a significant impact on the appearance of the bipoles in the fluoroscopic images. Finally, the visibility of some bipoles can be obscured by other catheters or other radioopaque objects.

The current implementation of the system is also limited by the need to manually associate each bipole in the fluoroscopic images with the corresponding electrogram signal. We are currently working on several approaches for automatically finding the location of the body of the catheters. Knowledge of the location of the catheter bodies would permit bipoles to be automatically associated with specific catheters.

Finally, the current version of the system is only capable of operating in two dimensions. Many cardiac electrophysiology procedures are performed using biplane fluoroscopy. In these cases, two different views of the heart are available to the clinician. Knowledge of x-ray camera geometry, combined with identification of catheter bipoles that are visible in both views, permits computation of the three-dimensional coordinates of the catheter bipoles. The three-dimensional coordinate reconstruction should assist in bipole localization (once the location of a bipole is determined in one fluoroscopic view, it's position is constrained to lie along a line in the other view). Three-dimensional reconstruction also has the potential to significantly enhance visualization of wavefronts moving through the manifolds of the heart. Our three-dimensional reconstruction work is being presented elsewhere at the meeting.[12]

ACKNOWLEDGEMENTS

This work is supported by a grant from the National Heart, Lung, and Blood Institute, Bethesda, MD.

REFERENCES

1 Man KC, Kalbfleisch SJ, Hummel JD, et. al., "The safety and cost of outpatient radiofrequency ablation of the slow pathway in patients with atrioventricular nodal reentrant tachycardia," *Am. J. Cardiol.*, 1993;**72**:1323-1324.

2 Kalbfleisch SJ, Calkins H, Langberg JJ, et. al., "Comparison of the cost of radiofrequency catheter modification of the atrioventricular nodal and medical therapy for drug-refractory atrioventricular node reentrant tachycardia," *J. Am. Coll. Cardiol.*, 1992;**19**:1583-1587.

3 Jackman WM, Beckman KJ, McClelland JH, Wang X, Friday KJ, Roman CA, Moulton KP, Twidale N, Hazlitt HA, Priori MI, "Treatment of supraventricular tachycardia due to atrioventricular nodal reentry by radiofrequency catheter ablation of slow-pathway conduction," *N. Engl. J. Med.*, 1992, **327**:313-318.

4 Calkins H, Sousa J, El-Atassi R, Rosenheck S, De Buittleir M, Kou WH, Kadish AH, Langberg JJ, Morady F, "Diagnosis and cure of the Wolff-Parkinson-White Syndrome or paroxysmal supraventricular tachycardias during a single electrophysiologic test, *N. Engl. J. Med.*, 1991;**324**:1612-8.

5 Boineau JP, Schuessler RB, Cain ME, Corr PB, Cox JL, "Activation mapping during normal atrial rhythms and atrial flutter," In Zipes DP, Jalife J, eds., *Cardiac Electrophysiology - From Cell to Bedside*, Saunders, WB: Philadelphia; 1990; 537-547.

6 Kim YH, Sosa-Suarez G, Trouton TG, O'Nunain SS, Osswald S, McGovern BA, Ruskin JN, Garan H, "Treatment of ventricular tachycardia by transcatheter radiofrequency ablation in patients with ischemic heart disease," *Circulation*, 1994;**89**:1094-1102.

7 Triedman JK, Saul JP, Weindling SN, Walsh EP, "Radiofrequency ablation of intraatrial reentrant tachycardia following surgical palliation of congenital heart disease," *Circulation*, 1995;**91**:707-714.

8 Davis LM, Cooper M, Johnson DC, Uther JB, Richards DA, Ross DL, "Simultaneous 60-electrode mapping of ventricular tachycardia using percutaneous catheters," *J. Am. Coll. Cardiol.*, 1994;**24**:709-719.

9 Kugler JD, "Catheter Ablation in Pediatric Patients," In Zipes DP, Jalife J, eds., *Cardiac Electrophysiology - From Cell to Bedside*, Saunders, WB: Philadelphia; 1995.

10 Ben-Haim SA, Gepstein L, Hayam G, Ben-David J, Josephson, ME, "A New Nonfluoroscopic Electroanatomical Mapping System," PACE (abstract), 1996;**19**:4, Part II:709.

11 Ben-Haim SA, Gepstein L, Hayam G, Ben-David J, and Josephson ME, "A New Method for Non-Fluoroscopic Catheter Based Endocardial Mapping," Marketing Brochure, 1995.

12 Dietz AJ, Kynor DB, Friets, EM, Triedman JK, Hammer PE, "Effects of Uncertainty in Camera Geometry on Three-Dimensional Catheter Reconstruction from Biplane Fluoroscopic Images," SPIE Medical Imaging Meeting, 2002.

Multiple isovalues selection by clustering gray values of the boundary surfaces within volume image

Lisheng Wang[1], Pheng-Ann Heng[2], Tien-Tsin Wong[2], Jing Bai[1]

[1] Institute of Biomedical Engineering, Department of EE&AE Technology, Tsinghua University, Beijing, 100084, P. R. China
[2] Department of Computer Science & Engineering, The Chinese University of Hong Kong, Shatin, New Territory, Hong Kong, P. R. China

ABSTRACT

In medical visualization, multiple isosurfaces are usually extracted from medical volume image and used to represent (approximate) the boundary surfaces of different structures in the image. In this paper, we will discuss the approximating problem of the boundary surface (contained within volume image) by isosurface. It is quite common that a medical volume image can contain multiple interesting structures; we present a novel approach for the selection of multiple isosurfaces to approximate the boundary surfaces of these multiple structures. With this approach, the discrete sampling points of the gray values of the boundary surfaces within volume image are computed first. Then by identifying appropriate clusters from the discrete sampling points and computing the mean of each cluster, we can determine the corresponding isosurfaces for approximating these multiple boundary surfaces.

Keywords: Boundary surface, approximating isosurface, threshold selection, clustering algorithm, isovalue, medical visualization, 3D segmentation, 3D edge detection.

1. INTRODUCTION

Extracting boundary surfaces of interesting structures within medical volume image is important in medical applications. For example, in computer-aided surgery, quantitative measurements need boundary surface; in computer-aided manufacturing, boundary surface is also needed when actual physical models or mold must be manufactured for surgical simulation or pre-surgical customization. Besides, boundary surface is very useful for the understanding, recognition, description, and measurement of its corresponding structure within volume image. Thus, extraction and modeling of the boundary surface within volume image is one of the most important research problems in medical volume image analysis. Usually, the boundary surface within volume image is too complex to be represented by its accurate mathematics. Thus, a polygonal surface model is usually extracted from volume image[1-5] as an approximation. In [1] and [2], contours (edge curves) are extracted first from 2D slices of medical volume image and then boundary surface is reconstructed from these contours. In [3], instead of detecting edge curve (contour) in each slice, the polygonal surface model of step-like boundary surface is directly extracted from volume image. In [4]-[5], 3D snake or deformable surface techniques are used to directly acquire an approximating surface of a boundary surface. However, the method for reconstructing boundary surface from contours cannot assure that complex boundary surface with many branches to be correctly reconstructed[6]. The method in [3] suffers the common problem of edge detecting technique that some of the detected edge (curve or surface) does not enclose an object completely when there is noise in the image or there is no obvious edge. Deformable surface techniques cannot detect and extract arbitrary boundary surfaces, or extract multiple boundary surfaces at the same time. Thus, by now, it seems that, most of the methods that extract polygonal surface model of the boundary surfaces from volume image based on edge matching techniques have some drawbacks in extracting closed, topology-correct boundary surfaces.

Comparing with the methods in [1]-[5], isosurface algorithm can extract smooth and closed isosurface with correct topology from volume image no matter how complex the extracted isosurface is[6-8]. Thus, isosurface algorithm is widely used in medical visualization for extracting closed polygonal surface model of the boundary surface from medical volume image. However, in most cases, the extracted isosurfaces are only an approximating surfaces of the given boundary surface. Thus, in order to decrease the error between the boundary surface and its approximating isosurface, we need to consider the problems: for a given boundary surface, what is its optimal approximating isosurface? How to compute its optimal approximating isosurface? These are fundamental problems to be solved in order to approximate the boundary surface by an isosurface. In medical volume image, usually multiple interesting objects/structures exist. Thus, multiple isosurfaces can be extracted to approximate these objects' boundary surface. This paper will address these issues, and propose a method for the selection of multiple isosurfaces from volume image.

Each isosurface is uniquely determined by its isovalue. Thus, the problem of multiple isosurfaces selection is actually the problem of multiple isovalue selection. Threshold selection methods are widely used in 2D image processing and have been extended to medical visualization for segmenting different regions or structures within volume image [9–10,16]. The main difference between the usual threshold selection and the isovalue selection studied here is as follows:

Threshold selection mainly considers the correct classification of discrete voxels of volume image. This is a problem in discrete space. It may have more than one solution. Namely, more than one threshold could serve as good threshold in the sense of correctly classifying voxels. However, the isovalue selection focuses on the approximation of boundary surface by the selected isosurface. Since boundary surface usually locates between sampling points rather than at sampling points, we need to approximate the boundary surface by interpolation in order to obtain sub-voxel accuracy. Essentially, this is a problem in continuous space. In principal, for the given boundary surface, its optimal approximating isosurface (and therefore isovalue) can be uniquely determined. While each optimal isovalue should be a good threshold, the converse is not true. Namely, many good thresholds that classify correctly discrete voxels may not be optimal isovalues.

This paper discusses the optimal approximating isosurface and its computation. The mathematics describing the optimal approximating isosurface is given, and its solution, which determines the optimal isovalue, is provided. This paper proves that, for the given boundary surface, the mean of the gray values of the points lying on the boundary surface is the optimal isovalue we seek. Based on these results, a method to compute the approximating isosurface for the given boundary surface within volume image is proposed. It first computes the discrete sampling points of the boundary surface from volume image. In the discrete sampling, the gray values of the points lying on each boundary surface will cluster around their mean. Thus, by identifying appropriate clusters from the discrete sampling, different clusters, which correspond to different boundary surfaces respectively, can be separated. By computing the mean of the each separated cluster, the isovalue of the approximating isosurface of each boundary surface is obtained. Thus, this method can be extended to the selection of multiple isovalues from volume image. Satisfactory results have been obtained by applying this method to extract approximating isosurfaces from CT medical volume image.

2. THEORETICAL ANALYSIS ON APPROXUMATING ISOSURFACE

In order to approximate the boundary surface within volume image, we first need to build the mathematical model for the boundary surface. In volume image, different structures usually correspond to different image intensity. Thus, boundary surface, which separates different structures from each other or from background, is the surface of which either side has great difference in the image intensities. Obviously, such boundary surface belongs to step-like edge (surface) and can be analyzed by edge detecting technique. Suppose volume image is sampled from a continuous three-dimensional function $f(x, y, z)$. Based on the edge detection theory, boundary surfaces of $f(x, y, z)$ are some continuous zero-crossing surfaces with high gradient value, i.e., they satisfy the following equation [3,10]:

$$\begin{cases} (1)\ l(x, y, z) = 0 \\ (2)\ \|\nabla f(x, y, z)\| \geq T \end{cases} \tag{1}$$

where, T is a predetermined gradient threshold, $l(x, y, z)$ represents the Laplacian operator of $f(x, y, z)$ and $\|\nabla f(x, y, z)\|$ represents the gradient magnitude function of $f(x, y, z)$. In this paper, our purpose is to select suitable isovalues such that their corresponding isosurfaces well approximate the boundary surfaces determined by Equation (1).

We first discuss the problem: what is the suitable approximating isosurface for a given boundary surface within volume image. Let $S(x, y, z)$ represents a given boundary surface of $f(x, y, z)$. Then it is a surface that separates an object from the background. Without loss of generality, suppose that the gray intensities of the object and the background are given as follows, respectively:

$$f(x, y, z) \geq N \qquad\qquad (x, y, z) \in \text{Object}$$
$$f(x, y, z) < M < N \qquad\qquad (x, y, z) \in \text{Background}$$

Then, each point $(x, y, z) \in S(x, y, z)$ has a gray value between the object and the background gray levels. Furthermore, the mean of gray values of points lying on $S(x, y, z)$ will be at a gray level between the object and the background gray levels. Thus, the mean of gray values of points lying on $S(x, y, z)$ is at least a good threshold in the sense of classifying voxels correctly. Let E_S represents the mean of gray values of points lying on $S(x, y, z)$, then

$$E_S = \frac{\int\limits_{S(x,y,z)} f(x, y, z) \, d(x, y, z)}{\int\limits_{S(x,y,z)} d(x, y, z)}.$$

where, $\int\limits_{S(x,y,z)} f(x, y, z) \, d(x, y, z)$ represents the integration of gray value function $f(x, y, z)$ over the boundary surface $S(x, y, z)$.

Generally, it is very complex to directly measure or estimate the approximating distance between $S(x, y, z)$ and any selected isosurface. Therefore, we study the approximation of $S(x, y, z)$ by isosurface from a different view. We will study such optimal approximating isosurface that approximates the gray values of the points lying on $S(x, y, z)$ with least square error. Let $I(r)$ represents the isosurface with isovalue r, defined as follows

$$I(r) = \{(x, y, z): f(x, y, z) = r\}.$$

Then the mathematics of the optimal approximating isosurface that approximates the gray values of the points lying on $S(x, y, z)$ with least square error can be presented as follows:

$$\min_r \int\limits_{S(x,y,z)} (f(x, y, z) - r)^2 \, d(x, y, z) \qquad (2)$$

This is an optimization problem. Its solution determines the optimal isovalue of $S(x, y, z)$, in the sense of approximating gray values of boundary surface $S(x, y, z)$ with least square error.

Let $f(r) = \int\limits_{S(x,y,z)} (f(x, y, z) - r)^2 \, d(x, y, z)$. To find the isovalue that minimizes $f(r)$, we differentiate $f(r)$ with respect to r and set the result to zero:

$$f'(r) = \int\limits_{S(x,y,z)} 2 \cdot f(x, y, z) \, d(x, y, z) - \int\limits_{S(x,y,z)} 2 \cdot r \, d(x, y, z) = 0.$$

We have

$$r = \frac{\int\limits_{S(x,y,z)} f(x, y, z) \, d(x, y, z)}{\int\limits_{S(x,y,z)} d(x, y, z)} = E_S$$

This fact shows that the mean of gray values of points lying on $S(x, y, z)$ is the optimal isovalue that approximates the gray values of the point lying on $S(x, y, z)$ with least square error. In fact, this result can be intuitively understood. We know that, if $S(x, y, z)$ can be well approximated by a specific isosurface, then the gray values of points lying on $S(x, y, z)$ will cluster around a gray value that equals to or be close to the mean of gray values of points over $S(x, y, z)$. See experimental results shown in Figure 3(2) and Figure 6(2), where histograms of gray values of one and multiple boundary surfaces are shown. Since gray values of points lying on each boundary surface cluster around their mean, if we select the mean as the isovalue of the approximating isosurface, then most of the points lying on the boundary surface will lie on or be close to the approximating isosurface. Intuitively, such approximating isosurface would be a good candidate of the approximating surface of the boundary surface. When we try to compute the approximating isosurface for the given boundary surface, we only need to compute the mean of the gray values of the points lying on the boundary surface.

We notice that, in 2D image processing, similar results has been pointed out by Katz[11,9] and Milgram et. al[13]. Katz states that since the pixels in the neighborhood of an edge have higher edge values, the gray level histogram for these pixels should have a single peak at a gray level between the object and the background gray levels. This gray level is, therefore, a suitable choice of the threshold value. Based on the fact, several thresholding techniques have been proposed in 2D image processing[12–16]. In these methods, edge points are first detected from image, and then threshold is deduced from the histogram of gray values of the edge points or from the histogram of the average gray value of each edge point. However, the edge points differ from the points lying on the boundary surfaces. The later usually locate between sampling points rather than at the edge points. Besides, they have the gray values between the object and background gray levels. Thus, essentially, the histogram of gray values of edge points and the histogram of the average gray values of each edge point both differ from the histogram of the gray values of points lying on the boundary surface. Furthermore, the threshold deduced from these two histograms usually is not the optimal isovalue.

In this paper, we try to compute the histogram of gray values of the points lying on the boundary surfaces within volume image, and deduce the isovalues of the approximating isosurfaces from the histogram.

3. COMPUTING DISCRETE SAMPLING OF GRAY VALUES OF BOUNDARY SURFACES

For discrete volume image, generally, its continuous sampling function $f(x, y, z)$ and the surface model of the boundary surfaces within it is too complex to be represented by an accurate mathematical expression. Thus, it is impossible to analyze the gray values of the points lying on boundary surface by an analytical method. Besides, it is impossible to compute accurately the mean of the gray values of the points lying on the boundary surface within volume image as well. Therefore, in the paper, we will compute the discrete sampling of the gray values of the boundary surfaces within volume image, and estimate the mean of gray values of the boundary surface by analyzing the computed discrete sampling.

We first introduce a method to compute the discrete sampling of the gray values of the boundary surface within volume image. It consists of the following two steps:

Step 1: compute the discrete sampling points of the boundary surfaces determined in equation (1).

Step 2: compute the gray values of the discrete sampling points obtained in Step 1.

Detailed explanation is given below.

In the paper, volume image is considered as the 3D sampling data sampled from the grid-points of the three-dimensional regular grids as shown in Figure 1. Here, adjacent eight grid points constitute a cell (grid or cube), and all such cells form the continuous volume occupied by volume image. Since the boundary surfaces within volume image are the continuous surfaces contained in the volume, they will divide the set of all cells into two classes: the cells that are intersected by the boundary surface — referred to as edge-cells, and non-edge cells. The boundary surfaces within volume image are contained in the set of edge-cells. Therefore, we can detect and extract the boundary surfaces from volume image by first detecting the edge-cells and then approximating the boundary surfaces in each edge-cell.

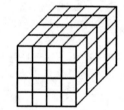

Figure 1. 3D regular grid

In [3], an approach is proposed to detect the edge-cells from volume image and approximate boundary surface in each edge-cell. Based on the fact that each edge-cell has at least three *edges* intersected by a boundary surface, all edge-cells are possible to be recognized by marching all cells of volume image and by checking whether there are at least three interacted *edges* in each cell. In [3], the *edge* intersected by boundary surface is detected by judging whether one *edge* satisfies the following rules:

(1) Its two vertices are a pair of zero-crossing points.

(2) Its two vertices both have high gradient values.

where, condition (2) is judged by thresholding the sum of gradient values of the two vertices of the *edge*. In each edge-cell, the boundary surface actually is the zero-value isosurface of Laplacian function of volume image. Therefore, we can extract the boundary surface by an isosurface algorithm[7,8] in each edge-cell. Generally, the accurate expression of the boundary surface is not known. Thus, in each edge-cell, boundary surface is approximated with several triangles. By approximating the boundary surface with polygons in each edge-cell, eventually the polygonal surface model of the boundary surfaces within volume image can be obtained.

We notice that, the vertices of the triangles included in the extracted polygonal surface model of boundary surfaces actually are the discrete sampling points of the boundary surfaces. Thus, by using the approach introduced in [3], we can compute discrete sampling points of the boundary surfaces within volume image. Because of noise in volume image, sometimes some small holes or small fragments might appear on the extracted polygonal boundary surfaces. However, since sampling points corresponding to the small holes or small fragments only occupy a very small percentage of the total discrete sampling points, all vertices of the triangles in the extracted polygonal boundary surfaces still constitute the valid discrete sampling points of the boundary surfaces within volume image.

It is known that, each computed discrete sampling point locates at one edge of an edge-cell. Its position is computed by interpolating the positions of the two vertices of the edge. Similar to computing the position of the discrete sampling point, the gray value of each discrete sampling point can be easily computed by interpolation as well. The simplest method to compute gray value of each discrete sampling point is to linearly interpolate the gray values of the two vertices of the edge at which the sampling point locates[7]. However, complex interpolation methods might decrease the error. In our experiment results, linear interpolation is used and the obtained results are satisfactory. For each discrete sampling point, two vertices of the edge at which this sampling point locates belong to the object or the background, respectively. Thus, the gray value of each discrete sampling point is at a gray level between the object and background gray levels. It follows that, the mean of gray values of the discrete sampling points of a given boundary surface is at a gray level between the object and the background gray levels.

By the method presented in this section, we can obtain the set of the discrete sampling of the gray values of the boundary surfaces within volume image. In Section 4, we discuss how the requested isovalues are deduced from the histogram of the gray values of those discrete sampling points computed from volume image.

4. SELECTION OF APPROXIMATING ISOSURFACES BY CLUSTERING ALGORITHM

We have noticed that, if a boundary surface $S(x, y, z)$ is well approximated by an isosurface $I(r)$, then the gray values of points lying on $S(x, y, z)$ will cluster around their mean E_S. The same property holds in the discrete sampling of the gray values of $S(x, y, z)$. Namely, the gray values of the discrete sampling points of each boundary surface will cluster around the mean of the gray values of this boundary surface. Based on this fact, we can estimate the mean of the gray values of the boundary surfaces within volume image by clustering the discrete sampling of the gray values of the boundary surfaces.

In the case of volume image containing only one object, we need only to deduce an isovalue from the discrete sampling points. In addition, there are such situations where volume image contains more than one object, but we are only interested in one given object. In these cases, we only need to compute the approximating isosurface for the solitary interesting boundary surface, and therefore, only an isovalue is needed to be deduced from the discrete sampling points. In later case, the discrete sampling points of the solitary interesting boundary surface must be computed or extracted solely. It can be realized by suitably selecting predefined gradient threshold T in Equation (1). In the above-mentioned two cases, there is only one cluster in the histogram of the gray values of the extracted discrete sampling points. Besides, in the histogram of the gray values of the extracted discrete sampling points, gray values will cluster around the mean of the gray values of the solitary interesting boundary surface. Thus, by computing the mean of the unique cluster in the histogram of the gray values of the extracted discrete sampling points, the isovalue of the requested approximating isosurface is obtained. Here, the mean of the unique cluster equals to the average value of the gray values of all discrete sampling points or nearly equals to the gray level at the unique peak in the histogram of gray values of the discrete sampling points (See Figure 3(2)).

In the case when the volume image contains more than one interesting object, we will approximate multiple different boundary surfaces within the volume image by different isosurfaces. Here, we need to compute multiple isovalues. Since the discrete sampling of the gray values of all boundary surfaces are mixed together, it becomes much more complex. It is not easy to separate the discrete sampling of the gray values of different boundary surfaces from each other. However, the discrete sampling of the gray values of each boundary surface will cluster around the mean of the gray values of this boundary surface. Thus, the discrete sampling of the gray values of each boundary surface will display itself implicitly by showing it as a cluster in the mixed discrete sampling of the gray values of all boundary surfaces. Therefore, different clusters, which represent the discrete sampling of the gray values of different boundary surface, will be displayed in the histogram of the gray values of the discrete sampling points of all boundary surfaces. By identifying appropriate clusters from the histogram of gray value of discrete sampling points of all boundary surfaces and computing the mean of each cluster, the mean of gray values of different boundary surface, which equals to the mean of one of the recognized clusters, is estimated. Usually, in the histogram of the gray values of the discrete sampling points of all boundary surfaces, the gray levels at different main peaks correspond to the means of gray values of different boundary surfaces (See Figure 6(2)).

After selecting multiple isovalues from the discrete sampling of the gray values of the boundary surfaces within volume image, the approximating isosurfaces of these multiple boundary surfaces are determined. Each approximating isosurface can be extracted from volume image by using any standard isosurface extraction algorithm, such as the Marching Cubes algorithm or other improved isosurface algorithms[6–8].

5. IMPLEMENTATION AND EXPERIMENTAL RESULTS

We have applied our method to medical volume images in order to approximate the boundary surfaces of the structures within volume images. In the implementation, we mainly consider the two cases.

5.1 Volume image containing only one object and one isovalue selection is needed

We consider CT volume image of a dry skull of an adult shown in Figure 2. It is included in the free demo of software 3DVIEWNIX developed by Medical Image Processing Group of Pennsylvania University. We thank for the use of the image. In the image, only one structure --- skull is contained. Since skull occupies only a very small percentage of the total volume image (See histogram of volume image shown in Figure 3 (1)), it cannot be "seen" from the histogram of volume image. However, by using our approach, we obtain the histogram of discrete sampling of gray values of the surface of skull as shown in Figure 3 (2). It has an obvious cluster and its mean, which is selected as the isovalue of the approximating isosurface, is easy to compute. The discrete sampling points of boundary surface of the skull and the approximating isosurface are shown in Figure 4.

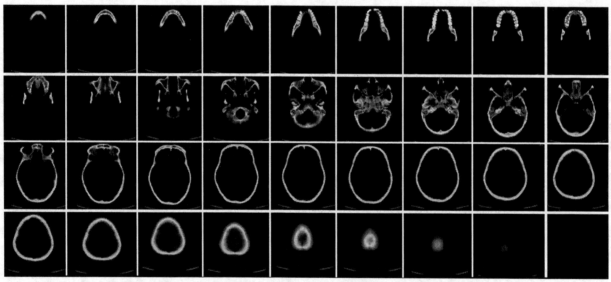

Figure 2. Slices of CT volume images of dry skull (128*128*68 8bits)

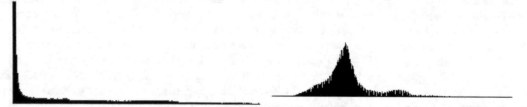

(1) histogram of volume image of skull.   (2) histogram of gray values of surface of skull.
Figure 3 Histogram of total volume image of skull and the histogram of discrete sampling
of gray values of surface of dry skull

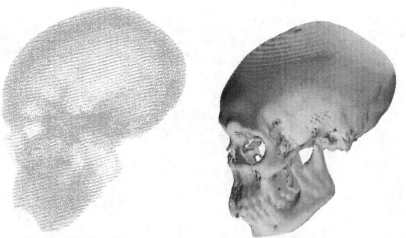

Figure 4. Discrete sampling points and approximating isosurface of boundary surface of skull

5.2 Volume image containing several objects and multi-isovalues are needed.

We consider CT volume image of head of a child shown in Figure 5. This image consists of two different structures: soft tissue and skull. We try to approximate boundary surfaces of skull and head by selecting two different isosurfaces. Since the skull occupies only a very small percentage of the total volume image, it cannot be "seen" or "recognized" from the histogram of total volume image. See Figure 6 (1). Thus, we directly compute discrete sampling of gray values of boundary surfaces within the image. See Figure 6(2), where, the histogram is displayed. Obviously, there are two obvious clusters, which correspond to the head surface and the skull surface respectively, exist in the histogram. By computing the mean of two clusters, isovalues of two approximating isosurfaces of head and skull are obtained. In

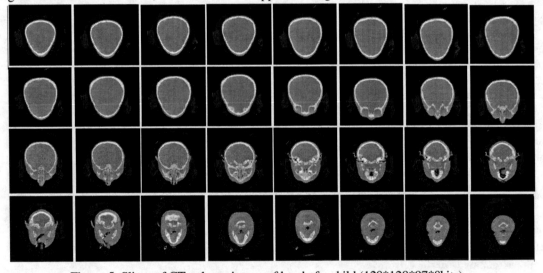

Figure 5. Slices of CT volume image of head of a child (128*128*97*8bits).

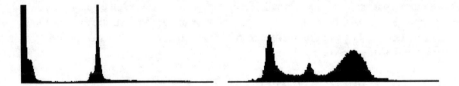

    (1) histogram of total volume image.   (2) histogram of gray values of boundary surfaces
Figure 6. Histogram of total volume image and the histogram of discrete sampling of gray values
of boundary surfaces within the volume image

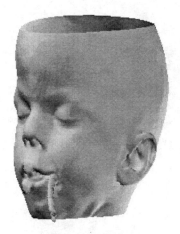 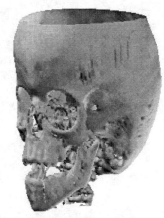 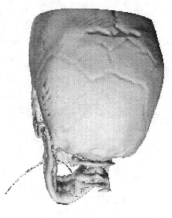

(1)approximating isosurface of head   (2)approximating isosurface of skull (front and back)

Figure 7. Extracted approximating isosurfaces of head and skull of a child

Figure 7, two extracted approximating isosurfaces are displayed. For the sake of comparison, discrete sampling points of the boundary surfaces within the volume image are displayed as well, see Figure 8. Experimental results presented in the section show that satisfactory results can be obtained if each boundary surface locates between two nearly homogeneous regions. The fidelity of the generated images comes close to the anatomical reality.

6. DISCUSSION

Our approach is mainly applicable to those medical volume images in which only several different structures are contained and each structure has similar gray values. In the case, each boundary surface separates two regions having nearly homogenous gray intensities respectively. Therefore, each boundary surface has distinct distribution of gray values and the cluster corresponding to each boundary surface can easily be recognized from the histogram of the gray values of the boundary surfaces by clustering algorithm. Thus, satisfactory results can be obtained in such cases. However, our approach cannot effectively process very complex volume images, such as the volume image mainly contains many small structures or the volume images in which the gray

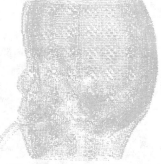

Figure 8. Sampling points of boundary surfaces of volume image

intensities of the background or the structures vary greatly. In the first case, there are too many small clusters in the histogram of gray values of the boundary surfaces to extract interesting clusters by clustering algorithm. In the second case, each boundary surface has largely varied gray values, and therefore usually cannot be well approximated by any selected isosurface. In the second case, the gray values of the points lying on the boundary surface have a very large variance. Generally, in the histogram of gray values of the boundary surfaces within volume image, for a given cluster corresponding to one boundary surface, the smaller its variance, the smaller error between the boundary surface and the computed approximating isosurface.

This paper proposes a method to select isovalue by analyzing the discrete sampling of the gray values of the boundary surface rather than by analyzing the histogram of total volume image. Thus, we can select approximating isosurfaces for such structures that only occupy a small percentage of the total volume image. Usually, such structures cannot be "seen" or "recognized" from the histogram of total volume image. In fact, the approximating isosurface of a given boundary surface is determined by the gray values distributing closely on either side of the boundary surface. We do not need to consider all gray values in volume image.

7. CONCLUSION

In medical visualization, isosurface is usually extracted from medical volume image and used to represent (approximate) the boundary surface of the structure in the volume image. Therefore, the approximating problem of boundary surface by isosurface is a fundamental problem in medical visualization. It focuses on the approximation of boundary surface by a specific isosurface. This paper discusses the problem, and proposes a novel approach for the selection of multiple isovalues from volume image. The proposed approach can efficiently process the volume images whose histogram exhibits several peaks of very unequal amplitude separated by a broad valley or whose histogram contains only one peak and a "shoulder". In these cases, interesting structures usually only occupy a small percentage of the total volume image, and they cannot be "seen" or "recognized" from the histogram of total volume image.

ACKNOWLEDGMENTS

The volume images used in the paper is downloaded via anonymous ftp from Chapel Hill Volume Rendering Test Data sets and the free demo of software 3DVIEWNIX. We are thankful for being allowed to freely download and use these data. This research is partially supported by the Chinese Postdoctoral Science Foundation and partially supported by the Hong Kong Research Grant Council (Project numbers: N -CUHK412/00 and CUHK 1/00C).

REFERENCES

1. D.Meyers,S.Skinner and K.Sloan, "Surface from contours", *ACM Trans on Graphics,*11(3), pp. 228-258, 1992.
2. M.W.Jones, M.Chen, "A new approach to the construction of surfaces from contour data", *Computer Graphics Forum*, 13(3), pp. 75-84, 1994.
3. P.A.Heng; L. Wang, T.T.Wong, K.S. Leung, J.C. Cheng, "Edge surfaces extraction from 3D images", *Proc. Medical Imaging 2001: Image Processing*, Milan Sonka; Kenneth M. Hanson; Eds. *SPIE* Vol. 4322, pp. 407-416, 2001.
4. G.Szekely, A.Kelemen, et.al, "Segmentation of 2-D and 3-D objects from MRI volume data using constrained elastic deformation of flexiable fourier contour and surface models", *Medical Image Analysis*, 1(1), pp. 19-34, 1996.
5. T.Mcinerney, D.Terzopoulos, "Topology adaptive deformable surface for medical image volume segmentation", *IEEE Trans Med Image*, 18(10), pp. 840-851, 1999.
6. T.T.Elvins, "A survey of algorithms for volume visualization", *Computer Graphics*, 26(3), pp. 194-199, 1992.
7. W.E.Lorensen, H.E.Cline, "Marching Cubes: a high resolution 3D surface construction algorithm", *Computer Graphics*, July, pp. 163-169, 1987.
8. G.M. Nielson, B.Hamann, "The asymptotic decider: resolving the ambiguity in Marching Cubes", *IEEE Proceeding of Visualization'91*, pp. 83-91.
9. P.K.Sahoo, S.Soltani, A.K.C.Wong, "A survey of thresholding techniques", *Comp Vision Graphics Image Processing*, 41, pp. 233-260,1988.
10. A. Rosenfeld and A. Kak Digital Picture Processing, Vols 1 and 2, Academic Press, 1982.
11. Y.H.Katz, "Pattern recognition of meteorological satellite cloud photography", Proceedings, Third symp.on Remote Sensing of Environment, pp173-214, 1965.
12. J.S.Weszka, R.N.Nagel, A.Rosenfeld, "A threshold selection technique", IEEE Trans *Computers*, 23, pp. 1322-1326, 1974.
13. D.L.Milgram, M.Herman, "Clustering edge value for threshold selection", *Comp Graphics & Image Processing*, 10, pp. 272-280,1979.
14. S. Wang, R.M. Haralick, "Automatic multithreshold selection", *Comp Vision Graphics Image Processing*, 25, pp. 46-67, 1984.
15. L.Hertz, R.W.Schafer, "Multilevel thresholding using edge matching", *Comp Vision Graphics Image Processing*, 44, pp. 279-295, 1988.
16. S.S.Trivedi, T.S. Herman G. T, J.K.Udupa, "Segmentation into three classes using gradients", *IEEE Trans Med Imag*, 16(2), pp. 116-119, 1986.

Identifying image structures for content-based retrieval of digitized spine x-rays

L. Rodney Long[*a], Daniel M. Krainak[b], George R. Thoma[a]

[a]National Library of Medicine, Bethesda, MD
[b]The Catholic University of America, Washington, DC

ABSTRACT

We present ongoing work for the computer-assisted indexing of biomedical images at the Lister Hill National Center for Biomedical Communications, a research and development division of the National Library of Medicine (NLM). For any class of biomedical images, a problem confronting the researcher in image indexing is developing robust algorithms for localizing and identifying anatomy relevant for that image class and relevant to the indexing goals. This problem is particularly acute in the case of digitized spine x-rays, due to the projective nature of the data, which results in overlapping boundaries with possibly ambiguous interpretations; the highly irregular shapes of the vertebral bodies, sometimes additionally distorted by pathology; and possible occlusions of the vertebral anatomy due to subject positioning. We present algorithms that we have developed for the localization and identification of vertebral structure and show how these algorithms fit into the family of algorithms that we continue to develop for our general indexing problem. We also review the indexing goals for this particular collection of digitized spine x-rays and discuss the use of the indexed images in a content-based image retrieval system.

Keywords: digitized x-rays, content-based image retrieval, spine, image segmentation

1. OVERVIEW

1.1 Indexing digitized spine x-rays

Our goal is the indexing of a collection of 17,000 digitized lateral cervical and lumbar spine x-rays collected by the National Center for Health Statistics (NCHS) as part of the second National Health and Nutrition Examination Survey (NHANES II), and the creation of an advanced query capability for accessing the indexed images that supports query by image example. The key biomedical features of interest for indexing have been determined by two workshops conducted at the National Institutes of Health, and include anterior osteophytes, disc space narrowing, and subluxation. For economic reasons alone, computer-assisted indexing is highly desirable. A hierarchical approach to such indexing that we have described elsewhere consists of high-level region classification, spine region localization, vertebra localization and identification, vertebral segmentation, and classification of the vertebrae by presence/absence of the biomedical features above. In this paper we describe approaches to anatomy identification in the images by means of automated and by means of interactive, computer-assisted methods. We compare the approach and results of two new algorithms with previous work[1]. Some of the same algorithms used for indexing the images may also be used to support query-by-example, since the example image requires the extraction of its relevant index features in order to search the database for images with similar features.

1.2 Image indexing in a content-based image retrieval (CBIR) system

The use of effective indexing algorithms is twofold: (1) the algorithms may be directly used to derive indexing information from the set of images in the database; this information then becomes part of the database, and becomes itself part of the data that may be queried; and (2) the algorithms may be used to derive indexing information "on the fly" from images that are input to the system as examples used to define the current query.

---

[*] long@nlm.nih.gov, phone 1 301 435-3208; fax 1 301 402-0341; National Library of Medicine, 8600 Rockville Pike, Bethesda, MD 20894

Medical Imaging 2002: Image Processing, Milan Sonka, J. Michael Fitzpatrick, Editors, Proceedings of SPIE Vol. 4684 (2002) © 2002 SPIE · 1605-7422/02/$15.00

An example of a CBIR system for a small database of NHANES II x-ray images has been created[5] as an initial test of data retrieval by any combination of health survey text data, vertebral dimensional data, and vertebral shape. This system is a small prototype suggesting the interface characteristics and functionality of a CBIR system for digitized x-rays. In this prototype, a MATLAB graphical user interface aids in the query for different aspects of vertebral data. Health survey data may be queried in combination with features such as anterior/posterior height ratio, anterior height, posterior height, and disc space. Query-by-example and query-by-sketch is supported. The query results are ranked by similarity to the example image or sketch. Query result images and other user-selected images may be displayed side-by-side for easy visual comparison. The system allows a sketch of the vertebra or an example vertebra including up to nine critical points: the six common morphometric points, the anterior midpoint, and the locations of anterior osteophytes. Shape similarity is based upon a least squares best fit model independent of rotation, translation, and scaling. Future work will include making the system independent of the nine critical points marked by radiologists and the inclusion of more complex shape matching algorithms.

2. ANALYSIS

By automated image content analysis, we refer to computer processing that outputs image content description with zero user intervention; when the user is allowed to input information to guide the analysis of image content, we refer to the processing as semi-automated, computer-assisted, or interactive.

2.1 Automated image content analysis

The type of image content of interest in this paper is the high-level semantic content corresponding to the mapping of specific image regions to descriptors used in the domain of biomedicine to label components of human skeletal anatomy. A sucessful automated analyzer would produce results that could be considered comparable to a human viewing the image and saying, "That [image object] is the C1 vertebra", " That [image object] is the spinous process on the back of the C3 vertebra". We take the point of view that labeling may meaningfully precede segmentation in the images, i.e., that we may meaningfully label parts of the image when the regions containing these parts are only localized by coarse boundaries. The uses of such labeling of regions include (1) the localization of regions of interest for further processing to refine object boundaries; and (2) the marking of significant regions to direct the user's attention in image display systems, such as medical education systems to display labeled anatomy.

2.2 Automated approach to anatomy localization

As remarked above, the process of anatomy localization for identification may be considered as distinct from, or only a rudimentary type of, segmentation: for our purposes, localization of a vertebral structure S means the computation of a simple closed polygon P that contains the structure, and identification means the association of a label with the polygon that correctly corresponds to the contained structure. Localization corresponds to the understanding of the image objects at a coarser level than segmentation, where object boundaries are determined in detail. Such localization/identification involves overcoming a number of difficulties, including detection of whether the computed P in fact contains the target structure S, contains S partially, contains other target structures partially or completely, and the problem of distinguishing, for the purpose of the correct assignment of anatomical labels, very similar and proximate structures. Our approach consists of (1) an initialization step to identify a beginning search curve fixed to the image anatomy at the back of the skull and extending to the top of the spine, and (2) curve analysis to locate and identify the first spine structure, the spinous process on the C1 vertebra, and (3) sequential localization and identification of the other vertebral structures of interest, including the vertebral faces.

Example output from the algorithm is shown in Figure 1 for four test cases. For these tests, the bounding polygon P was taken as a rectangle. Figure 2 is an example of a curve traced along the skull for one image, and illustrates the technique used.

2.3 Interactive image analysis

In an interactive image content analysis system, if the required user interaction is frequent, complex, and/or requires expert skills, the value of the computer assistance is diminished. The principle that we have followed is to attempt to mimimize the frequency and the complexity of the user assistance required, so that the algorithm may be successfully used with the only required human intervention being support at the level of a trained technician.

2.4 Interactive approach to anatomy localization

This algorithm has the goal of identifying the spinous processes of the vertebra and vertebral faces with the aid of user assistance. The specific instruction that we have for the user is, simply, "Draw a line from the skull area to the shoulder area that passes through the spinous processes." We believe that this instruction with a small number of examples of line drawing that show a line passing through the main part of the bodies of the spinous processes and including the dark gaps between the adjacent processes, will suffice to capture the required data.

2.4.1 Summary of algorithm to locate the spinous processes

The algorithm to locate and label the spinous processes is,

(1) compute the image grayscale profile along the user-defined line;
(2) compute the local minima of this profile;
(3) use a priori characteristics of the local minima within the spinous process gaps to filter out all of the local minima that do not fit the a priori local minima characteristics;
(4) apply a thinning procedure to reduce sets of multiple local minima between two spinous processes to a unique local minimum between each pair of spinous processes. The end result is, for each pair of spinous processes, a single point lying on the user-defined line, which is a local minimum for the region between the pair of spinous processes. We refer to this unique point as the inter-spinous process point for the two bounding spinous processes;
(5) calculate the location of a spinous process as the average of an adjacent (as they occur along the user-drawn line) pair of inter-spinous process points; we expect these points to bound a spinous process. Since skull position is known from the user-drawn line (that line, by requirement on the user, begins in the skull region), the spinous processes may be numbered anatomically correctly with process number one being the process following the first local minima (hence the process adjacent to the skull).

The algorithm input and output are illustrated in Figures 3 and 4. In Figure 3, the image is shown with the user-drawn line. This is the total user interaction with the image content analysis; after getting the input of the user line, the algorithm is completely automatic. In Figure 4, the algorithm output is shown: spinous processes 1-6 have been labeled, along with vertebrae C4-C6.

2.4.2 Details of the algorithm: identification of the inter-spinous process points

In this section we provide step-by-step details of the algorithm, beginning at the point that the user line has been input. The algorithm is explained with reference to the sample image shown in Figure 3.

(1) The image grayscale profile along the user line is computed. For the image and user line in Figure 3, this profile consists of N grayscale values, where $N \approx 1000$. From this profile of raw grayscale values, two smoothed profiles are computed; for each smoothed profile, the *ith* profile value consists of the mean grayscale value in a $\sigma - neighborhood$ of i (i.e. $2\sigma + 1$ grayscale values centered at i, where σ is a positive integer). Profile 1 is smoothed with a small σ in order to smooth out the effects of grayscale amplitude variations that occur over very small inter-pixel distances, due to noise, or very small variations in image structures that occur over this small scale, but which are irrelevant to the features that we want to detect, namely, the local minima due to the separation of the spinous processes; profile 2 is smoothed with a large σ in order to smooth out the all of the extrema (local minima and maxima) due to the spinous

process themselves: hence profile 2 is intended to capture the large scale trend of the grayscale along the user line, and preserves only the average behavior of the grayscale at this large scale. Figure 5 shows profiles 1 and 2 as they were computed for the user line from Figure 3.

(2) The local minima are computed along profile 1. Inspection of the profile 1 curve in Figure 5 shows a number of local minima; some appear in the skull region, some are on the bodies of the spinous processes (see the local minimum on spinous process 5, for example; this is marked with a ** in Figure 5); and some are in the spaces between the spinous processes. Since we are attempting to detect the spaces between the spinous processes, it is this last category that is of interest to us.

(3) We use the a priori assumption that the local minima corresponding to the spaces between the spinous processes will lie below the values of the locally-averaged grayscale (profile 2), while the local minima which correspond to grayscale "dips" that occur within the spinous process bodies will lie above this locally-averaged grayscale. Again, this separation is illustrated by spinous process 5 in Figure 5: profile 2 is seen to separate the local minimum within the <u>body</u> of spinous process 5, from the local minima that <u>border</u> spinous process 5. The local minima that remain as candidates for inter-spinous process points are those that lie below profile 2. These are marked with circles in Figure 5. ("Below" profile 2 means having a grayscale value less than profile $2 - \Delta_1$, where Δ_1 is a parameter of the algorithm). Two technical difficulties remain: (a) this set of local minima is may include local minima that are not between the spinous processes at all, but are actually in the skull region. (The skull region in these images may have significant grayscale variability, while the shoulder region is homogeneous to a high degree, and we do not have the same phenomenon of spurious local minima occurring there.) (b) also, the local minima that do correspond to inter-spinous process points are not unique: there may be more than one local minimum detected between a given pair of adjacent spinous processes. Both of these situations are illustrated in Figure 5.

(4) To deal with problem (a), a combination gradient and grayscale threshold test using a dynamically-computed grayscale threshold is employed to eliminate local minima in the skull region. First the location of the skull region is estimated by a two-step process. A mean grayscale value on the user line for the skull region is estimated by sampling grayscale on the user line from the region that with high probability corresponds to skull. Relying on the assumption that the user has drawn the line from skull to shoulder, the maximum grayscale value in the first half of the user line is found, and points in a small neighborhood of this maximum are assumed to lie in the skull region. The mean value of the grayscale for these points is the estimate SRG for skull region grayscale. Then, the most negative gradient on the smoothed profile 1 line is found: this should denote a strong edge pixel on profile 1. We search from the point in the direction of the beginning of profile 1 for the first zero gradient point. If this point passes a reasonability test for lying in the skull region, we take this point as the skull boundary. The reasonability test that we use is that the zero gradient pixel should have a grayscale value greater than $SRG - \Delta_2$, where Δ_2 is a program parameter; if the reasonability test is not passes we iteratively search profile 1 for the next largest gradient, search from that point to the beginning of profile 1 for the next zero gradient point, and test that point for grayscale reasonability. Once the skull boundary point has been determined, we discard any local minima that lie on the "skull side" of this point, as not belonging to an inter-spinous process region. To deal with problem (b) a second test is employed to eliminate multiple local minima between spinous processes, based on a priori assumptions about reasonable bounds on the distances between collinear points lying in distinct inter-spinous process spaces. If the Euclidean distance between two local minima is less than Δ_3, also a program parameters of the local minima is eliminated; the local minimum kept is the one for which the quantity that lies the furthest below profile 2.

Figure 6 shows the image with the user line and the final set of local minima marked with circles. These are the local minima determined by the algorithm to correspond the inter-spinous process points.

Note that spinous process 7 is visible in the image in Figure 6; in Figure 5 the part of profiles 1 and 2 that correspond to this spinous process has been manually marked, but Figures 5 shows that only one border of this spinous process has been detected; the local minimum lying closest to the shoulder is too small to be detected by the algorithm. Hence, spinous process 7 is undetectable by the algorithm for this image.

2.4.3   Details of the algorithm: identification of the vertebral faces

Following the identification of the spinous processes, the vertebral faces are identified. The approach that we took was to use the user line to orient a set of grids that we placed across the spine region. Then, for each of the local minima found above to lie between a pair of spinous processes, to search the grid for the paths of minimum grayscale, with the expectation that for the lower cervical spine vertebrae, which typically have visible background in the interveterbral spaces, we would be able to place a path that runs through this interveterbral space. These paths were expected to mark the separation between vertebrae and, since each path originates in an inter-spinous process space where we have labeled the spinous processes, we would be able to use the path information to label the particular vertebra. Figure 7 illustrates the grid concepts for the single grid associate with one inter-spinous process point. Figure 8 shows the grids for each of the inter-spinous process points for the example image from Figure 3. The parameters of the grids (width, height, and density) were set by informal methods, and are the same for all grids. The grid width ("across the spine") parameter was set based on sampling of typical spine widths in the images; similarly, grid height was based on inspecting image samples to determine heights that appeared likely to enclose the target area-the intervertebral space, when the grid is positioned with one edge along the user-defined line, with the center of that edge on an inter-spinous process point. Grid density was selected by running the algorithm over a range of densities and observing the resulting paths. The density used for the illustration in Figure 8 is much coarser than the densities actually used, and is shown here for illustration only. The grid width is set to an a priori value and then dynamically updated with information from the image: the a priori value was obtained by inspecting a small sample of images and manually estimating the distance across the spine, from the mid-spinous process region to the front of the spine. Once the grid is formed, this distance is refined, as follows: If the grid is of size $p \times m$, where the grid rows run parallel to the user-defined line, and the grid columns run normal to the user-defined line, then, for each grid k, and for each row i in that grid, we calculate the sum of gradient values

$$S_{ki} = \sum_{j}^{m} \nabla_{ij}$$

over the m columns of that row. We then sum S_{ki} over all of the grids to get

$$S_i = \sum_{k}^{n} S_{ki}$$

Finally, we calculate row i^* as the row for which S_i is maximized. The gradients are approximated as simple grayscale differences in the direction normal to the rows and computed so that a dark-to-light transition when moving in the direction of the arrow shown in Figure 9 results in a gradient with positive sign, i.e.

$$\nabla_{ij} = g_{i-1,j} - g_{i+1,j}$$

where g_{ij} is the grid's grayscale value at coordinates (i, j). We expect that the sum of the gradients calculated in this manner will be maximized for the grid line that lies closest to the front edge of the spine, where the dark-to-light grayscale transition is visually the strongest. Figure 9 shows the results of calculating this front edge line for the example image. Knowing this line provides an updated estimate of the search grid width that is based on actually data from the particular image being analyzed, and provides a linear estimate of the location of the front of the spine.

For each local minimum on the user line that we have identified as corresponding to an inter-spinous process point, we then calculate a path across the rows of the grid, beginning at the grid row 1 (on which the local minima lie) and ending on row f (the row that we have identified as nearest the front edge of the spine). The calculation of a path is posed as an optimization problem where the objective function is

$$O(P) = \sum_{P} g_{ij} + \lambda \sum_{P} \delta_{ij,kl}$$

where the path is specified as an ordered set of coordinates,

$$P = \{(i_1, j_1), (i_2, j_2), \dots (i_f, j_f)\}.$$

P is constrained to begin on the first grid row, at one of the local minima points (inter-spinous process points), i.e. $((i_1, j_1) = (1, j_q))$, where j_q is the grid column corresponding to the qth local minimum, and to end on the front edge grid row, i.e. $i_f = f$. The goal of the optimization is to minimize $O(P)$ over all possible paths on the grid. The first term on the right in the expression for $O(P)$ is just the sum of grayscale values along the path P; g_{ij} is the grayscale value at grid point (i, j) and is the cost associated with that grid point. The term $\delta_{ij,kl}$ is the transition cost associated with going from grid point (i, j) to grid point (k, l). We define this to be the Euclidean distance between the two points, i.e.

$$\delta_{ij,kl} \equiv \sqrt{(i-k)^2 + (j-l)^2}.$$

The term λ is a program parameter that we set to weight the relative importance of the two terms. The intent of the formulation is to find the path with the smallest cumulative grayscale while maintaining some degree of smoothness by weighting the second term to restrict the total path length. Figure 7 illustrates the concept of the optimal path determined by minimizing $O(P)$. The optimization problem over this grid is suited for a dynamic programming solution, and that is what we have implemented. Figure 10 shows solution curves computed for the lower inter-spinous process points (points 4-7) of the example image.

The final step in the algorithm is the localization of the vertebral faces. To achieve this, the posterior edge boundaries of the vertebrae are estimating by finding the grid row of maximum grayscale value, i.e. the brightest grayscale line. The procedure followed is essentially the same as for finding the grid row corresponding to the front edge of the spine, except that grayscale value, rather than gradient value is maximized. Figure 11 shows the bright edge line (maximum grayscale line) that was computed for the example image. Then, each pair of optimal paths determined to run through the interveteral spaces, the intersection of these paths with the front edge and bright edge lines are calculated; this yields four points that determine "corners" of the coarse vertebral segmentation. The diagonals determined by these corners are calculated, and the interesection of the diagonals is the point at which the vertebral label is placed. Figure 11 illustrates the diagonals and the placement of the intersection point.

3. IMPLEMENTATION AND RESULTS

We have implemented the localization/identification algorithms using MATLAB 5.3 on a Windows Pentium-class PC.

3.1 Automatic algorithm

The algorithm has currently been tested through steps (1) and (2) on 136 images of the cervical spine; for these images, P was taken as a rectangle. The results were evaluated by displaying the images with the region P as marked by the algorithm and answering the question, "Does P contain most of the body of spinous process 1?" With this procedure, 88% of these cases P were evaluated as containing the target shape, the spinous process on the C1 vertebra. A number of the failure cases were determined to be due to unexpected local minima in the search curve determined by the skull boundary, which in turn were due to small concavities in the skull shape. A difficulty with the current algorithm is that it does not incorporate any self-evaluation capability to estimate its success, and it does not estimate the target orientation within P, information that may be critical in used the results to move to other anatomy within the image. We are now researching smoothing methods to remove these irregularities, and are extending the algorithm to step (3), the full localization and identification of structures in the cervical spine. In this paper we provide complete results on the performance of the algorithm on all three steps.

This sequential localization and identification of structures is based on location of previously-determined structures, and a prior statistical data on the relative geometries of the vertebral structures. We have vertebral geometric data recorded under supervision of a board-certified radiologist for computation of the a priori statistics.

3.2 Interactive algorithm

For the initial evaluation that we have done, we have approached the evaluation of the interactive algorithm's performance by focusing on the three "trainable" variables below:

Δ_1 = factor to discriminate minima that lie below the local curve average ("true" inter-spinous points) from minima that lie above the local curve average (points that lie within the body of a spinous process)

Δ_2 = factor to determine whether a point meets grayscale reasonability criteria for lying in the skull region

Δ_3 = factor that sets the minimum allowed distance between two neighboring inter-spinous process points

The interactive algorithm was "trained" on these three parameters using a set of 20 images by repeatedly processing the 20 images while varying the parameters independently. In the first test run, a user line was manually drawn on the images; in subsequent runs, the same user line was used. The runs were evaluated by displaying the labelled images and visually judging whether the placement of the spinous process and vertrebra locations were within the visual boundaries of those respective objects, and whether the labeling was correct. Only labeling of C4 –C7 was attempted.

The results of these training were as follows: 13 (65%) of the images were processed correctly (all expected vertebrae and spinous processes were found and located correctly; 5 (25%) were processed partially correctly (two were correct, except for spinous process 6 being missed; 3 were correct, except for slight misplacements of the vertebrae locations); and 2 (10%) were failures (one failed due to incorrect identification of the skull edge; the other due to mis-identifying a local minimum that lay within the body of a spinous process as an inter-spinous process point).

The cases where spinous process 6 were missed were all cases where the shoulder-side boundary of this structure is only weakly visible in the image, resulting in a very small local minimum on the profile 1 curve; the detection of this miminmum is below the sensitivity of the current implementation. The cases where there were slight misplacements of the vertebrae locations are likely due to the characteristics of the grid model used to constrain the search for the coarse vertebral boundaries: we use a simple rectangular grid that does not model the geometry of the user line/spinous process/vertebral body configuration. The two failure cases require a refinement in the skull edge detection procedure and in the process of discriminating inter-spinous process points from local minima that may occur with the bodies of large spinous processes.

The major step that we anticipate in improvement of the algorithm is in incorporating a grid model that reflects where the intervertebral spaces lie with respect to the inter-spinous process spaces. If we may then couple the user line with this anatomy-based grid, we expect to locate vertebrae more accurately, and to test the locatability of higher vertebrae (C1-C3) with this method.

We have done only informal testing on aspect of the algorithm: the variability of placement of the user line, but in the tests run, the range of variability tolerated on the input line that produces visually invariant results in structure location and labeling are good. The main requirements are that the user line begin in the skull, end in the shoulder, and intersect the spinous processes in such a way that the inter-spinous process spaces are intersected. In all except one image, the lines could be drawn causally, subject to these constraints, with no geometric difficulties; in the one exception, the spine presentation had a curvature that required more careful line placement in order to meet the constraints. Rigorous testing with lines generated at random lengths and orientations, subject to these constraints, should expose any unforeseen difficulties due to user line placement.

The interactive algorithm is currently in a training and development phase which we will follow with testing on a set of images on which it has not been trained, to assess its expected performance.

4. CONCLUSION

We conclude by placing the work in developing these algorithms in the context of our total research and development work in indexing and retrieving the x-ray images. These algorithms, in combination with algorithms to accurately segment the spine vertebrae and to classify those vertebrae according to specific biomedical features of interest, form the basis for a projected future system that, with the proper biomedical validation, is intended to provide a method for the computer-assisted indexing of the entire 17,000 image collection. To date, our own efforts and those of our collaborators have resulted in (1) the establishment of an on-line, publicly accessible 17,000 image collection of digitized x-rays, (2) the creation of an ongoing research effort into the use of Active Shape Modeling for the vertebral segmentation of these images[2,3], (3) the creation of an ongoing research effort into the classification of the vertebrae by biomedical feature, based on shape characteristics[4], (4) our continuing development of high-level algorithms for image analysis, and anatomical localization and identification, and (5) the creation of a prototype system for the retrieval of the images by vertebral shape, based on query-by-example and query-by-sketch[5].

REFERENCES

1. Long LR, Thoma GR. Identification and classification of spine vertebrae by automated methods. Proceedings of SPIE Medical Imaging 2001, vol. 4322, pp. 1478-1489.
2. Sari-Sarraf H, Mitra S, Zamora G, Tezmol A. Customized active shape models for segmentation of cervical and lumbar spine vertebrae, Texas Tech University College of Elec. Eng. technical report, available at http://www.cvial.ttu.edu/~sarraf
3. Zamora G, Sari-Sarraf, Mitra S, Long R. Estimation of orientation and position of cervical vertebrae for segmentation with active shape models. Proceedings of SPIE Medical Imaging 2001, vol. 4322, pp. 378-387.
4. Stanley RJ, Long R. A radius of curvature-based approach to cervical spine vertebra image analysis. Proceedings of the 38th annual Rocky Mountain Bioengineering Symposium 37: 385-391, April 2001.
5. Krainak DM, Long LR, Thoma GR. A method of content-based retrieval for a spinal x-ray image database. Proceedings of SPIE Medical Imaging 2002, vol. 4685.

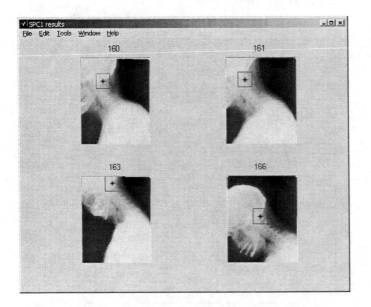

Figure 1. Examples of automated localization of spinous process 1 within a bounding box.

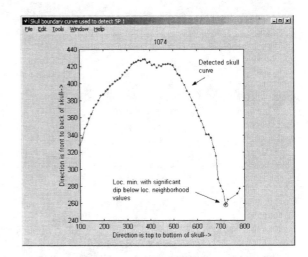

Figure 2 Example of the skull boundary curve used for the localization in one image. (Vertical and horizontal axes units are different.)

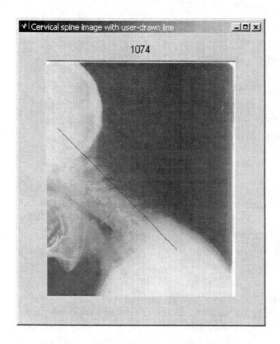

Figure 3 Input: cervical spine image with
user-drawn line.

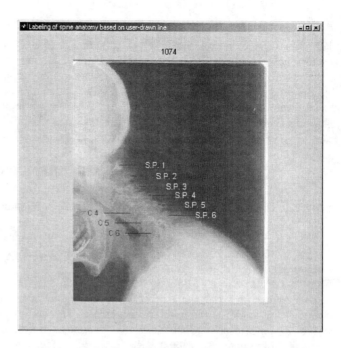

Figure 4. Output: labeled, located spinous processes
and lower vertebral faces.

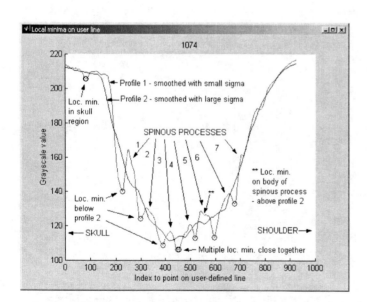

Figure 5. Illustration of concepts used to find the inter-
spinous process points.

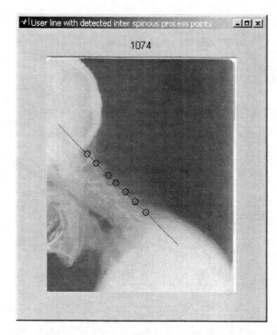

Figure 6. Results of finding the inter-
spinous process points.

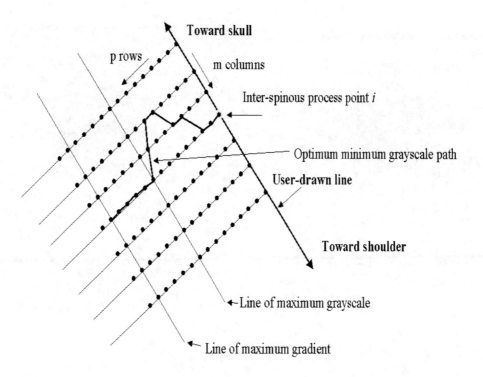

Figure 7. Illustration of concepts used to find the maximum gradient line, maximum grayscale line, and optimum minimum-grayscale path.
Illustrated for the grid associated with one inter-spinous process point.

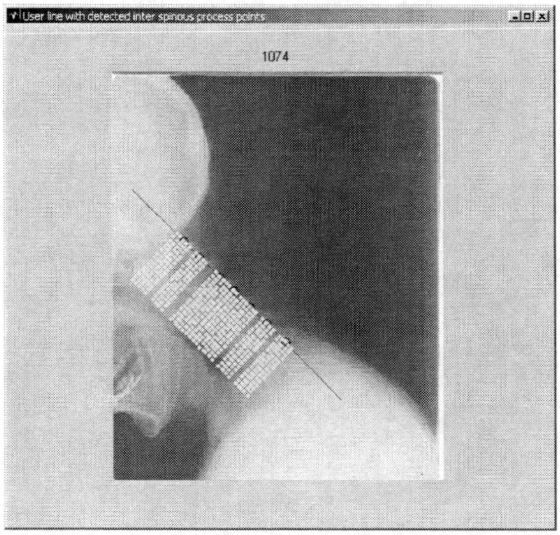

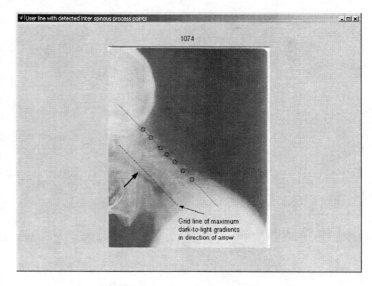

Figure 8. Grids for each of the inter-spinous process points.

Figure 9. The detected front edge grid line.

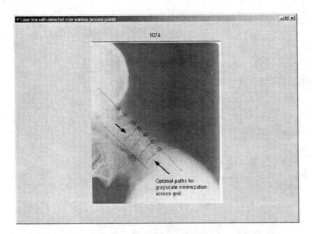

Figure 10. The optimal minimum grayscale paths
for the lower vertebrae.

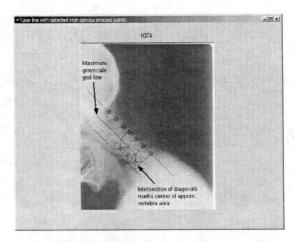

Figure 11. Diagonals formed by the "corners" of
the front edge/bright edge lines, and the optimal
minimum grayscale paths. Vertebrae faces are
labeled at the intersections of these diagonals.

Automatic localization and delineation of collimation fields in digital and film-based radiographs

Thomas M. Lehmann[*], Sascha Goudarzi, Nick I. Linnenbrügger,
Daniel Keysers[a], Berthold B. Wein[b]

Institute of Medical Informatics
[a]Chair of Computer Science VI
[b]Department of Diagnostic Radiology
Aachen University of Technology (RWTH), Aachen, Germany

ABSTRACT

Collimation field detection is an important pre-processing step for automatic image analysis of radiographs. However, most approaches are restricted to a small set of form archetypes or presuppose the presence of a shutter. Hence, existing methods are not applicable to large collections of radiographs from various modalities, such as obtained in the field of content-based image retrieval in medical applications. Based on analytical evaluation, the approach of WIEMKER et al. (Procs SPIE 2000; 3979:1555–1565) was selected, modified in order to reduce false positive detection, and evaluated on a large set of 4,000 radiographs (763 containing shutter edges) taken from daily routine including any kind of projective X-ray examinations. Eight subsets (each of 500 images) were compiled randomly. A set of 500 images was used to optimize the parameters and evaluated using the remaining 3,500 images. This procedure was repeated for all eight combinations. Using the initial approach, the specificity is 96.4% with a poor sensitivity of 44.1% resulting in an overall precision of 86.7%. All figures increase up to 98.5%, 55.6%, and 89.5%, respectively, if the algorithm also minimizes the variation of radiation density values outside the detected shutter area. In terms of sensitivity and precision, the results of optimization vs. evaluation for the same combination and of evaluation vs. evaluation for different combinations differed up to 13 and 9 percentage points, respectively. This indicates that still an insufficient number of images is used to allow complete generalization of the results.

Keywords: Radiation Field Recognition, Collimation Detection, Shutter Removal, Background Removal, Hough-Transform, Content-Based Image Retrieval, Software Evaluation

1. INTRODUCTION

Within a medical image, which has either been digitally recorded or secondarily digitized, not all pixels host information of diagnostic relevance. For example, patients are protected against unnecessary exposure to X-rays by use of radiopaque material, which is placed in between the beam pathways from the X-ray to the patient. This process is referred to as collimating and the radiopaque material is named collimator or shutter,[4] while the area under normal exposure is called the radiation field[13] or irradiation field.[4] Some modalities, e.g., fluoroscopy, have a non-rectangular aperture that covers parts of the screen. If film-based X-ray examinations are digitized, masking effects are also induced from the scanning process. In the following, we summarize all these different effects within the term "collimation field". Sometimes, a larger part of the film is shielded to be exposed separately in a second examination. This process is referred to as partitioning,[4] but is disregarded in this investigation.

Collimation field detection in radiographs is an important pre-processing step for automatic image analysis, indexing and retrieval.[11] Global measures of gray scale, texture, or structure are altered when the collimation field covers a substantial part of the digital image. Several methods for automatic segmentation have been suggested.[2,3,10,11,13-15]

---

[*] lehmann@computer.org; phone +49 241 80-88793; fax +49 241 80-82426; http://www.irma-project.org; Institute of Medical Informatics, Aachen University of Technology, Pauwelsstr. 30, D - 52057 Aachen, Germany.

Usually, the process of segmentation is comprised of two steps, localization and delineation. Localization addresses the question whether a shutter is present. Delineation determines the exact position and shape of the irradiation field. However, most approaches are restricted to certain assumptions, e.g. the collimation field must match a small set of form prototypes, have high-contrasted edges, is characterized by a certain grayscale, or, the algorithm is based on the simple hypothesis, that a collimation field is always present. In the latter case, only delineation is performed. Therefore, most existing methods are not applicable to large collections of radiographs from various modalities, such as obtained in the field of content-based image retrieval in medical applications (IRMA).[8]

In a recent approach, WIEMKER et al.[16] have proposed the automated recognition of the collimation field in digital radiographs by maximization of the Laplace area integral. This versatile approach does *not* assume that the collimation field

- is a substantial fraction of the overall input image,

- is in a near-central position of the input image,

- is in parallel with the image boundary,

- is rectangular or matches a certain set of shape primitives, nor that it

- is build from a restricted number of edges.

In addition, the algorithm of WIEMKER et al. can cope with locally missing shutter edge contrast and low gradients. However, the approach is rather based on the hypothesis, that a shutter is present. In other words, collimation fields are frequently detected in radiographs that are routinely exposed, although they are not present. In order to reduce false positive detection, we present a simple extension to the algorithm and rigorously validate the resulting method on a large set of radiographs, which have been taken from daily routine.

2. METHOD OVERVIEW

The automatic collimation field detection is done in sequential steps. At first, all images are reduced in size to strengthen image gradients and reduce computing time. A fixed dimension is selected regardless of the initial size and aspect ratio to emphasize shorter edges in non-quadratic collimation fields or image formats. Local gradients are computed by means of directed Sobel templates and stored in the accumulator array of the Hough transform keeping the orientation of edges. Local maxima are detected within the accumulator array and used to generate hypotheses of shutter edges forming convex radiation fields. A greedy depth-first search strategy is applied to avoid exhaustive search within the hypotheses search space. Hypotheses are evaluated concerning four criteria:

1. maximize the density gradient perpendicular to the shutter gradient;

2. maximize the radiation density inside;

3. maximize the enclosed area;

4. minimize the variation of densities outside.

Parameterization A and B use criteria (1,2,3) and (1,2,3,4), respectively. Note that variant A corresponds to the initial approach of Wiemker et al.,[16] while Criterion 4 is capable of reducing the number of positive collimator detection, which occurs frequently in skeleton radiographs from chest or skull if only the first three criteria are applied.

3. IMPLEMENTATION

3.1. Preprocessing and edge detection

Disregarding the aspect ratio, all images are resized to 128 x 128 pixels using linear interpolation.[7] This preprocessing not only allows significant code optimization but also strengthens local gradients at the frame of the collimation field, makes small local gradient masks applicable and emphasizes the shorter lines of rectangular radiation fields.

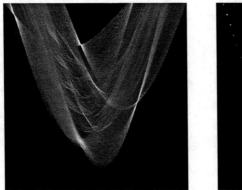

Fig. 1: Accumulator array of the Hough transform (left) and detection of local maxima (right).

In this work, the Sobel edge detection technique is applied yielding information about edge direction and magnitude. Next, a process is adopted from the Canny edge detection technique,[2] which is known as non-maximum suppression.[12] This step essentially locates the highest points in the edge magnitude data. It is performed by using edge direction information to check whether points are at the peak of a ridge. Given a region of 3 x 3 pixels, a point is at a maximum if the gradient at either side of it is less than the gradient at the center point.

3.2. Hough transform

The Hough transform[5] is applied to detect straight lines in the resultant edge image. In contrast to this initial implementation, where the source image is considered to be a binary image, edge magnitudes are used to weight the votes cast by a pixel in the edge image. The result is a set of line parameters in foot-of-normal parameterization together with the number of votes cast for each line representation. In addition, the Hough transform has been extended by a third dimension. Every edge point is classified according to its edge direction to give evidence to the orientation of the line that it contributes to. The part of a line that corresponds to a shutter edge candidate consists of many edge points, which all have almost the same edge direction. As a line crosses the entire image plane, there may be edge points on the line that do not belong to this shutter edge but to another edge resulting from anatomical structure or noise. It is not desirable that those edge points contribute votes to the line that represents the shutter edge candidate in the accumulator array. It is likely that in most cases, the edge direction of those points is different from that of points, which belong to the shutter edge candidate.

All edge points belong to one of two classes: edge points that point to one and to the other side of the line. Actually, both classes take votes from edge points with edge direction from a range of $180°$. On an ideal line, all edge points have an edge direction of $-\theta$ or $-\theta+180°$ according to the orientation of the line. A line can represent a gradient from bright to dark and vice versa. Thus the two classes are

- edge points with an edge direction in the range $-\theta \pm 90°$ and

- edge points with an edge direction in the range $-\theta+180° \pm 90°$.

Therefore, when an edge point casts votes to a line in the accumulator array defined by its direction θ and its normal distance ρ to the origin, it only adds votes to the class it belongs to, according to the edge direction and θ. This ensures that edge points having opposite directions, which suggests that they do not belong to the same connected edge, consequently do not contribute to the same class of the third dimension of the accumulator array.

Finally, this three-dimensional array is transformed into a two-dimensional array with votes and orientation assigned to each entry of the two-dimensional plane. This is achieved by determining the maximal votes of the third dimension for every point on the two-dimensional plane of the three-dimensional accumulator array. Those votes are assigned to the new two-dimensional array. The orientation is determined by the class where the maximum was found. Accordingly, the orientation can be either $-\theta$ or $-\theta+180°$. Note that the orientation of a line is defined in terms of edge direction. Thus, the orientation of a line represents the main edge direction of edge points on this line.

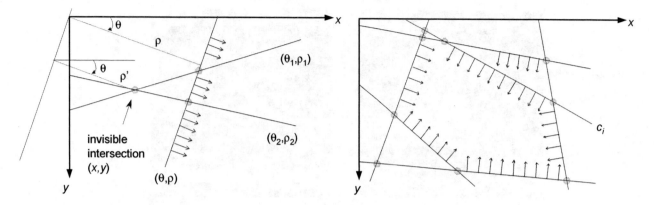

Fig. 2: Determination of invisible edges (left) and a set of shutter edges forming a hypothesis of the collimation filed (right), where the hypothesis c_i has just been switched on.

3.3. Maximum detection

Now, the resultant accumulator array is analyzed in order to find local maxima concerning votes in the Hough domain, which correspond to actual edges in the resized original image. This is achieved by grouping points into regions in the accumulator array, which represent separated lines. Accordingly, all points belonging to the same region correspond to the same line. The parameters (θ, ρ) of the line corresponding to a region equal the parameters of the maximum of that particular region.

First, a list of all points in the accumulator array with their parameters (θ, ρ), assigned votes, and orientation, is formed and sorted by votes with highest votes first. Thereafter, the list is explored from top to bottom. For each entry, it is checked whether it can be attached to an existing region, which is the case if its distance to the center of that particular region is smaller or equal to a certain region radius. For accumulator arrays of 180 x 180 cells, a radius of 10 cells has been chosen. If such a region is found, the point is attached to that region. Otherwise, a new region is created. A region is characterized by its center, which is the first point added to this region. This also is the region's maximum concerning the votes that are assigned to each point. The center and maximum does not change while new points are attached to the region. Accordingly, it is not necessary to keep track of the points that are added to a region. The total number of regions found can be influenced by adjusting the region radius. Figure 1 exemplifies an accumulator array and its corresponding local maxima.

3.4. Compiling hypotheses for collimation fields

The lines obtained in the previous step represent possible shutter edges. For accumulator arrays of 180 x 180 cells and a region radius of 10 cells, this list contains about 100 to 150 lines. The four image boundaries are added to this line list because image borders also are potential shutter edges. A collimation field hypothesis is a convex contour formed by several lines from the list of shutter edge candidates. A collimation field hypothesis is represented by a hypothesis vector

$$c = [c_1 ... c_N]^T \tag{1}$$

where each edge candidate can either be part of the hypothesis or not, i.e., be switched on or off. An entry of the hypothesis vector c_i is 1 if and only if the i-th shutter edge candidate is switched on, and 0 otherwise.

Given a set of lines that form a hypothesis, those lines have several intersections with each other. The actual contour of the region defined by a hypothesis results from the line segments between intersections that are not occluded by any other shutter edge candidate (Fig. 2). Here, the orientation of a line is taken into account. Let us consider an image with the shuttered area being bright. In this case, every shutter edge has an orientation that points toward the center of the image. Accordingly, a shutter edge candidate shields everything that lies in the direction opposite to the edge direction.

The set of line segments that are not occluded by any other shutter edge candidate is found by eliminating all invisible intersections, i.e., intersections that are covered by another shutter edge candidate. An intersection (x, y) of two lines (θ_1, ρ_1) and (θ_2, ρ_2) is obtained from

$$x = \frac{\rho_2 \sin\theta_1 - \rho_1 \sin\theta_2}{\cos\theta_2 \sin\theta_1 - \cos\theta_1 \sin\theta_2} \tag{2}$$

$$y = \frac{\rho_2 \cos\theta_1 - \rho_1 \cos\theta_2}{\sin\theta_2 \cos\theta_1 - \sin\theta_1 \cos\theta_2} \tag{3}$$

To determine whether an intersection is hidden by a particular shutter edge candidate (θ, ρ), the distance ρ' concerning the angle θ is calculated for the intersection (x, y) (Fig. 2). If ρ' is smaller than ρ of that specific shutter edge candidate, this intersection is invisible. For dark shutter areas or line orientations pointing from right to left, e.g., at right edges of a collimation field hypothesis with a bright shuttered area, invisible intersections are determined analogously. This process is executed for every pair of a shutter edge candidate and an intersection while effectively removing all invisible intersections. Line segments between remaining visible intersections form the contour of the collimation field hypothesis.

3.5. Evaluation of collimation field hypotheses using the Laplace area integral

Each hypothesis that was formed following the procedure described above, is evaluated by means of an objective function assessing four attributes of the hypothesis, i.e., the contour that is formed from the set of lines that represent the hypothesis:

1. the sum of the gradient over the contour;
2. the radiation density of the enclosed area;
3. the area that is enclosed by the contour;
4. the number of different gray-levels outside the contour.

The aim is to maximize the gradient over the contour, enclosed radiation density, and the enclosed area while minimizing the number of different gray-levels outside the contour.

The enclosed area is simply the number of pixels inside the contour. The radiation density of the enclosed area is the sum of the radiation at each pixel within the contour divided by the enclosed area. The radiation at a pixel depends on the brightness level at that particular pixel and the brightness of the shuttered area. If the shuttered area, i.e., the area where little radiation had passed through the object, is bright, gray-levels are logarithmically proportional to the radiation attenuation. If the area outside the contour is dark, gray-levels are in inverse proportion to radiation attenuation. The sum of the gradient over the contour can be calculated by the sum of the Laplace values within the contour.[16] This is known as the divergence theorem, which expresses the equivalence of a contour integral over a vector field and an area integral over the divergence of the vector field. Note that in a discrete domain, this theorem does not exactly hold true. However, the sum of the Laplace values within the contour is a reasonable approximation of the actual sum of the gradient over the contour. The number of different gray-levels outside the contour is evaluated by an analysis of the histogram of the shuttered area.

To speed up calculations, cumulative images of the original gray-level image and the image with Laplace values are calculated. Successively, a sum of pixels within the contour can be computed by subtracting pixels in the cumulative images that lie on left edges and adding pixels in the cumulative images that lie on right edges of the contour. The task of finding pixels that lie on left and right edges of the contour is not trivial. In this work, this is achieved by an adapted polygon filling algorithm. The original polygon filling algorithm[3] draws pixels on spans between left and right edges of a polygon. In this work, only the border pixels that lie strictly within the polygon, i.e., the contour, are considered and used as described above. Those border pixels are also used to calculate the enclosed area and to determine the area outside the contour, from which the histogram is evaluated.

3.6. Optimization by greedy depth-first search strategy

An exhaustive search of the hypothesis space of order $O(2^N)$ built from $N \approx 100$ shutter edge candidates cannot be conducted. Instead, a greedy depth-first search strategy is applied. WIEMKER et al.[15] have tested this approach for sufficiency by performing exhaustive searches of the hypothesis space for lower numbers N. The first hypothesis is the null hypothesis, i.e., only the image boundaries are turned on as shutter edge candidates. Then, all N shutter edge candidates are tentatively switched on, one at each time. The objective function is evaluated for every trial and the edge candidate yielding the highest result of the objective function is switched on permanently. This is continued in the next recursion, where again all of the $N-1$ remaining in-active edge candidates are tentatively switched on in addition to the first. Again, the candidate with the highest yield is then switched on permanently. This procedure is continued until none of the trials yields any increase in the objective function value.

After this single-track depth search, which does not fully explore any branches of the search tree, a restricted width search is conducted to check the consistency of the initial optimum hypothesis c. Let the preliminary optimum have K of the N shutter edge candidates switched on. Then, a greedy depth-first search is performed again with each of these K candidates switched on as the first shutter edge after the null hypothesis. If one of the K depth-first searches returns with a different edge set c' with K' edges turned on and an objective function value which is larger than the preliminary optimum, then this solution is adopted as the new preliminary optimum and the search starts again for all K' edges as starting points. Only if none of the K' depth-first searches returns with an objective function value higher than the preliminary optimum, the search terminates and the optimal edge set is fixed. Although the number of searching steps id not guaranteed to be small, in practice only a few searches need to be perform before termination of the algorithm.

This search is conducted twice. First, the shuttered area is considered to be dark. After that, the collimation field is looked at as being bright. Then, the maximum of the two runs is selected as the optimal edge set together with the information about the shuttered area's density.

3.7. Visualization

From this optimal edge set, the line segments between visible intersections of the shutter edges are determined. This contour is extrapolated to the initial size of the original input image, which has not been resized. This extrapolated contour is used to define a mask segment for the original image where points within and outside the contour are defined as valid and invalid, respectively. This mask is applied to further evaluation. In addition, the line segments can be used to draw the collimation field in the resized image for visualization purposes. Figure 3 shows successful delineation for rectangular, circular, and polygonal radiation fields.

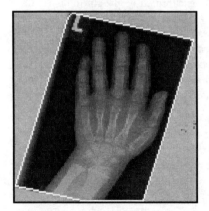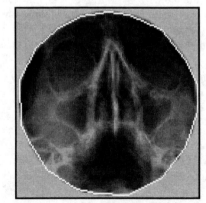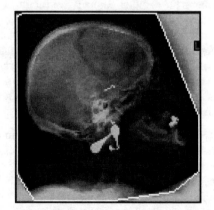

Fig. 3: Visualization of a rectangular (left), circular (middle), and polygonal (right) radiation field.

image subset	set of parameters	training			evaluation		
		sensitivity	specificity	precision	sensitivity	specificity	precision
0	A	0.46	0.97	0.87	0.46	0.96	0.87
	B	0.62	0.99	0.91	0.52	0.98	0.89
1	A	0.33	0.97	0.85	0.36	0.98	0.86
	B	0.47	0.98	0.89	0.56	0.99	0.90
2	A	0.53	0.97	0.88	0.52	0.95	0.87
	B	0.48	0.98	0.89	0.56	0.99	0.90
3	A	0.53	0.97	0.88	0.45	0.96	0.87
	B	0.74	0.98	0.93	0.61	0.97	0.90
4	A	0.48	0.97	0.87	0.46	0.96	0.87
	B	0.58	0.98	0.90	0.55	0.99	0.90
5	A	0.29	0.97	0.82	0.37	0.98	0.87
	B	0.49	0.99	0.88	0.56	0.98	0.90
6	A	0.56	0.97	0.90	0.45	0.96	0.86
	B	0.63	0.99	0.93	0.54	0.99	0.90
7	A	0.51	0.97	0.90	0.46	0.96	0.86
	B	0.55	0.98	0.91	0.55	0.99	0.90

Tab. 1: Results of cross-validation. The marked boxes are referred to from the body text.

4. EVALUATION

In total, 4,000 radiographs (763 with shutter edges) were randomly selected from clinical routine at the University Hospital, Aachen, Germany, including any modality of projective X-ray examinations. Note that a number of 4,000 references has been used by FDA (United States Food and Drug Administration) to validate software algorithms that screen normal head CT studies from studies that contain pathology.[1] Eight subsets (each of 500 images) were obtained randomly. A set of 500 images was used to optimize the parameters, i.e. the weights combining the criteria mentioned above. With respect to its application in content-based image retrieval, false positive location is to be avoided. Therefore during the manual parameterization, the specificity was tuned to be as large as 97% and 98% for parameter sets A and B, respectively. Note that a higher specificity was not possible for all eight sets of 500 training images. Using this sets of parameters, the evaluation was based on the corresponding 3,500 images. This process was repeated for all eight possible combinations of a 500 image subset and remaining 3,500 images.

5. RESULTS

For quantitative evaluation, only collimator segments covering more than 5% of the image area were considered as such. In case of any shutter segment, which has not been detected (false location) or any shutter segment, which has been detected although not present (false delineation), an error was recorded (Fig. 4). Table 1 summarizes the results. During the training phase, the sensitivity of variant B was up to 21 percentage points higher than that of variant A (see subset no. 3) although the specificity also was one or two points higher. Hence, the precision of variant A is always below that of variant B. Only for one case (see subset no. 2), variant A was superior to variant B with respect to the sensitivity. In general, these results were confirmed by the 3,500 reference images, which had not been seen during the training phase. Here, variant B was superior to variant A in all cases with respect to both sensitivity and precision. Nonetheless, if a high specificity of collimation field detection is enforced, the sensitivity is below 60% in almost all cases. The resulting overall precision is 86,6% and 89.9% for variant A and B, respectively.

6. DISCUSSION

Automatic delineation of collimation field is rather simple when the presence of shutter edges can be assumed, e.g. the algorithm is applied to a certain digital modality. With our approach, collimation fields are reliably detectable in any radiograph. The specificity of our algorithm is up to 99%. This figure is obtained from a rigorous evaluation that is based on 4,000 radiographs, which has not yet been reported for any method of collimation field detection.

Although only a very small number of parameters needs adjustment, i.e., the three relative weights combining the four criteria, and manual parameterization is performed using a very large number of 500 arbitrarily chosen images, the overall precision of training and evaluation decreases in two of the eight cases (25%) about as much as three percentage points (see subsets no. 3 and no. 6). Concerning the sensitivity of variant B, figures range about 9 percentage points from as low as 52% (see subset no. 1) up to 61% (see subset no. 3). In other words, the number of used images is still too small to allow absolute generalization of the results.[9] However, validation of algorithms for medical image processing is often based on a significant smaller number of images.

The proposed algorithm does not assume a certain set of form archetypes and detects shutters from any number of edges including curved shapes. Incorporating a Hough transform, the algorithm can cope with local missing shutter information. Overcoming a basic restriction of previous approaches, automatic collimation field detection now becomes available for a large range of applications such as content-based image retrieval in medical applications.

ACKNOWLEDGEMENT

This work was partly supported by the German Research Community (Deutsche Forschungsgemeinschaft, DFG) grant Le 1108/4-1.

REFERENCES

1. C. W. Brown, "Building a Medical Image Processing Algorithm Verification Database," *Proceedings SPIE Medical Imaging*, **3979**, pp. 772–780, 2000.
2. J. Canny, "A Computational Approach to Edge Detection," *IEEE Transactions on Pattern Analysis and Machine Intelligence* **8**, pp. 679–698, 1986.
3. S. N. C. Cheng, H.-P. Chan, L. T. Niklason, and R. S. Adler, "Automated Segmentation of Regions of Interest on Hand Radiographs," *Medical Physics* **21(8)**, pp. 1293–1300, 1994.
4. P. Dewaele, M. Ibison, and P. Vuylsteke, "A Trainable Rule-Based Network for Irradiation Field Recognition in AGFA's ADC System," *Proceedings SPIE Medical Imaging* **2708**, pp. 72–84, 1996.
5. R. O. Duda and P. E. Hart, "Use of the Hough Transformation to Detect Lines and Curves in Pictures,"

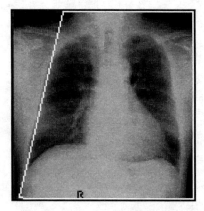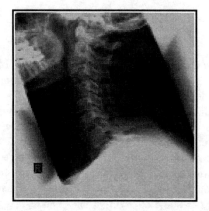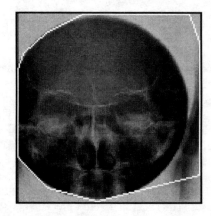

Fig. 4: False location (left) and false delineation (middle and right).

Communications of the ACM **15**, pp. 11–15, 1972.

6. J. D. Foley, J. F. Hughes, S. K. Feiner, and R. L. Phillips, *Computer Graphics: Principles and Practice*, Addison Wesley, second edition, 1995.

7. T. M. Lehmann, C. Gönner, and K. Spitzer: Survey: Interpolation Methods in Medical Image Processing. *IEEE Transactions on Medical Imaging* **18(11)**, pp. 1049–1075, 1999.

8. T. M. Lehmann, B. Wein, J. Dahmen, J. Bredno, F. Vogelsang, and M. Kohnen, "Content-Based Image Retrieval in Medical Applications: A Novel Multi-Step Approach," *Proceedings SPIE Medical Imaging* **3972**, pp. 312–320, 2000.

9. T. M. Lehmann, "From Plastic to Gold: A Unified Classification Scheme for Reference Standards in Medical Image Processing," *Proceedings SPIE Medical Imaging*, contents of this volume, 2002.

10. J. Lou and R. A. Senn, "Collimation Detection for Digital Radiography," *Proceedings SPIE Medical Imaging* **3034**, pp. 74–85, 1997.

11. Y. Lu and H. Guo, "Background Removal in Image Indexing and Retrieval," *Proceedings 10th Int. Conf. Image Analysis and Processing, IEEE Computer Society*, pp. 933–938, 1999.

12. M. Sonka, V. Hlavac, and R. Boyle, "Image Processing, Analysis, and Machine Vision," 2nd edition, Brooks/Cole Publishing Company, 1999.

13. H. Wang and B. G. Fallone, "A Robust Morphological Algorithm for Automatic Radiation Field Extraction and Correlation of Portal Images," *Medical Physics* **21(2)**, pp. 237–244, 1994.

14. H. Wang and B. G. Fallone, "A Mathematical Model of Radiation Field Edge Localization," *Medical Physics* **22(7)**, pp. 1107–1110, 1995.

15. R. Wiemker, S. Dippel, M. Stahl, and T. M. Buzug, "A Graph-Based Approach to Automated Shutter Detection in Digital X-ray Images," *Proceedings CARS'99 Computer Assisted Radiology and Surgery*, pp. 14–18, 1999.

16. R. Wiemker, S. Dippel, M. Stahl, T. Blaffert, and U. Mahlmeister, "Automated Recognition of the Collimation Field in Digital Radiography Images by Maximization of the Laplace Area Integral," *Proceedings SPIE Medical Imaging* **3979**, pp. 1555–1565, 2000.

17. J. Zhang and H. K. Huang, "Automatic Background Recognition and Removal (ABRR) in Computed Radiography Images," *IEEE Transactions on Medical Imaging* **16(6)**, pp. 762–771, 1997.

Knowledge-based Image Understanding and Classification System for Medical Image Database

Hui Luo[1], Roger. Gaborski[2], Raj. Acharya[3]

[1]Dept. of CSE SUNY at Buffalo, [2]Dept. of CS Rochester Institute of Technology,
[3]Dept. of CSE Pennsylvania State Univ.

ABSTRACT

With the advent of Computer Radiographs(CR) and Digital Radiographs(DR), image understanding and classification in medical image databases have attracted considerable attention. In this paper, we propose a knowledge-based image understanding and classification system for medical image databases. An object-oriented knowledge model has been introduced and the idea that content features of medical images must hierarchically match to the related knowledge model is used. As a result of finding the best match model, the input image can be classified. The implementation of the system includes three stages. The first stage focuses on the match of the coarse pattern of the model class and has three steps: image preprocessing, feature extraction, and neural network classification. Once the coarse shape classification is done, a small set of plausible model candidates are then employed for a detailed match in the second stage. Its match outputs imply the result models might be contained in the processed images. Finally, an evaluation strategy is used to further confirm the results. The performance of the system has been tested on different types of digital radiographs, including pelvis, ankle, elbow and etc. The experimental results suggest that the system prototype is applicable and robust, and the accuracy of the system is near 70% in our image databases.

Keywords: Knowledge-based, Medical image database, image classification.

1. INTRODUCTION

With the advent of Computer Radiographs and Digital Radiographs, image understanding and classification in medical image databases have attracted considerable attention. Accurate medical diagnosis often depends on the correct display of anatomical Region of Interest(ROI). the acquisition of CR and DR image and the final 'look' of a radiographic image is separated. This provides flexibility to users, but also introduces the difficulty in setting appropriate display parameters. To optimal render a CR image, it is reasonable to classify the images by its anatomical structures and then retrieve the corresponding tone scale function. The rapid convergence of medical imaging technology into digital acquisition and storage has made digital Picture Archiving and Communication System (PACS) grow at a significant rate. But, medical image classification and management systems, to date, have been primarily based on a few textual or numerical fields residing in standard relational database structures which is not sufficient to represent the information contained in images. There is reason to believe that the performance of medical image management system might be greatly improved if image databases can be organized and retrieved based on image content. To organize by image content implies the detection of anatomical structures in images as well as the understanding of their geometry. Thus the success of designing medical image understanding and classification system directly benefits medical imaging.

However, Image data is more structurally complex than other kinds of data. It is hard to let the computer automatically and efficiently analyze contents in images, since the way with which human beings capture the image content, group image features into meaningful objects and attach semantic descriptions to images through model matching has not been fully understood to automate the analysis procedure. In addition, segmenting an image into regions corresponding to individual objects, extracting features from the image that capture the perceptual and semantic meanings and matching the image with the proposed model based on the extracted features also make the analysis problem more challenging.

Various systems have been proposed in the recent literatures for content-based image classification and retrieval, such as QBIC [1], Photobook [2], Virage [3], Visualseek [4], Netra [5], and MAR [6]. These systems follow the same paradigm which treats an image as a whole entity and represents it via a set of low-level feature attributes, such as color, texture, shape and layout. As a result, all these feature attributes together form a feature vector for each image. The image classification is based on clustering these low-level visual feature vectors. Such clustering-based classification schemes are usually time-consuming and of limited practical use since little of the image object semantics is explicitly

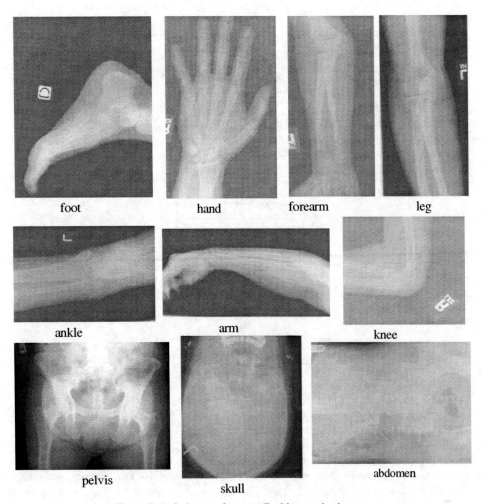

Fig 1: Sample images from medical image databases

modeled. Another difficulty with these schemes is that they generally do not apply to medical images.

We argue that understanding the entire content of an image may not be sufficient with such simple low-level feature extraction and matching algorithms in computer vision, since the fact that images have hierarchical structure is ignored. An experimental study conducted by Nishiyama et al [7] points out that human beings have two patterns in their visual memory when they view images. The first pattern is to roughly view the whole image and focus on the object outlines that are visually or semantically interesting. The second pattern is to concentrate on detailed attributes of specific objects within the image. Thus, to design an efficient and effective content-based medical image classification system, we need to appropriately combine such hieratical structure with feature extraction and match algorithms.

In this paper, we propose a knowledge-based image understanding and classification system for medical image databases. An object-oriented knowledge model has been introduced and the idea that content features of medical images must hierarchically match to the related knowledge model is used. As a result of finding the best match model, the input image can be classified. The implementation of the system includes three stages. The first stage focuses on the match of the coarse pattern of the model class and has three steps: image preprocessing, feature extraction, and neural network classification. Once the coarse shape classification is done, a small set of plausible model candidates are then employed for a detailed matching in the second stage. Its match outputs imply the result models might be contained in the processed images. Finally, an evaluation strategy is used to further confirm the results.

The rest of this paper is organized as follows: Section 2 briefly overviews the architecture of content-based medical image classification system. To address the system systematically, a detail description of coarse shape classification is presented in Section 3. Section 4 discusses how to implement a detail content identification on the processed images. Section 5 evaluates the match results. Then, the performance of the system is displayed in section 6, followed by the conclusion in section 7.

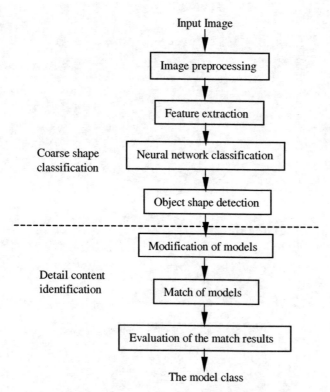

Input Image

Image preprocessing

Feature extraction

Coarse shape
classification

Neural network classification

Object shape detection

Modification of models

Detail content
identification

Match of models

Evaluation of the match results

The model class

Fig 2: Architecture of the classification system

2. SYSTEM OVERVIEW

The image classification problem of interest here can be defined as follows: Given an image, the system must derive appropriate descriptions of the image contents and classify it into one category of human body parts based on the detected contents. In this research, we work on CR images which include different body parts as shown in Fig 1 and assume that each input image belongs to one of pre-defined image categories.

To solve the problem, an object-oriented knowledge model [8] provides a powerful means for medical image understanding and classification. The key idea is that: content features of medical images must be hierarchically matched to the related knowledge model. The hypotheses used for the classification can be described as:

1) For each image category, the database system should maintain a knowledge model class which encapsulates all features relevant to this category and methods to detect these features from the processed images.

2) During classification, one knowledge model class can be assigned to an image only when the image features detected by the model class methods satisfy the pre-defined model "deformability" limits.

This strategy is likely to yield far better results than using generic strategies which classify an image with a set of low-level image features, since it exploits knowledge regarding not only the characteristics of one image category but also the ways to detect and recognize them.

What we propose here is a three-stage hierarchical image classification system. Fig 2 shows the architecture of the system prototype. The first stage focuses on the shape pattern of the model and ignores all finer details. To accomplish it, this stage performs the following functions: image preprocessing, feature extraction, neural network classification and object shape detection. The importance of this stage is to reduce the number of model candidates needed for detail matching and speed up the processing. Once the coarse shape classification is done, a small set of plausible model class candidates are then presented for a detailed matching in the second stage, in which the local features used to identify salient component objects in images are employed and incorporated with their spatial relation to discard those spurious match candidates. The output results imply a set of model which might be existed in the processed images. To further confirm them, an evaluation strategy is used to reject those unreasonable results and inference the most possible match models in the third stage.

3.   COASE SHAPE CLASSIFICATION

The classification in this stage focuses on the overall shape. However, incorporating scale, rotation and translation invariance in shape matching generally increases the computational requirements. So, the aim of this stage is to design a fast and robust scheme for shape classification.

3.1   Image Preprocessing
To speed up the processing, the first preprocess is to downscale the image size to equal to or less than 50x50 pixels, then we isolate the shape from its background by employing the maximum entropy thresholding technique[9]. The resulted binary image may contain speckles and misclassified regions, which can be easily removed using standard morphological operations.

3.2   Feature Extraction
A concise and quantitative description of the object shape is a challenging problem, especially describing a shape by a set of scale, rotation and translation invariant features. To achieve it, we extract a set of shape features from its histogram of the edge directions which is generated by applying the sobel edge operator on the binary images, and then quantifying its corresponding edge directions into 36 bins of $10°$ each. To explain it more clearly, some synthetic image examples are shown in Fig 3.

- The histogram of edge directions is invariant to translation in an image. Thus the position of the object in the image has no effect on its edge directions. This property can ensure that any features extracted from the histogram of edge directions are translation invariant.
- The use of edge directions is inherently not scale invariant. Two images identical in every aspect except their size will yield different number of edge points and hence result in two different histograms. In order to achieve invariance to scale, we normalize the histogram as follows:

$$H(i) = H(i)/n_e \qquad\qquad i \in [0,.....,35]$$

  Where $H(i)$ is the count in bin i of the edge direction histogram, n_e is the total number of edge points.
- A histogram of the edge directions is not invariant to rotation either. As shown in Fig. 3, these three images contain similar shapes with different orientations. Thus their histograms of edge directions are totally different. However, when we only consider the shape pattern of these histograms, they are same in that all of them have two peaks with $180°$ distance. If we can design a feature which only captures such information, the histogram of edge directions can be made invariant to rotation. To achieve this, we generate a set of edge direction histogram templates from some typical shapes extracted from our medical image databases as shown in Fig 4, and perform the match by first shifting the histogram templates, then computing the correlation between them and the edge direction histogram of the processed image. The shift operation of histogram templates can be seen as the rotation of their corresponding shape models.

Through carefully analyzing the characteristics of our medical image database and numerous experiments, we classify the edge direction histograms into three clusters: the one-peak cluster, the two peaks cluster and the more peaks cluster by evaluating the following nine features:

- *peakNum: the number of peaks in the histogram of edge directions*
- *peakDiffMax: the minimal distance between two nearest peaks*
- *degreeDisr: the total number of degree contained in the histogram of edge directions. This feature is helpful to describe the degree distribution of different shape.*
- *Model1,1w,2,3,4,8: the six maximal convolution values between the histogram of edge directions and six histogram templates*

Fig 4 shows the nine features of six typical shape extracted from the database and their corresponding images.

3.3   Artificial Neural Network Classification
Artificial Neural networks have been widely used in pattern recognition. In this research, a multi-layer feedforward neural network is used to classify the overall shape. There are nine input nodes in the neural network corresponding to the nine features detected from the edge direction histograms, and three output nodes in the output layer with respect to the three classification clusters. Here we choose one hidden layer with 14 nodes, since our experiment results show that only one hidden layer is good enough to discriminate the feature data. The decision rule is to assign an image to a class

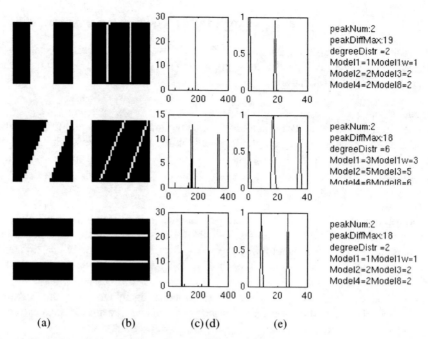

Fig 3: Illustration of the histogram of edge directions
(a): the original images
(b): the edge images of the original images
(c): the histogram of edge directions
(d): the quantified histogram of edge directions
(e): the nine scale, rotation and translation invariant features

corresponding to one output node with the highest value. To train the neural network, we use the back propagation learning algorithm. Once the network is trained, it can be used for the classification.

3.4 Object Shape Detection

Although the edge direction features give a concise description of the shape, it has a limited discrimination capability. In practice, it is quite possible that two or more different shape may share very similar nine shape features. This will introduce errors in the classification. Thus, the overall shape contour need to be extracted and used for verifying the classification.

Since the edge map of a binary image directly outlines the shape contour in the image, we choose it as the initial contour of the object, and then detect a finer contour using the snake model [10]. The obtained contour provides very useful information of the overall shape in the processed image, such as the size, location and orientation, which will be used to adjust the knowledge model for a more detail content identification in the next stage. Then, we verify each classification result by comparing the shapes of its related knowledge models with the overall shape in the processed image. If they are quite similar, we keep the original classification result; otherwise, we reject it.

4. DETAIL CONTENT IDENTIFICATION

Using the shape outline attribute for classification may lack sufficient discriminatory power. For example, two different body parts, such as ankle and elbow, may have very similar overall shape outlines, but they do have totally different bone structures. For further classification, it is necessary to integrate the information of the component objects in the knowledge model for a more elaborate matching. Thus in this finer classification stage, we emphasize the match of model component objects. The goodness of the matching is based on how many model component objects have been found in the images and how well their spatial relations satisfy the semantic graph defined in the model.

4.1 Modification of Models

The large variability of anatomical structures may influence the accuracy of model matching. In addition, the difference

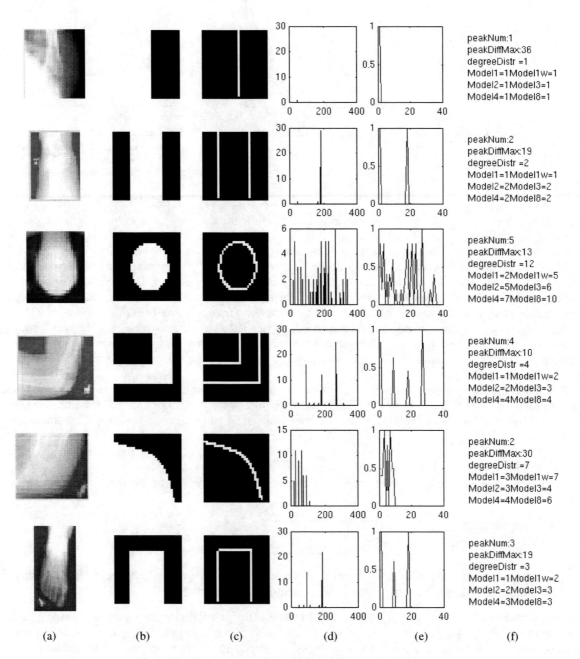

Fig 4: The histogram template and their corresponding images

    (a): The images have the typical shapes

    (b): The typical shapes

    (c): The contour images of typical shapes

    (d): The histogram of edge directions

    (e): The normalized histogram of edge directions

    (f): The nine features of typical shapes

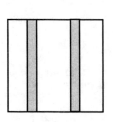 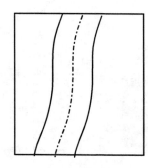 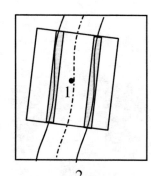

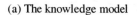

(a) The knowledge model   (b) The processed image   (c) Scale and rotate the knowledge model to match the processed image.
1: the model center
2: the fitted medial axis line

Fig 5: Illustration of matching a knowledge model to an image

of viewpoints, when radiographs are taken, may introduce the difficulties of appropriately locating the model in images. To solve these problems, we need to scale the model size as close as the real size of image objects, rotate it to correspond the image object orientation, and search for the most possible position to locate the model in images.

The size information is implied in the overall shape contour. To obtain it, we extract the medial axis of the contour by a medial axis transform [10] and estimate the size of the object from the contour. By comparing with the size of the knowledge model, a global scale ratio r_g can be derived. Regarding to the orientation, the medial axis actually provides enough information about the image object orientation. However, due to the size difference between the scaled model and the image object (in most cases, the scaled model is smaller than the image object), the matching is usually performed on parts of the image object. Thus the orientation can be determined by the orientation of medial axis in the overlap parts between the image object and the knowledge model. As for the model position, we define it as the coordinates of the model center.

The above information gives a coarse description of the image object situation. We can use them as the initial setting to adjust the model. But to further accurately locate the model into the processed images, we need to seek a set of most appropriate size ratio r, the position p, and the orientation angle α of the model by using a maximum a *posteriori* approach.

$$\langle r_{MAP}, p_{MAP}, \alpha_{MAP} \rangle = \arg \max_{r, p, \alpha} P(r, p, \alpha \mid \nabla I) \qquad (1)$$

where, ∇I is the gradient of the processed image. The maximum a *posteriori* can be computed from Eq. 2 using Bayes' rule.

$$P(r, p, \alpha \mid \nabla I) = \frac{P(\nabla I \mid r, p, \alpha) P(r, p, \alpha)}{P(\nabla I)}$$

$$= \frac{P(\nabla I \mid r, p, \alpha) P(r) P(p) P(\alpha)}{P(\nabla I)} \qquad (2)$$

Here, we assume that r, p and α are independent from each other. For computation efficiency, the normalization term $P(\nabla I)$ is discarded as it does not depend on the scale, position, or orientation.

Gradient Term: The first term $P(\nabla I \mid r, p, \alpha)$ in Eq. 2 computes the probability of seeing certain image gradients given the current shape model. Consider the relationship between the shape model determined by r, p, α and the gradient ∇I. If the shape model correctly locates in the processed image, we expect to see more image gradients in the overlap region, as shown in Fig 5 (c). More precisely, the closer between the image object shape and the model shape, the more image gradients correspond to the model edges. In order to make the model robust, we relax the shape constraint by extending the model shape edges width. Let $S = \{(x_{si}, y_{si})\}$ $i=1..n$ be a vector describing the points on the shape edges. We define the current model situation S^* computed from r, p and α as:

$$S^* = r \begin{bmatrix} \cos \alpha & -\sin \alpha \\ \sin \alpha & \cos \alpha \end{bmatrix} S + \begin{bmatrix} p_x \\ p_y \end{bmatrix} \qquad (3)$$

The best fit pose of the model may be found by maximize the gradient probability, which is modeled as:

$$P(\nabla I \mid r, p, \alpha) = \frac{\sum_{x=1}^{N} \sum_{y=1}^{M} S^{*}(x, y) \bullet |\nabla I(x, y)|^2}{\sum_{x=1}^{N} \sum_{y=1}^{M} S^{*}(x, y)} \qquad (4)$$

Scale Ratio Priori: The second term $P(r)$ in Eq. 2 is the scale ratio priori between the model and the image object size. Because of the variability of anatomical structures, the global scale ratio sometimes doesn't represent the real object size precisely. From our experience, searching around the global shape ratio r_g is quite possible to find a best fit shape ratio r. Thus the scale ratio priori can be modeled as a gaussian distribution over the global shape ratio r_g with variance σ_r.

$$P(r) = \frac{1}{\sqrt{2\pi}\,\sigma_r} \exp(-\frac{(r - r_g)^2}{2\sigma_r^2}) \qquad (5)$$

Pose Priori: For the position priori $P(p)$, we simply assume a uniform distribution over all positions in the image object.

$$P(p) = U(-\infty, \infty) \qquad (6)$$

This is reasonable, since the expected image object can appear at anywhere in the image, depending on how the radiologist takes the radiographs.

Rotation Priori: The last term $P(\alpha)$, the rotation priori, in Eq. 3 responds to the orientation of the medial axis of the image object in the overlap region. It is possible that the medial axis of the model sometimes doesn't align with the medial axis line of the overlap region very well. In such situation, a little bit adjustment would be very helpful for finding the best fit orientation. So the corresponding priori is designed as a gaussian distribution over the rotation range.

$$P(\alpha) = \frac{1}{\sqrt{2\pi}\,\sigma_\alpha} \exp(-\frac{(\alpha - \alpha_g)^2}{2\sigma_\alpha^2}) \qquad (7)$$

4.2 Match of Models

Once a knowledge model is correctly located in the processed images, we define a search region for each component object, and then perform a correlation match between the component object shape and image gradient. A component object shape is assumed to be found in the processed image only when its correlation value exceeds a pre-defined threshold which is derived from a number of experiments. Once all model's component object shapes are found in the processed image, their spatial relations will be checked by using the semantic graph match algorithm[8]. Our assumption used here is that: if the model finds its all component objects in the processed image and their spatial relations satisfy with the pre-defined spatial constraints, we say this model matches the processed image.

5.   EVALUATION OF MATCH

Evaluation of a match result is another important issue in the system. In this section, we discuss two topics related to the evaluation: 1) how to estimate the match accuracy between a knowledge model and a given image. 2) how to analyze the characteristics of the match results and use them to reject those unreasonable matches.

5.1 Confidence Level of Match

When evaluating a matched model, we are interested in how accurate the model can represent the image object. According to the hierarchical match strategy of the knowledge model, the match accuracy should be based on not only the match of its component object shapes, but also the match of its semantic graph. So the matching confidence level can be defined as:

$$Confidence\ \ Level\ (m) = \begin{cases} - & \exists c_{mj} < th & (1) \\ 0 & \exists \mu_{mj} = 0 \quad \forall c_{mj} \geq th & (2) \\ \dfrac{\sum_{j=0}^{n} \mu_{mj} \cdot c_{mj}}{\sum_{j=0}^{n} \mu_{mj}} & \forall \mu_{mj} > 0 \quad \forall c_{mj} \geq th & (3) \end{cases} \qquad (8)$$

Where, m is the model identity, n is the total number of the component objects in the model m. c_{mj} represents the match result of the j-th component object in the model m, and μ_{mj} describes the fuzzy membership[8] of a match position of the j-th component object in the model m. If any one of model component object shapes in the given model is unable to be found in the processed image, we declare this knowledge model fails to represent the processed image and reject it, as presented in Eq. 8 (1). If all model's component object shapes are found in the processed images, but their spatial relations don't satisfy with the model pre-defined spatial constraints, which means at least one of them lies outside of the pre-defined spatial position, we still think this model is not precise enough to represent the image and set its confidence level to be zero, as shown in Eq. 8 (2). Only when the model finds all its component objects in the processed image and their spatial relations satisfy with the pre-defined spatial constraints, we say this model can be used to explain the processed image and set its confidence level as Eq. 8 (3). By using this confidence level, we have a quantitative measurement of the matching between a knowledge model and the processed image.

6 SYSTEM EVALUATION AND EXPERIMENTAL RESULTS

The medical image database we used for our experiments consists of 50 foot, 50 wrist, 65 head, 60 leg, 50 ankle, 40 arm, 50 knee, 10 elbow, 40 pelvis, 30 skull, 20 abdomen CR images, summing up to a total of 465 images. The image size ranging from about 200x200 pixels (e.g. a hand radiograph) to 2500x2048 pixels(e.g. a pelvis radiographs) with 256 gray level.

To study the performance of coarse shape classification, we manually assign a category to each input image and use that as the target value, then divide these images into two sets: the training set and the testing set. In the training phase, the neural network is trained 200 iterations of the training data. The trained classification neural network is then put through the testing data. The output decisions are then compared with the target values. To measure the performance of a trained network in more detail, we perform a regression analysis between the network response and the correspond targets. The experimental results show that the overall correction percent is 92% and the correlation coefficient between the classification result and expected target is 90%. This is sufficient to demonstrates that the selected nine scale, rotate and translate invariant features have enough discrimination ability to classify the input images into one of the three categories.

Based on the characteristics of human body structures, most radiographs in our medical image database can be classified into cluster 2 (the two-peak cluster) such as leg, elbow, pelvis radiographs and etc. Thus, the detail content classification is mainly performed on the images belonging to this cluster. Table 1 lists the performance of the system on these images. Fig 6 displays some processed results.

Image categories	Image number	Process time/image	Number of image with Correct match	Correct percent
Elbow images	10	64 seconds	6	60%
Ankle images	50	58 seconds	36	72%
Pelvis images	40	80 seconds	30	75%
Knee images	50	45 seconds	41	82%
Wrist images	50	62 seconds	32	64%
total				70.6%

Table 1: the performance of detail content classification

Regarding to the process efficiency, the time-consuming processes in the coarse shape classification are the image preprocessing, feature extraction, and contour detection. Once the neural network is trained, the neural network classification is quite efficient. As for detail content classification, the computation cost is determined by the number of knowledge models needed for the detailed match and the complexity of knowledge models. For the five models in examples, the pelvis model is the most time-consuming one, as it has more component objects and its detection and match schemes are more complicated. Table 1 also lists the process time of each knowledge model. Since all these tests are performed using Matlab under SUN sparc 5 system with the main memory 250 MB, there is reason to believe that the performance of the system can be greatly improved if the whole process is programmed by C/C++. As the knowledge models are totally independent, another way to speed up the system is to design the match of each knowledge model parallel.

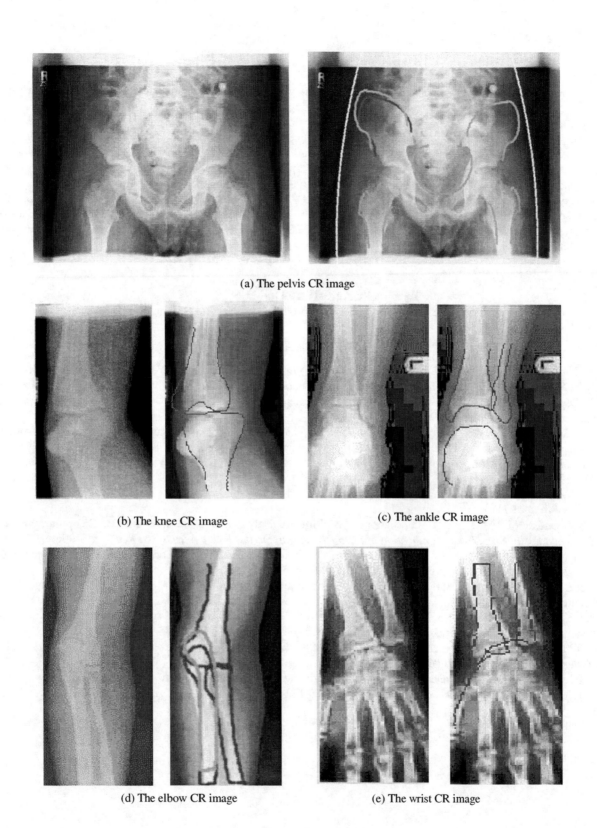

(a) The pelvis CR image

(b) The knee CR image

(c) The ankle CR image

(d) The elbow CR image

(e) The wrist CR image

Fig 6: The experimental results

7 CONLUSION

In this paper, we have presented a content-based medical image classification system. The system employs both global and local features to classify the input images by performing a three-stage processing. The first stage, coarse shape classification, focuses on the overall shape of objects in the processed images. Through the coarse shape classification, the input image is classified into one of three clusters. Once the coarse shape classification is done, a small set of plausible model class candidates are then presented for a detailed matching in the second stage, in which local features is used to identify salient component objects in images and incorporated with their spatial relation to discard those spurious match candidates. The output match results imply a set of model which might be existed in the processed images. To further confirm them, an evaluation strategy is used to reject those unreasonable results and inference the most possible match models in final stage. The performance of the system has been tested on different types of digital radiographs, including pelvis, ankle, elbow and etc. The experimental results suggest that the system prototype is applicable and robust, and the accuracy of the system is near 70% in our image databases

ACKNOWLEDGMENTS

The authors gratefully acknowledge the support of Eastman Kodak Company and NSF grant to Dr. Acharya.

REFERENCES

1. W. Niblack, R. Barber, and et al, "The QBIC project: Querying images by content using color, tecture, and shape" *Proc. SPIE Storage and Retrieval for Image and Video Databases*, Feb 1994
2. A. Pentland, R. W.Picard, S. Sclaroff. "Photobook: Content-based manipulation of image database". *International Journal of Computer Vision*, 1996
3. J.R. Bach, C. Fuller, A.Gupta, Arun Hampapur, et al. "The Virage image search engine: An open framework for image management" *Proc. SPIE Storage and Retrieval for image and Video Database*, vol 2670, pp. 76-87,1996.
4. J. R. Smith, S. F. Chang "Visualseek: A fully automated content-based image query system" *Proc ACM Multimedia 96*, 1996
5. W.Y. Ma and D.S. Manjunath, "Netra: A toolbox for navigating large image databases" *Proc IEEE Int. Conf. On Image Proc.* 1997
6. T.S. Huang, S. Mehrotra, and K. Ramchandran, "Multimedia analysis and retrieval system (MARS) project" *Proc of 33rd Annual Clinic on Library Application of Data Processing Digital Image Access and Retrieval*, 1996
7. H. Nishiyama, S. Kin, T. Yokoyama, Y. Matsushita "An Image Retrieval System Considering Subjective Perception" *Proc 1994 ACM SIGCHI Conf*, Boston, MA, April 1994, pp30-36
8. Hui Luo, R. Gaborski, R.Acharya " Knowledge Representation for Image Content Analysis in Medical Image Databases" *SPIE's International Symposium on Medical Imaging 2001* ,San Diego, California, February 2001
9   J.N.Kaper, P.K. Sahoo, A.K.C. Wong, A new method for gray level picture thresholding using the entropy of the histogram. *Computing Vision Graphics Image Processing*, vol 29, pp 273-285, 1985
10. Hui Luo, Qiang Lu, R. Gaborski, R.Acharya "Robust Snake Model" *IEEE Conference on Computer Vision and Pattern Recognition (CVPR2000)* Hilton Head Island, South Carolina , June 2000
11. J.F.Jeng, S. Sahni, "Serial and parallel algorithms for the medial axis transform" *IEEE Transactions on Pattern Analysis & Machine Intelligence.* vol 14, n 12. pp 1218-1224, 1992

Author Index